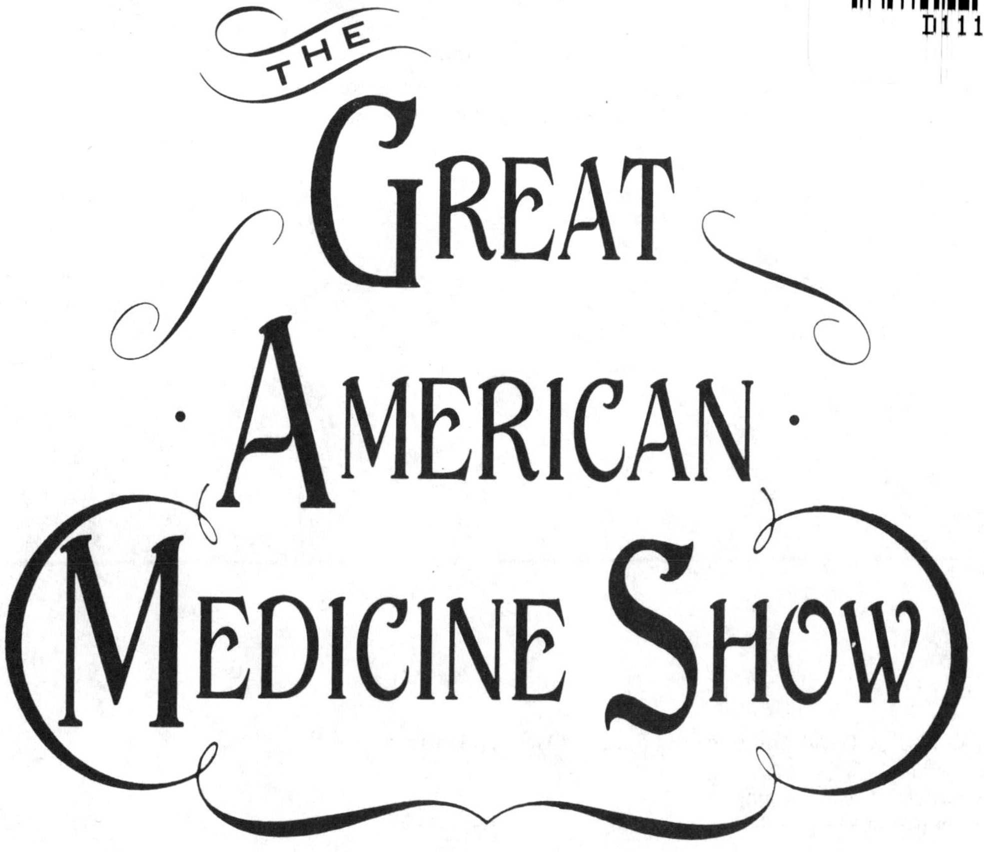

The Great American Medicine Show

BEING AN ILLUSTRATED HISTORY OF HUCKSTERS, HEALERS, HEALTH EVANGELISTS, AND HEROES FROM PLYMOUTH ROCK TO THE PRESENT

DAVID ARMSTRONG

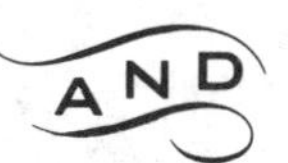

ELIZABETH METZGER ARMSTRONG

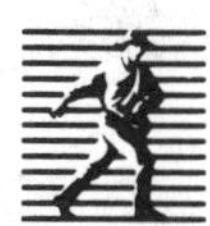

PRENTICE HALL
NEW YORK LONDON TORONTO SYDNEY TOKYO SINGAPORE

To our parents,
Christine and Richard Armstrong
and Sylvia and Ralph Metzger

First edition

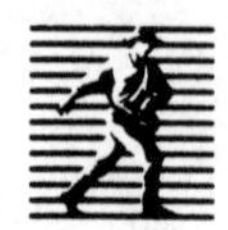

Prentice Hall

Simon & Schuster, Inc.
15 Columbus Circle
New York, NY 10023

Published by Prentice Hall

Manufactured in the United States of America

1 2 3 4 5 6 7 8 9 10

Library of Congress Cataloging-in-Publication Data

Armstrong, David.
The great American medicine show : being an illustrated history of hucksters, healers, health evangelists, and heroes from Plymouth Rock to the present / David Armstrong and Elizabeth Metzger Armstrong. — 1st ed.
p. cm.
Includes bibliographical references and index.
ISBN 0-13-364027-2 : $17.95
1. Quacks and quackery—United States. 2. Medicine shows—United States. I. Armstrong, Elizabeth Metzger.
II. Title.
R730.A75 1991
615.8′56—dc20

91-25496
CIP

Contents

ILLUSTRATIONS

PREFACE AND ACKNOWLEDGMENTS

The Great American Medicine Show is the result of three years of research and writing, of immersing ourselves in the health reform movements whose stories follow. Prime movers, like John Harvey Kellogg and William Keith Kellogg, Mary Baker Eddy, and Gloria Swanson, are well remembered. Others, like Samuel Thomson, Sylvester Graham, and Horace Fletcher, were famous long ago. Some of the movements we discuss, such as vegetarianism, homeopathy, temperance, and fitness, still represent serious alternatives to conventional lifestyles and medicine. Others, including patent medicines and phrenology, were sheer quackery and have deservedly died out. Whether serious or spurious, they are all part of the grand parade.

David thought of the idea of writing a history when he wrote a book of contemporary consumer reporting, *The Insider's Guide to Health Foods,* and became interested in how American health crusaders got from there to here. Liz's writing background and training in American social history made her a natural writing partner. We found working together remarkably easy. We divided up the chapters according to our interests. David couldn't wait to get his teeth into the writings of Horace Fletcher, the great masticator, and follow the traveling medicine shows, and Liz was eager to dip into mineral springs and water cures. We helped revise each other's drafts, traveled across the country together to track down illustrations and exhume musty historical volumes, and shared the anecdotes we uncovered. In all we dug into some 160 books and more articles, brochures, pamphlets, and advertisements than we care to count. We wrote and researched in seven states, the District of Columbia, England, and Ireland.

As we wrote, we renewed our respect for those millions of Americans whose historic drive for health and longevity has led to today's emphasis on exercise, nutrition, dieting, and preventive medicine. While we did not set out to prove a theory, our findings reinforced perennial American themes. Among them are the intimate connection between religion, reform, and health and the overriding optimism of American life, the belief that for determined individuals, anything—including self-cures against formidable odds—is possible. Indeed, we were struck by how often Americans have used health reform as a vehicle for reinventing themselves. As Yogi Berra once put it, ''It's déjà vu all over again.''

We could not have written this book without the encouragement and assistance of our families, friends, and colleagues all across the country. Our special thanks to our editor, Kate Kelly, whose enthusiasm never wavered, and her assistant, Susan Lauzau; our agent, Ellen Levine, whose skill and persistence helped make the book a reality; Michael Larsen and Elizabeth Pomada, for helping us develop the book proposal; Bernet Bai and Rodger Maerten, for providing us with a home base in the Midwest and driving Liz to Davenport, Iowa and Kirksville, Missouri for first-hand research; Bernhard Metzger, Karen Zander, and Elise and Victoria Metzger, for putting us up in Boston and giving us a taste of history by baking Graham bread; Barbara, Don, and Kelsey Yost, for giving us old home-remedy books; Margarette Armstrong, who donated Shaker literature on herbal medicine; Peggy Renner and Bob Nelson, for putting Liz up in Pasadena when she visited Aimee Semple McPherson's Angelus Temple; Karen Feldman, for the use of vintage dieting books and cookbooks; Jeanette Weinstock, for digging up information on homeopathy's early history in Pennsylvania; Jane Kinderlehrer, for taking us on a tour of Rodale Press; Ari and Jennifer Bai, for opening their home in Maryland to us during our illustration search in Washington, D.C.; and Shawn, Greta, and Jordan Elizabeth Bai, whose good humor gave us a lift when we needed it most.

The librarians and archivists who helped us during our many visits to the University of California at Berkeley, the University of California at San Francisco, San Francisco State University, the San Francisco Public Library, the Boston Public Library, and the St. Louis Public Library are too numerous to cite by name. We would, however, like to give special thanks to Jan Lazarus of the National Library of Medicine, Bethesda, Maryland; Ron Beer of the St. Louis Science Center, St. Louis, Missouri; Sue Rogers of the Kirksville, Missouri College of Osteopathic Medicine; Ruth Bondurant, who interrupted her Sunday activities to give Liz a private tour of the Still National Osteopathic Museum in Kirksville, Missouri; Glenda Wiese and Joy Mussmann of the David D. Palmer Health Sciences Library Archives, Palmer College of Chiropractic, Davenport, Iowa; Judy Chelnick, David Haberstich, and Deborra A. Richardson of the National Museum of American History, the Smithsonian Institution, Washington, D.C.; Richard J. Wolfe of the Francis A. Countway Library of Medicine, the Harvard Medical School, Boston, Massachusetts; Jim E. Detlefsen of the Herbert Hoover Library, West Branch, Iowa; June Griffiths of the Scott Andrew Trexler II Memorial Library, the Lehigh County Historical Society, Allentown, Pennsylvania; Pamela Brunger Scott, Managing Editor/ Operations, *San Francisco Examiner*; Judy Canter and the library staff of the *San Francisco Examiner*; Suzanne Locke and Steve Essaff of the photography department of the *San Francisco Examiner*; Pat Benton and Bill Redder of the St. Helena Hospital and Health Center, St. Helena, California; Diane Beckley of the Historical Society of Battle Creek, Michigan; Duff Stoltz of the Adventist Hospital, Battle Creek, Michigan; Alex Nichols of Sunshine Biscuits, Inc., Woodbridge, New Jersey; Kate Schellenback of the Bettmann Archives, New York, New York; Stevie Holland and Tom Logan of Culver Pictures, New York, New York; and the late Robert Rodale of Rodale Press, for sharing his ideas and visions on a soft summer day in Emmaus, Pennsylvania.

CHAPTER

· 1 ·

PILGRIMS' PROGRESS: EARLY AMERICAN MEDICINE

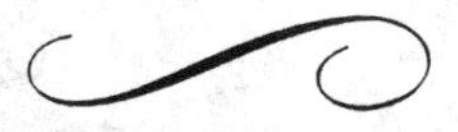

The times are ominous indeed,
When quack to quack cries purge *and* bleed.

WILLIAM COBBETT, 1799

George Washington lay dying. Barely able to swallow or breathe, the first President took to his bed at his Mount Vernon estate, attended by a team of physicians who hurried to his side through the winter chill.

Washington's doctors gave their illustrious patient the best care that orthodox eighteenth-century medicine could muster. They blistered his skin to draw off the fetid liquids that lurked within; applied poultices of wheat bran to his legs and feet to ease his discomfort; and administered calomel, a white, tasteless powder of mercury chloride, to empty his bowels and eliminate the toxins that were slowly killing the sunken father of the American republic.

The doctors also bled Washington on four occasions in fewer than 24 hours, piercing his skin with a sharp lancet and drawing off 32 ounces of troubled blood, letting the dark, thick liquid drain into cups assembled for that purpose. Washington's wife, Martha, opposed the bleeding (known technically as phlebotomy), fearing it would only weaken her husband further. But, whispering hoarsely to his doctors (he was also suffering from acute laryngitis), Washington himself asked to be bled.

All this was to no avail. Washington grew ever weaker and more wan. Finally, he asked to be left alone. On December 14, 1799, Washington died. He was 67 years old. Modern doctors, reading accounts of his fatal illness, think he expired from diphtheria or strep throat, given a lethal assist by the very treatments intended to save his life. Today, he would be treated with antibiotic drugs.

Antibiotics, however, would not be discovered for over a century after Washington's time. The "heroic" medicine practiced by his doctors—called heroic because physicians took extraordinary measures to intervene in the healing process and manage the patient's care—was strictly state-of-the-art. Washington's three attending physicians were among the top doctors of his day; one was trained personally by Washington's fellow patriot, Dr. Benjamin Rush, a signer of the Declaration of Independence and the most respected American medical man of the late eighteenth and early nineteenth centuries.

It was Washington's misfortune to live in an era when mercury poisoning and bleeding were at the cutting edge of health care. Even Washington's death did not dislodge the faith that mainstream doctors—called "regulars" in the parlance of the time—put in heroic medicine, although there was disagreement over how to apply heroic measures. Dr. James Craik, one of Washington's doctors, wrote that had they "taken no blood from him, our good friend might have been alive now. But we were governed by the

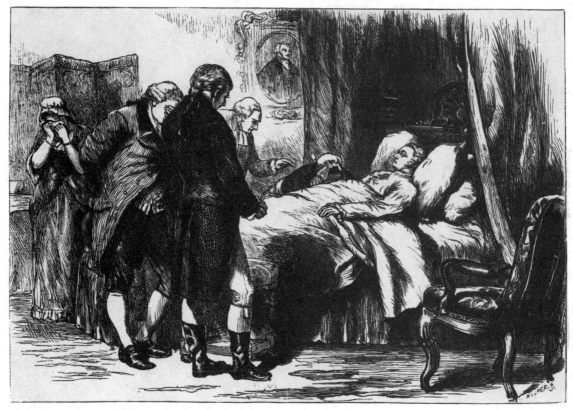

1. George Washington's doctors had to kill him in order to save him. *Culver Pictures.*

best light we had; we thought we were right, and so we are justified.''

Not everyone was so sanguine. William Cobbett, an English writer then living in America, devoted several issues of a newsletter to Rush, blaming Rush's theories for Washington's death. Rush, a serious and sincere man by all accounts, surely didn't mean to kill Washington or anyone else. But there was truth in Cobbett's screeds: the devastating bleeding and purging with mercury almost certainly hastened Washington's death, and it ensured the painful demise of an uncounted number of ordinary citizens as well.

Early Americans were well aware of the dangers of mainstream medicine and many people avoided any unnecessary encounter with regular doctors. That was not hard to do. At the time of the Revolution, just a quarter-century before Washington's death, only about 10 percent of the doctors in the original 13 colonies had formal medical education, and most of them were clustered in the larger cities.

It was there, in the new medical schools just beginning to emerge, that earnest young doctors were taught, with the best of intentions, how to kill their patients in order to save them.

SCHOOLS FOR SCANDAL

Until the eighteenth century, physicians in Europe and North America were more tradesmen than professionals, often splitting their time between mixing and selling medicines and cutting hair on the side to earn a little extra cash. Until 1745, British surgeons belonged to the same guild as barbers. But things were starting to change; by the early eighteenth century, pioneering medical schools were established in Europe, chiefly in Leyden, Paris, London, and Edinburgh.

The first medical school in colonial America opened in Philadelphia in 1762, when William Shippen, Jr. began giving lectures in midwifery. In 1763, he expanded his repertoire to include anatomical lectures ''for the advantage of the young gentleman now enjoined in the study of physic [medicine] . . . and also for the entertainment of any gentleman who may have the curiosity to understand the anatomy of the Human Frame.''

Even as medical schools were being established, they were viewed as mere supplements to real medical education: apprenticeship. The aspiring doctor served a master physician, called a preceptor, mixing medicines, keeping records, and, eventually, when the lessons began to sink in, helping the established physician treat patients. School was practically an extracurricular activity.

By the middle of the nineteenth century, dozens of medical schools had come into existence, but few were highly regarded, even in their own day, let alone by later observers. By 1910, when American medical reformer Abraham Flexner (1866–1959) wrote a seminal report on medical education, all but a few schools were considered diploma mills specializing in the production of quacks. Wrote Flexner: ". . . these establishments—for the most part they can be called schools or institutions only by courtesy—were frequently set up regardless of opportunity or need. Wherever and whenever the roster of untitled practitioners rose above half a dozen, a medical school was likely at any moment to be precipitated."

Typically, early medical schools required only a high school diploma and payment of a fee—*especially* payment of a fee—for enrollment. There were no other academic entrance requirements, no grades, and few examinations. A standard course of study lasted from 16 to 20 weeks. The primary method of instruction was the lecture, with the professor addressing his students from a far-off podium, a godlike figure handing down tablets of truth. There was little personal contact between student and professor, or between student and patient.

Even the casual standards of early medical education were too restrictive for democratic health reformers who proclaimed that in a free country, anyone should have the right to practice medicine. In the 1830s, a groundswell of sentiment called the popular health movement temporarily ended nearly all government regulation of health care, part of the wave of Jacksonian anti-elitism. By 1845, only three states still licensed medical doctors.

Medical schools didn't suddenly vanish when licensing laws were suspended. Even bogus schools still conferred respectability upon their graduates among gullible consumers. If anything, lifting restrictions bred still more schools, most of them privately owned and operated for maximum profit. Even university medical schools were largely autonomous of the institutions whose names they borrowed. Simply put, they were schools for scandal.

Few medical schools spent much money on their facilities. They had skimpy libraries, haphazard access to hospitals, and bare-bones clinical laboratories—even for students of basic anatomy. In such penurious circumstances, medical students were not above stealing bodies from graveyards to further their studies. This practice was more or less tolerated as long as students stuck to graveyards for paupers and blacks. When overeager students robbed graves in New York City's posh Trinity Churchyard in 1788, horrified townspeople rioted. After things simmered down, the task of procuring bodies was left to professional grave robbers, called, with a certain grim humor, "resurrectionists." They operated until 1854, when special legislation assigned unclaimed bodies to medical schools.

In the days of Washington and Rush, even hospitals were few and far between, and they were crowded, dirty, and restrictive. Two of the first American hospitals, in New York and Philadelphia, refused entry to unwed mothers and patients with venereal disease or other contagious illnesses. Supplicants had to be deemed "morally worthy" to be awarded a hospital bed.

THE GREAT UNWASHED

Ill-trained, uninformed doctors were not the sole source of health problems. Quite simply, the personal habits of early Americans were disgusting. People ate and drank themselves silly, and personal hygiene and public sanitation were virtually nonexistent, producing exactly the conditions that would have sent people packing to a good hospital, had there been one.

By and large, people lived in squalid circumstances that proved splendid breeding grounds for the great epidemics of yellow fever, typhoid, smallpox, and cholera that swept eighteenth- and nineteenth-century America. Night air was considered polluted by dangerous vapors, so sick rooms, and even ordinary bedrooms, were shuttered and stifling. Beds, even in comfortable homes, were infested with vermin.

On farms, where most people lived, outhouses were located in the garden or near the household well. Hard-to-clean clothes were caked with manure and worn until they rotted. Indeed, washable cotton clothing and bedclothes were major steps forward in the prevention of disease.

In the growing cities, housekeepers simply tossed garbage into the streets and emptied chamber pots the same way. In his autobiography, Rush writes that a friend of his, out for a late-night stroll during student days in Edinburgh, was unceremoniously drenched—"naturalized," as the townspeople put it—when a chamber pot was emptied on him from an upper-story window. There was, at all hours, horse manure in the streets; roaming, grunting pigs were turned loose to eat the garbage. Fresh water was hard to come by, especially on a citywide scale. Municipal water systems were unknown until 1830, when Philadelphia built one. New York finally followed suit in 1842, and Boston in 1848.

In city and countryside alike, the consumption of copious amounts of tobacco was an accepted way of life. Dipping snuff and smoking pipes were common habits among both sexes. Men also indulged in cigars and chewing tobacco, which was expectorated just about anywhere, at virtually any time. Foreign visitors routinely expressed amazement at the American propensity to spit. "In all the public places of America," wrote Charles Dickens, the inhabitants indulged in "the odious practise of chewing and expectorating."

Then there were the nation's bathing habits—or, rather, lack of bathing. Little privacy and precious little hot water were available in the first 50 years of the American republic, so bathing in private homes did not become common until households installed bathrooms. That did not happen fast enough for health reformers. In 1846, William Alcott wrinkled his nose and noted that the nation contained "multitudes who pass for models of neatness and cleanliness who do not perform this work for themselves half a dozen times—nay once—a year."

On the infrequent occasions when bathing was favored, the whole family washed up, one after another, in the same tub of water. The unfamiliar experience of scrubbing all over sometimes proved unnerving. As Elizabeth Drinker, one of Rush's patients, scribbled in her diary, "Nancy came here this evening. She and I went into shower bath. I bore it better than I expected, not having been wet all over at once, for 28 years past."

Eating habits were equally injurious to health. Early Americans, who performed hard physical labor and passed the winters in cold rooms, loaded up on fat and calories. They didn't worry about cholesterol; in the days when life expectancy was about 40, few people lived long enough to die from degenerative diseases. Americans, living in a naturally abundant country, ate plenty of food, but their meals were seldom nutritionally sound by the standards of later generations. People gorged themselves on greasy salt pork and, in the West and rural areas, on game. Little importance was put on fresh vegetables; indeed, New York City once banned their sale, as many vegetables—tomatoes are the best-known example—were believed to be poisonous.

Regardless of the bill of fare or where food was consumed, decorum at table was a rarity. Families were known to dip their spoons all at once into the same bowl, using forks to fix their meat on the plate and knives to convey food to their mouths, bolting their meals as quickly as possible. These habits persisted for a long time. At the turn of the twentieth century, a millionaire sportsman, one Horace Fletcher, forged a second career by urging eaters to slow down and chew their food thoroughly. It was, appropriately, called "Fletcherizing."

The gobble-and-go style and large, barely digestible meals were accompanied by drinking—and, again, the whole family was wont to join in. Americans were big drinkers, putting away twice as much hard liquor in 1820 as they downed in 1980. They swilled alcohol at every meal, including breakfast, and drank between meals when they felt like it, which was often.

Alcohol was associated with hospitality and was a popular ingredient in folk remedies. Men spent much of their social lives in taverns, drinking hard cider, applejack, and rum. (The upper classes favored sherry, rye, and Madeira.) Women discreetly sipped cider and patent medicines high in alcohol content.

Whiskey was valued nearly as much as money; in fact, it was used as money in backwoods economies. Barrels of whiskey were also familiar sights at community events such as barnraisings, weddings, bringing in the sheaves at harvest time, and elections—politicians were expected to provide free drinks at the polling booths. Even the Continental Army, in the teeth of the lengthy and discouraging war of independence from Great Britain, made time for daily rations of whiskey as a form of pay, although an Army surgeon general, the soon-to-be-famous Dr. Rush, said he'd really rather the men didn't drink so much.

BENJAMIN RUSH: DOCTOR DOOM

Even though he took the unpopular position of urging moderation in drink, Benjamin Rush (1746–1813) was, by any measure, the most important figure in early American medicine. A widely published author and influential teacher, Rush's views on medicine prevailed in mainstream circles from Revolutionary War days to the Civil War, nearly a century later.

Rush was a sturdy man of medium height, graced with aquiline features that combined with his serious mien to give him an appearance befitting a distinguished physician. His accomplishments, especially in politics and education, are still impressive nearly 200 years after his death. In addition to signing the Declaration of Independence, Rush helped to found several universities, spoke out against slavery and for the rights of women, and was an innovator in the humane treatment of the mentally ill at a time when

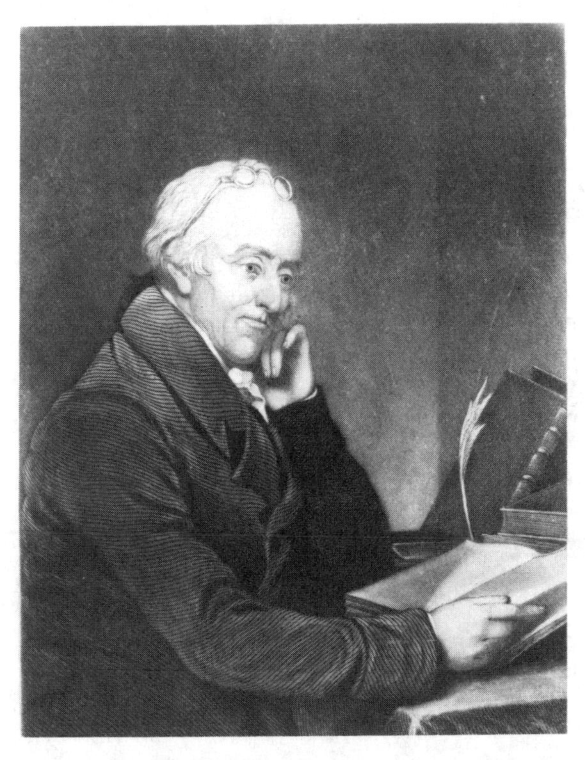

2. Dr. Benjamin Rush, the dominant medical man of the late eighteenth century. *National Library of Medicine.*

insane asylums chained and starved patients as a matter of course. He was a professor at the College of Philadelphia, the precursor of the University of Pennsylvania, and taught some 3,000 impressionable students in his years at the lectern.

Rush's teachings were products of Enlightenment rationalism. He was not a magus who dealt in amulets and charms, as were medievalist healers before him; he was a materialist. Rush believed, with his fellow products of the Enlightenment, that human beings could discover God's laws through applied effort.

This outlook was a sea change from medieval times and differed dramatically, as well, from the philosophies of religious traditionalists of his own era, who viewed disease as the bitter fruit of sin. When, in 1711, a primitive form of innoculation against smallpox was proposed in Boston, clerics opposed it, for fear that innoculation might work and thwart God's will. Not so Rush, who saw God's work in a more benign, harmonious light. (Rush personally innoculated Patrick Henry for smallpox years after the imbroglio in Boston.)

Yet while Rush's sensibility in some ways anticipated modern scientific medicine, nearly all the particulars of his system of medicine were wrong. Influenced by William Cullen, a prominent doctor who taught him at the Royal College of Physicians in Edinburgh, Rush believed that all disease sprang from a single, underlying cause, namely "morbid excitement caused by capilliary tension." Relieving that tension was Rush's rationale for copious bleeding.

The mercury-laden calomel, which Rush grandly called "the Sampson of the Materia Medica," poisoned his patients. Blistering merely inflicted unnecessary pain. Purging, the use of superlaxatives, dehydrated unfortunate patients. Even when Rush was right, he was wrong. As surgeon general, he urged the Continental Army to pitch its tents away from swampy ground, not to avoid disease-carrying mosquitos but to steer clear of vapors from decaying effluvia that he believed poisoned the air and spread sickness.

All these wrong-headed notions were products of the best medical education that Rush's era had to give. Born near Philadelphia, the son of a farmer/gunsmith father and a mother who ran a grocery with the grandiloquent but beguiling name Blazing Star,

COUNTRY COMFORTS

Not all of Dr. Benjamin Rush's treatments were frightening and strange. Some were amusing and strange, such as these selected "Directions for the Cure of Sundry Common Diseases Suited to Country Gentlemen in the United States," published in 1787:

Local inflammations tending to abcess:

Ripen them with a poultice made of bread boiled in beer or stale cider, and a few spoonfuls of strong lye with a little lard or oil and when ripe open it with a lancet, or a plaster made of flour, honey and the yolk of an egg.

Catarrh or Cold:

Bleed occasionally, if the pulse is hard or full. Abstain from eating meat and butter. Drink freely of bran and flaxseed hyssop teas. Take ten grains of niter [saltpeter] three or four times a day. When cough attends and is troublesome, take thirty or forty drops of laudanum [a tincture of opium] every night at bedtime.

Keep bowels open with the pills made of aloes and soap.

Headache:

Bleed if the pulse be full and tense. Take a purge, apply cold water to the head and go to bed.

Rush took his undergraduate degree at the College of New Jersey (now Princeton University). He read Hippocrates, the traditional father of Western medicine, in the original Greek; served an apprenticeship to a Philadelphia doctor; and sailed in the 1760s to Great Britain, where, supping with Oliver Goldsmith and Samuel Johnson, he was introduced to London society by Benjamin Franklin. For his thesis at Edinburgh, Rush made himself throw up and gamely analyzed the spilled contents of his own stomach, the better to study the mechanics of digestion.

When he returned to Philadelphia, Rush became a blazing star in his own right, winning the respect of his peers by championing familiars of heroic medicine such as bleeding. In the full flight of confidence, he didn't hesitate to drain up to four-fifths of a patient's blood, a technique made all the more discomfiting because Rush wasn't sure just how much blood the human body held.

Such sloppiness was all too characteristic of Rush and most of his contemporaries. Some of Rush's mistakes, viewed in the clear light of hindsight, were comical. After praising the healthful properties and taste of water from a Philadelphia spring, Rush had to beat a hasty retreat. The spring, it turned out, was contaminated; the taste Rush praised may have come from pollution.

Most of Rush's efforts were far less amusing, especially to his patients. After plunging with distinction into Revolutionary War politics, Rush returned to medicine, invoking his standard methods to treat the devastating yellow-fever epidemic of 1793, which killed 4,000 people in Philadelphia alone, nearly one-tenth of the city's population.

Yellow fever strikes suddenly, inducing chills and fever, dehydration, repeated vomiting, and, eventually, jaundice, giving victims their characteristic yellowish cast. The disease is caused by a virus and spread by mosquitos, a fact not discovered until 1900. Yellow fever survives in South American and African rain forests. It is treated by rest in a cool, well-ventilated room, a liquid diet, and fluid replacement.

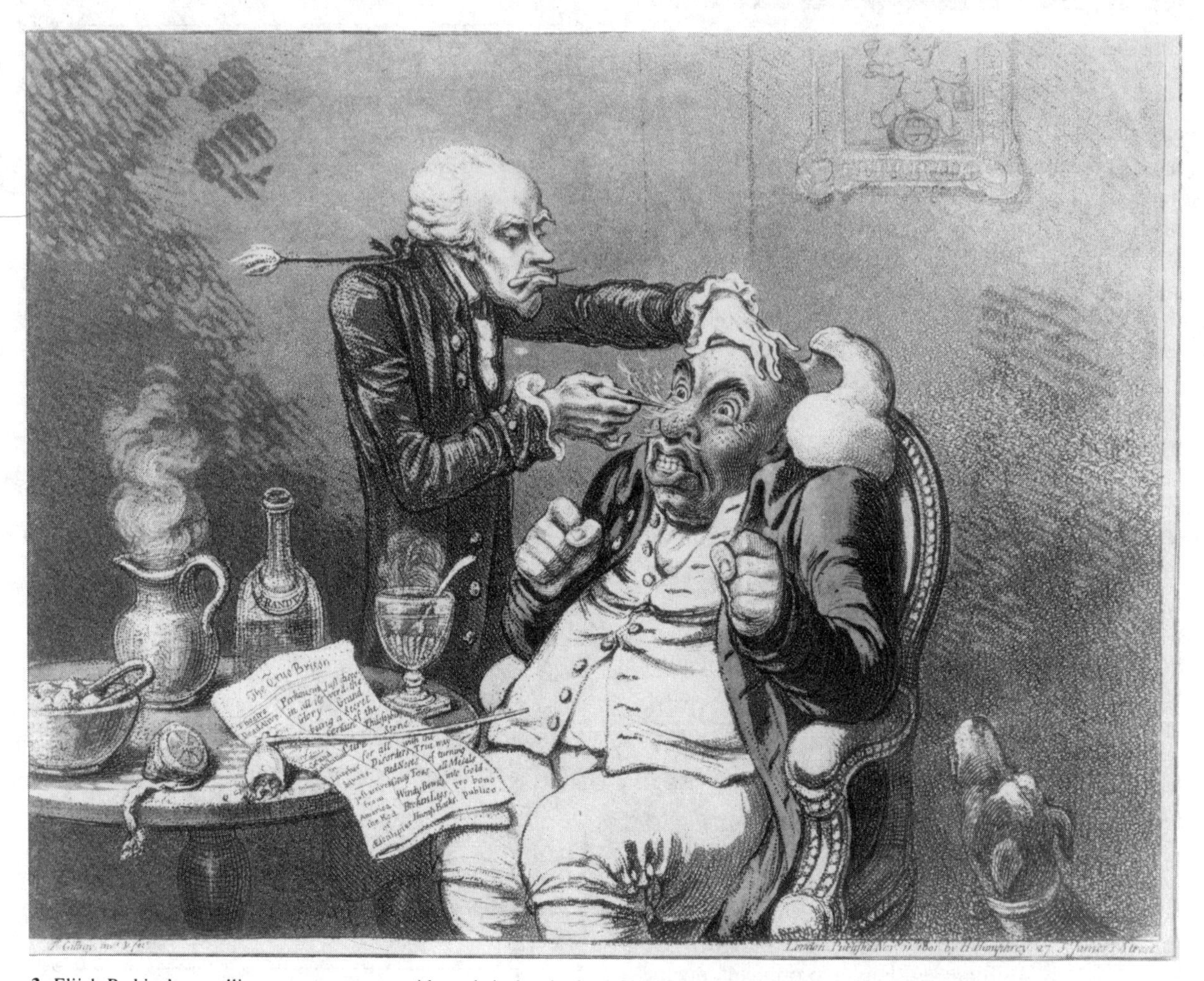

3. Elijah Perkins's metallic tractors were not without their drawbacks (1801). Drawing by J. Gillray. *National Library of Medicine*.

Two centuries ago, yellow fever was epidemic in the eastern United States. Superstitious early Americans were understandably terrified. They devised a number of ways to fend off the mysterious disease, firing cannons and muskets, soaking sponges in camphor and handkerchiefs in vinegar, carrying pieces of tar, and putting garlic in their shoes. They did not, however, drain stagnant ponds or overturn the barrels of rainwater that harbored mosquitos.

Rush fought the disease with his characteristic energy. Even in the best of times, he slept only four or five hours a night—always in an airtight room, usually with a nightcap. During the strain of the 1793 epidemic, he barely slept at all, calling on stricken patients all over the city and bravely risking his own health. As always, Rush prescribed purging and bleeding. The doctor and his assistants were so hard-pressed in the thick of the battle that they sometimes bled patients out of doors and because they didn't have enough cups, let the blood fall, thick and sweet, to the ground. This attracted more mosquitos.

Nothing he did worked. Rush's sister and three of his five apprentices died during the epidemic, which raged for three months and disappeared only with the onset of cool weather. Rush himself fell ill from exhaustion, his hands blackened by mercury, but survived the siege, living for another 20 years.

The failure of Rush's treatments darkened his reputation in some circles, but the doctor was still held in high regard by many. In 1794 and 1797, yellow fever struck again and Rush held fast to his ineffectual methods. Some grumbled that his treatments were brutal and defected to traditional herbal doctors and home remedies, but Rush became a grand old man of medicine, writing, lecturing, and shaping another generation of regular doctors between epidemics.

When he wasn't practicing medicine, Rush was busy taking his place in the pantheon of early American patriots. He carried on a lively correspondence with John Adams and Thomas Jefferson and was a close friend of each.

There were some annoyances, to be sure. In 1799, he sued William Cobbett for libel after the Englishman relentlessly attacked Rush's methods, acidly terming them "one of those great discoveries which are made from time to time for the depopulation of the Earth." Rush won the suit and his reputation as a distinguished physician seemed assured.

Rush died in 1813. He was 67, an advanced age for the time. Modern physicians, reading the old medical records, think he died from pneumonia accompanied by a tubercular cough. Nothing if not consistent, Rush asked his own physician to bleed him when the final crisis was at hand. After Rush passed away, Jefferson ruefully observed, "For classical learning, I have become a zealous advocate; and in this, as in his theory of bleeding and mercury, I was ever opposed to my friend Rush, whom I

ELISHA PERKINS'S TRACTOR PULL

Americans were just getting used to thinking of themselves as a people when their nationalistic fervor was joined by another, shorter-lived, enthusiasm: Perkinsism.

The namesake of the new force, Dr. Elisha Perkins (1741–1799), was no wild-eyed outsider. He was a Yale-educated surgeon who cofounded the Connecticut Medical Society. His fame came from metallic devices of his own invention that he dubbed "tractors," which, when rubbed over painful parts of the body, drew the pain to the extremities and finally out of the body altogether. He patented his tractors in 1797 and survived the indignity of being expelled from the medical society he helped start, which branded him "a patentee and user of nostrums."

Perkins's tractors, according to one account, "came in pairs, and consisted of two metal rods, some three inches long, made of brass and iron, rounded at one end, pointed at the other; half round on one side, flat on the other. With these implements, the patient was to extract the disease from his body by stroking the affected part first with one, then with the other tractor. The directions for use varied with the malady."

Convinced that he held the key to good health in his hands, Perkins hastened to New York City during one of the frequent epidemics of yellow fever. The tractors failed, however, to provide protection for Perkins or anyone else. The doctor fell ill and died of yellow fever in 1799.

Gone but not forgotten, Perkins inspired this contemporary verse, cited in an 1850 book, *Lessons from the History of Medical Delusions*, by Worthington Hooker, M.D.:

See pointed metals, blest with power to appease
The ruthless rage of merciless disease
O'er the frail part a subtle fluid pour,
Drenched with invisible galvanic shower,
Till the arthritic staff and crutch forego,
And leap exulting like the bounding roe.

greatly loved; but who has done much harm, in the sincerest persuasion that he was preserving life and happiness all around him."

A FEARSOME LEGACY

Jefferson's troubled tribute to his old friend could have been applied equally well to most regular American physicians before the Civil War. For although Rush was gone, his legacy, a fearful heritage of bleeding, purging, and poisoning, outlived him.

Despite ample evidence that they were killing patients, Rush's professional heirs were unassailable in their confidence. No major changes in treatment were needed, they believed, only fine tuning of their mighty medical engine. Wrote an unnamed "rural doctor" to a medical journal in 1843: "Few if any of the sciences are established upon a firmer basis than that of medicine. Its principles have their foundations in nature's laws and are consequently immutable."

Calomel remained in favor, usually combined with medicinal wine, laxative salts, opium, and castor oil. Used to cleanse the system of foul, bilious liquids, this poison caused patients to salivate uncontrollably, bleed from the gums, and evacuate the bowels without restraint. Often patients' stools were bloody, making mercury treatment in effect a form of bleeding. Patients suffered horribly, losing teeth and developing sores on the tongue and cheeks. Many, well aware of calomel's effects, dreaded the doctor's call. A popular verse went, "The doctor comes with free good will, but ne'er forgets his calomel."

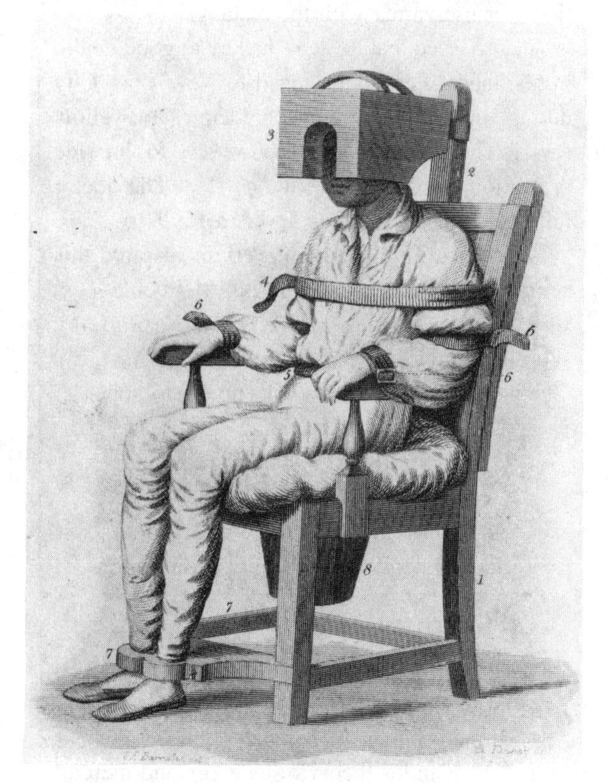

4. Benjamin Rush reckoned his tranquilizing chair would calm a body down (1811). *National Library of Medicine.*

Bleeding couldn't have felt much better, and it was prescribed for practically everything, including epilepsy and bruises from falls. The prestigious British medical journal *The Lancet* was named after the chief instrument used to draw blood, which replaced the earlier method of choice: sucking leeches. Children, even newborns, were not spared the lancet, as they, too, needed to lose the *materies morbi* infecting their tiny bodies. According to medical historian Harris L. Coulter, "Sometimes infants were bled from the jugular vein, since small veins were difficult to locate." The loss of large amounts of blood—and patients were bled copiously and frequently—fatally weakened some, denying an adequate blood supply to their vital organs.

Equally crude—if, in themselves, less lethal—were hot plasters used to induce sweating and blistering, popular not only among ill-equipped rural and frontier doctors in North America but also among top doctors in the cosmopolitan nations of Europe. When Britain's King George III suffered a manic-

FUN FACTS ABOUT LEECHES

- Until the middle of the nineteenth century, blood-sucking leeches were widely used to cure disease caused by bad blood—which, to physicians of the day, meant most any disease. Leeches finally passed from favor when doctors decided that using them was inexact: It was hard to tell just how much blood they drained from their unlucky host.
- Leeches are believed able to ingest up to 10 times their weight in blood.
- At its commercial peak, a nineteenth-century New York City firm imported 500 thousand leeches a year.
- In the late 1980s, leeches staged a modest comeback in medicine; an anticoagulant in their saliva was found to be useful in dissolving blood clots after microsurgery to reattach severed limbs.
- A Welsh firm headed by an American biologist sold some 100 thousand leeches to 150 hospitals for medicinal use in 1988. That same year, an American concern called Leeches USA, Ltd. sold the critters at a bargain price of six dollars apiece.

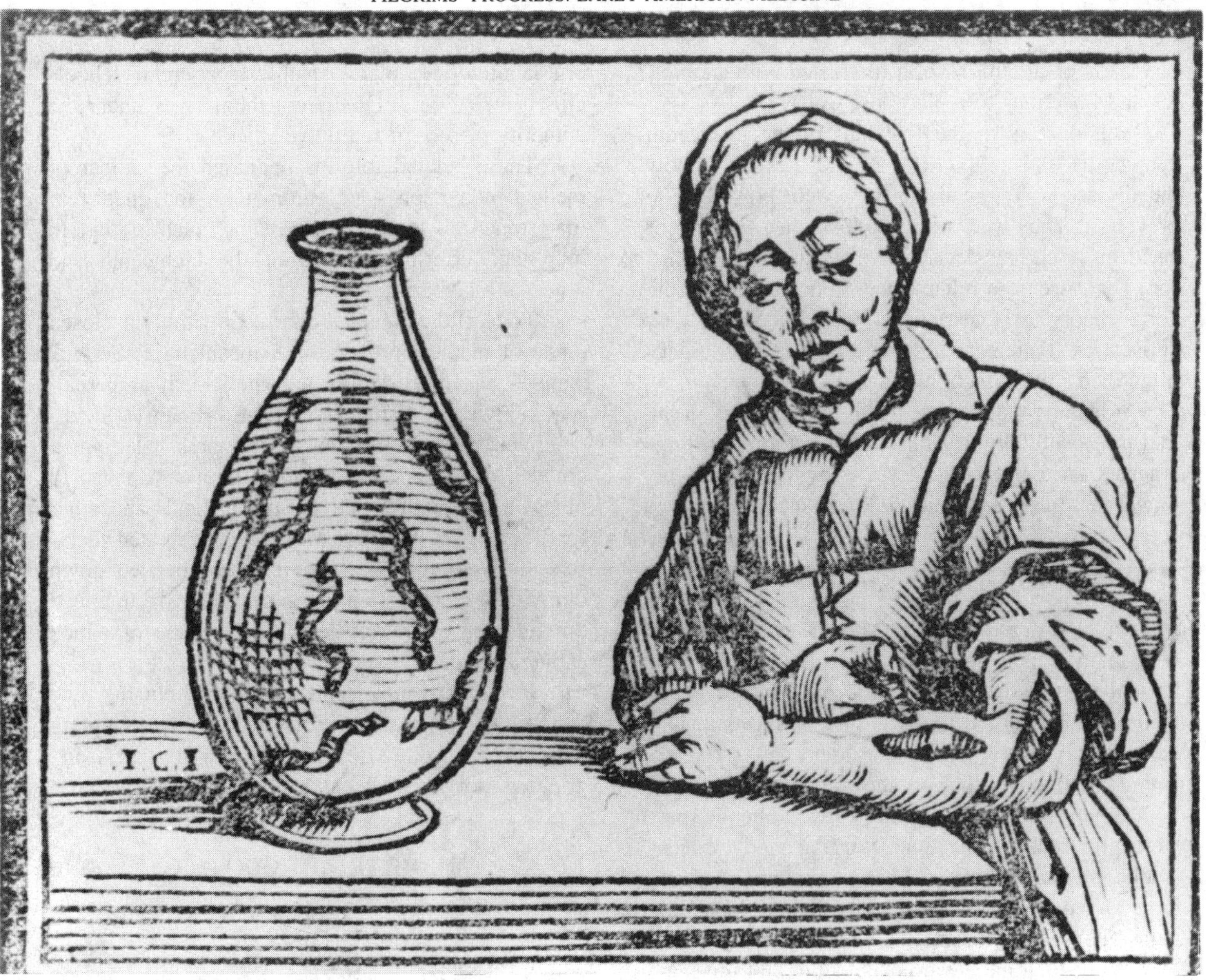

5. Blood-sucking leeches, as seen in this 1639 graphic, were commonly used to bleed patients. *National Library of Medicine.*

depressive fit in 1810, the monarch was forcibly strapped to a chair and his head was shaved and blistered.

In the early nineteenth century, the yellow-fever epidemics that raged over the fledgling United States were joined by another dreaded disease—cholera, which struck in 1832, 1849, and 1866. As with other diseases, religious fundamentalists saw cholera as God's judgment on a sinful, slothful people. When the disease swept through unsanitary slums, as it often did, the victims were blamed for bringing the curse on themselves by living physically and spiritually unclean lives.

People were as bewildered by the plague of cholera as they had been by yellow fever. Until the germ theory of disease was widely accepted in the late nineteenth century, scientists and physicians were unable to deduce the true cause of the disease: water and milk contaminated by a bacterium spread by flies. So they dreamed up fanciful causes to explain what they didn't understand.

One popular theory held that cholera was caused by a shortage of ozone in the atmosphere. This supposed shortfall, long before the actual decline of atmospheric ozone in the late twentieth century, was thought to be counteracted by sulphurous medications. So sulphur pills became the rage. Even sulphur candies were snapped up, becoming one of the first health-food fads.

Other suspected causes of cholera were more down-to-earth. When gummed postage stamps were introduced in Britain around 1840, rumor had it that licking the back of the stamps caused cholera. Methods used to combat the disease were equally bizarre. An Alabama doctor gained a measure of notoriety by giving cholera victims tobacco-smoke enemas.

Funny though these treatments may seem to later generations, cholera's effects, then as now, were no laughing matter. The disease, a severe gastrointestinal infection, induces vomiting, cramps, and diarrhea. Death is caused by dehydration. Today, cholera, restricted largely to overcrowded, unsanitary parts of the third world, is treated with antibiotics and injections to replace lost water.

But doctors in the first half of the nineteenth century had no antibiotics; nor did they know how the disease was spread, so they were powerless to prevent it. They were nearly as lost when surgery for accidents or chronic degenerative conditions was called for. There were no reliable anesthetics and, until the germ theory of disease was well understood, no antiseptics. Patients who struggled through surgery often died from infection or shock.

It is no wonder, then, that a popular view in the mid-nineteenth century held that doctors were nutcrackers used by angels for the swift and sure removal of souls from their corporeal shells.

REBELLION AND REFORM

In such a frightening climate, it is understandable why many people feared and distrusted physicians. Regular doctors were often criticized for their brutal methods and scorned for their shaky education. Understandably, many health consumers felt that alternative treatments, such as the gentle medicines of homeopathy and soothing water cures at bucolic spas, were preferable to bleeding, purging, and tobacco-smoke enemas. At least the alternatives, by and large, lived up to the first tenet of the Hippocratic oath: They did no harm.

While their patients were defecting, reform came slowly to the orthodox medical profession. The Johns Hopkins University medical school, established in 1893, finally provided the prototype of a modern, well-equipped school. Johns Hopkins required a college degree to enroll, provided student doctors with a good laboratory and a well-stocked library, and made regular work at the affiliated teaching hospital part of the course of study. The school, however, was not widely emulated for several decades. Even then, reform was spurred as much by exposure and fear of regulation as by a true desire to improve medical education.

In 1910, Abraham Flexner, a Johns Hopkins graduate (in education, not medicine), published a critical study, *Medical Education in the United States and Canada,* under the aegis of the Carnegie Foundation for the Advancement of Teaching. Visiting each of the 131 regular and irregular medical schools under review, Flexner wrote a devastating critique, exposing the schools for advertised but often nonexistent libraries and labs, lack of basic sanitation, abuse of academic standards, and ethical violations. Combined with gradually toughening state licensing requirements and the growing cost of installing modern laboratories, many small, commercial schools closed their doors. Others put themselves under the authority of recognized universities.

These belated reforms upgraded the caliber of medical education—and, ultimately, the quality of mainstream doctors. But they came much too late to help the suffering patients of the eighteenth and nineteenth centuries.

To fearful patients, the ferment within the closed circle of medical professionals meant little. So sick people consulted traditional healers such as herbalists, midwives, Native American shamans ("medicine men"), and other lay practitioners. Clergymen doubled as healers, a tradition that has survived to our own day with the laying-on of hands and other forms of divine healing. Many people treated themselves, swearing by family remedies handed down orally from generation to generation, or thumbed through dog-eared self-help books, some of which endured for decades.

In the early nineteenth century, about the time that regular doctors were unsuccessfully grappling with cholera, yellow fever, and other scourges, disgruntled individuals began to join forces.

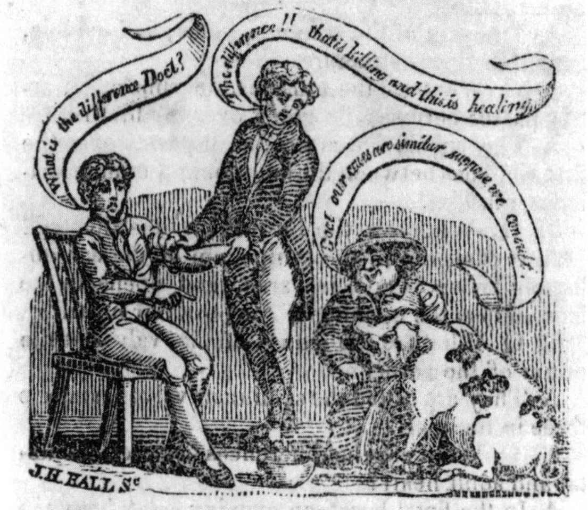
MEDICAL ANECDOTES.
What is the difference Doct?
The difference!! that is killing and this is healing
Doct our cases are similar suppose we consult.
J.H. HALL Sc
The *Doctor* takes the *life* to *heal*,
The *Butcher* does the *same* to *kill;*
The first *designs* the *breath should stay*,
The next *direct* the other way.
Should proof of this you wish to know,
See *plate* above, and *scrip* below.
Now form your minds, which of the two,
If sickness press, the work shall do.
Ratsbane, zinc, and vitriol too,
And mercury, to physic through;
We know these poisons they do give,
Are not their patients tough to live.

6. Not without reason, critics compared heroic medicine to simple slaughter. *National Library of Medicine.*

The Thomsonians, a short-lived movement that favored botanical medicine and self-care, enlisted fully one-sixth of the American public in the 1830s. The Grahamites trumpeted radical dietary reform, attracting legendary newspaperman Horace Greeley and Dr. John Harvey Kellogg, the cofounder of Kellogg's cereals. Phrenologists, who claimed to be able to diagnose illness and read character by measuring the skull, were popular figures. Temperance crusaders and their opposites, patent-medicine peddlers who dosed their nostrums with alcohol, drew broad followings. Unorthodox doctors called Eclectics tried a little bit of everything, even allowing patients to choose their own mode of treatment, surely the ultimate in populist medicine.

Still other movements and methods, some originating in the distant past, survive even on the verge of the twenty-first century. Vegetarians, homeopaths, fitness buffs, health-minded religious groups such as the Christian Science and Seventh-day Adventist churches, and ministers of the spine and bones such as chiropractors and osteopaths still exist and sometimes flourish. Taken together, they, like their bewigged and black-frocked ancestors, provide a vital if bewildering array of medical alternatives.

Sometimes worthy, sometimes wacky, nearly always colorful, idiosyncratic, and visionary, they are the masters of ceremony and the damsels in distress, the stage-door johnnies and the grand divas of the great American medicine show.

CRUDE BOYS AND JADED CLERKS

Low standards give the medical schools access to a large clientele open to successful exploitation by commercial methods. The crude boy or the jaded clerk who goes into medicine at this level has not been moved by a significant prompting from within; nor has he as a rule shown any forethought in the matter of making himself ready. He is more likely to have been caught drifting at a vacant moment by an alluring advertisement or announcement, quite commonly an exaggeration, not infrequently an outright misrepresentation. Indeed, the advertising methods of the commercially successful schools are amazing. Not infrequently advertising costs more than laboratories. The school catalogues abound in exaggeration, misstatement, and half-truths. The deans of these institutions occasionally know more about modern advertising than about modern medical teaching. They may be uncertain about the relation of the clinical laboratory to bedside instruction; but they have calculated to a nicety which 'medium' brings the largest 'return.'

—Abraham Flexner
Medical Education in the United States and Canada
Bulletin No. 4, 1910
Carnegie Endowment for the Advancement of Teaching

CHAPTER

· 2 ·

THE HERBALISTS: GREEN MEDICINE

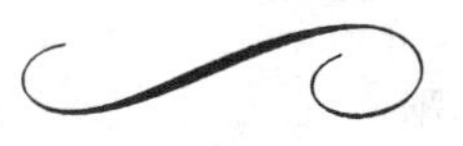

There is a wonderful science in Nature, in trees, herbs, roots and flowers, which man has never yet fathomed.

JETHRO KLOSS,
Back to Eden, *1939*

Inside the World Ginseng Center, on San Francisco's bustling Kearny Street in the heart of Chinatown, dried ginseng roots the size of a baby's fist are laid out in rows under display counters and stored in clear glass jars. The roots are positioned at eye level, like the impulse items in a supermarket. This is fitting, for the World Ginseng Center is a supermarket of modern and traditional herbal medicine, complete with such incongruous items as cigarettes, soft drinks, and advertisements for the California state lottery.

Despite all the add-ons, ginseng is clearly the main attraction. An herb long cherished in Chinese medicine, it is especially valued because ginseng's shape reminds observers of the human form, and the root is thus considered auspicious as a tonic and aphrodisiac. In fact, a lucrative trade in ginseng, which grew wild in colonial days, spurred some of the earliest contacts between North America and China, which couldn't get enough of the magical herb at home.

The impressive size, sparkling appearance, and steady patronage of this latter-day ginseng palace are testimony to the survival of herbalism in an era of heroic medicine and high technology.

The Asian, chiefly Chinese, brand of herbalism is one of four major traditions in American herbal medicine—the others being European, Native American, and the quirky, eclectic body of folk medicine that, over time, incorporated elements of the other three.

Botanists classify herbs as seed-producing plants that have flowers rather than woody stems. They generally die at the end of each growing season, then blossom again the following year. Modern commercial vendors use a somewhat broader working definition, counting as herbs parts of other plants sold for their aromatic or savory qualities.

Today, medicinal herbs, as distinct from seasonings for cooking, hold on to their popularity chiefly in ethnic enclaves of major cities, in backwoods hollows where technological change has not fully penetrated, and among the remnants of the back-to-nature counterculture that flourished in the 1960s and 1970s. In pills, powders, and tinctures, roots and bark, fresh leaves and prepared teas, herbs are sold in specialty shops, health-food stores, and nutrition-minded chain stores. It is not uncommon to find herbal dietary aids in suburban shopping malls, although they are a far cry from traditional herbal medicines.

Since the eighteenth century, ancient remedies and long-familiar plants have been tapped for valuable new medicines. Among them are malaria-fighting quinine (extracted from the bark of the Peruvian cinchona tree); digitalis, the heart medication derived from foxglove; cocaine, used as a local anesthetic after it was extracted from the leaves of the South American coca plant (and before it became a major source of drug abuse); opium, a powerful painkiller and sedative, taken from poppy seeds; the painkiller morphine, derived from opium; and salicin, the active principle in willow bark traditionally used to banish headaches, which led to aspirin.

Dr. James A. Duke, an economic botanist with the U.S. Department of Agriculture, writes, "Today, 75 percent of the world's population—the poor three-fourths—still relies on these plants and other tools of traditional medicine. Meanwhile, in the industrial world, at least 25 percent of our over-the-counter drugs derive from natural materials."

Certainly, our ancestors valued the healing properties of plants. There were no alternatives, save the bleed, blister, and purge techniques of the "regular" doctors.

SEEDS: EUROPE

Europeans used herbs long before their great migrations across the Atlantic. The names of most early healers went unrecorded, but by the fourth century B.C., the use of herbs had advanced far enough to be set down in writing by Theophrastos, a student of Aristotle.

Several centuries later, a Roman army physician by the name of Pedanius Dioscorides wrote a pioneering herbal, *De Materia Medica,* compiled in the first century A.D. By that time, the Roman legions had conquered much of the Mediterranean world and the Near East, taking their knowledge of plants and bagsful of seeds with them. The Romans were especially fond of garlic, which they regarded as a virtual panacea. They were not the first people to think so: The builders of the ancient Egyptian pyramids were given garlic rations to help them bear up under the work.

Galen (ca.129–ca.200 A.D.), a Greek-speaking native of Asia Minor who used herbs in his practice, was the most famous physician in Rome. After studying at Alexandria, the ancient seat of learning, Galen moved to Rome and became personal physician to the powerful emperor and Stoic philosopher Marcus Aurelius (121–180 A.D.). Galen built on the system of Hippocrates (ca.460–ca.370 B.C.). He adopted Hippocrates's theory of the four humors: blood, phlegm, black bile, and choler (yellow bile). According to Hippocrates's reasoning, if those liquid constituents of the body remained in balance, the body remained healthy; if disturbed, the body fell ill. Galen further classified medicines, most of them healing plants, according to their heat or coldness, dryness or moisture.

Galen's elaborate system and near-metaphysical way of looking at things enthralled medieval churchmen as well as his contemporaries. As a result, Galen may have been the most influential medical theorist of all time. Certainly, his system was the most long-lived. Galen's philosophy held firm for some 1,500 years, until European physicians added minerals—many of them actually poisons, such as mercury and antimony—to their satchels of Galenic botanical medicines.

Galen's system was strikingly different from the herbalism of unschooled tribal people. Traditional herbalists employed "specifics"—that is, they used a given plant to treat a specified disease, based on their own experience and observation. Barbara Griggs, a British historian of herbal medicine, observes:

> The generations of doctors who memorized Galen's near-numerical classifications soon learned to despise those simple healers who still used marshmallow for a severe case of diarrhea because it was usually successful in such cases, without having the faintest idea whether it was hot or cold or what, whether the patient suffered from an excess of phlegm or a deficiency of bile. Eventually, "specific" came to be a dirty word, meaning that the plant was administered in this uninstructed manner, rather than according to divine rules.

Galen was fond of complicated, costly medications with dozens of ingredients, including herbs and such exotica as viper's flesh. These medications—the most famous was theriac, which included opium, wine, and honey, as well as assorted herbs—were aged for maximum effect. Theriac already had 70 ingredients when Galen went to work on it; when he finished, it had more than 100. Regarded as a universal panacea for a very long time, it was still listed as a legitimate drug in western European pharmacopoeias in the late nineteenth century and must have been the most potent medication around, for good or ill.

Even these far-fetched medicines had practical uses, although they weren't necessarily what Galen and his followers expected. In 1775, the English physician William Withering (1741–1799) discovered digitalis by deducing the active ingredient in a medicinal brew containing no fewer than 20 ingredients. Withering got the recipe from an elderly woman in Shropshire who had kept it secret for years. He brewed tea from the foxglove leaf and used it to treat dropsy, bloating caused by fluid retention when the heart doesn't pump enough blood to the kidneys. Digitalis is still used to treat a fluttering, rapid heartbeat.

Traditional herbal-based recipes, whether a complex combination or a "simple," were usually passed on by word of mouth. When the oral tradition began to wane, Europeans revived the ancient tradition of herbals, jotting things down to preserve and disseminate information.

British herbals began appearing as early as the tenth century. Perhaps the most famous, Nicholas Culpeper's *Complete Herbal and English Physician,* was published in 1652 and republished in a pirated edition in New England in 1708. A classic volume that continues to be reprinted (though more for historical than medical reasons), Culpeper's book tied earthly cures to the movement of heavenly bodies. "He that would know the reason of the operation of the Herbs," Culpeper (1616–1654) wrote, "must look up as high as the stars."

In seventeenth- and eighteenth-century England, herbal gardens were cultivated in the congested heart of London for the edification of students and production of healing plants. The flowering patches were called "physic" gardens, from the Greek word that is also the root of *physician.* Some venerable gardens still exist, including the Chelsea Physic Garden, founded in 1673, whose directors allow tourists to venture behind its elegant brick wall on selected days.

Although Europe was home to many healing plants, the pursuit of new botanical medicines helped drive the exploration and colonization of the Americas. Cinchona, coca, sarsparilla, and tobacco were shipped back to Europe as valuable medicines, and the search for a fast passage to the Far East—the source of highly prized spices—drew many a wooden sailing ship from its snug European harbor.

A SURE CURE FOR THAT NAGGING COUGH

When European colonists landed in the future state of Virginia in the late sixteenth century, they discovered a curious and marvelous plant that they endowed with magical properties. The smoke, it was said, was magnetic; especially effective when inhaled, it cleared the lungs of impurities and was duly listed in the London pharmacopoeia in 1595 as a treatment for coughs.

The plant was tobacco (*Nicotiana tabacum*).

True, smoking tobacco wasn't a hit with everyone. England's King James I condemned it in 1604 as "a custome . . . daungerous to the Lungs, and in the black stinking fume thereof, neerest resembling the horrible Stigian smoak of the pit that is bottomlesse." Philadelphia's Benjamin Rush, writing in 1798, was scarcely more complimentary, linking tobacco with drunkenness and noting that it harmed the stomach, mouth, and nerves. However, the nineteenth-century phrenologist Orson Fowler considered tobacco an aphrodisiac.

By the 1980s, 54 million Americans smoked, chewed, or dipped tobacco products and some 390 thousand died annually of tobacco-related causes. The miracle weed hailed with so much hope four centuries earlier cost the U.S. economy an estimated 53.7 billion dollars in medical bills and lost workdays in 1984.

ROOTS: COLONIAL AMERICA

When explorers and adventurers from western Europe navigated safe passage across the Atlantic, they stumbled onto what were, to them, virgin continents. Wildlife, fish, and an intoxicating variety of plants grew in abundance. Everywhere, there was clear air and clean water, and there was plenty of space. Nowhere north of the Aztec capital of Tenochtitlan (present-day Mexico City) was there a city on the European scale where filth and pestilence could do its dirty work. There would be none for three centuries, until Europeans, their African slaves, and subjugated natives of the Americas built teeming cities and embarked on the Industrial Revolution.

The first European immigrants were impressed with the people they misnamed Indians, especially with their good health. The English writer John Josselyn, in his 1672 book *New Englands Rarities Discovered,* praised Indian medicine for its sensitive use of native flora.

Sadly, however, those favorable first impressions were not to last. Although North American colonists were often forced to rely on helpful Native Americans to survive, familiarity bred contempt. The new arrivals came to see themselves as superior and the Native Americans, for their part, were less willing to share what they knew with these strange, obnoxious newcomers.

Although many drugs in colonial Canada and the soon-to-be United States were botanicals (there were also animal and mineral drugs), only a few Native American remedies came into wide use among

New-Englands
RARITIES
Diſcovered:
IN
Birds, *Beaſts*, *Fiſhes*, *Serpents*,
and *Plants* of that Country.
Together with
The *Phyſical* and *Chyrurgical* REMEDIES
wherewith the *Natives* conſtantly uſe to
Cure their DISTEMPERS, WOUNDS,
and SORES.
ALSO
A perfect *Deſcription* of an *Indian SQUA*,
in all her Bravery; with a POEM not
improperly conferr'd upon her.
LASTLY
A CHRONOLOGICAL TABLE
of the moſt remarkable Paſſages in that
Country amongſt the ENGLISH.
Illuſtrated with CUTS.
By *JOHN JOSSELYN*, Gent.
London, Printed for *G. Widdowes* at the
Green Dragon in St. *Pauls* Church-yard, 1672.

7. Englishman John Josselyn wrote a pioneering American herbal (1672). *From John Josselyn,* New Englands Rarities Discovered, *reprinted by the Massachusetts Historical Society, 1972.*

Europeans. When, during the Revolutionary War, rebel physicians drew up a list of 48 plant remedies for the Continental Army, only three were derived from native plants. Most herbs and drugs were imported from Europe.

Those who couldn't afford to buy imported drugs, or who were frustrated by their scarcity, maintained backyard gardens; Paul Revere's eighteenth-century Boston home had an herb garden that was replanted in modern times for tourists trekking through the city's historic North End. Almanacs and newspapers printed recipes for medicines the way their modern counterparts print food recipes. Many people made their own drugs. Some also purchased them from physicians, who employed apprentices to make the medications—and made tidy profits on the side by selling the very same medicines they prescribed.

According to medical historian William G. Rothstein, writing in *Other Healers:*

> The botanicals were usually dried, ground into a powder or stored in leaf form. When needed, the leaves were brewed into a tea or a teaspoonful of the powder was added to some sweetened hot water and drunk by the patient. Occasionally, the powder was sniffed like snuff. Sometimes a number of drugs were combined according to a recipe, dissolved in water, vinegar, brandy or wine, and kept in bottles to be used as needed. The resulting medicine was often made more concentrated by boiling off most of the liquid. No matter how they were made, botanical medicines were often repulsively bitter to the taste, sometimes to the point of being nauseating. Occasionally, they were cooked with oils, fats or beeswax for long periods of time and used as ointments. Some botanicals were ground and mixed with a liquid and cornmeal or some other substance for use as poultices on wounds, burns or sores. The general preference was for drugs used singly known as "simples."

As American cities grew, swallowing cultivated land, herbal gardens and homemade medicines were supplemented by prepared medicines, some of them the patent medicines that gained their full measure of notoriety in the nineteenth century. But homemade medicines were not widely replaced for a long time.

Books such as *Primitive Physic,* a 1747 tome by evangelist John Wesley (1703–1791), were home favorites for 100 years. Wesley told readers how to treat their own illnesses with herbs and other drugs. This was powerfully appealing medicine to people too poor, too distant from the urban clusters, or too distrustful to put themselves in the hands of regular physicians.

BRANCHES: NATIVE AMERICAN HERBALISM

Traditional Native Americans were not the noble savages or perfect beings of myth, but they knew much about the healing properties of native plants. European colonists who were able to push beyond their own ethnocentrism learned a lot from them.

Perhaps the most spectacular recorded lesson came in 1535–36, when explorer Jacques Cartier found himself and his men ice-bound in the St. Lawrence River near the site of modern Montreal. To make matters worse, many of the Frenchmen had scurvy. Neither the Europeans nor the Native Americans knew the first thing about vitamin C, which wasn't discovered until the twentieth century; but the native people did know a good deal about scurvy.

Fortunately for Cartier's men—who, like other Europeans, thought that scurvy was caused by bad air—they were prevailed upon by local Natives to drink tea made from black spruce needles. They recovered. When John Josselyn wrote a century later, he noted that black spruce (rich in vitamin C) was commonly used by the Native Americans of New England. Even so, news of a cure for scurvy—which, among other things, causes the teeth to fall out—traveled slowly among European settlers, and the disease remained a scourge.

Generalizing about native North American medicine is difficult, since the tribes, speaking hundreds of different languages, were scattered over vast distances and lived in wildly varying climates. Virtually all Native Americans, though, believed in the efficacy of myth and magic. They danced, sang, and prayed, believing that spiritual energy charged healing materials—roots, bark, and tea—with power. Unlike modern-day doctors, they were not rational materialists. Rather, they believed in evil spirits and the power of animals to cause disease. To protect themselves, they carried amulets and charms. It is from these accouterments that derogatory stereotypes of medicine men and witch doctors come.

Central to Native American medicine was the Law of Similars, an element of sympathetic magic that native North Americans shared with traditional people in other parts of the world. Simply put, this is the belief that like cures like. Thus, a red plant would be good for the blood, a yellow plant for treating jaundice, and so on.

Unlike the immensely complicated remedies of Europe, most Native American medicines used one, two, or at most three ingredients. According to Barbara Griggs:

> As with most primitive cultures, emetics [to induce vomiting] and purges were strongly emphasized. . . . The Indians believed that all sickness was introduced via the digestive tract, and since many of their diseases must have been parasitic in origin, this was sound practical medicine. The sick man was thoroughly purged and vomited—early observers spoke of vomits strong enough to kill a horse—before a preparation of healing herbs was given to him. Then he was fasted before being put on a light diet of gruel made from grain and roots, until recovery was complete.

In addition to healing herbs, most Native American tribes made use of sweating in specially built sweat lodges, as well as occasional bloodletting—though they bled patients much less than did eighteenth- and nineteenth-century European Americans.

Despite their considerable knowledge and skills, traditional Indians were far from all-knowing, as latter-day champions of back-to-the earth movements would have it. Although adept at easing the trauma of childbirth, Native American cultures had spotty success with major surgery. Nature, which produced their *materia medica,* also shut off supplies with drought, flooding, insect armies, and storms.

Some failures were due more to social conditions than to natural causes. When Native Americans began to retreat before the advances of European colonists, they didn't know the flora and fauna of their new homes. Worst of all, they had no natural resistance or treatments for unfamiliar European diseases such as smallpox, which was sometimes deliberately introduced to their communities.

In spite of their problems, native North Americans initially impressed the first new arrivals from across the Atlantic. The Dutch in New Amsterdam, the Quakers in Philadelphia, and the Puritans in New England sang their praises, sometimes in spite of themselves.

Wrote an early Dutch settler: ". . . It is somewhat strange that among these barbarous people, there are few or none cross-eyed, blind, crippled, lame, hunch-backed, or limping men; all are well-fashioned people, strong and sound of body, well-formed, without blemish."

That observation was set down in 1624. Fifty-nine years later, William Penn wrote, "There are diverse Plants that not only the Indians tell us, but we have had occasion to prove by Swellings, Burnings, Cuts, etc. that they are of great virtue, suddenly curing the Patient. . . ."

Clearly, the Native Americans were doing something right. Their health and well-being—so unusual to Europeans who fled plague-swept cities—was due to the native people's use of healing plants, fresh air, and clean water, the abundance of open space, and their good personal hygiene. The Native Americans, who favored sweat baths, were much cleaner than the new arrivals. And their simple herbal cures were less lethal than the medicines of the colonists.

The historian Virgil J. Vogel notes that in 1618, just two years before the Pilgrims stepped ashore at Plymouth Rock, ". . . the *Pharmacopoeia Londinensis* . . . included mummy dust, human and pigeon excrement and stag's penis. As late as the eighteenth century, the materia medica of Herman Boerhaave included dragon's blood, oil of scorpions, troches of vipers, crab's eye and chalk."

The medicines bequeathed by native North Americans were generally less exotic and less harmful. Traders heading back to Europe filled their holds with sassafras, lobelia inflata (a vomit-inducing plant used to treat syphilis), petroleum (gathered from surface pools and used to soothe aches and pains), ginseng, and tobacco.

"More than 200 indigenous drugs . . . used by one or more Indian tribes have been official in the *Pharmacopoeia of the United States of America* for varying periods . . . or in the *National Formulary* . . ." reports Vogel, who counts "about four dozen drugs . . . native to South America" in the total.

In a curious way, Native Americans, though often held in contempt by white settlers, gained a reputation as healers. Thus the proliferation in the nineteenth century of "Indian" patent medicines (sold by non-Native Americans) such as Seminole Cough Balsam and Comanche Blood Strength-O; the Native American performers in traveling medicine shows; and "Indian" doctors who claimed to be natives or to have learned medicine from them.

Ironically, by the time these elements of popular culture became well-known, the societies that inspired them had been displaced or, in some cases, destroyed.

STRANGE FLOWERS: AMERICAN FOLK MEDICINE

Over time, the healing techniques of European colonists and Native Americans influenced each other, producing a new medicine practiced chiefly by housewives, farmers, and itinerant healers. This is the medicine of old wives' tales, strange-smelling preparations bubbling on cast-iron stoves and rites of spring whose origins are only half-remembered.

Folk medicine was—and is, in cultural corners where remnants survive—largely empirical and often improvised. Its early advocates didn't trust doctors or couldn't find or afford them. Some learned what they knew from the Native Americans, especially on the frontier, while others followed the precepts of popular, self-anointed white "doctors."

Early colonists such as John Tennent, author of the 1734 book *Every Man His Own Doctor*, advocated home remedies made from common herbs such as seneca snakeroot, which he recommended for gout.

In the early nineteenth century, advertising, then in its infancy, was used by pitchmen such as "Doctor" David Smith, author of *The Reformed Botanic and Indian Physician*, to play on the common—and justifiable—fear of regular doctors:

> . . . no longer suffer yourselves to be cut to pieces by the lancet or the two-edge sword of poisonous mineral drugs, which man's device has hatched up to pick your pockets and bear you to an untimely grave; for the God of Nations in early days supplied our ancient fathers with all the healing power arising from the Vegetable Kingdom. . . .

Among the healing techniques that Smith recommended was rubbing onions on the head to cure baldness and rubbing the head with vinegar to cure insanity.

Folk remedies, which calcified into habit and superstition, survive today in Appalachia, among African Americans of the rural South, in unassimilated Hispanic communities, and among the Pennsylvania Germans (popularly known as Pennsylvania Dutch, after *Deutsch*, the German word for *German*).

Long after the days of old Doc Smith, the Pennsylvania Dutch employed folk treatments, such as bitter-tasting herbs to purify the blood. Green plants such as watercress and lettuce were taken in

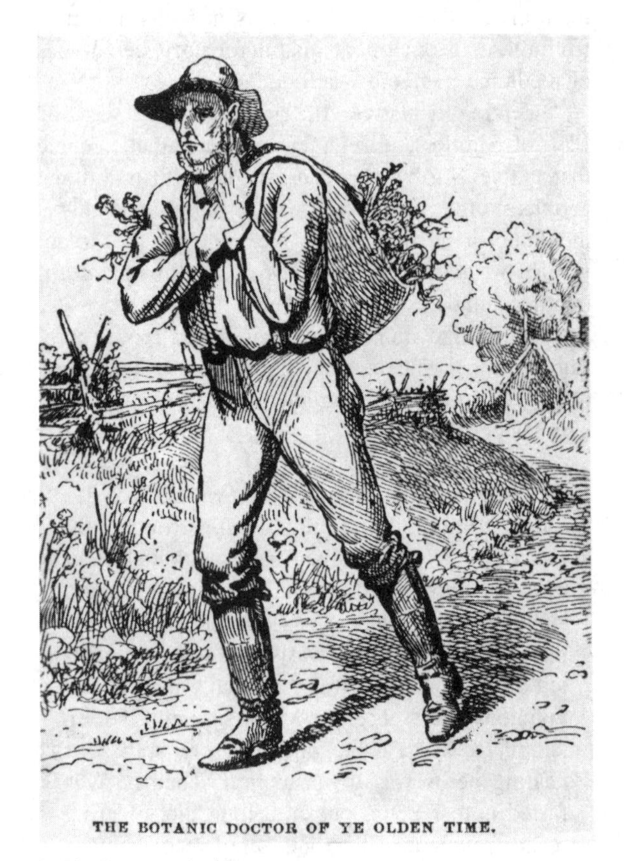

THE BOTANIC DOCTOR OF YE OLDEN TIME.

8. *The Bettmann Archive.*

BAD SEEDS AND EXTRAORDINARY ATTITUDES

Sure, George Washington grew marijuana hemp for making rope. And, yes, the active principle of marijuana, THC, is now used to treat glaucoma. But the fact is, marijuana (*cannibis sativa*) has long been the bad seed of the herb world. As such, it has received a bad press in sensational newspapers and magazines and such scare movies as 1936's *Reefer Madness*.

Health reformers, concerned that marijuana would lead to harder drugs and all-around wanton behavior, imparted their views in books of family remedies that sat on many a home night stand. The editors of *Health Knowledge*, a 1,527-page self-help volume published in 1919, characterized the effects of the disreputable herb in these words:

> In the state of intoxication, persons under its influence . . . show an excess of politeness, and 'salaam' to bystanders till exhausted, while still others become extravagantly merry, losing the sense of personality and assuming extraordinary attitudes. Finally, sleep comes in, attended by happy or amusing dreams of a sensuous nature.

the springtime, when the Pennsylvania Dutch also were known to practice a little blood-letting—just to clear things up, as sort of a spring house-cleaning for the body.

The Shakers, known for their simple, elegant furniture, were accomplished herbalists, too. The austere religious sect exported some 350 herb species as far away as Australia and sold herbs to domestic makers of patent medicines. The Mount Lebanon, Massachusetts Shaker village devoted 50 acres to herbs for medicines and garden seeds.

By the turn of the twentieth century, herbal folk medicine went into decline, spurred by advances in science, some of which drew upon the work of the old herbalists. Chemists learned to synthesize the active ingredients of plants in the laboratory, standardizing and sterilizing drug doses and stabilizing supplies. Combined with advances in surgery, radiology, and the discovery of vitamins and antibiotics, modern medicine leap-frogged traditional ways. Patients came to prefer dramatic, fast-acting drugs, instead of gentle but slow-acting botanicals, and chose antiseptic hospitals over low-technology home care when given a choice.

Still, the old ways never entirely disappeared. Jethro Kloss (1863–1946), a popular American folk healer and author, provided a living link between the twentieth century and the not-so-remote past with health retreats, soybean-based meat substitutes, and embrace of herbal medicine. All were disseminated in his "old-fashioned remedy book," *Back to Eden*, which Kloss self-published in 1939. The book, still in print in a paperback edition, is marketed by Kloss's heirs, who claim to have sold two million copies.

Kloss, called "the Walt Whitman of herbalists" in advertisements for his book in the 1980s, was a Wisconsin farm boy, the son of German immigrants. He was in poor health as a young man, but after sampling the red-clover tea recommended in Seventh-day Adventist founder Ellen G. White's books, Kloss regained his health. He worked for a time at the Battle Creek Sanitarium—John Harvey Kellogg's famous "San"—later opening places of his own, where he practiced hydropathic water cures and herbalism and made commercial health foods.

A devout Christian who named a son Eden and a daughter Promise Joy, Kloss acknowledged that he owed much of his knowledge to Native American lore and the herbalism that his parents brought from the Old Country. Apparently sincere but always controversial, Kloss championed lobelia, a Native American and Thomsonian favorite regarded as poisonous by the Food and Drug Administration, and detailed treatments for cancer and leprosy.

Back to Eden, which comes complete with mail-order forms and Kloss family pictures, also includes directions on "how to give a thorough Thomson emetic." With his nature-based philosophy, Kloss, whose book is available on the shelves of health-food stores, provides a direct link between the far-off 1830s and the far-out New Age of the 1990s.

CHINA AND AMERICA

Traditional Asian medicine—which, in North America, means Chinese medicine, the oldest and most widely traveled variety—is not widely known outside Chinese communities. Discriminatory racial barriers imposed by the white majority kept Chinese Americans in big-city ghettos and isolated agricultural towns until after World War II. Even now, cultural gaps keep some Chinese herbals and scholarly studies from being translated into English.

This is especially unfortunate, given that Chinese herbalism on both sides of the Pacific draws on a sophisticated and very old tradition, much of it strikingly different from Western medicine and that of North American natives.

The world's earliest known herbal, the *Pen-tsao,* a Chinese *materia medica,* is attributed to Shen Nung, the legendary Red Emperor, who supposedly lived some 5,000 years ago. The herbal included observations on 365 therapeutic plants. It was updated in the seventh century A.D., in a major effort that, according to Barbara Griggs, "occupied 2,000 scholars for . . . two years." In the 1590s, the *Pen T'sao Kang Mu,* a standard Chinese pharmacopoeia, further refined Chinese herbalism.

Nineteenth-century immigrants drew on this tradition and its allied elements, such as the Chinese notions of chi and yin and yang. Chi is the life force that flows along meridians and through organs tapped by needle-wielding acupuncturists. Yin is the feminine, passive form of energy; yang, the masculine, active form. Medicinal herbs are believed to have yin or yang properties.

Bruce Cost, a Caucasian author who writes about Asian cuisines and their cultural context, points out that many features of Chinese cooking were originally medicinal. Ginger, still often served with fish, was considered an antidote to shellfish poisoning. While fresh sprigs of coriander are now added to food for seasoning and eye appeal (or simply out of habit), the early Chinese used coriander to safeguard the diner from ptomaine poisoning.

Unlike many herbal traditions, Chinese herbalism has largely survived the passage of the centuries, both in its homeland and abroad.

In 1958, Mao Tse-tung declared that "Chinese traditional medicine and pharmacy are a great treasurehouse, and vigorous efforts should be made to explore them, and to raise them to a higher level." As a result, hospitals in the People's Republic of China prescribe herbal medicines, and acupuncturists work alongside Western-style medical doctors. Whether traditional medicine will survive the enthusiasm for all things Western in post-Mao China remains to be seen.

Certainly, it hasn't snuffed out tradition in North American Chinatowns, where signs advertising herbalists and acupuncturists jostle for space with M.D.s' shingles; sometimes, in fact, M.D.s also serve as herbalists and acupuncturists.

Although most Chinese herbalism remains within immigrant enclaves, China's time-honored enthusiasm for the ginseng root has spilled over into health-food stores associated with the New Age fusion of mysticism, money, and self-improvement that grew out of the hippie counterculture of the 1960s and 1970s. In addition to the solid root, ginseng tea (often sweetened with sugar to mask the bitter taste) and tinctures also line health-food store shelves.

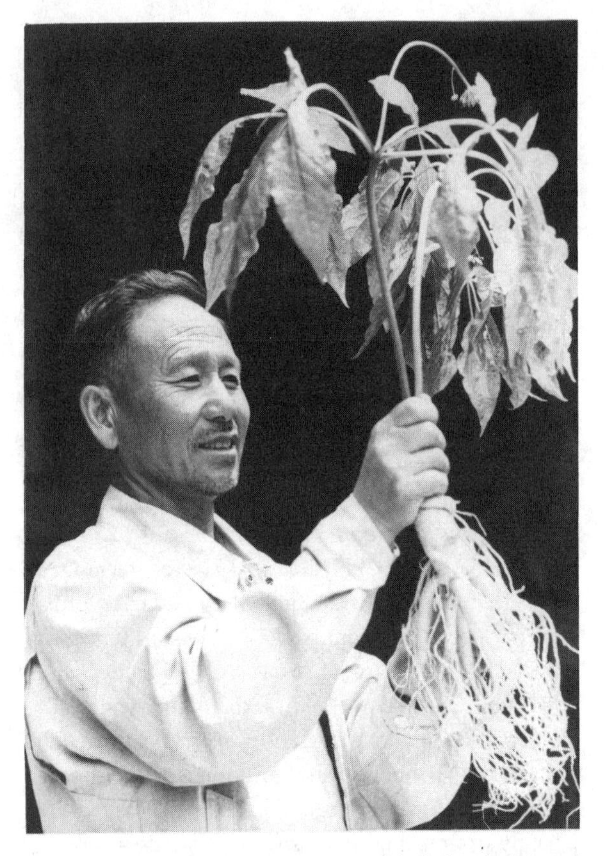

9. Ginseng has long been valued as a medicinal plant in Asia and North America. *UPI/The Bettmann Archive.*

America's interest in ginseng predates the late twentieth century by many years. Native North Americans used it as an aphrodisiac, among other things, and the root is well-known in American folk medicine. In colonial America, wild ginseng was picked for export to China.

According to William A. Embodein, Jr., author of a 1974 book entitled *Bizarre Plants:*

> American ginseng, christened *Panax quinquefolium* by Linnaeus in 1753 [Asian ginseng is *Panax ginseng*] was so prominent in Canada that by 1718, the Jesuits shipped the first boatload to Canton. . . . Boston sent its first load of ginseng to China in 1773 aboard the sloop Hingham; this load of 55 tons . . . possibly represented the most profitable cargo ever to leave colonial ports.

Gatherers of wild ginseng were common sights in eighteenth-century America. George Washington reported meeting them in the backwoods of Virginia, and Daniel Boone sold 15 tons of ginseng to a Philadelphia firm in 1788.

TODAY

Ginseng is still a big seller, both in Asia and in far-flung Chinatowns. Researchers in China and the Soviet Union have ascribed cures of nearly every malady imaginable to ginseng, which is now used chiefly as a tonic and nerve medicine. Since the FDA doesn't accept foreign test results, however, ginseng, like other herbs, is not legally recognized in the United States as a medicine. Officially, all the ginseng in the United States is used for making tea.

Chinese American herbal supermarkets go well beyond selling only ginseng. Many stock exotic botanical and animal materials that would be right at home in pharmacopoeias of centuries past. For example, the mail-order catalog of the Mayway Corporation, described in the *San Francisco Chronicle* as "the biggest wholesaler of Chinese herbs in North America," with offices in San Francisco and Hong Kong, lists among "its hundreds of entries scorpion at $28 an ounce, real musk for $375 an ounce and bat dung, a bargain for $3.50."

Modern Chinese American herbalists attract the disapproval of health authorities from time to time. In 1988, California public health officials warned

WITNESS TO A CENTURY

When Nathan Podhurst left his storefront shop, Nature's Herb Company, in 1989, an era departed with him. Podhurst, then 96 years old, had run the little firm, a nationally known herbal institution, since 1922.

The Austrian-born Podhurst was a licensed pharmacist. He stocked his archetypal mom-and-pop store, with its glass apothecary jars and metal tins full of dried herbs, with stand-bys such as cinchona bark—not malaria pills, but their botanical source.

"Those days when I started, you had to know everything," Podhurst told the *San Francisco Examiner*. "The composition of it, where it grows, when it's ripe. You had to be practically a botanist. . . . Now, you just have to be a merchant, know the business."

When Podhurst retired, he had worked at Nature's Herbs for 67 years, an unofficial national record.

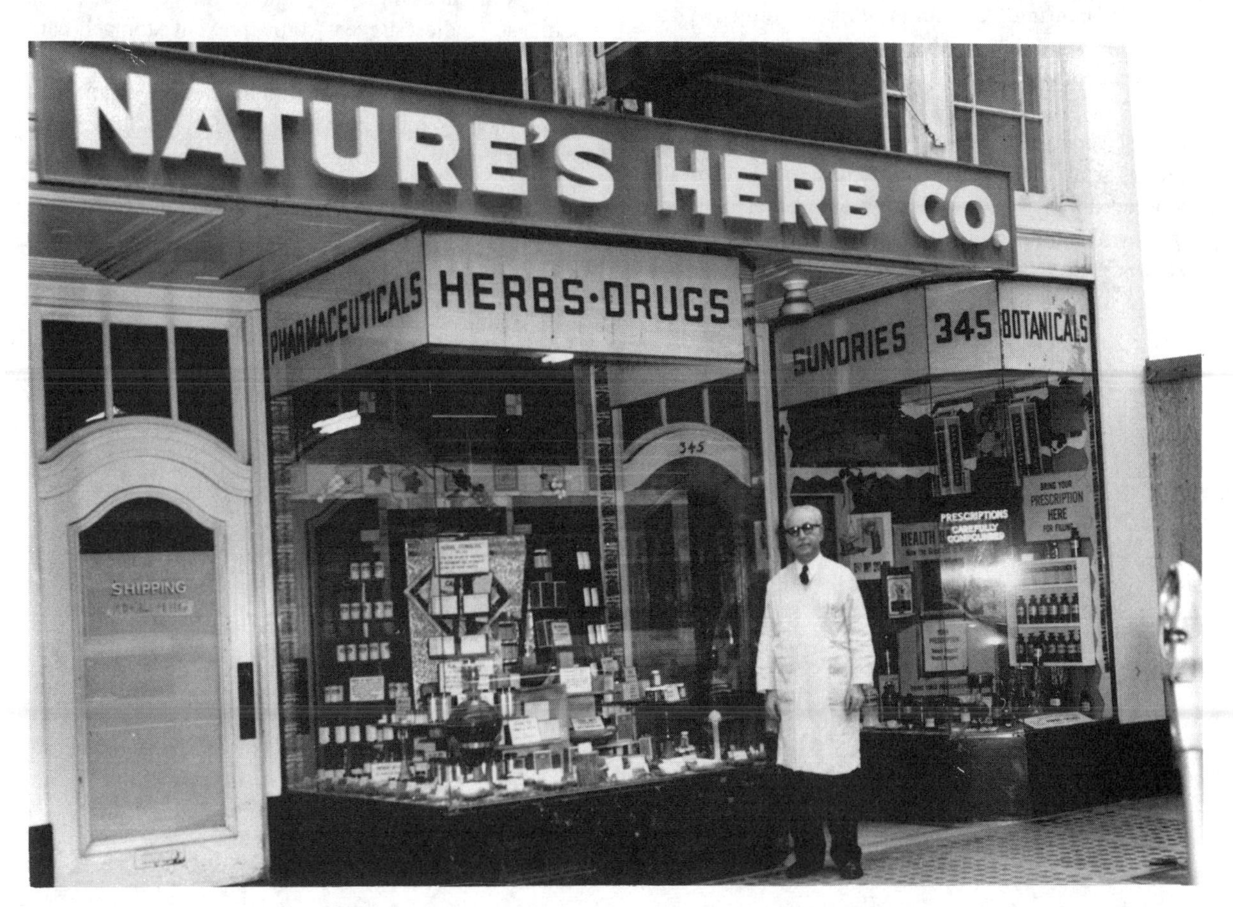

10. San Francisco herbal pharmacist Nathan Podhurst, photographed in the 1950s, was in business for 67 years. *San Francisco Examiner.*

Chinese herb-store owners that some prepared medications imported from China contain unlabeled poisons such as arsenic disulfide and mercury.

Along with an increasingly broad array of fresh and dried herbs for cooking, health-food stores and produce shops also stock a variety of herbal teas, a few of which have caused well-publicized allergic reactions in customers. American sales of herb teas accounted for 200 million dollars in 1987, several times the total at the start of the 1980s. Some teas and bulk herbs are surreptitiously used as medicines.

Some herbs left off the FDA's Generally Recognized as Safe (GRAS) list when it was drawn up in 1958, are illegal for any use. Sassafras, a favorite of Native Americans and colonial settlers, cannot be legally sold unless safrole—which the FDA considers a cancer-causing agent—is first removed. Lobelia is off-limits.

In the chain stores that anchor modern shopping malls, the word *herbal* is primarily a marketing buzzword, much like *natural* and *organic,* which have fuzzy or nonexistent legal definitions. Often, herbs are powdered, combined with other ingredients, and sold as stimulants (some containing caffeine) or diet pills. The FDA warns that herbal products can interact with prescription drugs. A few even contain unlabeled prescription drugs, according to the agency.

Diet pills, untested herbal stimulants, and botanical versions of Love Potion Number Nine are a far cry from the products of the healers of yore, who worked directly with locally grown plants, in attunement with ritual and myth. Nevertheless, herbal shortcuts are big sellers, testifying, in a roundabout and ironic way, to the staying power of herbal medicine.

HERB FUTURES

The future of herbal healing, at least as traditional practitioners know it, is uncertain. On the one hand, much of the world still relies on some variation of the ancient herbalists' art; on the other, the world is rapidly changing, as fast-lane lifestyles and the advance of medical science displace historic folkways.

Perhaps most important of all, the natural habitat for wild herbs is being burned, clear-cut, and paved. The destruction of Amazon Basin rain forests for ranching and farming threatens untold numbers of animal and plant species with extinction. A cure for cancer or AIDS could lie in a plant that the modern world has never heard of. Indeed, the USDA's James Duke reports that less than 2 percent of the Amazon's plants have been studied for medicinal use by outsiders. Recognizing the healing potential of endangered plants, the National Cancer Institute launched a five-year, three-continent search for new medicinal plants in 1988. By 1990, the institute was processing 10 thousand items a year, including herbs, algae, fungi, and marine organisms, in a dramatic race against time.

Increasingly valuable uses are being found for long-domesticated plants—onions, for example, which Chinese studies suggest could prevent stomach cancer (provided they are eaten steadily over a lifetime), and garlic, which international studies report can lower blood-serum cholesterol levels and reduce blood pressure. When it comes to herbs, the past may yet be a prologue.

Chapter 3

The Thomsonians: Every Man His Own Doctor

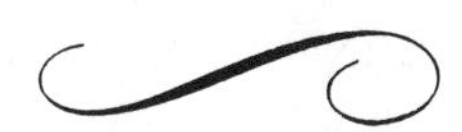

The moment you blend the simplicity of my discoveries with the abstruse sciences such as chemistry . . . that have nothing to do with medicine . . . the benefit of my discoveries will be taken from the people . . . and, like all other crafts, monopolized by a few learned individuals.

SAMUEL THOMSON, 1836

Samuel Thomson was losing control. The founder and namesake of an immensely popular health movement, the self-taught healer who scorned educated physicians as "learned quacks," the herald of a utopia where free men and women would cure each other's ills with a few simple herbs and billowing clouds of steam, was being attacked—attacked!—in the very convention he had assembled to sing his praises.

Thomson, a dynamic man of humble origin, was used to controversy, but only outside the Thomsonian ranks. Why, just a few years earlier, his followers in South Carolina declared his birthday a holiday and raised this toast: "The Healing Art—Its most enlightened advocate, the son of nature, Dr. Samuel Thomson."

But to the newly dissident Thomsonians, the old man was arrogant and headstrong. He believed his system could not be improved upon. His rebellious followers insisted the movement needed professional Thomsonian doctors, hospitals, medical schools, and literature. This enraged the founder, who favored "the study of patients, not books—experience, not reading."

To Thomson's restless followers, the patriarch was in the way; they would have to defy him. Defy him they did. One of Thomson's ablest supporters, Alva Curtis, led a walkout at the 1838 convention in Philadelphia, splitting the Thomsonian movement and effectively ending it as a social force.

Aghast, Thomson dissolved the assembly and resolved never to call another. He retired to his Boston home and watched his dwindling following squabble over what was left of the movement that, at its height, enlisted one in six Americans.

Thomson died five years later, in 1843, far removed from the limelight. His obituary rated all of four lines in the *Boston Daily Advertiser,* less than an item on the same page about a 14-year-old who accidentally shot himself, and an announcement of an upcoming barbecue. Thomson, like Thomsonianism, was well and truly dead.

DOWN ON THE FARM

Samuel Thomson's origins held no portent of his stormy life. He was born on an Alstead, New Hampshire farm in 1769, the son of strict Baptists. Although he was disabled—the boy was born with a club foot—Samuel's father put him to work in the fields at age five.

The unschooled child of nature recalled his early years in his autobiography, *A Narrative of the Life and Discoveries of Samuel Thomson,* published in 1822, after he had become well-known. Written with the help of literate associates, the graceful, simple book went through 13 editions.

Thomson's *Narrative* explains how he came upon *lobelia inflata,* later to become the cure-all in his system of medicine. Young Sam, it seems, found the plant growing wild in the fields. Curious, he chewed the pods and experienced a sudden and not altogether pleasant reaction: he vomited. As he grew up, the little jokester induced his boyhood pals "merely by way of sport" to chew lobelia, and laughed when they vomited.

Thomson learned about other plants from "an old lady by the name of Benton. . . . The whole of her practice was with roots and herbs, applied to the patient, or given in hot drinks, to produce sweating. . . . We became very much attached to her; and when she used to go out to collect roots and herbs, she would take me with her, and learn me their names. . . ."

Young Thomson's regard for healing plants grew even stronger when, at age eight, "the widow Benton" cured him of "the canker-rash." Thomson had rather less esteem for regular practitioners of physic. When his mother was dying, the attending physician "gave her disease the name of galloping consumption, which I thought was a very appropriate name . . . for they are riders . . . and they galloped her out of the world in about nine weeks."

Despite his antipathy for doctors, Thomson nearly apprenticed to a local physician, but wasn't accepted because he had virtually no formal education. Although he was often called "doctor" by his followers in later years, the title—like the "doctor" bestowed on fellow health-crusader Sylvester Graham, a clergyman—was honorary.

In his early twenties, Thomson took over the family farm; he married a local woman and fathered eight children. More misfortune with regular physicians followed. When a doctor of physic made no progress with the canker-rash of his two-year-old daughter, Thomson picked the child up, held her over steaming water (with a cloth wrung out with cold water to shield her eyes), and effected a cure.

About this time, the frustrated farmer decided he could cure his family better than could the doctors with their fancy degrees. He lumped physicians with lawyers and clergy as parasites. In *Learned Quackery Exposed,* an 1824 book he wrote in verse, Thomson observed:

> On lab'rers' money Lawyers feast,
> Also the Doctor and the Priest;
> Although their offices are three,
> They will oppress where'er they be.

Like other ordinary people of his time, Thomson feared the bleed, blister, and purge methods of the physicians. Of mercury-laden calomel, he observed, not illogically, "Poison given to the sick by a person of the greatest skill will have exactly the same effect as it would if given by a fool."

By his mid-thirties, after practicing on his family, Thomson decided that he could cure the sick as well as anyone. "I had no need of learning," he wrote, "for no one can learn that gift."

In a few years, Thomson built a reputation as a healer in his native New England by his use of herbs and steam. As his practice grew, he attracted the critical attention of regular doctors, who derided him as an unlettered quack.

One hostile physician, a Dr. French, brought charges against Thomson in 1809 for allegedly killing a patient by poisoning him with lobelia. Thomson rejoined that the man had left his bed too soon and wandered off into the winter cold, bringing on his own demise. Awaiting trial, Thomson languished for six weeks in an unheated cell that he shared with a child molester. Conditions were so filthy that his cellmate said of the resident lice, "there were enough of them to shingle a meeting-house."

Thomson finally stood trial, symbolically enough, in Salem, Massachusetts, home of the infamous witch trials of the seventeenth century. The celebrated botanist Manasseh Cutler (1742–1823) testified that the plant that the prosecution introduced into evidence as lethal lobelia was, in fact, harmless marsh rosemary, and the case was dismissed. When Thomson and his pals adjourned to a nearby tavern to celebrate, a tableful of doctors who had been drowning their sorrows stalked out.

Buoyed by the trial results, his fame spreading, Thomson became more aggressive. He called on the

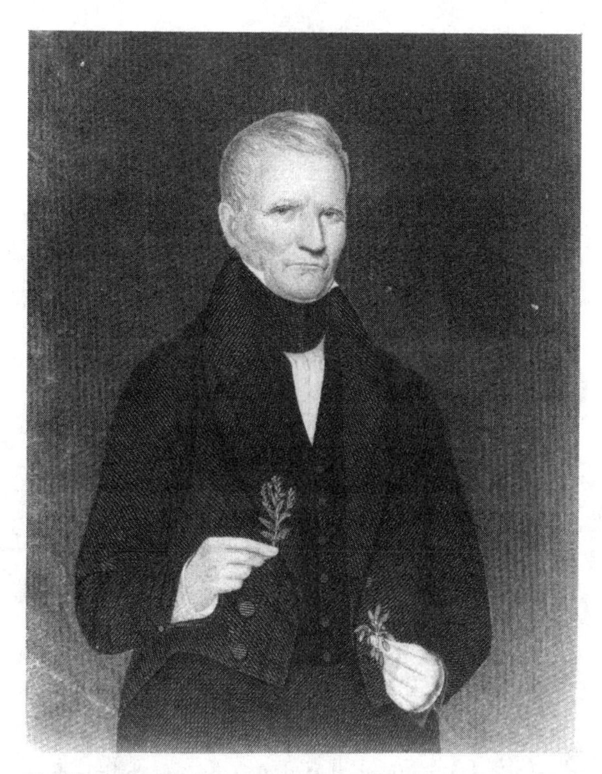

11. Skeptics derided Samuel Thomson as a "puke doctor," but millions of Americans swore by his remedies. *National Library of Medicine.*

elderly Benjamin Rush in the last year of Rush's life, and was received politely by the famous bleed-and-purge doctor. A Harvard professor of medicine, Benjamin Waterhouse, wrote Thomson a courteous note and Thomson represented the letter as an endorsement of his treatments, which he began to formalize into a system. In 1818, the one-time country bumpkin moved to cosmopolitan Boston, where he proceeded to market his system and spark a movement.

"PUKE DOCTORS AND STEAMERS"

Thomson set out the essential elements of his treatments in *Learned Quackery Exposed*, when he wrote:

> Let names of all disorders be,
> Like to the limbs joined on a tree;
> Work on the root, and that subdue,
> Then all the limbs will bow to you . . .
> My system's founded on this truth,
> Man's Air and Water, Fire and Earth,
> And Death is cold, and life is heat,
> These temper'd well, your health's complete.

Shorn of Thomson's poesy, the passage means that plants are beneficial because they grow toward the sun, the source of heat, light, and life. Minerals, by way of contrast, are harmful because they come from the ground, which is cold, signifying illness and death. Thomson's therapeutics were aimed at restoring body heat directly with plants and plant-derived drugs and indirectly with emetics, enemas, and purges to cleanse the body and prepare the way for heat to return.

Thomson used 60 to 65 herbs and drugs, including ginseng, peppermint, turpentine, camphor, and horse radish. His favorites, however, were lobelia, used to induce vomiting and cleanse the innards; *capsicum minimum* (cayenne pepper, now used mostly in spicy cooking) to raise the temperature; and steam vapor baths to raise a sweat. Thomson held that lobelia induced less severe vomiting than other emetics, with less harmful side-effects, although, as the modern scholar Joseph Kett has observed: "After all, when one vomits, one vomits; it is often difficult to distinguish grades of unpleasantness."

After 1825, copies of Thomson's self-help book, *New Guide to Health*, were bound into his autobiography. Although the subtitle of *New Guide* bragged of "a plan entirely new," this was far from the case. Native North Americans used lobelia, popularly known as Indian tobacco, and had long made use of steam baths and sweat lodges. The earth, air, fire, and water of Thomson's philosophy had been put forward by, among others, the Roman physician Galen, whose theories had held sway in Western medicine for 1,500 years. Very little of Thomson's system was original.

One aspect of Thomsonian medicine, however, that was unique was his "courses" of treatments, numbered one through six, and the combinations in which his botanical medicines were given. Thomsonian courses included powders, tinctures, syrups, enemas and infusions, with No. 1 alone consisting of lobelia teas, baths, and rubdowns, among other things. When the patient wasn't busy vomiting, he was sipping herbal teas, often served scalding hot. Other courses included complex combinations of botanicals, not the "simples" of traditional herbal healers.

A Thomsonian cure was no day at the beach. Although it did not include the toxic mineral drugs of the regulars, and probably caused less harm than, say, mercury, the heavy doses of up to 30 ingredients, hot steam baths, and scalding teas were rugged indeed, especially when spread out over a period of days.

Did Thomsonian remedies work? There is surprisingly little in the historical literature about this obvious question. Even standard doctors conceded that Thomson's treatments might help colds and some fevers, but Thomson and his growing battalion of foot soldiers in the war against disease claimed far

RED-HOT IDEA

Cayenne pepper is known in the late twentieth century as a fiery addition to spicy foods. In the nineteenth century, Thomsonians employed it for a somewhat more novel purpose: They gave cayenne enemas to the sick. One can only wonder about the effectiveness of the technique—it has presumably been years since anyone tried it—but, administered with bayberry teas, lobelia, and other powerful agents, cayenne must have made an impression on our forebears.

bigger victories. They claimed to have cured thousands in the great cholera epidemics of 1832 and 1834, but surviving records of documented cures are scanty.

Regular doctors derided Thomsonians as "puke doctors and steamers" and pointed out that otherwise harmless plant drugs could have narcotic and intoxicating effects in large doses. They also bristled at Thomson's blunt appeal to the resentment that uneducated, powerless people felt toward educated doctors. The *Boston Medical and Surgical Journal* (precursor of the prestigious *New England Journal of Medicine*) fumed that Thomsonianism appeals "to the worst passions of the human heart, and by catering to the most vicious, low, and groundless prejudices of mankind."

Despite, or maybe because of, the fierce opposition of regular doctors, Americans flocked to Thomsonian medicine in the early decades of the nineteenth century. Thomson, seizing the moment, patented his system in 1813. The patents (which were renewed twice, lapsing in 1852) ensured that money from his medicines and Thomsonian infirmaries that were beginning to spring up went to him.

THE ENTREPRENEUR

Although Thomson was a self-assured and sincere healer, his greatest gift was packaging and promotion. And while his patented "Improved System of Botanic Practice" championed self-reliance, Thomson controlled the supplies of drugs and knowledge of how to use them.

In 1811, two years before he obtained his first patent, Thomson began selling "family right certificates," which gave buyers a 16-page instructional booklet and membership in "Friendly Botanic Societies." The price was 20 dollars, a large sum at the time. An additional two dollars bought separate copies of Thomson's autobiography. Thomson employed agents to market the system.

Although they were initially expensive, family-right certificates enabled buyers to cut down on their doctor bills. The certificates also allowed members to buy unadulterated domestic drugs. Thomson bragged that his medications were true-blue American, not English imports. He combined this patriotic pitch by appealing to nascent feminism. Thomsonian home treatments allowed women to practice medicine on men, but held feminism within bounds by keeping it in the family—and sidestepped the ticklish question of whether women should allow themselves to be examined by male physicians. By 1839, Thomson said he had sold 100 thousand family-right certificates, for a combined total of two million dollars.

Thomsonian agents marked up the medications that the founder compounded and sold to them wholesale, taking a percentage of the retail price. By 1837, there were 167 authorized agents in 22 states and territories. Still, not all was well. Renegade agents cheated the founder, marketing new, "improved" medications that they sold as Thomsonian drugs, and even wrote their own books. Thomson responded by firing some agents and suing others. He regularly issued broadsides and edicts, but to little avail. Unauthorized agents, knowing a lucrative thing when they saw it, kept turning up.

Thomsonian drugs proliferated, reaching regular drug stores in addition to Thomsonian dispensaries and infirmaries. A Dr. J.W. Chapman, advertising in the *Boston Courier* in 1843, proclaimed that he "invites all invalids to give it a trial, being well assured that if any system on earth can cure, it is the Thomsonian." Another Thomsonian advertised that his treatments posed "not the least danger to the most feeble constitution."

Evidently, many accepted those proclamations with full faith and credit. The governor of Mississippi estimated that fully one-half the population of his state subscribed to Thomsonianism. In Ohio, it was about one-third. The movement claimed three million adherents, one-sixth of the American people in 1839.

Thomson's appeal was even cross-cultural. A Philadelphia Thomsonian magazine reported in 1839 that part of the Cherokee nation had adopted Thomsonianism and ordered a store of medications "before leaving the place of their birth, to secure the best means in their knowledge to guard and preserve their health." The mass migration of 1838 is remembered as the Trail of Tears; many perished despite their apparent conversion to Thomsonianism.

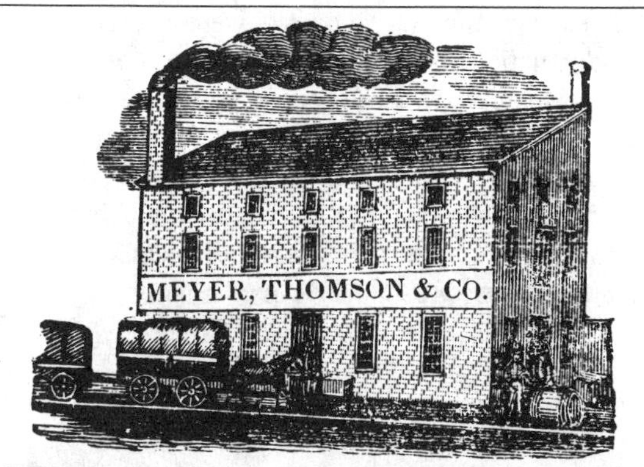

WHOLESALE & RETAIL
THOMSONIAN
BOTANIC MEDICINE STORE.

The subscribers have the largest and most valuable collection of

BOTANIC MEDICINES

in the United States, comprising all the compounds and crude articles recommended by Dr. Samuel Thomson, part of which is as follows:

African Cayenne	Lobelia,—do. Seed
Balmony	Nerve Ointment
Barberry	Nerve Powder
Butter Nut Syrup	Pond Lily
Cancer Plaster	Poplar Bark, coarse and fine
Clivers	Prickly Ash
Composition	Raspberry Leaves
Conserve of Hollyhock	Slippery Elm
Cough Powder	Woman's Friend or Females' Bitters
Ginger	Unicorn Root
Golden Seal	Wake Robin, &c. &c. &c.
Gum Myrrh	

12. Thomsonian remedies were widely advertised, as seen here. *National Library of Medicine.*

Perfect it wasn't, but Thomsonianism was indisputably popular, and its commercial success laid the foundation for a political movement.

THOMSON AND JACKSON

From Thomsonianism's growing numbers came a movement of do-it-yourself health crusaders determined to dislodge conventional medicine and shake society in the process. "The people," declared a journal boldly named the *Philadelphia Botanic Sentinel and Thomsonian Medical Revolutionist,* "could not be more deceived by any set of men than they are by the old physicians. They profess to know and do what they neither understand or have power to do. The people will not much longer bear this imposition."

Thomsonianism as a social and political movement tapped the discontent of the common man, especially in the rural South and West (the present Midwest), where book-learning was scarce and self-reliance often a necessity. Thomsonian literature was written in plain English and its practitioners didn't put on airs. As sociologist Paul K. Starr observed, "The Thomsonians viewed knowledge as an element in class conflict."

Thomsonianism was part of the broader movement under President Andrew Jackson that mobilized working people against privileged elites. As Thomson condemned physicians, clergymen, and lawyers, Jacksonians condemned the rich, whom they considered parasites on the body politic. Thomsonians prized practical, hands-on knowledge; many allied themselves with the Workingmen's Party, which opposed paper money and banks.

Thomsonians joined with other health reformers in the popular health movement, aimed, in part, at breaking the regulars' legal monopoly on the practice of medicine. Thomson's son John is said to have pushed a wheelbarrow holding a 31-foot-long petition demanding the end of medical licensing onto the floor of the New York state legislature. In the 1840s, all but three states struck down licensing laws; those who broke the law were seldom punished anyway.

Thomson himself made the most of this visceral and intellectual link to Jacksonianism. Since his second patent, granted in 1826, came during Jackson's presidency, Thomson claimed that Old Hickory personally endorsed his system; more likely the President, who didn't directly run the patent office, didn't know the New England health crusader from Adam.

In the 1830s, when Thomsonianism reached its peak, the movement had its own lecture circuit, infirmaries, health practitioners, network of Friendly Botanic Societies, and publications, all established in the teeth of fierce opposition. The *Philadelphia Botanic Sentinel and Thomsonian Medical Revolutionist* confided in its editorial columns that "when we struck off the first number of Vol. I of the *Sentinel,* the name of a Thomsonian had the sound of 'mad dog.' "

Later, with its newfound popularity, the *Sentinel* wrote up successful cures and printed accounts of the master himself, including his treatment of one poor soul with a remedy still popular today: hot chicken soup.

The *Sentinel* modestly called Thomsonianism "the best ever introduced for the reversal of disease." A near-religious fervor was not uncommon. "Next to the Christian religion," gushed a letter writer, "[Thomsonianism is] the greatest boon that has ever been granted by indulgent heaven to the sons and daughters of affliction."

The reception from conventional medical publications was less adulatory. The *Boston Medical and*

Surgical Journal denounced Thomsonianism and attributed its popularity to the natural human desire to save a buck and favor the underdog.

Criticism from the outside was to be expected; but Thomson's troubles didn't stop there. Just as the founder was plagued by renegade agents who tried to take over his business, so was he pressured by ambitious lieutenants who wanted to hijack his political movement.

SCHISM

The Thomsonians held yearly conventions from 1832 to 1838. The first, held in Columbus, Ohio, was called to crow about the Thomsonians' apparent success in treating cholera. The last, the Philadelphia gathering of 1838, ended by breaking the heart of the founder, by then a wizened man of 69.

Alva Curtis (1797–1880), editor of the *Thomsonian Recorder*, headed a growing and clamorous faction that called for more training, even formal medical schools, to advance the Thomsonian system. The old man, of course, was dead-set against such heresy. He believed his system complete; it needed only fine-tuning, not overhaul. Some healers were especially gifted, true, but they were not to become professionals. In Thomsonian theory, practitioners would treat the sick for 8 to 10 years, teach their peers everything they knew, and then retire.

It was not to be. Thomson's ever-bolder critics decided that it would be foolhardy to limit themselves to the prejudices of one man, especially a man so evidently lacking in breadth of vision, formal education and personal charm. Even a friend described Thomson as "coarse in manner." Another complained that he was "dictatorial of temper." Many criticized his exclusive hold on Thomsonian drugs, a charge he vainly tried to refute by arguing that quality would suffer if he didn't personally control supplies.

No matter what he said or did, the tattoo of criticism continued. It even kept on after his death, when the famed phrenologist Orson Fowler examined Thomson's skull and proclaimed him petty and stubborn.

Finally, in 1838, with the founder's denunciations ringing in their ears, Curtis and his allies walked out. They established the Independent Thomsonian Botanic Society and a medical school and infirmary in Columbus. Eventually, they dropped Thomson's name and became known as Physio-Medicals.

The Physio-Medicals made no lasting contributions to medicine. They did soften the rigors of classic Thomsonianism and accepted modern medicines such as quinine, but they were poorly trained and dogmatic. As late as 1907, a professor in a Physio-Medical school confidently declared that the germ theory of disease was poppycock. Curtis himself abandoned the sect and the Physio-Medicals dwindled in number as a more dynamic brood of Thomson's rebellious children, the Eclectics, stormed the battlements of established medicine.

THE ECLECTICS

Spurred by the charismatic Dr. Wooster Beach (1794–1868), the Eclectics broke ranks with the Thomsonians earlier than the Physio-Medicals, and far more successfully.

Beach, a conventionally trained medical doctor, believed himself to be of a higher class than the unlettered Thomson—although, like the patriarch, Beach studied with an herbal healer before starting his own system. Described as aristocratic, "a tall, heavy-browed, swarthy-complexioned man," Beach was eager to put his theories into practice. In 1827, he opened the United States Infirmary in New York City.

Beach was familiar with Thomsonian botanical practice, but determined to go beyond it. He and his followers considered themselves open to good ideas from any source. Trying a little bit of this and a little bit of that, Beach earned the soubriquet "eclectic"; it stuck to him and his system.

In 1830, in Worthington, Ohio, Beach opened the first degree-granting medical school in American botanical medicine, preceding the Physio-Medical schools by a decade. The Eclectic institutions made history in another more important way, too, breaking with standard medical schools by admitting women and blacks.

Responding to skeptics' dismissals of Eclecticism as a peculiar pseudo-system, the *American Eclectic Medical Review* rejoined that, yes, Eclectics were peculiar, "in that we select our remedies from every school of practice and from all sources with impartiality; peculiar, in that we reject bloodletting and all other measures which are extremely depletive and exhausting; peculiar, in that we object to mercury, arsenic and other mineral poisons; and peculiar, also, in that we are actively discovering and developing numerous remedies of inestimable value, from the fields and forests of our own country."

But while the Eclectics rejected conventional heroic medicine, they were drug-happy in their own right. Their herbal-based remedies, given in often-massive doses, were trying, and the consequences of their complex, compounded drugs were difficult to predict.

In 1847, the Eclectics introduced a new wrinkle, when John King (1813–1893) developed what he termed "concentrated" medicines made with the resinous materials of plants. King's drugs were suspended in a base of the emetic *podophyllum* (May apple root), which seemed only fitting in an age when people believed that induced vomiting was good for everything.

Concentrated medicines were easier to use than crude plants and had the cachet of modernity. In the 1850s, Eclectic concentrated medicines were sold in standard drug stores as well as Eclectic pharmacies. By the 1860s, the Eclectics used some 350 drugs, up from the 60 to 65 of Samuel Thomson's time only a quarter-century earlier.

Concentrated medicines eventually were discredited, however. Many contained inert ingredients; others were adulterated. Complained a disillusioned practitioner in 1859:

> The manufacture of botanic medicines has become a lucrative business; and unprincipled men, disregarding the direful consequences, are adulterating our most sanative preparations. It is not uncommon to find, in our wholesale drug stores, lobelia seed adulterated with tobacco, pulverized capsicum with logwood, ginger with corn meal, cream of tartar with alum, jalap with sawdust, etc.

The Eclectics' stock dropped for a time, but shot back up when John Scudder (1829–1894) joined forces with King to produce new botanical remedies that tasted good and were administered in much smaller doses than traditional Eclectic and Thomsonian drugs. Scudder and King, in turn, hired a gifted chemist, John Uri Lloyd, to make sure that the medications were pure. In time, the traditional herbal doctor, with his steaming teas and bitter-tasting roots, seemed downright old-fashioned.

The Eclectics stayed on the cutting edge of alternative medicine for more than 50 years. By the dawn of the twentieth century, there were just under 5,000 Eclectic doctors, about four percent of American physicians. Nevertheless, Eclectics ranked behind both regulars and homeopaths in number, income, social standing and education.

Regular doctors had, by then, regained much of the status and legal standing they lost in the Thomsonian wave of the 1820s, 1830s, and 1840s. The regulars had abandoned the worst excesses of heroic medicine. Moreover, scientific advances were quickly being incorporated into mainstream medicine, making outsiders like the Eclectics look more and more like garden-variety crackpots.

This unflattering image was underscored in 1910, when Abraham Flexner's report *Medical Education in the United States and Canada* documented filthy laboratories, inadequate libraries, and poor academic standards, especially among Eclectic colleges. Within a few years, most Eclectic schools closed their doors.

GO TO MED SCHOOL, YOUNG MAN

The first commencement of the Eclectic Medical College of the City of New York, held on February 16, 1867 at the Cooper Institute, was addressed by, among others, Horace Greeley. Greeley was, of course, the famous editor of the crusading *New York Tribune*, credited with capturing the spirit of his age by proclaiming "Go West, young man."

Greeley was almost as pithy in his talk to the Cooper Institute, described by an Eclectic journal as a "capacious hall . . . crowded to overflowing with a brilliant and unusually intelligent [a redundancy, but why quibble?] and evidently interested audience, many of whom were ladies."

Said Greeley:

> I look upon the establishment of an Eclectic Medical College in this city as a protest against abuses and as an evidence of reform. It is a palpable expression of a desire for free thought. . . .
>
> I see no reason why I should not call on my neighbors or friends of the allopathic, homeopathic or Eclectic schools to advise for my child when it is sick. Yet the intolerance of existing professional rules is such that I cannot do so without risking a wrathful refusal. . . .
>
> I see no reason why forty or fifty rich or lucky physicians in New York should take the cream of practice here and all of the influential positions, and all of the prominence, under arbitrary rules made by themselves.

American Eclectic Medical Review, March 1867

LEGACY

The Eclectics are remembered for speeding the development of laboratory-made drugs and the demise of crude plant medicines. A number of their preparations made their way into various editions of the *U.S. Pharmacopeia* in the late nineteenth century, and one of the sect's schools, the Eclectic Medical Institute, in Cincinnati, held on until 1939. An Eclectic Medical Association, its thinning ranks filled by diehard old-timers, persevered until the 1960s, when it, too, faded into history.

Samuel Thomson, the godfather of nineteenth-century American botanical medicine, is virtually forgotten, his name familiar only to scholars and habitués of musty libraries. Although Jethro Kloss lauds Thomson and his cure-all, lobelia, in his 1939 book *Back to Eden,* few have actually read Thomson and virtually none of his remedies survives intact.

The patriarch of a movement that once commanded three million followers leaves almost no physical traces, even in his adopted city, Boston. Thomson's home at 46 Salem Street, where he died in 1843 at age 74, was razed. The site is a few steps off the tourist Freedom Trail, in a parking lot under an interstate highway. Where this grand eccentric once mixed his potions and brooded about his enemies, motor oil forms pools on a macadam surface and the wheels of progress speed by overhead, heedless of the history buried below.

THESE BOOTS ARE MADE FOR SHOPPING

After Eclecticism succeeded Thomsonianism, the new botanical medicine spread from its American home to Great Britain. There, the president of the Midland Botanic and Eclectic Association, Jesse Boots, of Nottingham, got the notion that even "scientific" Eclecticism could be improved upon.

Wrote Boots: "I had an idea that the herbalist and chemist at the time was very much out of date. . . . I thought the public would welcome new chemists' shops in which a gentler and better variety of pharmaceutical articles would be obtained at cheaper prices."

How right he was. Boots's idea caught on, and so did his shops, which now girdle the United Kingdom. Although it has long ceased to be an Eclectic business, Boots's roots are not completely forgotten. In 1989, a Boots shop on London's trendy King's Road, in Chelsea, had mounted a window display advising customers to speak with the pharmacist about special herbal pharmaceuticals available for purchase.

CHAPTER

· 4 ·

HOMEOPATHY: THE LAW OF SIMILARS

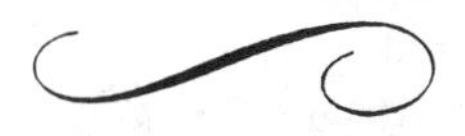

Through the like, disease is produced, and through the application of the like, it is cured.

HIPPOCRATES, fourth century B.C.

The pharmacists inside the colonial-style red brick building in Berkeley, California were busily filling prescriptions for a short line of customers from the clinic next door. In the back, head pharmacist and proprietor Michael Quinn carefully measured a drop of sarsaparilla into a vial of grain alcohol, topped it with a cork stopper, and rapidly pounded the vial 10 times on his laboratory table. He then diluted a few drops of this mixture into a second vial of alcohol, then a third, and then a fourth vial, each time diluting and then pounding the solution on the table. By the twelfth dilution, according to Quinn, not a single sarsaparilla molecule was left.

As the pounding echoed through the wood-paneled room, Quinn smiled with satisfaction. He had come a long way since his days as a San Diego pharmacist, specializing in intravenous medicine. Now running the only modern-day American homeopathic pharmacy adjacent to a homeopathic clinic, he was at long last following his dream: He was operating a homeopathic pharmacy where he would mix his own remedies, following the time-honored methods of homeopathy's founder, the German physician and theorist Samuel Christian Hahnemann (1755–1843).

If Hahnemann's ghost were to visit Berkeley's Hahnemann Medical Clinic and Pharmacy today, he might be flattered that his followers chose to name their institutions after him. He would no doubt enjoy meeting (and giving advice to) his modern-day colleagues who, like himself, turned to alternative methods of healing after becoming disillusioned with conventional medicine. Always one to respect efficiency, he would be impressed with Quinn's computer-run "potentizing" (diluting) machine, designed to dilute and "succuss" (pound) remedies up to 10 thousand times in 36 hours. After touring the clinic next door, he would be delighted with the renewed interest in homeopathy, after its near-demise in America in the 1950s.

THE FIRST HOMEOPATH

The basic premise of homeopathy goes back to the days of Hippocrates in the fourth century B.C. and was put into practice by ancient civilizations and Native American peoples long before Hahnemann popularized it in modern times. However, the late-eighteenth-century physician was the first to test systematically the theory that a sick person can be cured if given minute doses of a substance that causes similar symptoms in a healthy person. Hahnemann called it "the law of similia," and his method of healing "homeopathy," from the Greek words *homoios* (like) and *pathos* (suffering). He coined the term "allopathy" (opposite suffering) for the conventional (also known as "regular," "orthodox," or "heroic") medicine of his day, a term still used by Hahnemann's modern-day followers to describe conventional medicine's attempt to suppress or stabilize symptoms.

Although treated as quackery in this country for much of its history, homeopathy is today a popular form of treatment in many parts of Europe and Asia, particularly in India, where there are 120 homeopathic medical schools and more than 100 thousand homeopathic practitioners. In the 1980s, Britain's Queen Elizabeth II's personal physician, Dr. Ronald Davey, was a homeopathic doctor with degrees in both orthodox and homeopathic medicine. And in the Netherlands, homeopathy is one of the most widely used forms of alternative medical treatment. Yet Europe was not always so friendly to either homeopathy's microdoses or its founder.

Trained in allopathic medicine and fluent in eight languages, Hahnemann gave up his medical practice while still in his twenties and turned to translating medical and pharmaceutical texts and writing in order to support his wife, Henriette, and growing family, which eventually numbered seven children. For Henriette, a pharmacist's daughter, it was bad enough that her principled young husband refused to accept payments from his dying patients. But after he stopped practicing medicine altogether, she never forgave him. For the disillusioned Hahnemann, there was no alternative. He was too horrified by the results of conventional remedies to continue the standard methods he had learned as a medical student in Vienna. These included removing large quantities of blood from the patient, assisted by live leeches or suction cups, purging, blistering and administering lethal doses of arsenic and other "fever powders."

By 1790, Hahnemann, then in his thirties, had alienated not only his long-suffering wife, but most of his former colleagues, whose methods he bitterly criticized in his writing. A man ahead of his time, Hahnemann not only preached the need for preventive medicine, baths, pure air, and personal hygiene, but, like his American contemporary Dr. Benjamin Rush, advocated humane treatment of the insane. Barely able to make a living, the ever-restless Hahnemann moved his family from town to town, across the German landscape, from one drafty house to another, where he spent most of his waking hours bent over his writing desk.

THE QUININE EXPERIMENT

One day, Hahnemann was hard at work translating the highly acclaimed pharmaceutical text *Treatise on the Materia Medica,* written by the eminent Scottish physician William Cullen, whose near-religious ferver for the cure-all of bleeding patients was carried to extremes by Dr. Rush.

As he scratched away at his translation, Hahnemann grew more and more disturbed. When he got to Cullen's prediction that the cinchona bark used in quinine, a popular cure for malaria, works by fortifying the stomach, Hahnemann threw down his pen in disgust. Not satisfied merely to scribble his response in the margin of the text, he set out to prove the master was mistaken by scientifically testing Cullen's theory. Setting the standard for testing all homeopathic remedies for the next 150 years, Hahnemann used only a healthy subject for this experiment: in this case, himself.

Hahnemann first ordered a supply of quinine from Leipzig, then proceeded to take four drams (one-half ounce) twice a week. Taking meticulous notes, foreshadowing the homeopathic practitioner's penchant for detailed recording of patient complaints and ailments, he described the results: "My feet, my fingertips, at first became cold. I grew languid and drowsy; then my heart began to palpitate, and my pulse became hard and small; intolerable anxiety,

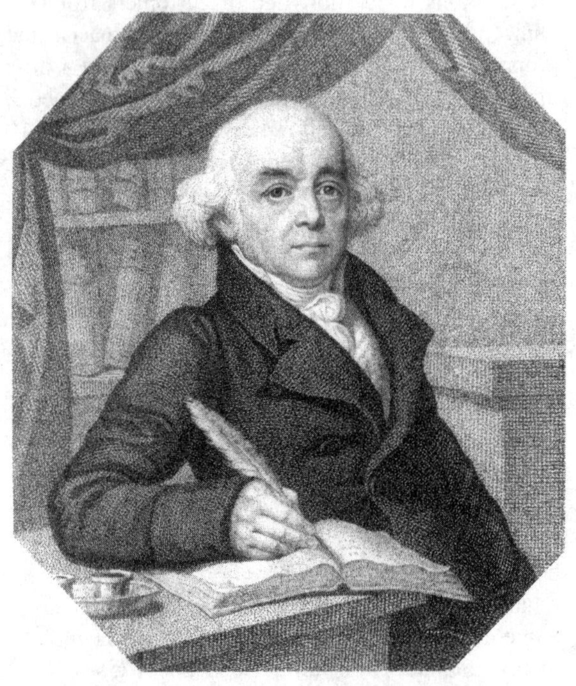

13. Homeopathy's founder, Samuel Hahnemann, was an influential, though much maligned, scientist. *National Library of Medicine.*

trembling, prostration through all my limbs. Then pulsation in my head, flushing of my cheeks. . . ." Hahnemann, a healthy man, was experiencing a fever. He found that the symptoms lasted two or three hours but would cease when he stopped taking the quinine.

Cullen was wrong, Hahnemann decided. It was not quinine's astringent quality that cured fever. *Fever cures fever!* Although Hahnemann did not go public with his finding for another six years, his quinine experiment became known as the first homeopathic research experiment, or "drug-proving."

"LAW OF INFINITESIMALS"

In the early nineteenth century, Hahnemann continued to expand and publicize his theory. Taking voluminous notes, he experimented with new drug provings, using himself and his family and friends as subjects. Not until 1810 did he officially go public with his discoveries in the first volume of his first important work, the *Organon of Homeopathic Medicine.* A year later, he published the first volume of his drug-provings repertory, *Materia Medica Pura.* In true Hahnemannian style, his repertory listed not only every remedy he tested and the symptoms it caused, but the names of every subject used in each experiment along with his or her reactions.

Hahnemann argued that the body has its own natural healing power. He also wrote that practitioners must test and administer only *one* remedy at a time, carefully tailored to fit each individual's needs. Just as no two people have the same kind of headache, so no two individuals should receive the same headache remedy. (Headaches, in fact, have been among the leading complaints among homeopathic patients. The 1877 homeopathic repertory of symptoms and their remedies, written by the American James Tyler Kent, devoted more than 80 of its 1,500 pages to headache remedies alone.)

Perhaps the most controversial aspect of Hahnemann's theory was his "law of infinitesimals." Here he argued that the more diluted the dose, the more powerful the remedy. Such multi-diluted remedies could only be produced by combined serial potentizing and succussing, like the process demonstrated by Berkeley's Michael Quinn. Although Hahnemann himself did not dilute solutions higher than 30 times and his precise recommendations in this area are unclear, many of his nineteenth-century American followers diluted their solutions as much as 100 thousand times. They became known as the "highs" for "high potency" practitioners. Their tradition of single, highly diluted remedies is continued today by the so-called "classical" homeopaths, who insist that they are closer to Hahnemann's instructions and don't consider the "low-potency" combination remedies sold in many health food stores to be truly homeopathic.

Hahnemann's emphasis on single, diluted remedies was ridiculed by members of the German allopathic medical establishment. In contrast, their heroic prescriptions called for spoonful after spoonful of up to 200 ingredients in a single medication. But the most extreme reactions came from the apothecaries, whose incomes were threatened by doctors who insisted on preparing and dispensing their own medicine.

Fortunately for Hahnemann, he would live long enough to see homeopathy not only accepted in Europe but spread to America, where it would both threaten and alter conventional nineteenth- and twentieth-century medicine beyond his dreams. After Henriette's death, he also lived long enough to marry one of his patients, a titled Frenchwoman whose influence helped win him a royal ordinance with permission to practice homeopathic medicine in Paris, where he lived happily for the rest of his days.

By the time Hahnemann died at the age of 88, he was a wealthy and respected physician, whose theories were accepted by many of the most prominent citizens in Europe and the United States. He left behind more than 70 original works on medicine and chemistry and 10 volumes of drug provings, including 99 provings tested on his own body.

HOMEOPATHY, AMERICAN STYLE

While Hahnemann was busily expanding his repertory of homeopathic remedies in Germany and France,

ALL IN THE FAMILY

Hahnemann insisted that homeopathic remedies be made only from natural ingredients. According to one of Hahnemann's many biographers, Martin Gumpert, Hahnemann enlisted his entire family in the gathering of these ingredients. In all seasons of the year, he sent his flock of children into the fields to gather henbane, sumach, deadly nightshade, and other flowers. With expert hands, the Hahnemann children cut away the bark of young branches, collected roots, plucked leaves and laid out flowers to dry. No child was exempt from work, and all work was carefully inspected by the doctor.

his followers in the United States were successfully transporting his theories across the Atlantic. Success came easily, for nineteenth-century Americans were ready for alternatives to the heroic treatments they endured throughout the pre-Civil War years. Homeopathy, introduced in the 1820s in eastern Pennsylvania, the Middle West, New England, and New York, was one of the first alternatives to compete seriously with conventional medicine. By the 1840s, homeopathy would also draw the most virulent response from the medical establishment toward any of the medical "heresies."

According to a leading historian of American homeopathy, Harris L. Coulter, American doctors singled out homeopathy for attack because a large proportion of homeopathy's converts were allopathic doctors. The leading American homeopaths, among them Dr. Hering, made a special effort to proselytize among both medical students and established physicians. As modern-day homeopathic educator and publisher Dana Ullman puts it, "This was no David and Goliath. It was Goliath against Goliath. The homeopaths were medical doctors. They couldn't be called untrained sloths."

Nor could conventional doctors take homeopathy's lay converts too lightly. In the nineteenth century, homeopathy drew applause from educated, influential, and wealthy Americans in the Northeast and Midwest, many of whom were also active in the anti-slavery, temperance, vegetarian, and women's rights movements of the day. Among its more famous adherents were William James, Henry Wadsworth Longfellow, Nathaniel Hawthorne, Harriet Beecher Stowe, Daniel Webster, Louisa May Alcott, William Cullen Bryant, and Lincoln's Secretary of State, William Seward.

CONSTANTINE HERING'S "DOMESTIC KIT"

In Henry James's classic work *The Bostonians,* one of the leading characters is a female homeopathic doctor named Dr. Prance. Women were among homeopathy's earliest and most consistent converts. Many mothers used homeopathy for their children while the adults continued with their allopathic physicians. Much to the horror of some of homeopathy's most consistent critics, their own wives could be counted among the converted.

It did not take long for Hering to understand the needs of female consumers in his adopted country.

THE ALLENTOWN ACADEMY

In Allentown, Pennsylvania, the "Father of American Homeopathy," German immigrant Dr. Constantine Hering, along with the Swiss immigrant Dr. Henry Detwiller, founded the first homeopathic medical school in America. Called the Nordamerikanische Academie der Homoeopathischen Heilkunst (North American Academy of the Homeopathic Healing Art), the school opened on April 10, 1835, Hahnemann's eightieth birthday, but closed its doors six years later because of enrollment problems. This was hardly surprising, since all its courses were conducted in German. Today the modern Allentown School District's administration building has replaced the old Allentown academy, and a commemorative plaque honors the site of the "first homeopathic college in the world." Hering went on to Philadelphia to found the Homoeopathic Medical College of Pennsylvania. Later called Hahnemann Medical College (today's Hahnemann University), it became the center of homeopathic training in nineteenth-century America.

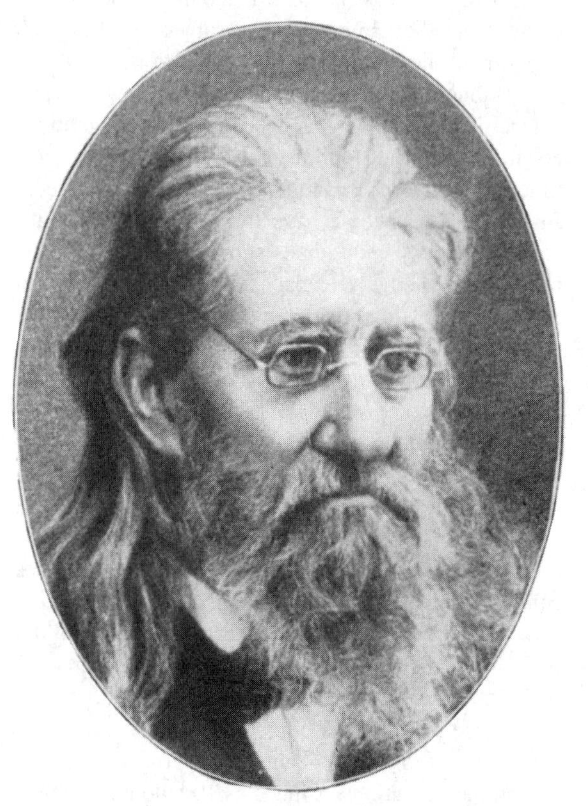

14. Philadelphia's Constantine Hering introduced homeopathy to the United States. *From Moses King,* Philadelphia and Notable Philadelphians. *New York: King, 1902. National Library of Medicine.*

Catching on quickly to the art of American marketing, he devised what he called the "domestic kit," containing medicines identified by number with specific instructions according to symptoms. This domestic kit, a natural extension of the American mother's home remedy tradition, was in large part responsible for the spread of homeopathy beyond the cities and into the West.

HEROIC MEDICINE DECLARES WAR

In 1844, when homeopaths founded the first national medical society in the United States, the American Institute of Homoeopathy, it was a signal for the allopaths to take the offensive. The first step for the regulars was to form their own national organization. In 1846, they organized the American Medical Association. The new AMA's first order of business was to cleanse itself of homeopaths, by kicking out all homeopaths from its local medical affiliates. The AMA succeeded in every state except Massachusetts. (In the 1870s, Massachusetts, too, gave way. By that time there were only eight homeopaths left in the state AMA organization.)

The next step was to create what became known as the "consultation clause," stating that any doctor who consulted with a homeopath or other "nonregular" practitioner would lose his or her membership in the AMA, thus preventing the accused doctor from legally practicing medicine. The consultation clause was eventually dropped, but not before its enforcement was carried to bizarre extremes. One Connecticut doctor lost his membership in his local AMA for consulting with a homeopath, who happened to be his wife.

The AMA's offensive was assisted by volumes of essays and hours of public lectures denouncing Hahnemann and his theories. The most famous American to speak out against homeopathy was poet and physician Oliver Wendell Holmes, whose two 1842 lectures, "Homeopathy and Its Kindred Delusions," delivered to the Boston Society for the Diffusion of Useful Knowledge, were widely read throughout the country in a hot-selling pamphlet. Ridiculing homeopathy's microdoses, Holmes predicted that "after its [homeopathy's] novelty has worn out, the ardent and capricious individuals who constitute the most prominent class of its patrons will return to visible doses, were it only for the sake of change."

Yet another widely read treatise was the *History of Medical Delusions*, published in 1850 by Dr. Worthington Hooker of Connecticut. Hooker ridiculed homeopathy's miniscule doses, but directed his major attack on homeopathy's founder and his followers, who, he stated, elevated Hahnemann to the "undeserved" position of medical hero. Asserting that Hahnemann had "literally added nothing" to medical theory, Hooker accused his followers of charging "heroic" fees for their infinitesimal doses. Feeding into the anti-foreign ferment of the times, Hooker argued that homeopaths associated with "dishonorable men and especially with irresponsible foreigners."

In spite of conventional medicine's attack, homeopathy enjoyed enormous popularity in America from the mid-nineteenth to early twentieth centuries, particularly in the urban areas of New York, Pennsylvania, Massachusetts, and the Midwest. Homeopathy enjoyed an upswing during the three devastating cholera epidemics of the nineteenth century, when statistics showed that homeopathically treated patients suffered fewer deaths than those treated in allopathic hospitals. Some life insurance companies even offered a 10 percent discount to homeopathic patients, in the belief that they lived longer.

By 1900, there were 22 homeopathic medical colleges in the United States and more than 15 thousand homeopathic practitioners, about one-sixth of the American medical profession. At the turn of the twentieth century, homeopathic doctors finally earned respectability in conventional medical circles, helped by the regulars' new fears of and attacks on the new medical "quackeries" of osteopathy and chiropractic.

DECLINE

Yet by the 1930s only one homeopathic medical school still existed in the United States, Philadelphia's Hahnemann Medical College, which held out until 1945 when it dropped homeopathy from the required curriculum. By the 1950s, not a single homeopathic school remained and fewer than 200 physicians in the United States were practicing Hahnemann's principles. What happened?

The decline of homeopathy in the United States was a complex process, a result of trends in both American conventional medicine and homeopathy.

Much to the relief of the American populace, by the end of the Civil War allopathic doctors had discarded many of their most obviously barbaric heroic practices, a trend that brought back skeptical patients who had defected to alternative medicine.

Once allopathic medicine regained strength in the medical arena, the AMA was able to take the upper hand. Its vehicle was, once again, licensing, but its weapon this time was Abraham Flexner's 1910 report *Medical Education in the United States*

REMARKS

ON

THE ABRACADABRA

OF THE

Nineteenth Century;

OR ON

DR. SAMUEL HAHNEMANN'S

HOMŒOPATHIC MEDICINE,

WITH PARTICULAR REFERENCE TO

DR. CONSTANTINE HERING'S

"CONCISE VIEW OF THE RISE AND PROGRESS OF HOMŒOPATHIC MEDICINE,"
Philadelphia, 1833.

BY

WILLIAM LEO-WOLF, M.D.

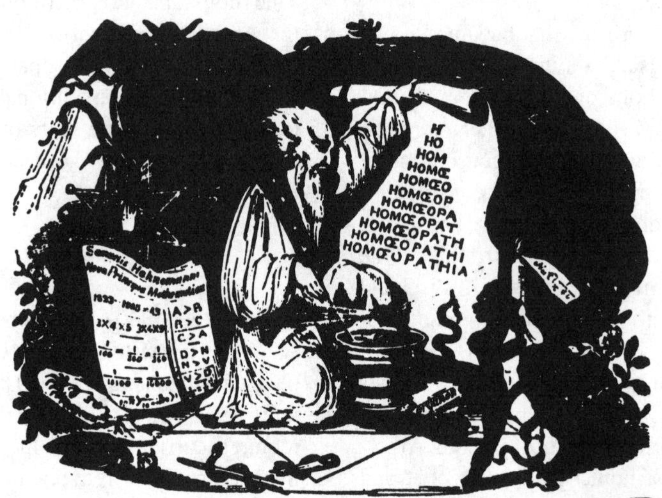

When thus ripe lies are to perfection sprung,
Full grown and fit to grace a mortal tongue,
Thro' thousand vents impatient forth they flow,
And rush in millions on the world below.—POPE.

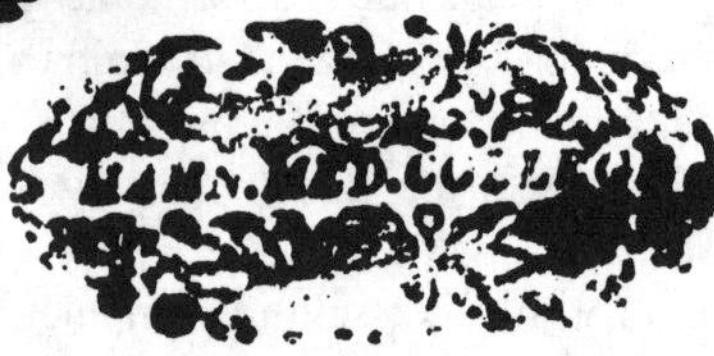

NEW-YORK:
1835.

PUBLISHED BY CAREY, LEA AND BLANCHARD, IN PHILADELPHIA.

15. Mainstream medical writers came down hard on homeopathy. *Countway Library, Boston.*

and Canada, sponsored by the Carnegie Foundation for the Advancement of Teaching.

The Flexner Report gave nearly universally low ratings to the homeopathic schools. These ratings, based on the allopathic training model, essentially controlled not only which graduates could take the new licensing exams (only those from highly rated schools), but what kinds of courses medical schools offered so that their graduates could pass the exams. Since conventional medical courses offered in homeopathic colleges necessarily took priority, the homeopathic curricula suffered. Simply put, the Flexner Report devastated formal homeopathic education in the United States. Many would-be homeopaths simply gave up, reverting to the modern, quick-fix remedies their patients now expected.

RENAISSANCE?

Conventional American medicine and the pharmaceutical industry still do not accept homeopathy's premise that practitioners may mix their own remedies. Allopathic doctors still oppose homeopathy's single-dose, individualized remedy, born of laborintensive patient interviews. Unlike homeopaths in Europe and Asia, American homeopaths are not taken seriously by most American medical students and doctors, who know little or nothing about homeopathy's principles. Dana Ullman blames America's unique "technology macho. . . . The more high-tech you put into something, the more value it must have, but if something [like homeopathy] has been around a long time, that's not considered 'medical progress.' "

Yet homeopathy is making a modest comeback in the United States. A small but growing number of health consumers, most of them well-educated, living in or near large urban areas, are, once again, searching for alternatives to orthodox medicine. And, like the first popular health movements of the 1830s, 1840s, and 1850s, this modern-day consumer rebellion draws from an eclectic mix of new-and-old remedies and movements—women's health, massage therapy, acupuncture, biofeedback, vegetarianism, water cures, physical fitness, and homeopathy.

Today many health-conscious consumers' first introduction to homeopathy is through the low-potency remedies sold in health-food stores. Over-the-counter remedies have been legally available in the United States since 1938, when Congress created an official *U. S. Pharmacopoeia* for homeopathic medicine as an amendment to the Pure Food and Drug Act. In the tradition of Hering's home remedy kit, these remedies continue to be the most visible form of homeopathic treatment in the United States. In 1988, the Food and Drug Administration issued guidelines for over-the-counter homeopathic remedies, including the requirement that they must be sold only for conditions the consumer recognizes as "self-limited," such as headaches or colds.

The number of homeopathic doctors is slowly growing. Approximately 2,000 medical doctors practiced homeopathy in the United States in the late 1980s, about 1 out of every 285 physicians. These did not include an additional 2,000 homeopathic health professionals, such as dentists, podiatrists, and chiropractors, who use homeopathic remedies as part of their treatment. Although there are no longer homeopathic medical schools in the United States, American doctors travel to Athens, Greece to study with George Vithoulkas, widely regarded as the world's leading homeopath, at the Athenian School of Homeopathy. Others study at training centers in the United States and in homeopathic "study groups."

The legal status of homeopathy in the United States is still tenuous, and many state medical boards look askance at doctors who use homeopathic methods.

DOWN MEMORY LANE

For a man who was so meticulous, Hahnemann was never able to give scientific evidence for why his highly diluted remedies worked. Yet controversial experiments in the 1980s in France, Italy, Israel, and Canada, organized by the French immunologist Jacques Benveniste at the University of Paris, may validate Hahnemann's theory of microdoses. These experiments attempted to show that an antibody so diluted that no antibody molecule could be present actually changes the internal structure and chemistry of white blood cells. According to Benveniste, this phenomenon is possible because water has a "memory" of substances it once contained, even after these substances are no longer present.

His debunkers, a team organized by the editor of the journal *Nature,* included, besides the editor, a professional magician and a self-appointed investigator of scientific fraud. After duplicating Benveniste's experiments, this odd trio challenged his findings, claiming that his experimental design was flawed.

Only three states in 1991—Nevada, Arizona, and Connecticut—licensed homeopathists. Moreover, modern-day homeopathic doctors suffer from the same kind of legal headaches as did their nineteenth-century predecessors.

In 1985, George Guess, an M.D. practicing homeopathy in Asheville, North Carolina, suffered a legal setback when the North Carolina Board of Medical Examiners found him guilty of "unprofessional conduct" and ordered him to stop using homeopathic medicines in his practice. By 1989 Guess had won legal victories in two lower court decisions, but the North Carolina Supreme Court reversed those decisions, making it illegal to practice homeopathy in the state. Guess's case is not yet closed, however. In 1991 the ACLU filed a class action suit, arguing that consumers have a right to receive unorthodox medical treatment.

As Dr. Guess would attest, homeopathy is not entirely out of the woods; yet as a small but growing number of patients can confirm, neither is it entirely out of mind.

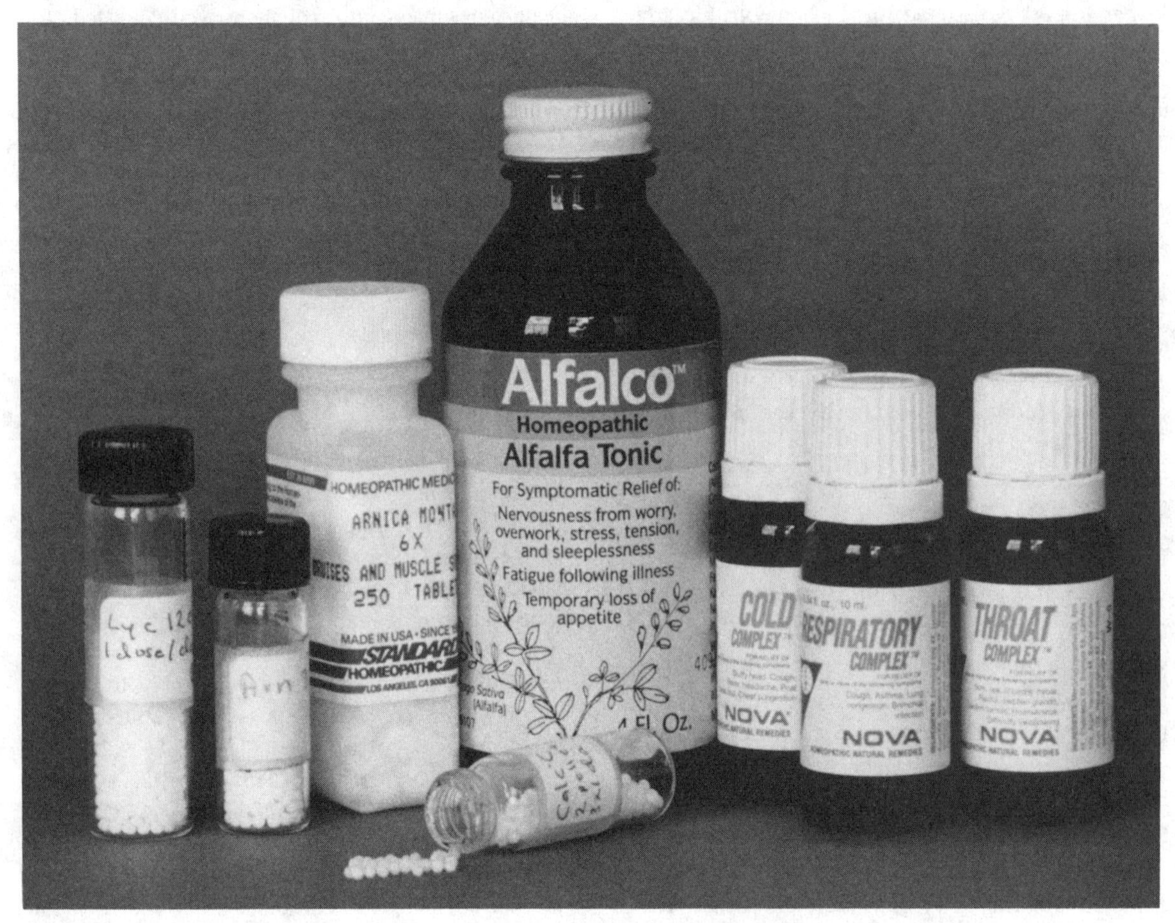

16. There is a modern homeopathic remedy for every ailment. *Photograph by Karen Preuss.*

CHAPTER
· 5 ·

TEMPERANCE: EXORCISING DEMON ALCOHOL

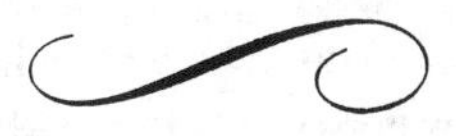

The drunkard does not merely die to society, he clings to it, like a gangrenous excrescence, poisoning and eating away the life of the community.

EDWARD HITCHCOCK in the Journal of Health, *1830*

Sophisticated city speakeasies and backwoods stills; soft-spoken "substance abuse" counselors and hatchet-swinging anti-saloon commandos; the high-spirited flappers of the Jazz Age and the down-and-out denizens of Skid Row; less-filling "lite" beers and near-lethal bathtub gin; Eliot Ness and Al Capone; the wets versus the dries.

Some of the most powerful symbols of American popular culture have come from two centuries of struggle between health-minded reformers and the unwilling objects of their attention: the makers, sellers and consumers of alcoholic beverages.

Over the years, temperance has taken many forms, ranging from the mild moral suasion of early reform groups to their angry offspring, the prohibitionists. Social and political changes paralleled changing ideas about alcohol itself: from hearty approval in colonial times to worries about drinking's effects on character and productivity and, finally, to the now-widely accepted idea of alcoholism as a disease.

Only slavery, war, and immigration (with which temperance was linked) have polarized Americans more. And only anti-alcohol forces, out of all the health reform movements that have shaken the nation, have managed to produce amendments to the United States Constitution: namely, the Eighteenth Amendment, which instituted Prohibition, and the Twenty-first Amendment, which repealed it.

Very little of this commotion was foreseen. Back in colonial America, when even the Pilgrims lingered over their beer, and decent, hard-working people threw back eye-openers at breakfast, the very idea of putting an end to drinking was inconceivable.

"GOD'S OWN CREATURE"

"Drink is in itself a good creature of God," wrote the Puritan preacher Increase Mather in 1673, "and is to be received with thankfulness, but the abuse of drink is from Satan."

Mather's observation crystallizes the ambivalence that many, then and now, feel about drink. Even so, the Puritans, contrary to their reputation for joylessness, liked to drink. The Pilgrims made a dark, bitter-tasting brew, a vitamin-rich porter that kept well at sea and helped them endure the lengthy Atlantic crossing on the Mayflower. Once on land, the new arrivals made more beer and hard apple cider and fermented wine from local berries and fruits. Like Mather, they believed in moderation—

temperance, in the true sense of the word—not abstinence from alcohol.

In the early days, when people made their own at home, alcoholic beverages were considered liquid foods. Rye and corn whiskey, after all, come from grain; wine from fruit; and beer from barley, so this was not an entirely illogical conclusion.

Moreover, alcohol was cherished for its medicinal value. It was widely used as an ingredient in soothing cordials and potent patent medicines. It was employed as a painkiller before the development of anesthetics and to relax apprehensive patients, bring down fevers, warm chilly bodies and even to treat the universal complaint of early America: dyspepsia, or indigestion.

Indeed, alcohol was initially regarded as a wonder drug, and bore the name *aqua vitale* (''water of life'') when it was first isolated by chemists. The Pilgrims believed that alcohol strengthened the heart. Among their sure-fire cures, according to food historians Waverly Root and Richard de Rochemont, were ''yellowmint in whiskey flavored with cherry bark'' for the blood; ''heated white whiskey with sugar'' for coughs; for measles, straight whiskey would do.

Alcohol was present in copious amounts for weddings, funerals, and even ordinations. Open jugs of the hard stuff were made available for shoppers. Barbers gave their customers a swig or two. An eye-opening morning jolt recalled the blood from the extremities, where it pooled during the night. Everyone imbibed beer and cider at the family table, including small children. The colonists' love for distilled liquors is evident in the intoxicating name accorded them: ardent spirits.

Tavern owners were men of consequence and taverns were lively social centers; newspapers were available there; politics and business were conducted there; and polling stations were located there.

At election time, candidates provided free liquor to voters, who came to expect it as their due. When George Washington ran for Virginia's colonial legislature in 1758, nearly all of his recorded election expenses went for alcohol. The custom known as ''treating'' reached an all-time low in 1829, when boozy revelers at Andrew Jackson's inaugural ball nearly wrecked the White House; the party finally ended when the servants stopped serving free liquor.

Booze wasn't just for special occasions. Laborers, soldiers and sailors considered alcohol part of their pay. Drinking was believed to be crucial for feats of strength, to weather long stretches at sea and combat lassitude. When alcohol rations were cut off in 1640s Boston, angry laborers conducted one of the first strikes in North America. The crisis weathered, workers resumed their breaks at 11 A.M. and 4 P.M., not for coffee or tea but for drinks. The morning libations were called ''eleveners.''

Although early Americans savored drinking for pleasure and relied upon alcohol as medicine, there were other practical reasons for the popularity of alcohol. Well water and milk were often impure. Slow transportation prevented frontier farmers from getting their crops to the cities; rather than let grain rot in the fields, they distilled it and shipped liquid grain. Indeed, so important was this trade that when the fledgling federal government moved to put an excise tax on whiskey, it triggered the Whiskey Rebellion of 1794. President Washington was forced to raise a militia against fighting-mad western Pennsylvania farmers to enforce the tax.

Alcohol had long been central to the colonial economy. It was part of the notorious triangular trade of molasses, slaves, and rum. Rum and whiskey were commonly used to barter with the Native Americans, who had high regard, but low tolerance, for ''fire water''—some of it poisoned by European colonials. Indeed, alcohol figures prominently in the sad early history of American race relations.

All this led to a staggeringly high intake of alcohol. Root and de Rochemont, writing in 1976, reported that early Americans had a consumption rate ''roughly double our own,'' putting away some 5.8 gallons of pure alcohol per capita in 1790. Despite their powdered wigs and starched collars, early Americans were party animals.

Amidst all the hard-drinking hilarity and wheeling and dealing, dissenting voices, quiet at first, were raised. In 1773, the Methodist minister John Wesley advocated the radical step of forbidding the distillation of whiskey. The following year, the Quaker reformer Anthony Benezet wrote an anti-alcohol pamphlet called ''The Mighty Destroyer Displayed,'' and the battle was joined. Clearly, the ''good creature of God'' was being relegated to the Devil's medicine chest.

DEMON ALCOHOL

The more Americans drank, the faster America fell apart, or so it seemed to the autocratic planters, intellectuals, and merchants who ran the country in its infancy. Between 1790 and 1830, alcohol consumption jumped to an all-time high of 7.1 gallons of pure alcohol per capita a year. The old-line elite feared that drunken revels such as the historic blowout at Jackson's inaugural ball were ill omens, heralding even worse debauchery to come.

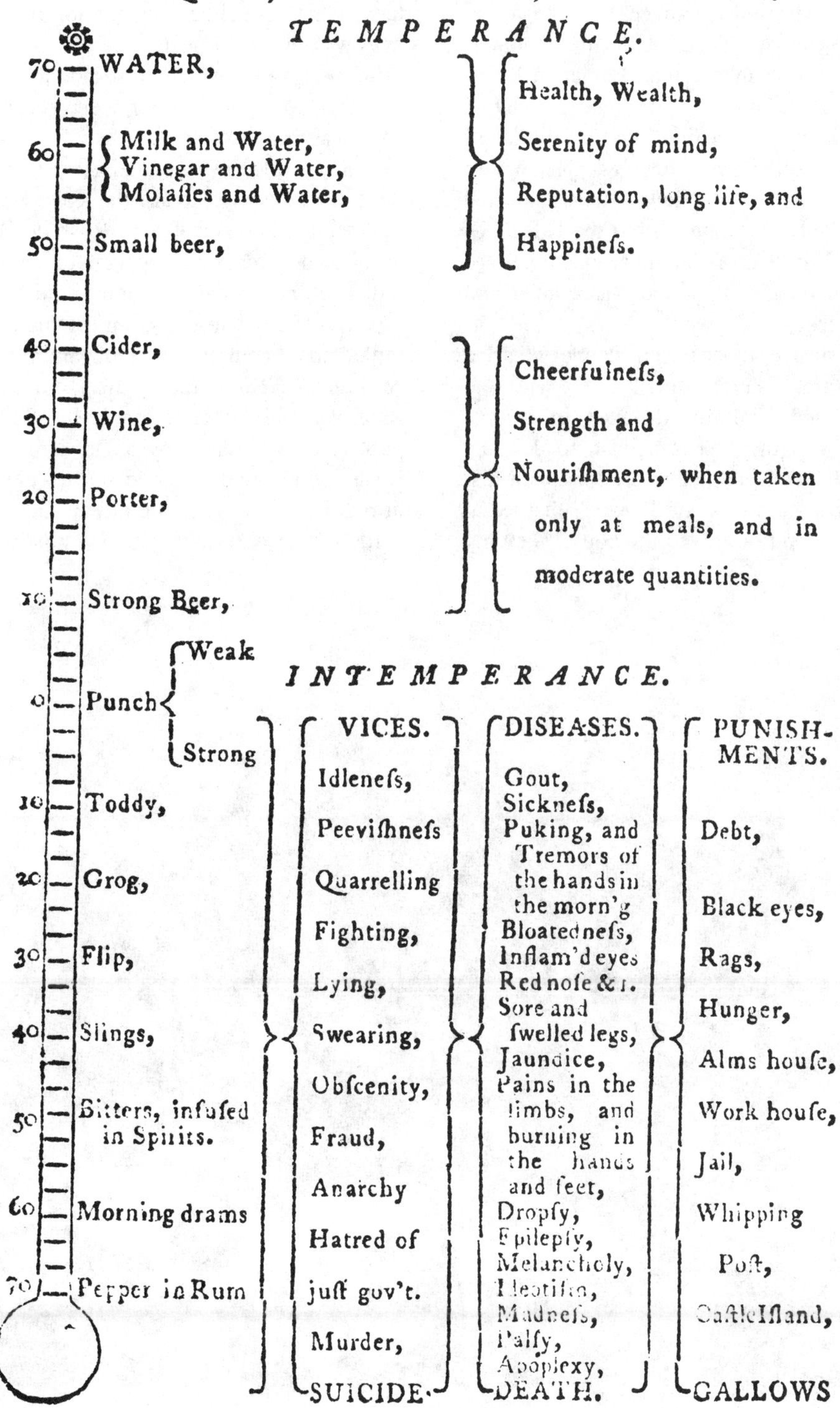
A MORAL and PHYSICAL THERMOMETER:

Or, a *Scale* of the *Progreſs* of TEMPERANCE and INTEMPERANCE.

LIQUORS, with their EFFECTS, in their uſual Order.

TEMPERANCE.

70 WATER,

60 Milk and Water, Vinegar and Water, Molaſſes and Water,

50 Small beer,

Health, Wealth, Serenity of mind, Reputation, long life, and Happineſs.

40 Cider,

30 Wine,

20 Porter,

10 Strong Beer,

Cheerfulneſs, Strength and Nouriſhment, when taken only at meals, and in moderate quantities.

0 Punch — Weak / Strong

INTEMPERANCE.

10 Toddy,

20 Grog,

30 Flip,

40 Slings,

50 Bitters, infuſed in Spirits.

60 Morning drams

70 Pepper in Rum

VICES. Idleneſs, Peeviſhneſs, Quarrelling, Fighting, Lying, Swearing, Obſcenity, Fraud, Anarchy, Hatred of juſt gov't. Murder, SUICIDE.

DISEASES. Gout, Sickneſs, Puking, and Tremors of the hands in the morn'g, Bloatedneſs, Inflam'd eyes, Red noſe & f. Sore and ſwelled legs, Jaundice, Pains in the limbs, and burning in the hands and feet, Dropſy, Epilepſy, Melancholy, Ideotiſm, Madneſs, Palſy, Apoplexy, DEATH.

PUNISHMENTS. Debt, Black eyes, Rags, Hunger, Alms houſe, Work houſe, Jail, Whipping Poſt, Caſtle Iſland, GALLOWS

17. Benjamin Rush devised an exact measurement for the evil effects of alcohol. *From Benjamin Rush,* An Inquiry Into the Effects of Spiritous Liquors on the Human Body. *Boston: Thomas and Andrews, 1790. National Library of Medicine.*

They decided to mobilize. The temperance movement that resulted "demonized alcohol," write scholars Linda A. Bennett and Genevieve M. Ames, ". . . and became the largest enduring middle-class mass movement of the 19th century."

Even before the nineteenth century, however, temperance advocates received intellectual ammunition from no less a personage than Benjamin Rush, signer of the Declaration of Independence, friend of Jefferson and Franklin, leading light of Philadelphia's medical establishment. In 1784, just before the Revolutionary War wound down, Rush published a pamphlet entitled "An Inquiry Into the Effects of Ardent Spirits." It was a damning indictment of alcohol's assault on the body and was quoted and reprinted for decades.

By ardent spirits, Rush meant alcohol distilled from fermented grain, sterner stuff than the wine and beer he considered healthful if taken in modest amounts. Rush was the first American to describe systematically habitual and heavy drinking as a disease. He termed it "a disease of the will" that led to physical addiction and destroyed the body. The only cure for addiction, he concluded, was abstinence.

In Rush's view, alcoholism progressed in distinct stages and led to dropsy, diabetes, epilepsy, palsy, and upset stomach. To illustrate his argument, Rush produced a "Moral and Physical Thermometer," which matched consumption of specific beverages with stages of health and disease. The healthiest drink was water, which corresponded to "health and wealth." Wine and porter were acceptable. Ardent spirits were the worst.

Some of Rush's statements in his influential work were fanciful, to say the least. Referring to one intemperate imbiber of rum, Rush described how the unfortunate creature happened to let loose a belch rather too near a candle flame—and exploded.

By 1829, when a group of medical doctors in Philadelphia commenced publication of the biweekly *Journal of Health,* the medical model presented by Rush was gaining acceptance. In 1830, the *Journal* published an address by a Dr. Hosack, who, with Rush, proclaimed water to be the most satisfactory drink of all (thus ignoring the dismal sanitation standards of the day) and, citing Sir Isaac Newton and

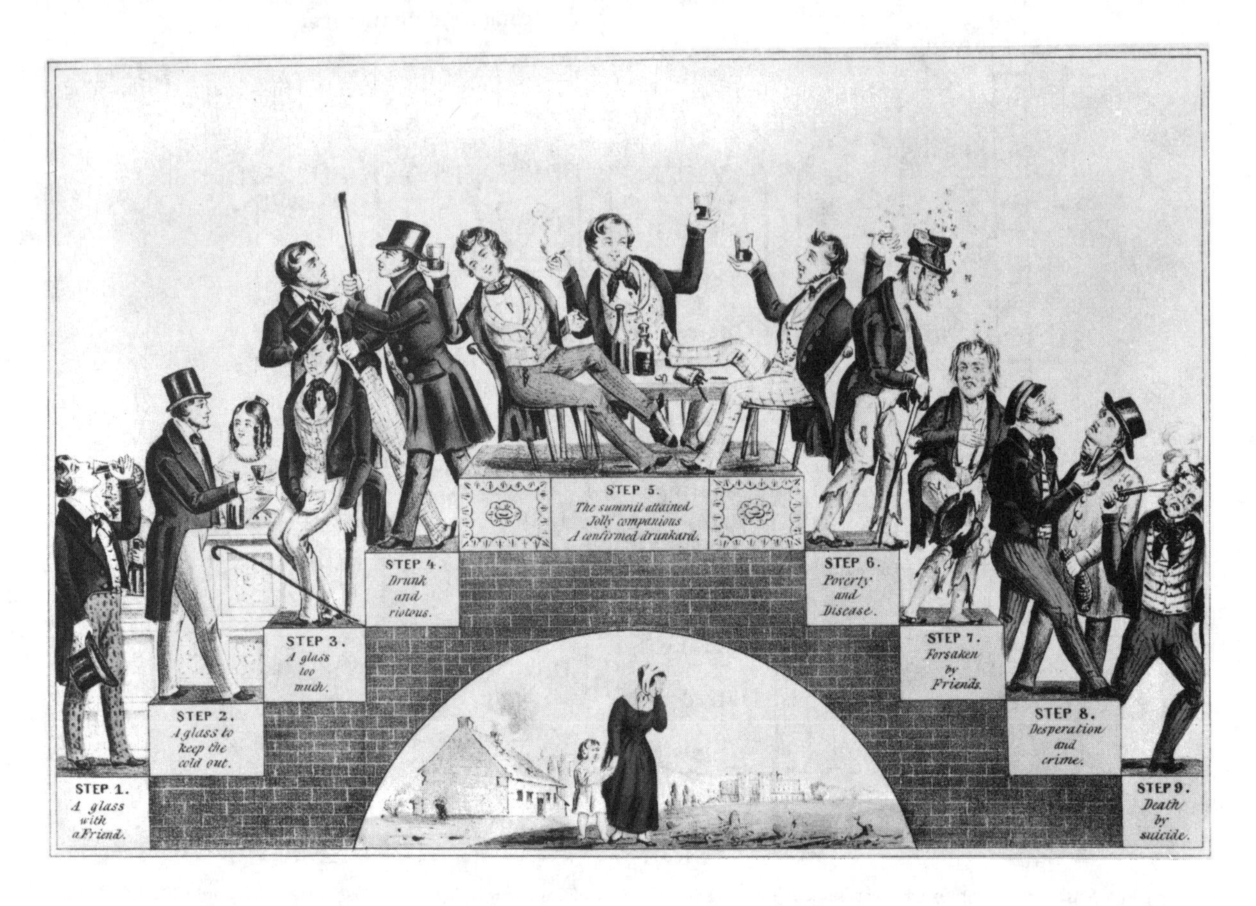
STEP 1. A glass with a Friend.
STEP 2. A glass to keep the cold out.
STEP 3. A glass too much.
STEP 4. Drunk and riotous.
STEP 5. The summit attained Jolly companions A confirmed drunkard.
STEP 6. Poverty and Disease.
STEP 7. Forsaken by Friends.
STEP 8. Desperation and crime.
STEP 9. Death by suicide.

18. That first sip leads inexorably to suicide, so said temperance workers. *Courtesy of the Library of Congress.*

other intellectuals, said to sip water as an example of what exorcising demon alcohol could do for the mind.

Throughout the Jacksonian era, Philadelphia remained the center of the embryonic temperance movement, boosted by its resident physicians, abstaining Quakers, and Presbyterian clergy. The first national temperance convention was held in that city in 1833. Even earlier, in 1830–31, the Reverend Sylvester Graham, working as a lecturer for the Pennsylvania Society for Discouraging the Use of Ardent Spirits, worked out of Philadelphia.

Graham, who became famous for his stern opposition to sex and his advocacy of vegetarianism, focused his temperance work on the physiological effects of alcohol. Graham believed that alcohol, being unnecessary for life, wears out the body. Therefore, it is best avoided. The argument must have been convincing; just outside Philadelphia, in the town of Chester, there were eight temperance hotels in Graham's day.

It was fitting that Graham was a man of the cloth, for organized religion supplied much of the intellectual firepower, not to mention the foot soldiers, for the holy war against demon alcohol. The Christian soldiers were armed with a newfound belief in the perfectibility of Man. Sin was choice, not destiny. By diving into medicine and politics, one could do the work of the Lord on Earth.

Medical and religious forces joined up early. Rush sent 1,000 copies of his "Inquiry" to a Presbyterian convention in Philadelphia in 1811.

In 1826, the Reverend Justin Edwards helped form the American Temperance Society, an early and important national organization. It was a big year, for almost simultaneously the Reverend Lyman Beecher, a Congregationalist, published *Six Sermons on Intemperance,* in which he argued that even moderate drinking was harmful. Only abstinence would ensure personal salvation and social stability.

There was a frankly unsavory underside of the temperance movement. It had a nativist, Know-Nothing constituency that was dead-set against immigration, especially from Ireland and Germany. Early Irish immigrants were mostly young, single men who did irregular, dangerous, dirty work for low pay and whiled away the hours drinking whiskey in saloons, which they used as social and cultural centers. German immigrants were more established and family-centered, but they enjoyed tippling, too, preferring lager in beer gardens and beer halls where they took in Sunday concerts.

Old-line Americans thought matters were taking a scandalous turn. Referring to polling places in taverns and the proliferation of dram shops, which sold cheap spirits by the glass, the *Journal of Health* warned of "our liberties bartered for a dram." The *National Philanthropist*, published in Boston, took as its motto "temperance drinking is a down-hill road to drunkenness." The editor of the *National Philanthropist* was the famous abolitionist William Lloyd Garrison, whose brother died a drunkard.

Most early temperance societies were just that: temperate. They didn't try to eliminate the sale of alcohol, which they called "the traffic," only to regulate it. But, as the struggles of the wets and the dries grew more strident, the live-and-let-live attitude hardened.

REFINED AND VIRTUOUS FEMALES

Edward Hitchcock, writing in the *Journal of Health* in 1830, noted:

> The powerful excitement which intoxicating liquors produce destroys a relish for the simple and noiseless pleasure of home, and virtuous, temperate society; and a love is created for places of public resort, such as the grog shop and the tavern. Here also men can indulge in the grossness of manners, which is the natural consequence of stimulants and narcotics, and which induces the dram-drinker, the wine-bibber, the smoker, the chewer, and snuff-taker, to avoid the society of refined and virtuous females.

THE DRY TIDE

The growing movement for abstinence from alcohol was a dry tide washing over the nation. Although it is remembered as a stuffy movement of prim naysayers, the temperance groundswell actually mixed progressive and reactionary ideas. Nativist sentiment against stereotyped whiskey-drinking Irish and beer-swilling Germans infused the temperance ranks, but so did more liberal-minded notions.

Temperance reform was often closely linked with the first wave of American feminism. Women who endured beatings and abandonment by drunken fathers and husbands swelled the ranks of reform. Women sometimes drank heavily, too, being especially fond of cordials and patent medicines, but this problem was seldom publicly discussed.

Temperance advocates adopted an ambitious social agenda which included the elimination of poverty, crime, immorality, and insanity, much of which they blamed on liquor. Many prominent people subscribed to temperance, among them Horace Greeley, Henry David Thoreau, Henry Wadsworth Longfellow, Henry Ward Beecher, and Horace Mann. They worked in what historians call "the stewardship tradition," the benevolent guidance of the nation by its old-line elite.

Temperance was also championed by the emerging industrialists, men who saw that the changeover from seasonal farm work and hard physical labor to the precision factory jobs of the Industrial Revolution required sobriety. Alcohol rations would not do in this brave new world.

By the 1830s, the temperance movement had nearly completed a radical turn away from moderation and toward abstinence. Temperance societies nominated their own candidates—dries, of course—for public office, and more and more members "took the pledge," that is, they swore to abstain from alcohol. Dries, who numbered one and a half million in 1830, wrote the letter "T," for total abstinence, next to their names on membership rolls and so created a new word: "teetotaler."

Under the leadership of the Boston-based American Temperance Society, which endorsed abstinence in 1837, teetotalers inundated the land with tracts, pamphlets, newspapers, and lectures. The ATS recruited women on the grounds that temperance would promote healthy, happy families and rein in even moderate tipplers. Just as there was no such thing as being a little bit pregnant, there could be no compromise with demon alcohol.

Temperance crusaders proved to be masters of political organizing, using state-of-the-art technology to disseminate their views. In his book *Sobering Up America,* Ian R. Tyrell writes, "Daniel Fanshaw, the printer for both the New-York City Temperance Society and the American Tract Society, was the first to introduce machinery into the New York book publishing business, even before regular commercial publishers did."

The most important precursor of Alcoholics Anonymous, a self-help group called the Washingtonians, was founded in May 1840—in a Baltimore tavern, ironically enough. Named after the nation's first president, the Washingtonians seeded local chapters and created a women's auxiliary called, of course, the Martha Washingtonians.

All this activity spawned a temperance counterculture, complete with songs, bands, theaters, literature, and festive social events. Alcohol-free concerts, fairs and picnics, designed to provide alternatives to the grog shops, were common in antebellum America.

The temperance counterculture produced hit shows and bestsellers. "Ten Nights in a Barroom," Timothy Shay Arthur's novel (later also a play), was melodramatic—a little girl, timorously entering a smoky saloon to retrieve her besotted father, is killed when a snarling bartender beans her with a shot glass—but it was immensely popular. The standard textbook *McGuffey's Reader* carried lines such as: "O, water for me/Bright water for me/And wine for the tremulous debauchee."

Critics, who dubbed the purists "ultras," were not amused by the movement's growing strength. In his grumpy but entertaining 1838 book *Humbugs of New-York,* David Meredith Reese, a physician, railed against the ultras of the metropolis. Reese assailed the notion that sacramental wine should be replaced by nonalcoholic beverages and observed of temperance advocates that "many of them go as far as to repudiate the very name of temperance societies, and assume that of total abstinence societies. . . ."

In the 1840s, soon after Reese wrote, legally sanctioned abstinence became reality in much of the nation through local and state laws, leaving moral suasion, which had never worked well enough to suit some teetotalers, to the pantywaists and go-slowers. Promoted by evangelical Christians and temperance societies, many municipalities went dry in the 1840s. But it wasn't until 1851, when Maine went dry, that statewide prohibition caught on.

So-called Maine laws spread across North America. By 1855, 13 states and territories and two Canadian provinces instituted prohibition. But while they were easy to pass, Maine laws proved difficult to enforce. Immigrants and their supporters opposed them, as did well-heeled liquor sellers. Then, too, professional police were rare in those days, so getting tough with liquor vendors was easier said than done. By the end of the Civil War, only 10 years after the high-water mark of state prohibition, most of the Maine laws were repealed.

JOHN BARLEYCORN MUST DIE

But the struggle was not over. The postbellum drive for an alcohol-free America got a major push in 1874, when the Women's Christian Temperance Union was founded. Headed by Elizabeth "Mother" Thompson, the WCTU commenced pray-ins in saloons, exhorting barkeeps to close their shops and patrons to take the pledge. Their efforts were known as "the women's crusade."

In their book *Drinking in America,* Mark Edward Lender and James Kirby Martin observe that the WCTU "represented the first mass entry of women into American reform work and politics." After its

THEATRE!

BENEFIT

And last appearance but one of the Celebrated American Comedian

YANKEE LOCKE!

ON THIS OCCASION WILL BE PRESENTED W. W. PRATT'S MORAL LESSON, ENTITLED

TEN NIGHTS IN A BAR-ROOM.

YANKEE LOCKE will appear in his original character of **SAMPLE SWITCHELL**, as performed by him with great success in all the principal cities in the United States.

NOTICE—This Thrilling Drama has been taken, scene by scene, from T. S. Arthur's celebrated story, bearing the same title. The representations of "Ten Nights in a Bar-Room!" have been witnessed by over 100,000 persons—heads of families, members of churches, all interested in the propagation of the great doctrines of Temperance, have borne testimony to the excellent effect produced by the life-like delineations of

FOLLY, MISERY, MADNESS AND CRIME.

Caused by the Brutal, Disgusting, and Demoralizing Vice of Drunkenness.

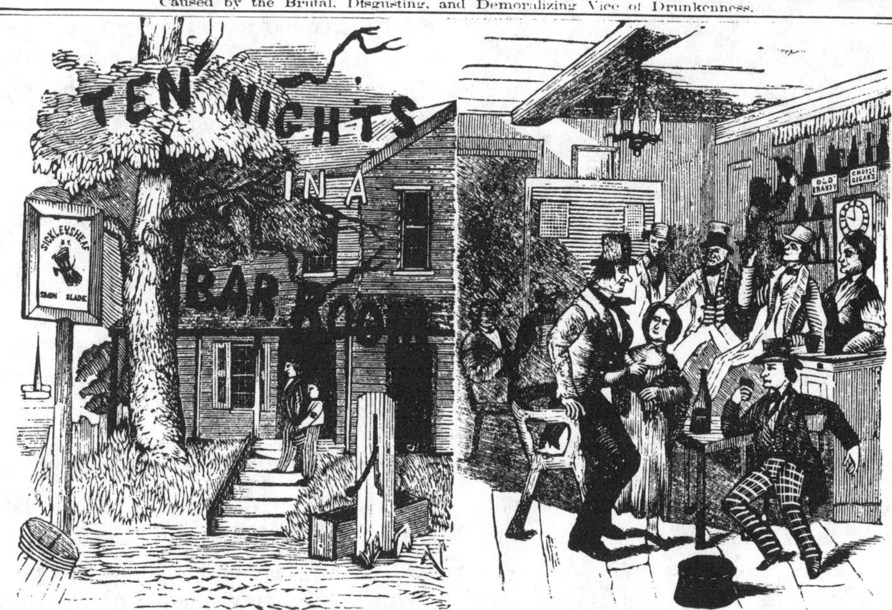

FRIDAY EVENING, DECEMBER 29th, 1865,

WILL BE PRESENTED THE MORAL DRAMA, IN 4 ACTS, ENTITLED,

TEN NIGHTS in a BAR ROOM

SAMPLE SWITCHELL, A genuine Yankee, in favor of Temperance, but drinks his regular Daily Allowance, **YANKEE LOCKE.**

Joe Morgan, the Inebriate..........Mr C J Fyffe
Simon Slade, the Landlord..........Mr H C Page
Mr Romaine, the Philanthropist..........Mr Geo Fisher
Willie Hammond, the Pride of the Village...S Bloomingdale
Harvy Green, a Fast Young Man..........Mr R B Richards
Frank Slade,..........Mr D Cameron
Mrs Morgan, the Drunkard's wife..........Mrs M A Pennoyer
Mehitable Cartwright, Sample' Sweetheart...Miss J. Fisher
Mrs Slade..........Miss Jane Parker
Little Mary Morgan, the Angel Child..........Little Nellie

Synopsis of Scenery, Incidents; Etc.

ACT I.—SCENE 1.—Hammond's residence, his interview with the new landlord of the "Sickle and Sheaf," Sample's description of his lady-love, the romantic maiden, the anxious mother. SCENE 1.—Interview between Mr Romaine and the Yankee, Sample's ideas of moderate drinking. Return of the landlord Simon, his brilliant idea of the future. SCENE 3.—Interior of the Sickle and Sheaf, the ex miller and the happy landlord, arrival of the pride of the village, the young squire, the landlord's wife. "We shall never, Simon, be as happy again as we were at the old mill," the gambler's intimacy with Willie Hammond, poor Joe Morgan, the inebriate, his account of his past life and that of his friend, Simon Slade, Arrival of little Mary in search of her father; darkly shadowed is the sky that hangs gloomily over her young life; departure of the inebriate and his child; quarrel between Green and Willie; timely arrival of the Yankee. "Lay there till the cows come home."

ACT II.—SCENE 1.—The young spendthrift—Return of Mehitabel from the villiage post office—Her account of the Black Knight of the Enchanted Castle—Sample's ideas of abolition—The Yankee and the Philanthropist. SCENE 2.—Sample's description of the communion gin. SCENE 3.—Simon Slad's progress in tavern keeping—The landlord's enterprising son, Frank—Joe Morgan's unwelcome visit to the Sickle and Sheaf—The quarrel between the landlord and his drunken customer—The tumbler and the fatal blow—Arrival of little Mary—"Father, father! they have killed me!" SCENE 4.—The Yankee and the Gambler—Cross questions—Sample's definition of the word "Gentleman"—The treat—The Yankee's desire for Green's future happiness. SCENE 5. The drunkard's home—The patient wife besides the bed of her suffering child—Joe Morgan's promise—Little Mary's anxiety for her father's good—Frightful delirium of the poor inebriate—"Come here, this is little Mary's room, nothing can hurt you here." Affecting Tableau.

ACT III. SCENE 1. Sickle and Sheaf, the landlord and his son, Mrs. Slade's account of her interview with little Mary, Sample and the young squire on a time, the Yankee's story about uncle John and the poor house, the fight and death of Willie Hammond. SCENE 2. Escape of Green, the Yankee in pursuit, "Wonder if I have got the nightmare," the arrest, "come, old fellow, it's time you pass in your check." SCENE 3. Joe Morgan's wretched home, the wife and mother watching by her suffering one, "I'll never drink another drop of liquor as long as I live." The dying child.

We shall meet in the land where the spring is eternal,
Where sadness never cometh, nor sorrow nor pain—
Where the flowers never fade in that clime always warm
We shall meet, and our parting shall be never again.

DEATH OF LITTLE MARY.

ACT IV. SCENE 1. The meeting of Sample and Mr. Romaine after a lapse of five years, Sample a Teetotaller, His quaint description of matters and things that have transpired at Cedarville Arrival of Mehitable—Sample popping the question—His idea of measuring calico—Comic Song—"Farewell to rum and brandy"—SCENE 2. Representing the Sickle and Sheaf in a state of decay. Appearance of Simon Slade—The wonderful transformation of the once happy miller.—Frank's progress in dram drinking—the quarrel between father and son—Death of Simon Slade—"Frank Slade, you have murdered your father!" SCENE 3. The happy home of Mr Morgan—Arrival of Mr Romaine and others—Resolutions—The wife's joy Sample Switchel, and his new suit with Mehitable.

A drunkard no longer—that is over,
Free, disenthralled, I stand a man once more.

EPILOGUE AND HAPPY TERMINATION.

THE ENTERTAINMENT WILL CONCLUDE WITH THE MUSICAL FARCE OF

A LOAN OF A LOVER!

Capt. [illegible]..........[illegible]
Mynheer Swyzel..........Mr George Fisher

PRICES AS USUAL.

19. "Ten Nights in a Barroom" was a melodramatic and popular entertainment in the Civil War era. *Courtesy of the Library of Congress.*

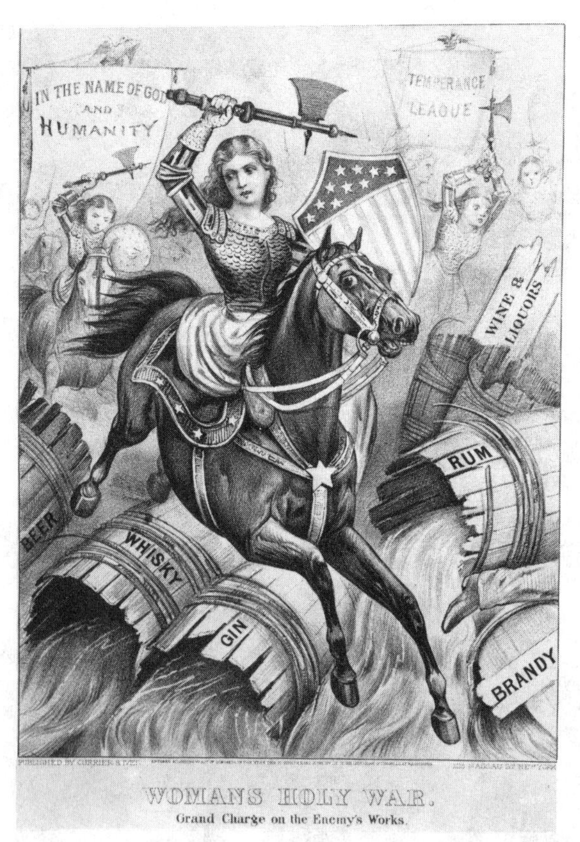

20. Currier and Ives depicted more than pretty landscapes at the height of the temperance battles (1874). *Courtesy of the Library of Congress.*

prime target, which was, of course, drinking, the WCTU took aim at tobacco, obscenity, gambling, and intercollegiate sports, not forgetting to promote the middle-class Americanization of immigrants, female suffrage, anti-rape laws, and world peace.

Politically savvy, the WCTU formed a coalition with the National Prohibition Party, founded in 1869. (It is a curious historical footnote that the Prohibition Party nominated as its presidential candidate in 1904 one Silas C. Swallow.)

The WCTU increased its influence under the leadership of Frances E. Willard (1839–1898), dean of women at Northwestern University and now the only woman represented in the Statuary Hall of the U.S. Capitol. Advancing the "politics of the Mother Heart," the WCTU fought for "home protection" from the ravages of drink.

The WCTU's best-known member, or at any rate its most notorious, was Carry Nation (1846–1911), head of a Kansas chapter, who captured the national limelight as a destroyer of saloons. Nation employed hatchets to chop long mahogany bars into splinters, a process she called "hatchetization." She also made adroit use of rocks wrapped in paper, which she called "smashers." Her weekly newspaper was, with impeccable logic, called the *Smasher's Mail*.

Although she was caricatured in her day and ours—and Nation was almost a self-caricature—she had her serious and enlightened side. Nation espoused sex education and equal rights for women; she opposed wife-beating; she frowned on smoking; she saw alcoholism as a disease and was, herself, the widow of an alcoholic.

She was born in Kentucky before the Civil War as Carry Moore, into a family of eccentrics; her mother believed herself to be Queen Victoria. An aunt was even odder; she thought she was a weathervane.

As a child, Carry was sickly, experiencing strange, powerful dreams and visions, which continued throughout her life. As an adult she was far from frail, however. Standing nearly six feet tall, stout and fierce-looking in her severe bonnet and plain, round eyeglasses, Carry Nation was strong enough to rip a door off a saloon ice chest and pick up an iron cash register and hurl it into the street.

Journalists (who persisted in misspelling her first name as Carrie) could no more resist writing about her than they could put off exposing a politician's "love nest," complete with the obligatory underage showgirl. Nation understood this, and played her role as an avenging angel to the hilt. She was a forceful public speaker, touring England and North America, and delighted in providing reams of colorful newspaper copy, becoming one of the twentieth century's first media darlings.

Nation began her attack on saloons in Kansas, where she lived after leaving her native Kentucky. Kansas was officially dry, but enforcement was slack. In 1900, Nation busted up her first saloon, a place in Kiowa—but only after hearing a voice which she believed to be God's telling her it was all right. She shattered bottles, glasses, and mirrors with bloodcurdling ferocity.

Nation was a master of the riposte. On another attack—her missions took her all over America—she stood accused of defacing private property. "Defacing? Defacing?" Nation shot back. "I'm defacing nothing. I am destroying!"

Despite her extremism, Nation was an inspiration to America's dries, who were on a roll again after repeal of the first state prohibition laws. As the *Smithsonian* magazine put it in 1989, "Carry Nation is the grandmother of our recent concern about the excessive use of drugs in general. . . ."

America's three-century hangover prompted calls for quick, sure cures—the medical equivalent of Nation's hatchets—even as the political wars intensified. The most famous cure was propagated in the

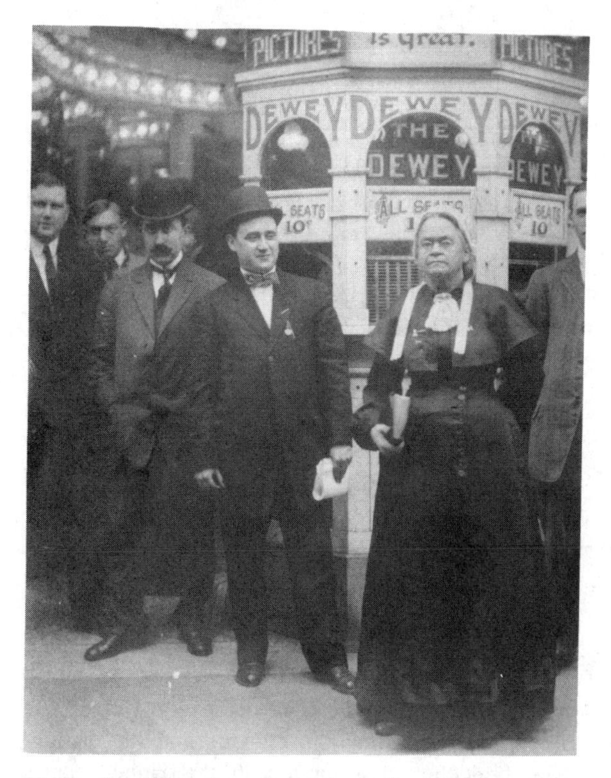

21. The formidable Carry Nation fought for temperance with a Bible and a hatchet. *Kansas State Historical Society.*

late nineteenth century by Dr. Leslie E. Keeley (1834–1900), an enterprising physician who claimed that he could dry up alcoholism with his "gold cure."

Keeley theorized that alcoholism poisoned the nerve cells, causing physical addiction. Remove the cause and you could regenerate healthy cells. To accomplish this, Keeley marketed a proprietary medicine called "Bichloride" or "Double Chloride of Gold," which he sold via mail-order and at sanitaria that bore his name.

Keeley never revealed his formula. Laboratory tests showed only traces of gold in the product, which was said to purge toxins by increasing elimination. Indeed, Keeley's critics charged that his medication could damage the kidneys.

Keeley patented his bottles, which he gave a curious, almost triangular shape and closed with sealing wax, urging that they be destroyed after use so no inferior product would sully the containers. He formed Keeley Leagues, which met in annual national conventions in the 1890s. There was a Keeley Day at the Chicago World's Fair of 1893.

The doctor opened a Keeley Institute in Dwight, Illinois in 1891 to treat alcoholics and drug addicts, later seeding franchises elsewhere. "The billboards and wall-sized signs [of] a Keeley Institute were almost obligatory for a city to be up-to-date from the 1890s to the First World War," wrote scholar H. Wayne Morgan.

No shrinking violet, Keeley wrote advertisements that proclaimed: "ABSOLUTELY CURE ANYONE—It stands at the head of medical agencies, the peerless alleviation of human suffering, the magic destroyer of the alcoholic appetite, and the true deliverer from the wily snares of liquor."

In a pamphlet peppered with personal testimonials, Keeley wrote, "It is as rational, from a medical point of view, to treat drunkenness by expostulation, pledge-signing, reproaches and legislation as it formerly was to treat insanity by incantation, exhibitions of the bones of saints, and the laying-on of hands." This modern man of science was less than scientific, however, when he announced that "we are so perfect in our methods that a mistake cannot occur."

SANITARIUM TREATMENT.

Under Dr. Keeley's personal care, a limited number of patients are received at Dwight. All cures made in from eight to twenty days, without pain or nervous shock.

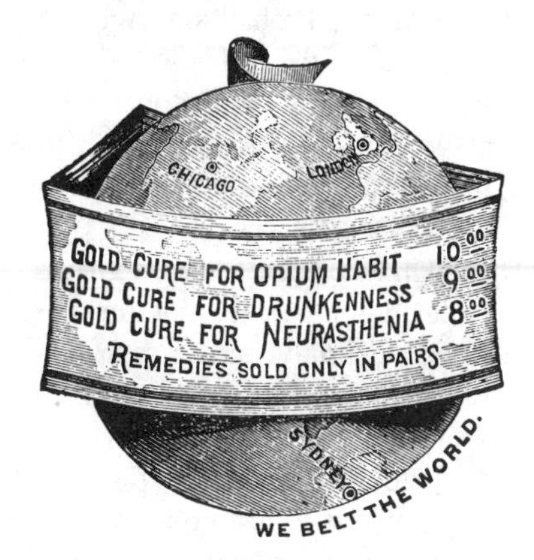

Course of treatment at Dwight, limited to three weeks. Terms and dates made known on application. Confidential correspondence solicited.

THE LESLIE E. KEELEY CO.

DWIGHT, ILLINOIS.

22. Keeley's substance-abuse remedies were ballyhooed in no uncertain terms. *National Library of Medicine.*

Keeley's domineering personality, modern disease-model of alcoholism, and the pleasant surroundings at his institutes proved to be a winning combination. Some 400,000 Americans took the Keeley cure by 1918. Church groups endorsed Keeleyism and the U.S. Army used it to treat drunken doughboys. But Keeley's methods gradually fell from favor after his death in 1900, and political pressure grew ever stronger to remove the source of alcoholism —booze itself—rather than waste time fiddling with cures.

Prominent Americans such as John D. Rockefeller, Henry Ford, and William Randolph Hearst jumped on the prohibition bandwagon for medical and moral reasons and because they believed banning booze would upgrade industrial efficiency. The dry tide even reached across the Atlantic. A World War I law that mandated afternoon pub closings (so that munitions workers would go back to work sober) endured in England from 1915 until 1988.

With that kind of momentum, it was just a matter of time until nationwide prohibition became a reality. The time came on January 1, 1919.

THE NOBLE EXPERIMENT

Nationwide prohibition—Prohibition with a capital "P," as it came to be known—triggered a 14-year revolution in American life. The authorizing legislation, the National Prohibition Act (known as the Volstead Act, after the Minnesota congressman who sponsored it), passed on October 28, 1918, over President Woodrow Wilson's veto. It took effect as the Eighteenth Amendment, after the necessary 36 states ratified the new law.

The tough federal law outlawed the sale—though, in an interesting loophole, not the possession—of unauthorized alcoholic beverages. Sacramental wines were excepted, as was liquor used for medicinal purposes and prescribed by a physician. But prison terms of up to five years and fines as high as 10 thousand dollars were in store for smuggling ("bootlegging") outlawed commercial liquor.

Prohibition was the major, albeit temporary, triumph of the stewardship tradition. It represented the political peak of 150 years of calls for temperance, then abstinence, then legal sanctions. Prohibition was dubbed "the noble experiment," a tag line that has endured, with unintended irony. It is attributed to Herbert Hoover, who referred to Prohibition as "an experiment noble in purpose and far-reaching. . . ."

Almost immediately, the radical new law created unintended consequences. Consumption of homemade wine went way up. "From 1925 to 1939," according to *Drinking in America,* "Americans drank more than 678 million gallons of home-fermented wine, three times as much as all the domestic and imported wine they drank during the five years before Prohibition; this figure does not include the wine made from backyard vineyards, from dandelions, currants, cherries and other fruits. . . ."

In a way never intended by champions of Prohibition, the ban made drinking seem wild, crazy, hip, and daring. The concealed flask of spirits, the midnight knock at the speakeasy door, and the nip of fiery liquors in the rumble seat of a sporty roadster became symbols of defiant fun. All of a sudden, drinking, until then seen as a cause of illness, weakness and failure, was, through a cultural alchemy, transformed.

Despite its reputation as a spectacular failure that was widely ignored, especially by organized crime, Prohibition succeeded on several fronts. The rise in home distilling and brewing notwithstanding, overall alcohol consumption in the United States dropped by between one-third and one-half. Historian John C. Burnham writes that alcohol-related hospital admissions fell and there were fewer arrests for drunkenness. Cirrhosis of the liver killed fewer people. Social workers reported reduced drinking problems among the urban poor.

Even so, opposition to Prohibition grew stronger, setting in motion a dialectic that would eventually overturn the law. As late as 1930, Senator Morris Shepperd of Texas scoffed, "There's as much chance of repealing the Eighteenth Amendment as there is for a hummingbird to fly to Mars with the Washington Monument tied to its tail."

He was wrong. Morris and his fellow dries underestimated the determined, sophisticated opposition to their favorite constitutional amendment. Organized labor, after the Great Depression hit home in 1929, looked to a revitalized liquor industry for badly needed jobs, and businessmen hoped for a revived tax on legal alcohol coupled with lighter income taxes.

President Franklin D. Roosevelt, after only a month in office, amended the Volstead Act in 1933 to permit the sale of beer with 3.2 percent alcohol. That first step became a gallop on December 5, 1933, when, with enthusiastic popular support, the Twenty-first Amendment was passed, overturning the Eighteenth Amendment and ending the Noble Experiment.

BOOTSTRAP TEMPERANCE

Repeal took the wind out of traditional temperance organizations, reducing their membership and political clout. Some states and localities remained officially dry, but the push for reform shifted back to the private sector, with its self-help groups and medical researchers.

The largest and most important self-help organization, Alcoholics Anonymous, was launched shortly after repeal of Prohibition. Founders William Wilson (1895–1971), a stockbroker, and Dr. Robert Smith (1879–1950), a surgeon, met in Akron, Ohio in 1935, and each resolved to help the other solve his drinking problem. The tiny group that formed around them took the name Alcoholics Anonymous in 1939.

Religiosity plays a key part in AA's regimen, as it did in so many nineteenth-century temperance societies. Fully 6 of AA's 12 steps to recovery refer to faith. AA has inspired an estimated 200 groups that use 12-step programs to fight the likes of gambling, compulsive shopping, drug use, overwork, and binge-and-purge eating. As for AA, the organization operated in more than 100 countries at the start of the 1990s.

While AA revived and refined earlier self-help concepts, the medical model of alcoholism as a disease, introduced by Benjamin Rush in 1784, also underwent a revival. Medical authorities began to treat alcoholism again on a significant scale in the 1940s, about a decade after Prohibition ended. The World Health Organization adopted the medical model in 1952, with the AMA following in 1961. Medical scientist E.M. Jellinek, who endorsed the idea that alcoholism is a physical addiction, not just a psychological failing, drew up a chart of alcohol-related afflictions in 1952 that looked not unlike Rush's old "Moral and Physical Thermometer."

Today, the disease model is widely accepted. Alcoholism is believed to be the result of a combination of physiological and genetic factors. As of 1988, there was a staggering total of 7,000 treatment facilities in the United States, using a variety of techniques to help drinkers sober up.

THE NEW TEMPERANCE

The concern for health and fitness that swept much of the Western world in the 1970s and 1980s produced a powerful groundswell against the abuse of alcohol. Fueled by anger over drunk driving, worry over lost productivity, and the billions spent for care of alcoholics, the diffuse movement that resulted can fairly be termed the new temperance.

The institutions of the old temperance play no central role. The Prohibition Party is an election-day curiosity. The Anti-Saloon League is gone. In 1989, a *Smithsonian* magazine writer even came across a lively bar in Kiowa, Kansas, hard by a memorial to Carry Nation.

The Women's Christian Temperance Union still exists, counting 50 thousand members in 72 countries. The WCTU's influence in American politics is much reduced, but its dedication to the fight is undiminished. In a 1983 feature story, the *San Francisco Examiner* interviewed a WCTU member who insisted, following her nineteenth-century forerunners, that "Jesus was the great physician. He would never have condoned alcohol, something that dulls the brain. It's sacrilegious to use fermented wine in communion."

The legions of new temperance advocates were very much on the job at the dawn of the 1990s. Private, nonprofit institutions such as Mothers Against Drunk Driving, the Center for Science in the Public Interest, and the National Council on Alcoholism spearheaded the movement.

Private groups got a boost from the public sector in the 1980s, when C. Everett Koop, President Ronald Reagan's surgeon general, urged the end of "happy hours" for discounted drinks, advocated higher taxes on alcoholic beverages and called for restraint in advertising, as well as stepped-up public service announcements about the dangers of drinking. Moreover, Congress, in 1988, required that health-minded warning labels be placed in "a conspicuous and prominent place" on every container of beer, wine, and liquor.

Concerned about its tarnished public image, the alcohol industry multiplied its public service announcements about "responsible" drinking and, on at least one occasion, put its money where its mouth was. Canada's Joseph E. Seagram & Sons gave 5.8 million dollars to Harvard University for medical research into alcoholism.

Almost simultaneously, distillers and vintners launched aggressive counterattacks against the new temperance. Opponents of heavy drinking were caricatured as "neo-prohibitionists" by California winemaker Robert Mondavi, though that is a misnomer since few reformers advocate an outright ban.

Industry in the late 1980s also emphasized the brighter side of medical research. Vintners pointed out that moderate wine-drinking may decrease the risk of heart attacks by raising high-density lipoprotein in the blood. Indeed, in some countries, notably

Italy and France, wine has never lost its reputation as a vital, health-giving beverage—a reputation that extends to beer in Ireland, where the leading brewer extolls its dark, creamy stout with this simple line: "Guinness is good for you."

In America, the history of drinking (though not of temperance) surfaces in advertising campaigns. In 1989, the Associated Press reported that the Beer Institute, a Washington, D.C. trade organization, planned a campaign in which "one ad will use early American paintings to show how beer was brought to America on the Mayflower, was used to celebrate the first Thanksgiving and was part of the daily ration for soldiers in the American Revolution."

Of course, in some places the past has never completely vanished. Kansas didn't legalize liquor by the glass in public bars until 1987, after 107 parched years. Utah and West Virginia still restrict liquor in public bars, perhaps anticipating the day when the rest of the nation, its dry instincts whetted once more, heads back to the future.

SOBERING FIGURES

- The Centers for Disease Control report that 105,095 Americans died from injuries or disease linked to alcohol in 1987.
- Alcohol is involved in about half of hospital emergency-room admissions.
- Alcohol is expected to cost the U.S. economy 150 billion dollars a year in absenteeism and reduced efficiency by 1995.
- Men are the heaviest drinkers, knocking back about three times more alcohol than women who, studies show, get drunk faster than men. Young people ages 18 to 34, people with annual incomes above 35 thousand dollars a year, and Southerners drink more than other Americans.
- U.S. membership of Alcoholics Anonymous grew from 750 thousand in 1978 to 1.6 million in 1988.
- From 1980 to 1989, American consumption of wine dropped from 3.18 gallons per person to 2.11 gallons; beer from 36.85 gallons to 33.7; and distilled spirits from 3.02 gallons to 2.16.
- In 1989, Anheuser-Busch announced it would boost spending for its "responsible drinking" commercials from 8 million dollars a year to 30 million dollars, following the U.S. Surgeon General's criticisms of alcohol advertising.
- The alcohol beverage industry spent two billion dollars on advertising in 1988.

CHAPTER · 6 ·

SYLVESTER AND THE GRAHAMITES: "PUT BACK THE BRAN"

Every farmer knows that if his horse has straw cut with his grain, or hay in abundance, he does well enough. Just so it is with the human species. Man needs the bran in his bread.

REVEREND SYLVESTER GRAHAM, circa 1835

One March afternoon in 1837, a gentle preacher by the name of Sylvester Graham sparked a riot in Boston. Graham was famous for preaching the then-incendiary gospel of regular exercise, fresh air, weekly bathing, and meatless and liquor-free meals. Even more radical, he demanded that millers put the nutritious bran back into their popular white bread.

When word got out that Graham was in town, a mob of 200 men surrounded Boston's Amory Hall, where the minister was scheduled to lecture on "physical education" to an all-female audience. Finding the door blocked by the revelers, the frightened but determined women pushed their way into the hall, "followed," according to Boston's *Evening Transcript,* "by a still greater number of the mob."

As both camps waited for Graham to arrive, the rioters degenerated into a chorus of hissing, barking, and crowing, followed by a finale of "Graham! Graham! Graham!" Perhaps warned of the hazardous welcome awaiting him, Graham never showed up for his lecture. Thanks to the timely arrival of the city marshall, the mob was dispersed and Graham's supporters were quickly escorted from the hall.

A century and a half later, the health-minded minister who stirred such passions is remembered chiefly as the namesake of the Graham cracker. Yet for a brief period in the 1830s, Sylvester Graham stood in the spotlight as a popular, much sought-after lecturer, who filled meeting halls up and down the East Coast with his speeches on dietary and hygienic reform.

Long after Graham's death in 1851, his followers, the "Grahamites," who included such luminaries as Dr. William Alcott and his first cousin Bronson (father of author Louisa May), feminist and cookbook author Catherine Beecher, and John Harvey Kellogg of cornflake fame, would continue to spread the gospels of vegetarianism, water cures, fresh air,

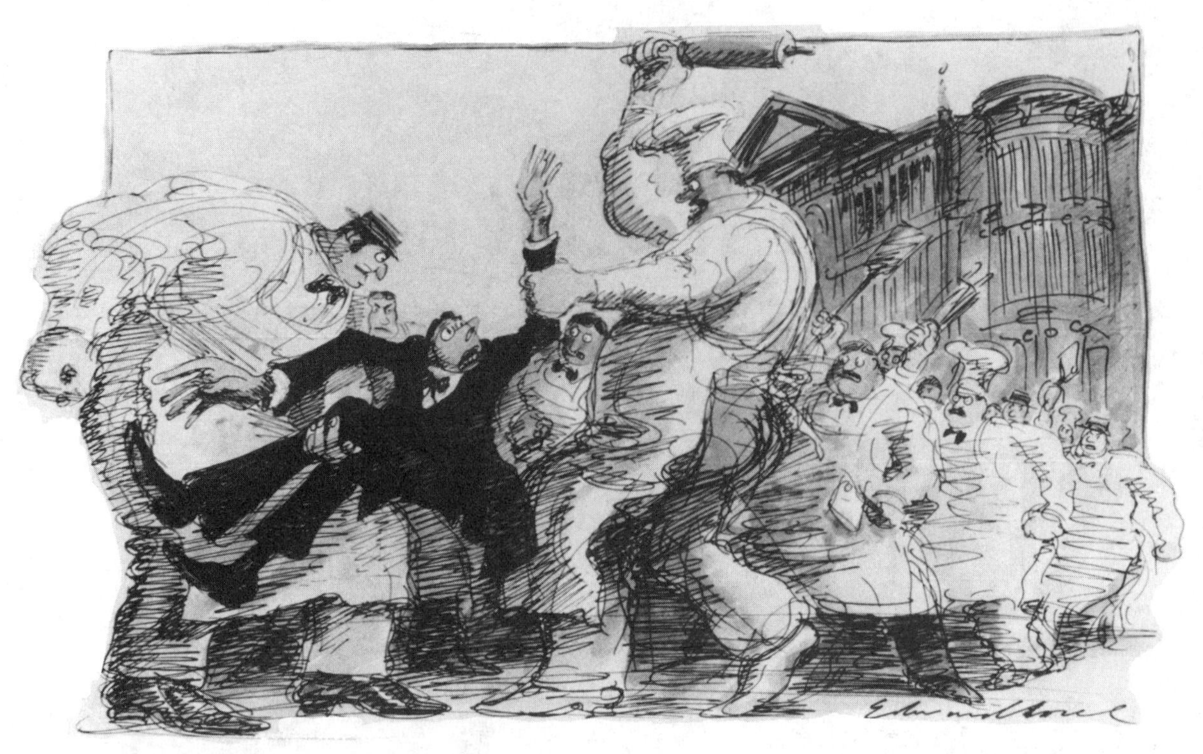

23. Not everyone took kindly to Sylvester Graham's injunctions against red meat and white bread. *Drawing by Edward Sorel.*

exercise, temperance, and "bran bread." And, while the modern-day varieties of Graham crackers sold in supermarkets and health-food stores are a far cry from the chewy, coarse, whole-wheat bread Graham popularized in his day, Graham can be credited with being the first to preach that you are what you eat.

THE SEVENTEENTH CHILD

Sylvester Graham was born in 1794 in the Connecticut River Valley town of Suffield, Connecticut, not far from the Massachusetts border. He was the seventeenth child of a successful minister named John Graham. Both Graham's father and immigrant Scottish grandfather preached the gospel of the Great Awakening, the Protestant revivalism that spread through New England in the eighteenth century.

The youngest child of his father's second marriage, Graham seems to have spent a depressed and lonely youth, no doubt aggravated by the death of his 72-year-old father when Graham was only two. According to the probate court, Graham's mother was "in a deranged state of mind" after her husband's death, and so the court appointed a guardian for Sylvester and two older siblings.

Although the records vary in detail, young Graham spent his late teenage years boarding with one older sister after another until he and his mother finally settled in Newark, New Jersey to live with an older brother.

In Newark, Graham gained a reputation as the town dreamer and rebel. According to one local resident, Graham was "an eccentric and wayward genius," who wiled away his time reciting poetry, unsuccessfully wooing women, writing letters to the newspaper, and trying to court the town's leading citizens. A bachelor, without any idea what he would do with his life, Graham never quite fit into Newark's society.

When he was 29 years old, Graham decided it was time to get an education, and he enrolled in a preparatory school run by Amherst College. Perhaps it was his age or his unconventional ways—he was a nondrinker at a time when temperance was not yet fashionable among educated folks—or his tendency to antagonize others by his forceful personality, but Graham soon found himself on the outs with his classmates. After only one semester, Amherst expelled him after he was falsely accused of assaulting another student.

Despondent over his failed academic career, Graham ended up in Compton, Rhode Island, where he rented a room at the house of Oliver Potter Earl, a sea captain with two young daughters. Graham had a nervous breakdown soon after moving in, and the sisters nursed him back to health. By the following fall, he had married the older of the two, a girl named Sarah.

The responsibilities of marriage seem to have propelled Graham into choosing a career. Not surprisingly, he decided to become a Presbyterian minister. And, not surprisingly, he did not want to go back to school for his training. Instead, he studied privately with the local parish minister who had officiated at his wedding. By the time he was ordained and returned to New Jersey to begin his first real job, Graham was 34 years old.

Yet Graham's stint as a New Jersey minister was short-lived. During the two years when he was first a guest preacher in Belvidere and then minister of a congregation in Bound Brook, Graham managed to get himself into trouble once again. This time he earned the wrath of his congregation in Bound Brook by speaking out for temperance, which in those days meant cutting hard liquor from one's diet and cutting down on, though not eliminating, beer and wine. But all was not lost. Graham had his first real taste of pecuniary success—10 dollars for his work in Belvidere and 300 dollars in Bound Brook, enough to rent a 10-room house. And his temperance sermons gave him a reputation that would set him in the direction of fame, if not fortune.

FROM MINISTER TO PROFESSIONAL REFORMER

Graham's New Jersey temperance sermons brought him to the attention of reformers in nearby Philadelphia, where the medical community dominated the temperance movement and gave the Pennsylvania temperance organizations a health-oriented focus. The City of Brotherly Love had been the birthplace of the movement in the 1780s and was now, in the early nineteenth century, the leading center for a growing American temperance movement. Just as his luck in New Jersey ran out, the Pennsylvania Society for Discouraging the Use of Ardent Spirits (later shortened to the Pennsylvania Temperance Society) offered Graham a job. Perhaps recognizing his talent for arousing a crowd, the organization hired him as a traveling lecturer. Graham would finally find his true calling—that of a professional lecturer and reformer. For once his timing was perfect. In those days, fans swarmed into lecture halls to hear their favorite celebrity reformers.

The moody young preacher was an instant hit. Taking what was then a radical position, he was among the first to speak out against fermented drinks as well as distilled liquor, a departure from the accepted position of the late Dr. Benjamin Rush and his followers. Particularly in the working class suburbs of Philadelphia, Graham was able to mesmerize the crowds with graphic descriptions of the ill effects on the body of "every liquid more stimulating than water." Borrowing arguments from both French temperance theorists and Philadelphia's temperance doctors, Graham constructed what became known as the "physiological" argument against drinking, in language that the lay listener could understand. Simply put, he told his audiences that drinking was "disturbing to the body and detrimental to the health."

While Graham perfected his temperance lectures in Philadelphia, he took advantage of the city's state-of-the-art medical libraries to immerse himself in thick volumes of technical works on human physiology. The more he read, the more he became convinced that temperance in drinking was only one of the keys to health and longevity. After one year, he severed his connections with the Temperance Society and struck out on his own as a kind of freelance lecturer, touching on a wide area of health reforms that would become known as the "Graham System."

Night after night Graham packed the halls of Pennsylvania, New York, and southeastern New England with his lectures on all aspects of daily living. While he spoke primarily on temperance and food reform, he also preached control of sexual appetite and laid out a strict regimen of frequent exercise, weekly bathing, and fresh air. He called his lecture

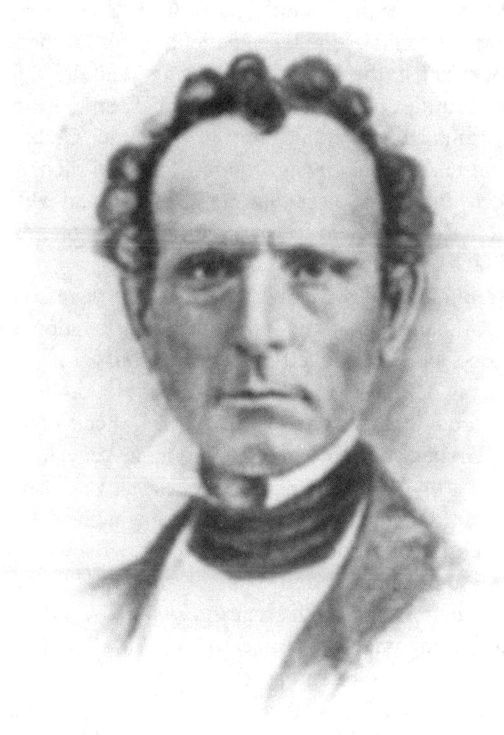

24. Sylvester Graham was known for much more than the Graham cracker. *National Library of Medicine.*

series "the Science of Human Life," which in 1837 was published in two thick, ponderous volumes.

"A PROPERLY FUNCTIONING STOMACH"

Dietary reform was Graham's major grist, and the subject that would make him famous. Once again, his timing was perfect. When cholera swept through the East and Midwest in 1832, the first of three cholera epidemics that hit the United States in the nineteenth century, Graham found the perfect rationale for his recommendations. For cholera, according to Graham, was the obvious result of his contemporaries' abominable eating habits, a greasy, heavily spiced fare of salted beef and pork, pickles, sweet potatoes, and white bread, washed down with large quantities of raw whiskey.

Eyeing the groaning boards of his day with disgust, Graham warned his audiences that a healthy stomach is essential to good health. "Every affection and every disturbance of the stomach influences, in a greater or less degree, every organ and every function of the body." Long before the discovery of vitamins, minerals, and cholesterol, Graham insisted that diet and health are directly connected.

An early believer in the power of preventive health, he begged his audiences to immunize themselves against the deadly cholera by changing their drinking and eating habits. At a time when many doctors urged their frightened patients to fortify themselves against the disease by eating and drinking large quantities of meat, wine, and brandy and blamed fresh fruits and vegetables for the epidemic, Graham warned his listeners away from all forms of alcohol, tobacco, mustard, spices, tea, coffee, meat, and white bread and urged them to eat large quantities of fresh fruits and vegetables.

Although he recommended a strictly vegetarian diet, Graham did allow for a small daily ration of "roasted beef or boiled mutton without gravy or seasoning" for anyone who had trouble dropping carnivorous habits completely. A man ahead of his time, Graham did not believe in cooking vegetables, or in warm food in general, since heat was also a stimulant. Graham was also set against what he called "concentrated" food, including butter, cream, molasses, sugar, honey, and soups.

Graham's anti-flesh arguments were directly tied to his strong views on other matters of the flesh. Masturbation, "the great evil," was particularly dangerous; even sex within marriage should be carefully curbed. Yet his recommendations were consistent with his larger system of health maintenance. Graham believed that eating meat, particularly pork, resulted in hot tempers and sexual excess and that sexual excess led to increased consumption of the deadly meat and rich foods. Just as dietary excesses irritated the stomach and weakened the individual, so too much sex or even *thinking* about sex predisposed the individual to disease.

Sexual abstinence was as important as a healthy diet. Using cholera "statistics" from India, he argued that even the benefits of a meatless diet could be outweighed by what he claimed were the Indians' "intemperate" sexual habits and overly spicy food. While such views might sound bizarre to today's readers, many nineteenth-century physicians and lay people sincerely believed that the higher cholera rates among poor people, blacks, and immigrants were caused by overindulgence in spicy foods and sex. Moderation was the rule for married couples—sex no more frequently than once a month.

GRAHAM BREAD TAKES CENTER STAGE

Graham's obsession with dietary reform and hygiene was consistent with his fellow antebellum reformers' criticism of urban life, as hordes of Americans moved from the countryside and small towns into the rapidly growing, industrializing cities.

Graham was primarily distressed by what he saw as the decline of urban food, which he argued was so adulterated that it was unfit to eat. He claimed that milk, for example, was "highly charged with

YOUR DOCTOR RECOMMENDS

In the April 1831 issue of the *Journal of Health,* America's first consumer health magazine (begun in 1829), the allopathic doctor–editors encouraged their readers to lighten up on breakfast fare. Although their recommended menu most likely did not meet with Graham's approval, it was revolutionary for the times. They suggested a "soft boiled fresh egg, slice of the lean part of cold beef or mutton, a portion of cold roasted fowl, or even a beef-steak properly cooked." They had "no objections to coffee, when not too strong, and taken in moderation, with a sufficient amount of pure milk and sugar, although we have much stronger objections to tea, especially green tea." They recommended "good chocolate" as an "excellent substitute for coffee."

the odor and taste of filth . . . and, when the cows are fed on the vile dregs of distilleries and other improper substances, their milk is anything but wholesome." Graham was evidently not far off base. Commercial milk in nineteenth-century cities was often tainted with chalk, plaster of Paris, and molasses to make it look richer and whiter. Nor was the adulteration of food a uniquely American phenomenon. In London, one concerned citizen named Frederick Accum discovered that the city's lovely green pickles got their vivid color from copper and that red lead gave Gloucester cheese its rosy glow.

Graham argued that bread was the "ideal food," and so he saved his most vehement attack for the new, fashionable, commercially baked white bread, made of "superfine" (highly refined) flour. In his own lifetime, Graham had watched bread-baking move from the fireplaces of America's rural kitchens into the commercial bakeries of the cities, and from a tough-crusted, whole-wheat loaf to a soft, white, thin-crusted product. "Put back the bran!" cried Graham, arguing that "bran adds to the nutritiousness of the bread, increases its digestibility, invigorates the digestive organs and preserves the general integrity of their functions."

Mourning the commercialization of bread, Graham recommended that bread-making return to the ovens of America's wives and mothers, that it be made only from coarsely ground "unbolted wheat meal" and served stale, after it was at least 24 hours old. Here women's role was crucial. In his *Lectures on the Science of Human Life* Graham argued that "it is the wife, the mother only . . . she alone it is who has the maturity of judgement and skillfulness of operation which are the indispensable attributes of a perfect bread-maker."

Graham could not have known that the new, mechanized milling process that quickly removed the wheat germ from the flour was robbing the flour of most of its protein, minerals, niacin, and other B vitamins. Knowledge about nutrition would not be discovered until the early twentieth century. Yet Graham realized that some foods do have more natural nutritional value than others, and that food processing frequently removes nutrition. Although he figured out that fiber was important in one's diet, it took until the twentieth century for nutritionists to recognize its importance.

Many physicians laughed at Graham, claiming that the coarse "Graham" bread (also known as "dyspepsia bread" because it was supposed to help cure indigestion) was itself actually indigestible. And the commercial bakers shouted that they were only giving their urban customers what they wanted—an inexpensive product that was pleasing to the eye, did not quickly spoil, and tasted delicious with stacks of butter.

Graham's early lectures instantly swept him into national prominence. When the cholera rumors first swelled, he delivered the first of more than a dozen "lectures on cholera" before 2,000 fascinated New York City listeners. From there he went on to Albany, then back to New York, where he spoke to standing-room-only crowds.

After the disease temporarily subsided, Graham continued lecturing on food and hygiene reform. By the mid-1830s, he was traveling the lecture circuit through Massachusetts, Rhode Island, Maine, New York, New Jersey, and Pennsylvania. The accounts of the day picture him as a tireless speaker who had the ability to spellbind audiences with his advice and stories on just about every topic related to health. While fending off unfriendly mobs during his March 1837 tour in Boston, Graham managed to deliver lectures on diet, masturbation (known euphemistically as his "lecture to young men"), and hygiene as well as comparative anatomy, physiology, and biblical interpretations of diet.

Graham was one of the first American health reformers to reach a mass audience through lectures. When he went on the road, it was a time when lectures were the major form of entertainment in the United States, much like movies are today. He also was one of the first to publicize his cause in the new popular press through announcements for his lectures and essays. During his 1837 stay in Boston, for example, Graham defended his record and theories to "the citizens of Boston and the Public General" in the *Boston Courier*. The paper explained to its readers that "at the request of the writer, who thinks himself a wronged and injured man, we have consented to allow him use of our columns to present his case." While the editors explained that they had never heard Graham lecture, "we must be permitted to say that we have always doubted whether any public good has resulted from his operations."

Graham's listeners either loved him or hated him, took in his every word or wrote him off as a complete quack. Ralph Waldo Emerson referred to Graham as "the prophet of bran bread and pumpkins." Others labled him "Father Fiber." Following one of Graham's cholera lectures, one New York writer warned that all the Grahamites would die if they followed his regimen. After reading a copy of Graham's published *Lectures to Young Men on Chastity,* a horrified Bostonian wrote to the *Boston Courier,* "I could not put it into the hands of the very class of readers for whose improvement it professes to be designed for—young men; not one of whom, unless he is already half-corrupted, could read it without a blush.'' Even Graham's dear wife Sarah ignored his recommended regimen and kept a well-stocked supply of the rich foods and meats Graham abhorred. She was also known to take a nip of gin or wine now and then.

Yet, for all those who laughed at his theories, there were many who came away from his lectures determined to change their habits. Graham would hear from these converts in the form of testimonials, moving, heartfelt letters describing how dramatically the Graham system had changed their lives.

By the time Graham was 43 years old, he was weakened by an exhausting nonstop schedule of lectures and tired of the endless debates surrounding his theories. His overbearing manner turned away many would-be sympathizers, and his obsession with masturbation, ''the solitary vice,'' alienated many New England liberals. In late 1837, the father of the Graham cracker retreated with Sarah and their two children, Henry and Sarah, to Northampton, Massachusetts, not far from the town where he was born. Here he bought the first and only house he ever owned. The locale was a logical choice for the weary minister. At the time, Northampton was a popular health resort, famous for its water cures.

Graham spent the final years of his life bathing in the town's springs, tending his vegetable garden and bombarding the newspaper with letters complaining about the decay of urban life and the evils of flesh-eating. Just before he died on September 11, 1851, at the age of 57, the fragile minister, who had suffered from ill health all his life, could be seen wandering through the streets in his bathrobe on the way to his daily swim. After trying and then rejecting the local allopathic doctor's regimen of opium enemas, cherry wine, and meat, Graham tried a strict diet of rice in a last desperate attempt to save his life. Although the *Northampton Courier* only briefly mentioned its famous citizen's death, the reform-minded *Phrenological Journal* honored him as ''the great pioneer of dietetic reform.''

''YOU MUST BE A GRAHAMITE''

The debates over the Graham system lingered long after Graham removed himself from the spotlight and long after he died. In the Northeast, ''Grahamism'' became synonymous with a regimen of meatless meals, coarse whole-wheat bread and abstinence from wine, beer, and liquor. Anyone who declared himself or herself a vegetarian was immediately assumed to be a Grahamite.

SYLVESTER GRAHAM'S ''HIT LIST''

meat	fish
white bread	beer
wine	distilled liquor
sexual excess	masturbation
tobacco	mustard
spices	tea
coffee	butter
cream	soup
molasses	sugar
honey	stuffy rooms
uncleanliness	sedentary habits
warm food	

The Grahamites selectively borrowed from Graham's principles of hygienic and dietary reform and made them palatable to a small but growing minority of health-conscious Americans who were eager to improve their daily regimen. Graham thus set the stage for those who preached vegetarianism, hydropathy (water cures), Saturday night bathing, physical exercise, and abstinence from alcohol, coffee, and tea. Grahamism was also adopted by American phrenologists, those who believed that character was reflected by the shape of the skull.

Grahamite institutions and ''societies'' (clubs) sprang up in the Northeast and Midwest. In 1833, the first Graham boarding house was started in New York City. The boarding house served a strict diet of organic, unsifted bread that had been baked 12 hours before serving, vegetables, milk, oatmeal, barley gruel, and water. The proprietors forbade tea, coffee, tobacco, liquor, and chocolate and encouraged their guests to drink as much rainwater as possible. The guest list included some of the day's leading abolitionists such as William Lloyd Garrison, Horace Greeley, and Arthur Tappan.

Other abolitionist leaders also counted among the most visible Grahamites. Henry Stanton attended the 1839 Grahamite American Health Convention, and Sara Grimke, a leading Southern abolitionist, was a firm believer in gymnastic exercise and moderation in diet and sex.

America's leading phrenologists, Orson and Lorenzo Fowler, whose New York City publishing house printed and distributed hundreds of books on phrenology, water cures, physiology, vegetarianism, and temperance, adopted Grahamism and published many of Graham's lectures.

The New England Grahamites were a particularly active bunch. In 1836, Boston abolitionist David Cambell and his wife opened a Graham boarding house at 23 Brattle Street ''for those who have adopted the Graham rules of diet at home and do not like to depart from those rules when in this city on business.'' From 1837 to 1839 Cambell also served as editor of the weekly *Graham Journal of Health and Longevity*. (Boston's Brattle Street, today underneath the modern City Center, was demolished in the early 1960s.)

The *Graham Journal* (Graham had no affiliation with its publication) published excerpts from Graham's writings, articles on health, and testimonials from converts to the Graham system. It ran ads for a health bookstore on Cornhill Street, a health-food store that specialized in grains and beans, with ''Graham flour constantly on hand,'' and the Cambells' own boarding house. The journal also announced the monthly meetings of the Boston-based American Physiological Society, a club organized by Graham's followers and led by John Benson, a wealthy merchant and Graham convert, and Dr. William Alcott, one of the most active leaders of the American vegetarian movement.

Many of the most ardent Grahamites were women, attracted to Graham's recommendations on family diet, preventive health care, and dress reform, which in those years meant loose, comfortable clothing instead of the popular waist-squeezing corsets.

Testimonials from women made up a large percentage of those sent to the *Graham Journal*. One letter from ''Mrs. Sigourney'' also addressed the effects of ''tight lacing'' on women's health. The writer warned women against the ''tyranny of fashion,'' asking them to protect themselves against injuries inflicted by ''compression of the vital parts . . . too numerous to be here recounted.''

Some of the most illustrious nineteenth-century female reformers preached the Graham system. Catherine Beecher recommended ''bread made of coarse flour . . . the most healthful kind'' in her 1873 book *Miss Beecher's Housekeeper and Healthkeeper*, although she included recipes for ''fine flour'' as well as ''unbolted flour.'' And Ellen Harmon White, spiritual leader and founder of the Seventh-day Adventist Church and founder of Battle Creek, Michigan's Western Health Reform Institute (later taken over by John Harvey Kellogg), placed Graham bread on the top of her list of recommended foods. The ''San,'' as Kellogg's famous health retreat became known, and the water-cure establishments so popular both before and after the Civil War were actually expanded versions of the Graham boarding houses. Both combined Graham's vegetarianism with hydrotherapy. Both provided their clientele with a retreat from the ''bad'' habits of urban living.

THE OBERLIN EXPERIMENT

Educators and college students were among the most eager Grahamites. Williams College students organized a Graham club for health and hygiene discussions; in its July 6, 1839 issue, the *Graham Journal* published a notice from Connecticut's Wesleyan University that eight students had formed a club to ''live according to the Graham system.'' The students agreed to stick to a strictly vegetarian diet and eliminate condiments from their meals. ''We used unbolted wheat flour, Indian corn meal, rice, beans and potatoes, all prepared in the plainest and simplest diet. . . .

THE

GRAHAM JOURNAL

OF HEALTH AND LONGEVITY.

HE THAT STRIVETH FOR THE MASTERY, IS TEMPERATE IN ALL THINGS.—Paul.

VOL. III] BOSTON AND NEW YORK, SATURDAY, OCT. 12, 1839. [No. 21.

OPINION OF A SCOTSMAN OF GRAHAM'S WORK AND SYSTEM.

SIR: Having just completed the reading of Graham's Lectures on the Science of Human Life I am disposed to express to you my opinion concerning the work and the great principles it advances. In my judgment it is a work of great merit and will benefit mankind immensely at some future period, and not a little at present. But alas! man is ignorant of his own nature and relations, and is little inclined to become truly and thoroughly acquainted with himself, and therefore he must suffer the penalty of his transgressions and be made little wiser for his afflictions.

Graham and his lectures may be scoffed at and derided by those who follow the fashions of the deluded world, and do not incline to investigate and judge for themselves in matters of this kind, yet I cannot doubt that the time will come when the name of Graham will be classed with the names of the great and good, and that his labors will greatly benefit generations yet unborn.

In many respects my own experience and observation fully corroborate the doctrines taught in the lectures, yet I am not one who may properly be considered a broken down invalid who has had his health greatly improved by the Graham system, but I may say that I have been brought up a Grahamite from the cradle, until I came to this country in 1836. I was born in Scotland. My father rented a small farm, the produce of which, consisted of oats, barley, potatoes, turnips, cabbage, cattle, hens, milk, eggs, butter, cheese, &c. We were fed on oats, barley, potatoes and milk. The rest was sold to pay the rent. I lived in Scotland full thirty years and during all that time I suppose I did not eat so much flesh-meat, nor drink so much tea and coffee as I did the first fourteen months after my arrival in this country. Flesh-meat, tea, coffee, sugar, molasses, pepper, mustard and other spices, vinegar, &c. were not used at all in my father's house except perhaps in cases of sickness, or some extraordinary occasion.

With regard to eating too much, Mr Graham is certainly correct. It is indeed a besetting evil in man:—at least I have found it so. One of the early admonitions I received from my father was, not to

25. The seminal *Graham Journal of Health and Longevity* was packed with personal testimonials. *Countway Library, Boston.*

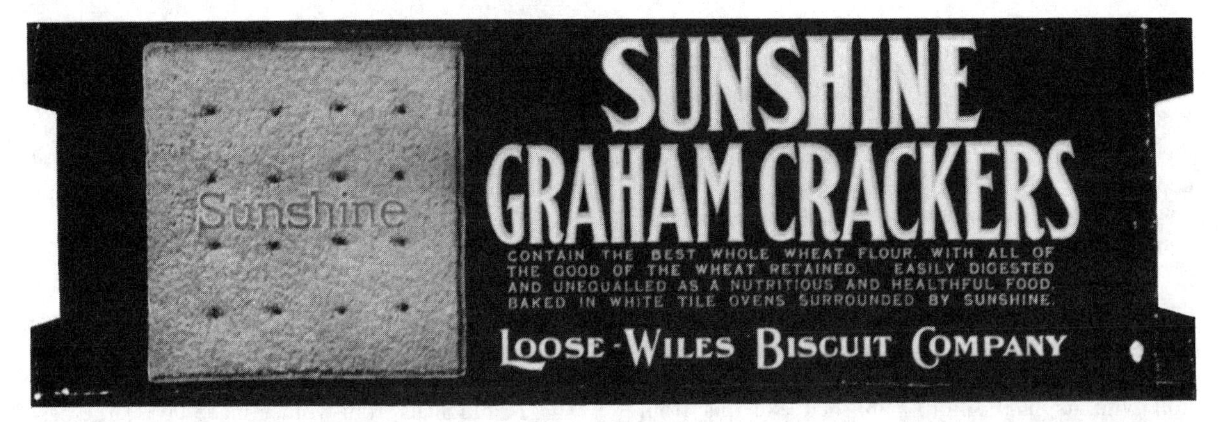

26. In their early years, Graham crackers were advertised as a healthy, wholesome snack (1917). *Sunshine Graham Crackers used with permission of Sunshine Biscuits, Inc., Woodbridge, NJ 07095.*

We feel less inclined to sleep after dinner than when gorged with beef and gravies, and are better prepared to pursue our studies."

But the most famous Grahamite college experiment of all was at Oberlin College, in Ohio. Ever since its beginnings in 1833 as the first American coeducational college, Oberlin had taken an active role in the reform movements of the day, particularly abolitionism, women's rights, and temperance. Adopting Graham's physiological reforms was a logical extension of this tradition.

Oberlin's original rules stipulated that the food be "of plain and holesome [sic]." Coffee and tea, highly seasoned meats, wine, beer, tobacco, and rich pastries were prohibited. All students were required to study physiology. Female students and faculty wives agreed to boycott tight lacing and wear practical footwear in the rain and cold. They also formed the Female Society of Oberlin for the Promotion of Health, while the men organized the Oberlin Physio-

DEAR MR. GRAHAM

. . . I enjoyed good health until I was married, which took place in my eighteenth year. Soon after this my health began to fail and continued to decline for a considerable time. I became very weak, and subject to turns of fainting, and frequently fainted away while engaged in my domestic concerns, and sometimes two or three times a day. My head ached incessantly and often with great violence. . . . I used to have a doctor, as often, on an average, as once a fortnight or three weeks, and took a great deal of medicine, but without anything more than a momentary relief. . . . Miss Burr, one of your most faithful disciples, first converted me to your system, and then took me with her to hear your lectures at Mulbury Street, and afterwards to Clinton Hall, early in the spring of 1832. I immediately abandoned my tea and coffee, the latter of which I was very fond of, and gradually got into your whole system strictly. Now I can work about my house during the day, and take long walks for pleasure without feeling fatigued. I am now full of health.

from Sarah Van York,
New York City, to the
Graham Journal of Health,
January 17, 1833

LOOK, MA! NO MEAT!

Cold water, milk and wheat will make the sum almost entirely of our articles of food. Bread and butter or bread without butter, bread and milk—and milk toast—compose the variety of our breakfasts and suppers. We have not had what you could call a meal of meat since we have been here. Twice we had a few mutton bones—just enough to set the appetite, once we had a little fish, and a little dried beef several times. We frequently have what is called Graham pudding made of wheat just cracked, and boiled a few minutes in water. Boiled Indian puddings sometimes, and Johncakes—this makes the sum total of our living—a splendid variety I assure you . . . If only I could have a little coffee and a mouthful of meat now and then.

Letter from an Oberlin College
student to his parents, August 1836

logical Society. Students were required to bathe regularly, even in winter, and even though they had to carry the water from outdoor pumps to their rooms.

A SHORT HISTORY OF THE GRAHAM CRACKER

In the 1860s, a Grahamite named James Caleb Jackson was the first to bake and sell Graham crackers. Jackson was best known for Our Home on the Hillside, a popular water-cure establishment near Dansville, New York. Jackson wanted to find a way to create a simple version of Graham bread, a healthy cracker that could be packaged and preserved for an unlimited time and sold to his patients. First he mixed Graham flour and water, then baked this mixture and pressed it into sheets. He then broke up this concoction into bite-sized pieces, and baked it again. Jackson ended up, not with Graham crackers, but with something he called "Granula," America's first cold breakfast cereal. Granula, a forerunner of today's granola, was a commercial bomb.

Large American food companies took off where Jackson gave up. National Biscuit Company (now Nabisco Brands) began manufacturing Graham crackers in 1898, joined in the 1910s by Loose-Wiles Biscuit Company (now Sunshine Biscuits, Inc.). By that time the Graham cracker was earning its reputation as a healthy after-school snack for kids, especially when combined with a glass of milk. Known as "the ideal wartime energy food," the cracker maintained its healthy reputation through World War II and beyond. In the 1950s, food companies began to expand their Graham cracker lines, adding honey, cinnamon, cheese, and even chocolate to their crackers, and then crushing them to cash in on the popularity of Graham cracker pie crust.

In the late 1980s, small health-food companies competed with Nabisco and Sunshine for the baby boomer market that grew up on Graham crackers and milk, but demanded a sugar-free, preservative-free cracker. Health Valley, in California, manufactured several varieties of Graham crackers, including popular Oat Bran Graham Crackers, containing "no cholesterol," and Amaranth Graham Crackers, "made with the mystical grain of the Aztecs."

Oberlin's bout with Grahamism might have taken a different turn had it not been for Oberlin founder Charles Finney's decision to invite professional Grahamite David Cambell to refine and run the college's Graham system. When Cambell left his editor's chair at the *Graham Journal* in 1839 and removed himself and his family to Ohio, Oberlin's Grahamism took what some parents and students felt was a rather extreme plunge. This was particularly evident in the dining hall, where the portions were noticeably smaller after Cambell's arrival and students and staff were forbidden to eat any meat whatsoever. (Previously, a meat table had been provided for an additional fee.) Diners were not allowed to use spices, including salt and pepper. When one teacher brought his own pepper shaker to the table, he was ordered removed from the dining hall. Later, when the teacher was dismissed from his position at the college, some believed the firing was related to his dining room offense.

The college's staff and students were either ecstatic or horrified by the changes. One Quaker student wrote home that after he began taking daily baths and eating Graham bread, "my mind immediately burst from its debasement and reassumed its pristine vigor. . . . Faith takes the place of darkness, and happiness of gloom and misery." But one hungry student walked nine miles to the town of Elyria, where he sat down to a large, un-Grahamlike meal at a tavern. He then continued walking, all the way to Cleveland's Western Reserve College, where he promptly enrolled.

Although the townspeople in Oberlin joked that they could spot an Oberlin student by his or her "leak, lean, lantern-jawed visage," many parents hardly saw it as a joking matter. When rumors of mass starvations began to reach home, the trustees asked Cambell to resign. In 1845, Finney officially renounced his belief in dietary reform and, as one disappointed Grahamite groaned, "they rushed with precipitous and confused haste back to the flesh pots."

ARE *YOU* A GRAHAMITE?

Grahamism has survived, although not under the minister's name. After the 1830s, Americans' dietary and hygiene habits began to improve. Alcohol consumption declined, as temperance crusaders took up the pitch of total abstinence. Per capita meat consumption also began to decline, as Americans shed their fears of fresh fruit and vegetables and began to eat more balanced meals. After the Civil War, consumer demand for fruits and vegetables was assisted by the invention of refrigerated railroad cars and mechanized canning. Saturday night bathing became part of family ritual long before indoor plumbing and modern-day showers, and regular exercise was gradually accepted as important for health and longevity.

By the 1980s, Graham's warnings about diet were taken seriously by the American scientific community, as the public was asked to cut back on caffeine, salt, meat, fat, and cholesterol. Confirming Graham's warnings linking caffeine and overstimulation, the January 1990 *Archives of Internal Medicine* published a report linking coffee-drinking to increased sexual activity. (The researchers urged consumers to interpret the results with restraint.)

Health-conscious consumers were also responding aggressively to Graham's warning to "put back the bran." Bran, in fact, was making a comeback, and in a big way. No longer relegated to senior citizens' morning cereal or special diets for those with chronic constipation problems, bran, particularly combined with oat flour, was being touted as a way to cut one's cholesterol count. Encouraged by Robert Kowalski's best-selling book *The Eight-Week Cholesterol Cure,* consumers gobbled up oat bran bread, cookies, cereal, and muffins and rushed to supermarkets and health food stores to stock up on oat bran flour, causing a severe shortage of and inflated prices for the precious flour.

As oat bran flour moved to the front shelves, Graham flour was getting harder and harder to find. Even in those stores that still stock it, you'd be hard-pressed to find someone who knows exactly what Graham flour is. (Modern-day Graham flour is wheat flour in which the outer bran layer is coarsely ground. Additional bran is frequently added.) And, should you be curious enough to ask the staff if they have ever heard of Sylvester Graham, you'll probably be answered with smiles and shrugs.

CHAPTER · 7 ·

VEGETARIANISM: "HOG VERSUS HOMINY"

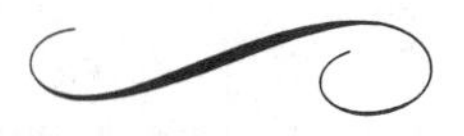

Away with your beef and your mutton!
Avaunt with your capers and sauce!
For Beefsteaks I don't care a button;
Veal cutlets—I count them as dross;
Lamb stew, chicken salad, don't mention;
With my stomach roast pig don't agree;
From such messes I practice abstention—
Farinacea's the forage for me!

"Song of the Vegetarian"
Tune: "Columbia"
The Vegetarian Magazine,
February 15, 1900

On a warm, sunny afternoon in the late 1980s, a hungry lunch crowd stood in line inside the entrance of a San Francisco vegetarian restaurant called Greens, run by the area's Zen Center. "Do you have a reservation?" the host asked the first couple in line who, like many of the waiting hopeful, had spent the morning at a nearby crafts fair. When it turned out they had not, he apologetically turned them away. Meanwhile, those wise enough to have called ahead were happily feasting on such delectables as pita sandwiches filled with hummus, peppers, cucumbers, olives, and feta cheese; marinated tofu sandwiches; garden salads made with vegetables fresh from the Zen Center's nearby farm; vegetable curry; mesquite-grilled vegetables; and vegetarian pizzas, tostadas, and pasta dishes.

Housed inside a former military base looking out on San Francisco Bay and the Golden Gate Bridge, Greens has been filled to capacity since it opened in 1979. According to the *Vegetarian Times*, a monthly magazine based in Oak Park, Illinois with a monthly circulation of 160 thousand, nearly 1,000 restaurants in the United States were busily serving up vegetarian dishes to customers in the late 1980s. They included everything from gluten Bar-B-Que Twist at Chicago's Soul Vegetarian East and soy hot dogs at Detroit's Cafe Martinique to tofu cheesecake at Madison, Wisconsin's Country Life and organic oatmeal at Hollywood's 24-hour I Love Lucy, drawing such regulars as actors Olivia Newton-John and Peter Falk.

After a long history as America's culinary stepchild, vegetarianism has matured into the forefront of the nation's food consciousness. By the 1980s, vegetarians were no longer seen as long-haired kooks munching on bean sprouts and peanut butter sandwiches. Mainstream America, frightened by warnings linking poor diet and ill health, began cramming refrigerators with beets and carrots and stocking shelves with vegetarian bibles and cookbooks, such as Frances Moore Lappé's international best-seller *Diet for A Small Planet; The Greens Cookbook; The New Laurel's Kitchen* by Laurel Robertson, Carol Flinders, and Brian Ruppenthal; Molly Katzen's *Moosewood Cookbook, The Enchanted Broccoli Forest,* and *Still Life with Menu;* and *Diet for a New America,* by Baskin-Robbins heir John Robbins. And while still only a small fraction of Americans consider themselves vegetarians—about 4 percent of adults in the late 1980s, although the exact number is difficult to calculate—there is no question that vegetarianism has come of age.

"BEHOLD THE VOICE OF THE DUMB"

Although American vegetarians have traditionally switched to meat-free diets with visions of promised health and longevity, much of the long history of vegetarianism in both Eastern and Western cultures has been based on religious and ethical arguments.

Long before the modern health-food movement, long before the nineteenth-century American reformer William Alcott was arguing that "a vegetable diet lies at the basis of all Reform, whether, Civil, Social, Moral or Religious," the "father of vegetarianism," the sixth-century B.C. Greek mathematician Pythagoras (of geometry fame), equated meat-eating with "the murder of animals." He argued that animals had the same right as humans to live out their lives.

Like many of his contemporaries, Pythagoras believed in reincarnation and used it to bolster his arguments for vegetarianism. According to one story, Pythagoras once stopped a man from beating a dog because he said he heard an old friend's voice in the dog's howls. Three centuries later, the less-well-known Neoplatonist Porphyry continued Pythagoras's humanitarian argument. By the early nineteenth century, when the vegetarian movement first took root in England, vegetarians were called Pythagoreans.

Modern English writers took up the cause from a variety of angles. From the late seventeenth to the early nineteenth century, English vegetarians argued for a kinder, gentler diet. Food writer Thomas Tryon, citing the "voice of the dumb," defended the rights of animals, while physicians George Cheyne and William Lambe outlined some of the earliest health-linked arguments, advancing the then-unpopular belief that a vegetarian diet was more digestible than one based on flesh. (Lambe went so far as to argue that a meatless diet could cure tuberculosis.) It took vegetarian Frank Newton to convert his famous friend Percy Bysshe Shelley to vegetarianism, resulting in Shelley's widely read pamphlet *A Vindication of Natural Diet,* initially a footnote to his poem "Queen Mab." Before Sylvester Graham ranted against our carnivorous civilization, Shelley argued that man's health had been destroyed by animal food.

As in Eastern cultures, spirituality has played a major part in the English vegetarian movement. In 1817 this strand of vegetarianism found its way to the United States, via one Reverend William Metcalfe, a leader in England's vegetarian-based Bible Christian Church. The Bible Christians, originating in Manchester and created by a minister named William Cowherd, claimed that a vegetarian diet alone was sanctioned by the Bible. "They shall not hurt nor destroy. . . . He that killeth an ox is as if he slew a man," he argued. By the time Cowherd's friend Metcalfe brought his flock to Philadelphia, where he started a church on North Third Street, near Gerard Avenue, American health reformers were ripe for the vegetarian cause, which by the 1840s became the cornerstone of the American popular health movement.

SOME CELEBRITY VEGETARIANS

George Bernard Shaw, novelist, playwright, and social critic; Bronson Alcott, father of author Louisa May Alcott; Casey Kasem, radio deejay, voice of "American Top 40"; Madonna, singer; Michael Jackson, singer; Richard Wagner, composer; Cesar Chavez, labor activist; Upton Sinclair, author; Cicely Tyson, actress; Paul McCartney, musician and composer; Steven Jobs, head of Next, Inc. and former chair of Apple Computer; Mary Pickford, actress; Tony LaRussa, manager of the Oakland Athletics.

From *Vegetarian Times,* December 1988, and *The Book of Lists,* by Irving Wallace, David Wallechinsky, and Amy Wallace

EAT VEGGIES, BE HEALTHY

Sylvester Graham, William Alcott, Et Al.

William Metcalfe organized the first vegetarian group in America, along with the country's first vegetarian

ARE YOU A VEGETARIAN?

CARNIVORE: Your diet is based on meat and fish.
OMNIVORE: You eat a mixed diet of vegetables, fruits, grains, etc., plus meat and fish, dairy products and eggs.
PYTHAGOREAN: You're a vegetarian living in the nineteenth century, most likely refraining from meat and fish, but eating dairy products and eggs.
LACTO-OVO VEGETARIAN: You don't eat meat or fish, but you do eat dairy products and eggs. Since the late nineteenth century, lacto–ovo vegetarians have formed the majority of the vegetarians in the United States.
LACTO VEGETARIAN: You don't eat meat, fish, or eggs, but you do eat dairy products.
VEGAN (pronounced VEE-gun): You eat no fish or animal products, including eggs and dairy products. In addition, you do not use any animal products at all in your clothing or personal hygiene products, makeup, etc. Vegans have been organized in England since 1944, and in the United States since 1960.
FRUITARIAN: Your diet is based on fruit, supplemented by squash, eggplant, tomatoes, peppers, seeds, and nuts.
SPROUTARIAN: Your diet is based on seeds, fruits and raw vegetables.

Based on definitions in
Vegetarian Times, December 1988

magazine, *The American Vegetarian.* Between the 1817 founding of Metcalfe's church and 1850, when American vegetarians formed their first national organization, vegetarian leaders gradually relegated humanitarian and spiritual concerns to the backburner, adopting the more secular tone of America's current vegetarian movement. Beginning in the 1830s, movement leaders began arguing from the "physiological" (health-related) point of view, based on the principles of Presbyterian minister Sylvester Graham, America's first prominent health-food reformer, and the physician, educator, and writer Dr. William Alcott.

Although there is some debate as to who influenced whom, the records show that Graham was hired as a traveling temperance lecturer for Metcalfe's church in the early 1830s, just about the time he was formulating his ideas on dietary reform, and that Metcalfe, in turn, became active in the larger health-oriented vegetarian movement.

Soon Graham struck out on his own, lecturing around the Northeast on "right living," a guide to health and longevity. While the "Graham system" was a mixture of cries for temperance, warnings against sexual excess, and pleas for exercise, fresh air, dress reform, and cleanliness, the most important area of Grahamism was diet. And while Graham is chiefly remembered for the Graham cracker, he, along with Alcott, was the first American to stump for "physiological vegetarianism," linking vegetarianism to health.

William Alcott and others extensively refined Graham's principles, adding large doses of science to the Graham system that to today's readers may seem bizarre. Not until the twentieth century did nutritionists discover that vegetables were both high in fiber and low in saturated fat. Alcott postulated that meat "atoms" were less stable than vegetable atoms because meat decomposes more quickly than vegetables in the body, thus linking a longer lifespan with a vegetarian diet. Digestion was a key point for the physiological vegetarians. As James C. Whorton

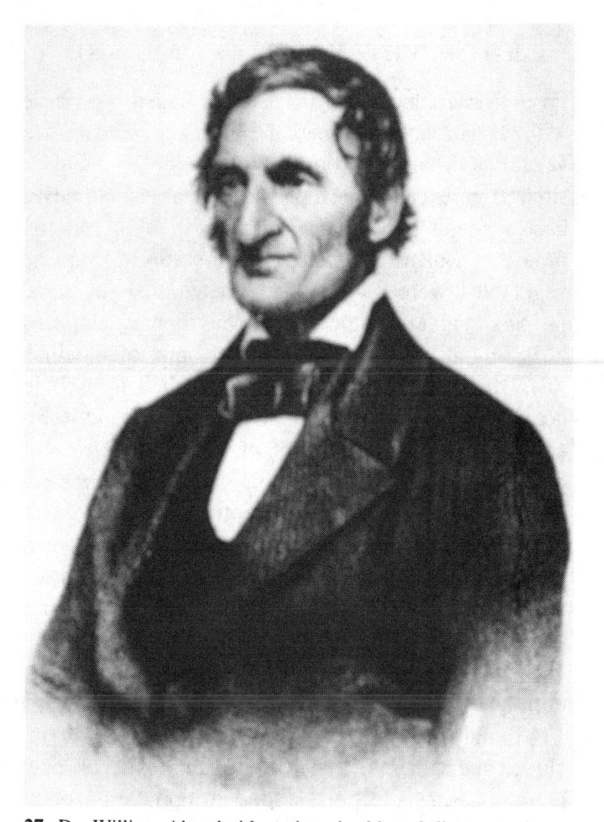

27. Dr. William Alcott's ideas about health and diet were almost as stern as his visage. *From* Memoirs of Teachers, Educators, and Promoters and Benefactors of Education, Literature and Science. *Second Edition. New York: F.C. Brownwell, 1861.*

writes in *Crusaders for Fitness,* a major study of nineteenth-century health-reform movements, "slow digestion is good digestion" became an axiom of vegetarianism.

Although vegetarianism as a separate movement remained relatively small in pre-Civil War America, most of the larger, better-organized health-reform movements adopted vegetarianism. In the spring of 1850, the first meeting of the American Vegetarian Society was held at New York City's Clinton Hall, business address of the famous phrenologists Orson and Lorenzo Fowler. That meeting and subsequent ones read like a "who's who" of antebellum reformers —hydropathists Russell Trall and Joel Shew, Dr. Thomas "free love" Nichols, Lucy Stone, Amelia Bloomer, Susan B. Anthony, Harriet Beecher Stowe, Dr. James Caleb Jackson, and Horace Greeley. After the Civil War, second-generation phrenologist and temperance reformer Harriet Fowler wrote a 79-page booklet called *Vegetarianism: The Radical Cure for Intemperance,* in which she recommended a lacto-ovo vegetarian diet of beans, peas, lentils, eggs, cheese, macaroni, Indian corn meal, garden vegetables, and fruit to squelch one's desire for strong spirits.

WHOLE WORLD TEMPERANCE CONVENTION VEGETARIAN BANQUET, METROPOLITAN HALL, NEW YORK CITY

September 1853

BILL OF FARE

Vegetable Soups

Tomato Soup
Rice Soup

Farinacea

Graham Bread
Mixed Fruit Cake
Fruited Bread
Apple Biscuit
Wheat Meal Cakes
Moulded Rice
Corn Blanc Mange
Moulded Farina
Moulded Wheaten Grits

Vegetables

Baked Sweet Potatoes
Stewed Cream Squashes

Pastry

Mixed Fruit Pies
Pumpkin Pies

Fruits

Melons
Apples
Peaches
Pears
Grapes
Pineapples

Cooked Fruits

Plum Jellies
Baked Apples

Relishes

Coconut Custard
Fruited Ice Cream

Beverage

Pure Cold Water

The Water-Cure Journal,
October 1853

HOLD THE VEGGIES, PLEASE

Early American vegetarian leaders had to do battle with a national meat-eating habit and disdain for vegetables that few consumers or allopathic (mainstream) physicians questioned. Vegetables had never been a major part of the American diet. In colonial times, as Robert Shaplen wrote in 1956, "fruit and vegetables were so little in demand that the local farmers scarcely bothered to grow them." Colonial New Englanders served vegetables only to embellish main dishes, much like cranberry sauce is used in holiday turkey feasts today. Waverly Root and Richard de Rochemont, authors of *Eating in America,* point out that "New Yorkers shunned vegetables until well into the nineteenth century." What vegetables were served were limited to potatoes and cabbage, never leafy green vegetables. When cooked, vegetables tended to be boiled, often for hours at a time, and served in small portions.

This dietary pattern remained much the same until about 1900, according to Calla Van Syckle in a 1945 study of American food consumption. "It included meat in relatively large quantities, with beef predominating and pork second in popularity; potatoes, cabbage, onions, and other fresh vegetables in season and in moderate amounts. . . . A diet high in meat, sweets, and white flour foods represented a traditionally high standard of living to the immigrants from the British Isles, Ireland, Northern European and Scandinavian countries who made up the bulk of our population."

The majority of allopathic physicians followed the conventional belief that vegetables were more difficult to digest and that meat was essential to strength because it was most like human flesh. After 1860, this meat-stamina connection took the center stage as physical fitness and spectator sports became popular. In the late nineteenth century, meat-eaters also argued that what separated humans from other primates was our "broader" (that is mixed) diet, in opposition to the vegetarians' evolutionary argument that the "natural" diet of all primates was flesh-free.

One notable exception before the Civil War was the group of Philadelphia physicians who created the *Journal of Health* in 1829, the first American health magazine aimed at consumers. Along with encouraging their readers to adopt temperance habits and to bathe and exercise frequently, the editors jumped into the dietary issues of the day. They fell short of recommending complete abstention from meat, opting, instead, for a mixed diet of meat and vegetables "as the one most friendly to the human constitution, and the best adapted to preserve it in a proper state of health and vigour." However, they also defended vegetarianism: "As a general rule, it will be found that those who make use of a diet consisting chiefly of vegetable matter, have a manifest advantage in looks, strength and spirits, over those who partake largely of animal food: they are remarkable for the firm, healthy plumpness of their muscles, and the transparency of their skins."

Vegetarians eagerly trumpeted their successes. In 1855, the London *Vegetarian Messenger* reprinted a two-page letter that appeared in *American Vegetarian* from Dr. A.W. Scales, offering a personal testimonial of his conversion to a vegetable diet. Two years earlier Scales had renounced his flesh-eating habits, after his weight jumped to 240 pounds. (He was down to 190 pounds when he wrote the letter.) "My obesity had become a loathsome burthen [sic], which incommoded every function, and made me a stupid, indolent, short-winded, panting, eating animal." After reading, among others, the works of Sylvester Graham and William Alcott, the doctor not only switched to a vegetarian diet but prescribed it to all his patients. Scales wrote that he now enjoyed "the rational enjoyment of the powers of life, more than I ever possessed while using a flesh diet—the great adulterator of all that is noble or good in man."

PASS THE VEGETABLES, PLEASE

In spite of the carnivorous habits of the majority of Americans, vegetarians continued to hold their own in the late nineteenth and early twentieth centuries. In the 1870s, Reverend Henry Stephen Clubb, who inherited the Bible Christian Church leadership after William Metcalfe's death and would keep it going into the early twentieth century, revitalized the national organization, calling it the Vegetarian Society of America. He also started a new magazine called *Food, Home and Garden*. Clubb's church continued to add a spiritual tone to the American vegetarian movement, which, by the early twentieth century, would be largely dominated by Ellen G. White's vegetarian Seventh-day Adventists.

In the Midwest, Chicago's vegetarians started *The Vegetarian Magazine,* reflecting both the humanitarian and physiological principles of the movement. The magazine also had a particular reverence for the role of wives and mothers, dedicating a special "Of Interest to the Housewife" section that included recipes and menu-planning tips.

The magazine's vegetarian recipes were part of a larger cookbook trend that has continued to this day. In addition to Ella (Mrs. John Harvey) Kellogg's *A Vegetarian Cookbook from Battle Creek,* vegetarians could order books like *Meatless Dishes,* "containing an interesting sermon on salads," and *American Vegetarian Cookery.*

The Vegetarian Magazine also supported the growing women's suffrage movement, proudly announcing a meatless luncheon served in 1903 for the Brooklyn, New York Woman Suffrage Association. The menu listed an interesting assortment of dishes, including a nut roast with tomato sauce, "Saratoga chips," and "Apple pie à la Battle Creek."

Beginning in the 1850s, groups of vegetarians tried to organize colonies in Kansas, Missouri, Arkansas, California, Oregon, and Mexico. The most famous attempt was the abortive octagon settlement in "Kanzas," organized by the Vegetarian Kanzas Emigration Society in the mid-1850s. In an article in the April 1855 *Water-Cure Journal,* the organizers explained that "by going to Kanzas in such a company, they would be preserved from all temptation to depart from the principles they so highly value, and by united effort they may become the means of inducing thousands to adopt a system of diet they so highly value." The organizers may have had problems attracting enough interested vegetarians, for the following month, they welcomed friends "who approve of the plan of settlement, but are not prepared at once to adopt the vegetarian practice." Their only requirement was abstention from intoxicating beverages.

Hopes for forming vegetarian colonies continued into the early twentieth century. The February 15, 1900 issue of *The Vegetarian Magazine* published a letter from a reader recommending colonization in Mexico. "I know a county that has a large tract, with which favorable terms could probably be made. Here olives, oranges, lemons, beans, corn and cotton all pay well, with cheap labor." Later that year the magazine printed an article encouraging its readers to colonize in Zeitonia Heights, Missouri, 120 miles from St. Louis, in an area "destined to become a great fruit growing country."

By the turn of the twentieth century, American vegetarians had established a number of organizations

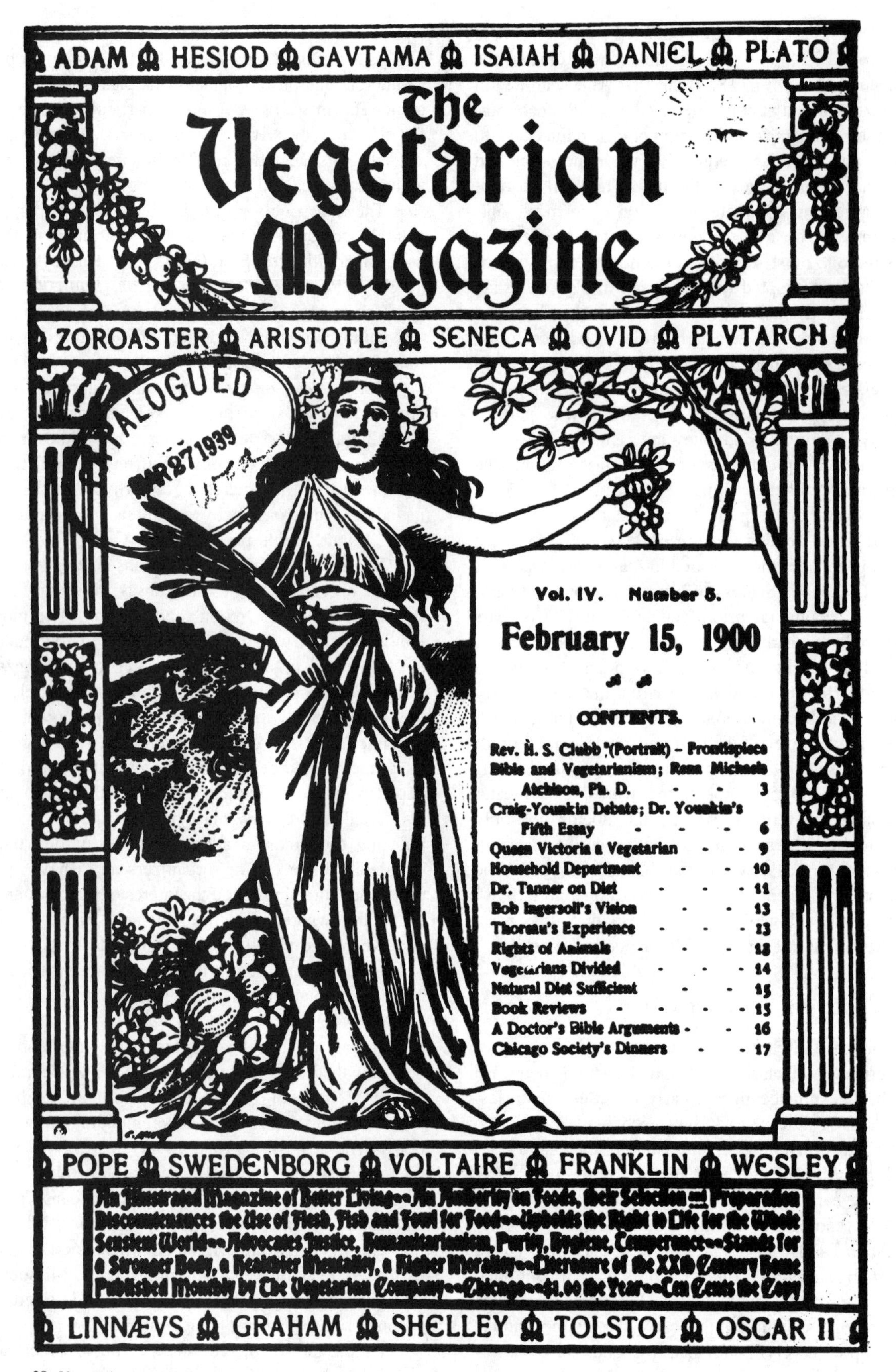

ADAM ♣ HESIOD ♣ GAVTAMA ♣ ISAIAH ♣ DANIEL ♣ PLATO

The Vegetarian Magazine

ZOROASTER ♣ ARISTOTLE ♣ SENECA ♣ OVID ♣ PLVTARCH

Vol. IV. Number 5.

February 15, 1900

CONTENTS.

POPE ♣ SWEDENBORG ♣ VOLTAIRE ♣ FRANKLIN ♣ WESLEY

An Illustrated Magazine of Better Living--An Authority on Foods, their Selection and Preparation
Discountenances the Use of Flesh, Fish and Fowl for Food--Upholds the Right to Life for the Whole
Sensient World--Advocates Justice, Humanitarianism, Purity, Hygiene, Temperance--Stands for
a Stronger Body, a Healthier Mentality, a Higher Morality--Literature of the XXth Century Home
Published Monthly by The Vegetarian Company--Chicago--$1.00 the Year--Ten Cents the Copy

LINNÆVS ♣ GRAHAM ♣ SHELLEY ♣ TOLSTOI ♣ OSCAR II

28. Vegetarians and their publications laid claims to classical roots (1900). *Countway Library, Boston.*

with varying interests, among them, groups in Philadelphia, Chicago, New York, and St. Louis. Animal rights advocates joined the Society for the Prevention of Cruelty to Animals and read *Our Fellow Creatures*, the official magazine of the International Kindness to Animals Society. On the spiritual side, there was Annie Besant's mystical Theosophists and, of course, the Seventh-day Adventists, whose spiritual leader, Ellen G. White, first adopted a meat-free diet as part of her church's creed after a vision in 1863.

ON THE OFFENSIVE

But it was fellow Adventist Dr. John Harvey Kellogg of cornflake fame, Sister White's chief physician at her Battle Creek Sanitarium in Michigan, who took over the major secular vegetarian battle at the dawn of the twentieth century. As Kellogg, along with his younger brother Will, was rapidly turning Sister White's sanitarium into the secular, world-famous "San," headquarters for America's first cereal and health-food empire, he was also wasting no time writing and lecturing for the vegetarian cause.

Always the practical one, Kellogg took an eclectic approach to the subject, emphasizing religious, physiological, or humanitarian reasons, according to the makeup of his audience.

For the health-minded, he argued that cereal, not fish, was "brain food" and refuted "20 delusions about flesh food," arguing, for example, that "man is not naturally a flesh eater" and meat is filled with poisons. In 1923, long after the passage of the 1906 Pure Food and Drug Act, Kellogg warned, "the people of the United States have little or no protection against the use of diseased meats."

For the humanitarian-inclined, Kellogg brought forth ethical arguments, pointing out the commonality between "these lower creatures" and humans. "But although the sheep goes dumb to the slaughter, do not its eloquent eyes appeal for mercy? Do not the bleating of the calf, the bellowing of the bull, the cackling of the frightened geese, the gobbling of the reluctant turkeys, and the cries of hundreds of other creatures that we call dumb . . . rise in eloquent protest against the savagery?"

To his religious audiences, Kellogg cited biblical references to vegetarianism: "We are assured that St. Matthew lived upon seeds and hardshell fruits and other vegetables without touching flesh."

Others joined ranks with the king of cornflakes in a new, more aggressive "muscular vegetarianism," to borrow James C. Wharton's phrase, as scientific evidence began linking a meat diet to cardiovascular disease. Athletes took the term "muscular" more literally, testing their skills to show the world that vegetarians were no wimps. In 1896, the Londoner James Parsley led his newly formed vegetarian athletic and cycling club to a first prize win in the all-England hill-climbing race.

On this side of the Atlantic, Olympic swimming

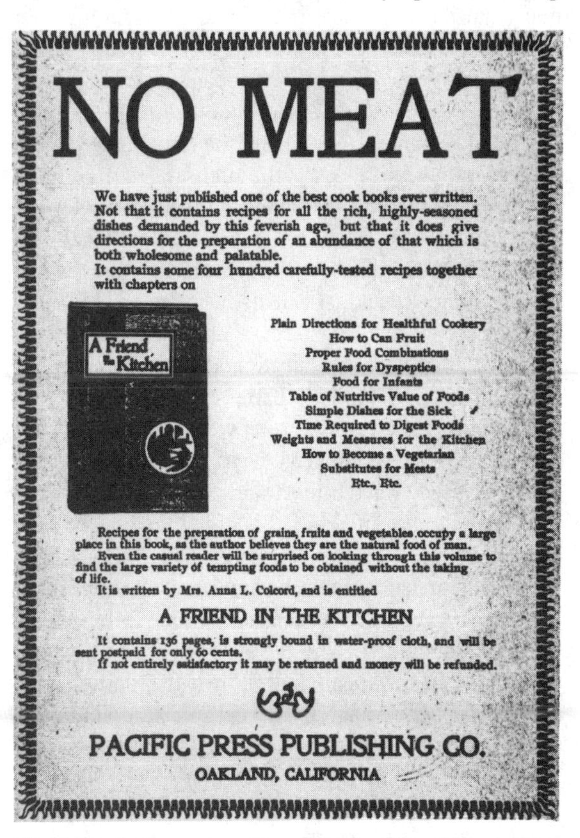

29. No hamburger recipes were to be found in this vegetarian cookbook (circa 1898). *From* Vegetarian Magazine, *August 15, 1900. Countway Library, Boston.*

A VEGETARIAN'S GUIDE, 1900

To assist its readers, *The Vegetarian Magazine* listed in its June 1900 issue more than 20 restaurants and guest houses. Vegetarians in New York had their pick of five restaurants, among them the Physical Culture Strength Food Restaurant on Pearl Street and the Straight Edge Kitchen on Seventh Avenue. Battle Creek, Michigan customers could dine at the Hygienic Dining Hall on Main Street. Chicagoans could relax at one of the era's most well-known vegetarian restaurants, the Mortimer Pure Food Cafe on Washington Street.

champ Johnny Weissmuller came to Battle Creek to dedicate the San's new 120-foot pool, and promptly adopted Kellogg's vegetarian diet. Vegetarian Margarita Gast broke the women's cycling record on a diet of fruit, zwieback, raw potatoes, and claret. And at the first public meeting of the St. Louis Vegetarian Society in 1903, Professor J.E. Mizee, director of the Broadway Gymnasium in nearby Illinois, demonstrated his strength by having a volunteer drop a 50-pound stone on his stomach from a height of six feet. According to *The Vegetarian Magazine,* "the members of the press who were present were deeply impressed by this refutation of the oft-made assertion that the vegetarian diet will not give nourishment enough for the performance of arduous physical strains."

"A CHICKEN IN EVERY POT"

Inspired by Upton Sinclair's *The Jungle,* the Pure Food and Drug Act of 1906 helped to publicize one of the main vegetarian arguments, that eating meat was no better than ingesting poison; yet few Americans stopped eating meat. During World War I, many cut back on meat out of wartime scarcity, but only as an emergency measure. As in the period after World War II, most Americans looked forward to the days when they could once again fill up their lunch and dinner plates with the foods they were used to. And while research, such as Van Syckle's 1945 study, showed that many Americans no longer ate mountains of pork and beef at every meal and that many, particularly in urban areas, were beginning to prefer breakfast cereals in the morning, most did not see vegetarianism as a healthier alternative. In the 1920s, although nutritionists began to emphasize "protective foods," namely milk, vegetables, and fruit, vegetables and fruits were generally of the canned variety. (Chickens were still considered a luxury, raised, for the most part, for eggs.)

Vegetarians in the 1920s fell into one of two categories: the Seventh-day Adventists, who singlehandedly carried organized American vegetarianism into the 1960s; and "eccentrics," like followers of Bernarr Macfadden, whose *New York Daily Graphic* preached vegetarianism and published a daily health column by vegetarian Dr. Herbert Shelton alongside stories describing executions of mass murderers.

One of the lowest points for the secular vegetarian movement in America was the late 1940s to the early 1960s. "The Depression did not teach us anything," explained Jay Dinshah, who started the American Vegan Society in 1960. After so many years of denial, Americans welcomed the glut of automobiles, new homes, and hearty, meat-filled meals. In 1956, the United States Department of Agriculture (USDA) came out with the "Basic Four Food Groups," still the basis of nutrition education. The "vegetable–fruit" group was relegated to one-quarter of the pie, the others being "milk," "meat," and "bread and cereals." According to the *Vegetarian Times,* "the USDA embarked on a public nutrition program to spread the message of this new, easier approach to good diet. One of the effects was a rise in meat-eating in the late fifties. . . ."

VEGGIES ON THE RISE

In 1977, Senator George McGovern presented his "Dietary Goals for the United States" before the Senate Select Committee on Nutrition and Human Needs. His report urged Americans to cut back on animal fats, refined carbohydrates, and salt. A little more than 10 years later, the Surgeon General's "Report on Nutrition and Health" advised Americans to reduce their consumption of fat and cholesterol and eat more whole grains, fresh fruits, and vegetables. Although many vegetarian activists criticized both reports for their allegedly watered-down final versions, Americans began to take notice. Many were just plain scared.

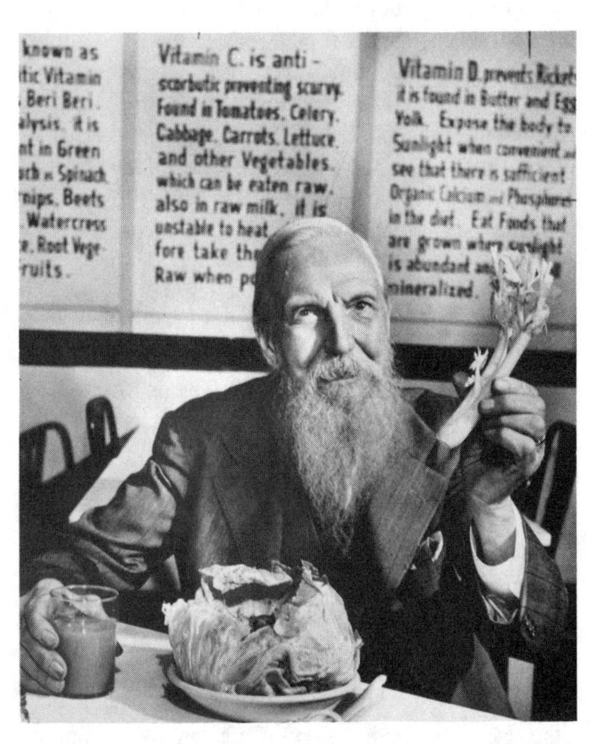
known as
Beri Beri.
Watercress
Vitamin C. is anti-
scorbutic preventing scurvy.
Found in Tomatoes, Celery,
Cabbage, Carrots, Lettuce,
and other Vegetables,
which can be eaten raw,
also in raw milk, it is
unstable to heat
Vitamin D prevents
it is found in Butter and
Yolk. Expose the body to
Sunlight when convenient
see that there is sufficient
in the diet. Eat Foods that
is abundant

30. John Maxwell, the Vegetarian Party's 1948 U.S. presidential candidate, got four votes. *Photograph by Hank Walker,* Life *Magazine, April 26, 1948. © Time Warner Inc.*

By 1986, the *San Francisco Examiner* was describing the boom in retail sales of tofu and other soy foods, showing "a heightened awareness of the importance of diet. Health-conscious baby boomers have been leading the way by exercising more and eating lighter foods." The following year *Prevention* magazine ran a story called "What Doctors Are Learning from Vegetarians," in which the writer cited a 21-year study that followed the health of 25,600 Seventh-day Adventists. The study showed that the Adventists' risk of dying from diabetes was only half that of the general population. "Looking even closer, researchers found that, especially for men, diabetes was listed more often on the death certificates of meat-eating Adventists than on those of vegetarians." Two years later, U.S. Surgeon General Dr. C. Everett Koop, in his "Report on Nutrition and Health," specifically linked diet to heart disease, stroke, cancer, obesity, diabetes, and high blood pressure, warning consumers that the main culprits were saturated fats and cholesterol found in animal protein.

The revitalized American vegetarian movement's emphasis has been almost exclusively on health, heralding a new phase of "physiological" vegetarianism that would have pleased Sylvester Graham and William Alcott. Vegans like Jay Dinshah were not altogether pleased, since, as he argued, ethical issues such as animal rights tend to be ignored.

The 1970s also saw the rebirth of nationwide vegetarian organizations. In 1973, Dinshah, back-to-the-lander Scott Nearing (who lived to be 100), and others started the North American Vegetarian Society, to help seed grassroots groups. By the late 1980s, the *Vegetarian Times* listed more than 160 vegetarian organizations across the United States and Canada, including groups for animal rights and secular as well as religious organizations. One of the most successful was the Baltimore-based Vegetarian Resource Group, which started as a local organization. In the late 1980s, the group was publishing the *Vegetarian Journal* and counted more than 3,500 members throughout the country. As for those "four food groups," by 1991 one group of physicians advocated putting that sacred cow out to pasture. The Physicians Committee for Responsible Medicine recommended a diet based on whole grains, vegetables, legumes, and fruit.

JOHN MAXWELL FOR PRESIDENT

In the late 1940s, as most Americans were devouring their meatloaf and pork chops, a few vegetarian souls tried to publicize the vegetarian cause on the national level. Two of these were John Maxwell, owner of a Chicago vegetarian restaurant, and Symon Gould, editor of the *American Vegetarian* and a New York City bookseller. The two formed the American Vegetarian Party in 1948, just in time to run for president and vice president. Although their ticket received only four votes that year, the American Vegetarian Party ran presidential candidates every four years until 1960.

Vegetarian Times
July 1988

WARNINGS FOR A SMALL PLANET

In 1971, a 27-year-old Californian named Frances Moore Lappé came out with a book called *Diet for a Small Planet*, considered a classic of the modern vegetarian movement. Lappé took the then-radical position that raising grain-fattened animals was not only wasteful, but unnecessary for meeting daily nutritional needs. As an alternative, she presented a guide for "making the most of plant protein" and offered a "nutritionally sound alternative to a meat-centered diet." Her book sold more than four million copies in six languages and, with a special tenth-anniversary edition, continues to sell exceptionally well. It is credited with breaking the meat-eating habits of many a carnivore. As of 1990, Lappé was working on a revised edition of *Diet for a Small Planet* to celebrate her book's twentieth anniversary.

CHAPTER 8

PHRENOLOGY: BONEHEAD MEDICINE

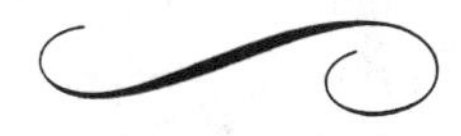

1. Have a healthy stomach.
2. Have a clear conscience.
3. Engage in some useful pursuit.
4. Pay attention to the requirements of the body, exercise, bathing, clothing, etc.
5. Indulge in no bad habits.
6. Keep your temper.
7. Keep down an envious or jealous spirit.
8. Avoid controversy.
9. Read the PHRENOLOGICAL JOURNAL.

From "How to Be Happy"
American Phrenological Journal, *March 1875*

Visitors to New York City in the 1840s found one of the hottest attractions located inside a large brick building called Clinton Hall at the corner of Beekman and Nassau streets, showplace of American phrenology.

Day after day this combination museum, examination room, gift shop, lecture hall, and publishing house drew throngs of the curious, visitors who gaped in hushed silence at the hundreds of casts, busts, and paintings of deceased citizens; who listened in awe to lectures on vegetarianism and temperance; who came away with overpriced mementos, a head chart or phrenological bust "showing the exact location of all of the organs of the brain." While the crowd slowly wandered through the museum, the more adventurous stood in line for a phrenological reading by one of the famous Fowler brothers, who examined the grooves and bumps of each visitor's head and described its owner's talents and shortcomings and dreams.

Most of us in the late twentieth century have a hard time understanding the popularity of a movement like phrenology. Yet phrenology, the nineteenth century's pop psychology, permeated our language, literature, culture, business life, and just about every major popular health-reform movement of the time. Following Horace Greeley's advice "to avoid accidents, trainmen should be hired on the basis of the shapes of their skulls," employers required phrenological charts for prospective workers. To have been phrenologized was a sign of status, and many a citizen proudly displayed his or her character chart fashionably framed on the wall.

Throughout the mid- and late nineteenth century, phrenologists helped to educate the American public about the popular health movements of the day, including Grahamism, vegetarianism, dress reform, water cures, physical fitness, and octagonal-shaped buildings, in their highly successful, long-lived *American Phrenological Journal*. In a uniquely American spirit of optimism, phrenologists advertised that, through self-knowledge, one could lead a healthy and happy life.

"SCIENCE OF THE MIND"

Phrenology was introduced into the United States in 1832 by a Viennese physician named Joseph Spurzheim, student and disciple of phrenology's creator, Dr. Franz Joseph Gall.

Gall developed his theories in the late eighteenth century while a medical student in Vienna. Observing his fellow students, he noticed that those who had good memories tended to have large foreheads. Gall further postulated that there is a direct correlation between personality and the shape and size of one's brain. However, the brain is not one single organ, he argued, but is divided into 37 separate physical "organs." Each organ corresponds to a different "mental faculty" or "propensity" such as "secretiveness," "firmness," or "destructiveness." Gall argued that the size of each organ determines the power of its corresponding mental faculty.

Gall's was essentially an optimistic theory, for he emphasized that we are not necessarily stuck with predetermined character traits. With proper exercise and control, we can change the size and shape of these 37 organs and thus control our personalities. In practical terms, we can consciously develop our virtues and inhibit our vices. Herein lay the appeal of his theory, particularly to reform-minded and optimistic Americans of the pre-Civil War years drawn to his promise of transformation through self-knowledge.

While Gall originated the theory, Spurzheim actually coined the term "phrenology," calling it "the science of the mind."

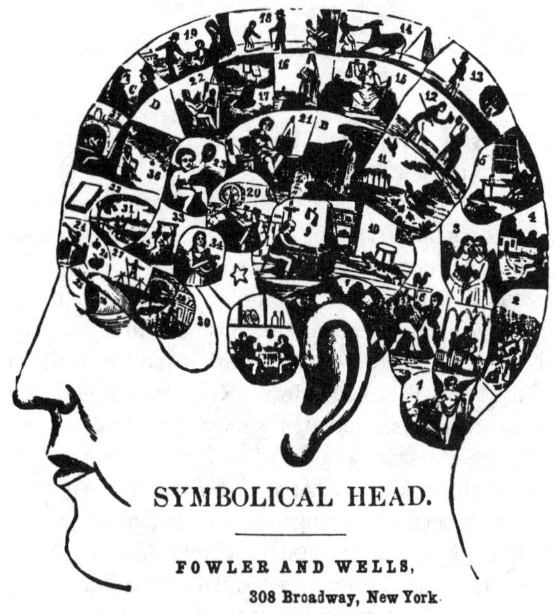

SYMBOLICAL HEAD.
FOWLER AND WELLS,
308 Broadway, New York.

31. The mind was no puzzle for phrenologists, or so they thought. *From* American Phrenological Journal, *June 1889. Countway Library, Boston.*

PHRENOLOGIZING THE WHALE

"It is plain, then, that phrenologically, the head of this Leviathan, in the creature's living intact state, is an entire delusion. As for his true brain, you can then see no indications of it, nor feel any. The whale, like all things that are mighty, wears a false brow to the common world."

Herman Melville
Moby-Dick or, the Whale, 1851

"TO PHRENOLOGIZE OUR NATION"

Phrenology had a head start in the United States via one Dr. Charles Caldwell of Kentucky's Transylvania University, whom many credit with being the true "father of American phrenology." Caldwell had met both Gall and Spurzheim in Europe. He also wrote the first book on the subject to be published in America, called *Elements of Phrenology*. More than 40 phrenology societies sprang up before 1830, the first one in Philadelphia in 1828. However, most were small debating societies, modeled after those in Britain.

Spurzheim, a tall, distinguished-looking physician, was an instant hit during his two-month tour of America in the fall of 1832. Hundreds crowded into his lectures, pulled off their wigs and caps and unpinned their hair in the hopes of being analyzed by the doctor as he demonstrated his theories to his captivated audiences. Then, on November 10, Spurzheim suddenly died while lecturing in Boston. According to the *American Phrenological Journal,* "on the occasion of his funeral, many of the business houses in that city closed their doors."

Spurzheim's brain was carefully preserved in alcohol in a laboratory at Harvard's medical school, and his theories quickly spread throughout America. His death only intensified interest in the new, mysterious science. By the time George Combe visited the

YOU ARE HOW YOU'RE SHAPED

Phrenological theory identified four basic temperaments. Most likely they were precursors of the twentieth century divisions of ectomorph, mesomorph, and endomorph.

TEMPERAMENT	PHYSICAL TRAIT	PERSONALITY
Vital	broad chest, round, full form	love of sensual pleasure, strong impulses
Muscular	prominent muscles harsh features	toughness, tendency to prostrate other functions
Active	sprightliness, ease of motion	bright intellect
Nervous	shortness of form, delicate health, large brain	excitability, impulsive

American Journal of Phrenology, January 1856

United States in the late 1830s, he found a phrenology fad that was already becoming a national phenomenon.

Although it initially appealed only to the elites in the East and Midwest, by the 1850s phrenology had spread to small-town America, aided by that uniquely American character, the traveling "bump doctor," close cousin of the mountebank or medicine-show doctor. For a price, these "professors of phrenology" made their living lecturing, selling books and charts, and analyzing the heads of their audiences, all for a fee. If Europe created phrenological theory, America created what became known as "practical phrenology," phrenology applied to every aspect of life, from choosing mates or careers to raising children.

Much of phrenology's appeal in the United States was its promise that anything was possible, that each individual had the power to reform, to control his or her own destiny. In 1839, in their introductory statement to the first issue of *The American Journal of Phrenology and Miscellany,* the editors specifically made a distinction between "monarchial countries where society is clearly divided into *classes*" and the United States, where "knowledge here is every man's birthright." For the new nation in the throes of Jacksonian democracy with the motto "every man his own doctor," phrenology's appeal was its availability to everyone.

THE FOWLER FAMILY

America's most practical and successful phrenologists were the Fowler clan—Orson, Lorenzo, and Charlotte Fowler and Charlotte's husband, Samuel Wells. Their children would carry phrenology into the early twentieth century.

Orson Fowler, a talented writer and lecturer, began his phrenological career while finishing a degree in theology at Amherst College. When he was not burying his head in his studies, he was immersed in the writings of Gall, Spurzheim, and Combe and demonstrating the new science on his friends. One of his successful converts was his friend and classmate Henry Ward Beecher. The other two were his siblings Lorenzo and Charlotte.

The Fowler brothers were America's first itinerant phrenologists, delivering lectures and feeling the hollows and hills of their compatriots' heads throughout New England, New York State, and the Midwest. In the tradition of traveling medicine shows, the brothers were true entertainers. They never failed to add drama to their demonstrations, which brought in audiences and often converted the most die-hard skeptics. They whipped out thick tape measures for measuring each customer's head; read heads while blindfolded; took turns examining the same head while the other brother left the stage. Physicians in the audience tried to trick the Fowlers by dressing like beggars. Through it all the brothers never lost their sense of humor or their mission.

The Fowlers' reputation for bumpology drew some of America's leading citizens to their lectures and doorsteps. The brothers phrenologized health reformer Samuel Thomson, abolitionists Theodore Weld and Arthur Tappan, the poet John Greenleaf Whittier, humorist Mark Twain, and the young Clara Barton, whose parents were concerned with her extreme shyness and thought a phrenological analysis would give them some clues. (After completing his analysis, Lorenzo Fowler told Clara's parents that Clara would make a good teacher.)

The brothers learned early that their clients demanded a record of their phrenological examinations. At first they produced a customer's phrenological chart on a slip of paper. This was soon replaced by a large sheet of paper, then a pamphlet, and finally a 200-page book for their Clinton Hall patrons.

Eventually the Fowlers retired from full-time traveling road shows and moved on to more stationary instruction and entertainment. Foremost in their minds was the creation of a phrenological "cabinet," a rapidly growing collection of busts, casts, and portraits of deceased citizens from all walks of life, many of which had been donated to the Fowlers by European phrenologists.

After first locating their cabinet in Philadelphia, the Fowlers, along with Charlotte and Samuel Wells, moved their operations to New York City, where they set up the famous Fowler and Wells firm in Clinton Hall. In addition to featuring the cabinet, their main attraction, they published America's first phrenological magazine, the *American Phrenological Journal*; the *Water-Cure Journal*, hydropathy's leading American publication; and health reform and phrenological books. They also lectured, started a school they called the American Phrenological Institute, and analyzed the heads of citizens from all over the world.

HEADY BUSINESS

The monthly *American Phrenological Journal* became the most direct way to spread the word about phrenology throughout the country. In the first year of the journal, the editors explained their purpose—"to preserve from oblivion the most interesting of the numerous facts confirmatory and illustrative of phrenology." In the new mass-media America, the journal quickly became the bible of American phrenology with one of the longest histories of any nineteenth-century magazine, publishing from 1838 to 1911.

The journal was successful because it adapted to the times. Begun while the firm was still in Philadelphia, the *American Phrenological Journal and Miscellany*, as it was called then, was initially a scholarly-looking magazine that published transcriptions of American and English lectures and debated phrenological theory. The editorial content and design appealed to a small, educated audience and was acknowledged by even mainstream medical editors. The prestigious *Boston Medical and Surgical Journal*, precursor of the *New England Journal of Medicine*, congratulated the *American Phrenological Journal* on its debut: "It is really an excellent publication, with which we could not well dispense. It keeps constantly improving in the character of its materials —a property not always characteristic of all the periodicals abroad."

By the time the journal published its last issue in 1911, the publication (now called *Phrenological Journal and Science of Health*) had undergone a series of changes in name, cover design, and editorial content to appeal to a mass audience. Practical phrenology was the editorial catchword, and throughout its history the journal provided its readers with large doses of practical advice. It had added illustrations, advice columns, a personals column, and lively news items.

Fowler and Wells were always thinking up gimmicks to bring in new subscribers. One was the journal's free "Character Sketches," begun after the Civil War. New subscribers were invited to submit two photographs, a front and a side view, along with a stamped, self-addressed envelope and one dollar for a year's subscription, in exchange for a phrenological analysis to be published in the journal.

W.D. Salisbury from England was described as having a "sensitive, nervous organization with good intellectual abilities and would be very reliable in any position of trust. Drawing, designing, or constructive work would suit him best." E.W.E. from Kansas was told "you are almost too wide awake for this century, but will be in your element in the twentieth."

In the 1880s, another method for increasing the journal's circulation was the Plaster of Paris Phrenological Bust giveaway, "so lettered to show the exact location of each of the Phrenological organs." Potential subscribers were told "parents should read the JOURNAL that they may better know how to govern and train their children."

Advertisements were a major way to spread the gospel. After Fowler and Wells started the American Institute of Phrenology in the 1860s to meet "the increasing demand among the American people for correct information in regard to Phrenology, physiognomy, and the proper means of maintaining health and vigor both of mind and body," the Fowlers used the journal to advertise the school's course of study.

The expanding list of the firm's publications department, including books on religion, animal mesmerism, health reform, women's rights, and how to build an octagonal home, always appeared in the journal. In keeping with the Fowlers and Wells philosophy of "every man his own phrenologist," the firm took out full-page ads in the late 1880s for such do-it-yourself phrenology books as *Fowler's Self Instructor in Phrenology*, "nearly 200 pages with 100 new illustrations, including a chart for the use of Practical Phrenologists."

REFORM THROUGH SELF-KNOWLEDGE

A knowledge of one's strengths and weaknesses was only the first step on the road to transformation. Armed with a personal phrenological chart, one also had to decide what route to take. For phrenologists, reform meant health reform, for a major tenet of

ADVERTISEMENTS. 1

JUST PUBLISHED. **NEW EDITION.**

Fowler's Self Instructor

In Phrenology.

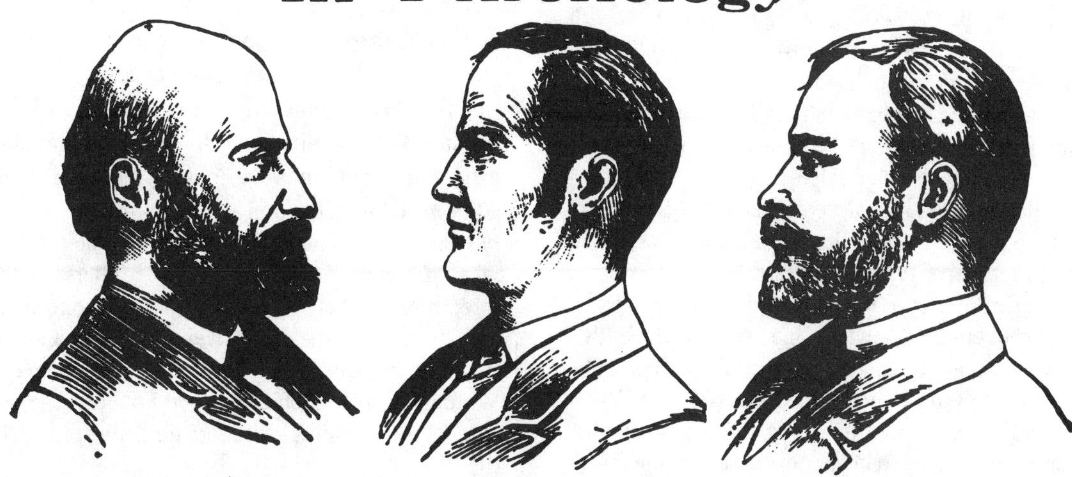

LARGE. SMALL. LARGE.

The Self Instructor in Phrenology and Physiology, with more than 100 new illustrations, including a chart for the use of Practical Phrenologists. By O. S. and L. N. Fowler. Revised by Prof. Nelson Sizer. Nearly 200 pages, 12mo, cloth, $1.00; paper cover, 50c.

The object of this manual is to teach inquirers the organic conditions which indicate character and talent. In order to make it accessible to all, its facts and conditions are condensed, and elaborate arguments are avoided.

In the preparation of this work, an arrangement was made to analyze each of the faculties, and describe them in seven degrees of development, including the most palpable combinations of the faculties, and the characters naturally resulting from such combinations.

All the engravings illustrating the faculties and temperaments have been drawn and executed expressly for this work, and will nowhere else be found, special pains being taken in each engraving to indicate the location of the organ described, by a dash or star; hence, beginners can thus learn how to locate the organs, and the book will become really a Self-Instructor.

It may be safely said that there is no book on Phrenology which has such accurate and specific indications of the location and appearance of organs when large and small.

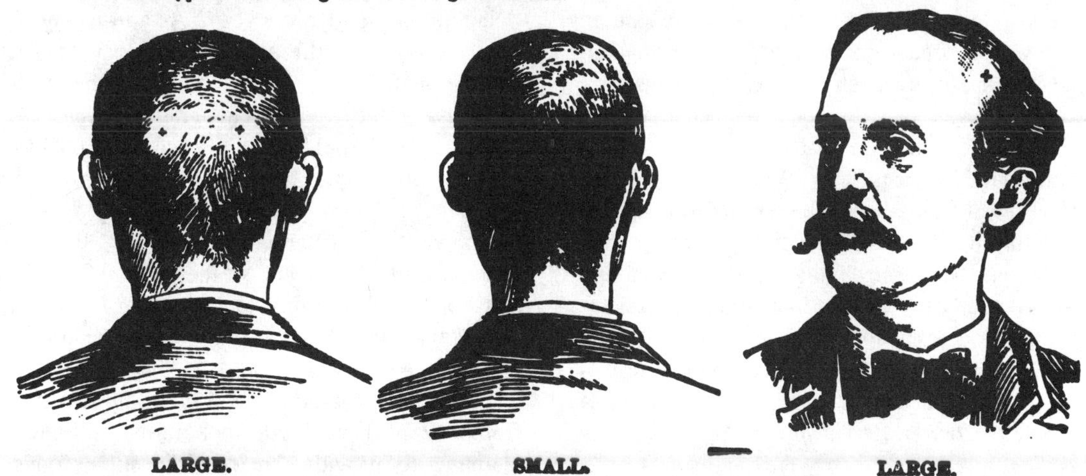

LARGE. SMALL. LARGE.

It is probable that more than 250,000 copies of former editions of this work were sold. And this is certainly better than it ever was before, having been thoroughly revised. Sent by mail, postpaid, on receipt of price, $1.00 in cloth; 50c. in paper binding. Address

FOWLER & WELLS CO., Publishers,

775 Broadway, New York.

32. Fowler and Wells promoted do-it-yourself phrenology. *From* American Phrenological Journal, *December 1889. Countway Library, Boston.*

phrenology was that the brain is intimately connected to the body and that we must pay close attention to our physical health.

The Fowlers were among Sylvester Graham's staunchest supporters. The firm published transcriptions of Graham's lectures as well as his books, and Graham used Clinton Hall's auditorium for several of his lectures on "physiological reform." In its early issues, the *American Phrenological Journal* created a special section on physiology, in which the editors described the evils of alcohol, coffee, tea, and tobacco and recommended daily servings of Graham's whole-wheat, unsifted bread. In their lectures and writings, the Fowlers also used Gall's description of the cerebellum as the center of lust to warn their audiences of overdeveloped "amativeness," the phrenological term for sexual desire.

American phrenology had strong ties to the temperance movement. Fowlers and Wells helped the cause with their publication of a series of booklets called "Whole World Temperance Tracts." The Fowlers' commitment carried into their teachings, requiring that their students take a course on "Temperance Teaching and Reform" before they could graduate. Lorenzo and Lydia Fowler took the crusade with them to England, where their daughter Jessie would become the honorary secretary of the British Women's Temperance Association.

The phrenologists also supported the American vegetarian movement in no uncertain terms. Samuel Wells was a founding member of the American Vegetarian Society, which was organized at Clinton Hall. Before the Civil War, the firm helped advertise a number of planned utopian vegetarian settlements in Kansas, whose organizers dreamed of creating octagonal vegetarian towns on the Western plains.

Orson Fowler had a special interest in health-related architecture and originated the short-lived octagon house fad before the Civil War. Fowler claimed that this "ideal shape," the closest one to a sphere, would assure its inhabitants' health by bringing light and fresh air into their living quarters. Although Fowler eventually lost interest in his dream, octagon-shaped homes quickly sprang up in New York State and the Midwest, made by builders who had probably read one of Fowler's most popular books, *A Home for All; Or a New, Cheap, and Superior Mode of Building*.

Hydropathy was also high on the Fowlers' list of reforms. In addition to taking over the publication of the floundering *Water-Cure Journal* in 1848, the Fowlers advertised water-cure establishments in the *American Phrenological Journal* and published most of the major books on hydropathy in America. Lorenzo Fowler was particularly interested in the water cure and taught courses at Russell Trall's Hydropathic and Physiological School in New York.

Lydia Fowler was largely responsible for pushing the firm into actively supporting dress reform for women. Along with his motto, "Total abstinence or no husbands," Orson Fowler warned his audiences, "Natural waists or no wives." As anti-lacing societies were organized throughout the country, the *American Phrenological Journal* attacked the evils of compressing the organs as a "gradual suicide."

The firm's publishing arm churned out dozens of books on health-related topics, books called *Food and Diet, Tobacco,* and *The Science of Swimming.* In support of vegetarianism, in 1890, the journal advertised two books hot off the press, *The Scientific Basis of Vegetarianism* and *Fruits and Farinacea*.

Fowler and Wells also advertised health-related products, some with rather dubious claims. In the December 1889 issue of the journal the Health Food Company of New York took out a full-page ad, claiming to provide "readily digestible foods for each and every diseased or enfeebled state of the body." Included on its list of products were whole-wheat gluten, cereal coffee, peeled wheat flour, lactic wafers to "relieve all stomach and bowel troubles in babies and young children," and gluten suppositories, "of great value in constipation and piles."

PHRENOLOGIZING THE POET

In 1849, a 29-year-old printer and bookseller named Walter Whitman was phrenologized by Lorenzo Fowler at Clinton Hall. Fowler noted that the young man's head showed a character that "fought with tongue and pen. . . . You have a good command of language, especially if excited." That day marked the beginning of a business relationship between the future poet and the Fowlers. Initially, Whitman arranged to buy and sell Fowlers and Wells publications. In 1855, the phrenologists published and distributed Whitman's first edition of his collection of poems, called *Leaves of Grass*. Unfortunately, Whitman's book did not take off. First advertised at two dollars, within three months the price was reduced to one dollar and eventually the book went out of print. Although the poor sales appear to have damaged Whitman's relationship with the Fowlers, the poet saved his phrenological chart until the end of his life.

A BUMPY ROAD

Phrenology was not without its critics. As "practical phrenology" swept through the United States, bumpology was lampooned by the medical establishment as well as the more theoretically minded British and American phrenologists, horrified by what they saw as the cheapening of Gall's science.

In 1833, one of America's leading magazines, *North American Review*, argued that phrenology was still an unproved science and "a quackery which succeeds by boldness." Five years later Dr. David Meredith Reese wrote an antireform book called *Humbugs of New-York*, in which he devoted a long chapter to phrenology, "the science falsely so called . . . among the prevalent and prevailing humbugs of the day." Reese shook his finger at those "great names" in the scientific community who called phrenology a "science." He saved his anger for the traveling bump doctors, whom he accused of flattering their clients for pecuniary reasons alone. "Thus when an illiterate, stupid, indolent, and conceited knave is told by the phrenologist that the development of his 'organs' indicate that he is, or may become readily, a linguist, a philosopher, and a saint, he lays the flattering unction to his soul and forthwith pays his fee and departs with his 'character' in his pocket. . . . Phrenologists are keen enough to discern that flattery is a correct coin among their dupes."

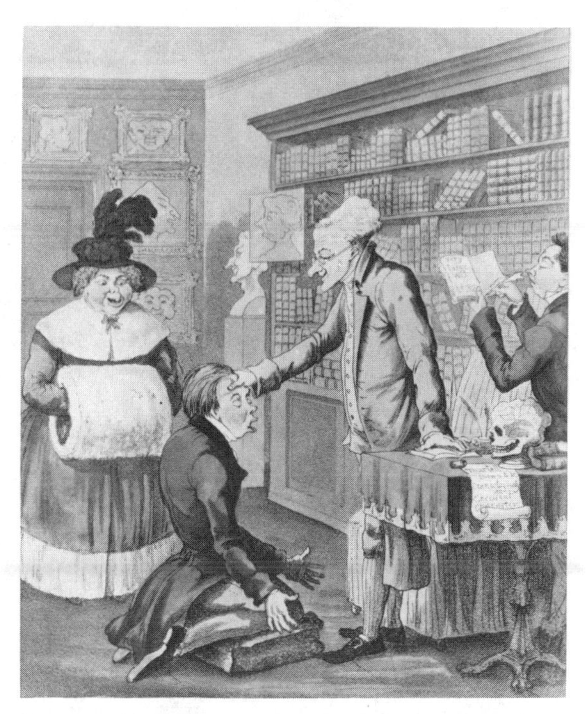

33. Nineteenth-century artists had a field day poking fun at bonehead medicine. *Caricature by George Cruikshank (1826). National Library of Medicine.*

By the 1860s, the Fowler and Wells firm had undergone major changes as its partners' needs changed. Orson moved on to other interests, most notably a mammoth octagon house he designed and built in Peekskill, New York. He eventually moved to the Boston area, where he became obsessed with "sex education," an interest that did not please the more strait-laced Samuel Wells. Lorenzo and his physician wife, Lydia, emigrated to England with their children, where they continued their phrenological work in London and worked with the English temperance movement. Lydia, who followed Elizabeth Blackwell as the second woman to graduate from a medical school in the United States, continued her health work in London. That left Samuel and Charlotte Wells to continue the work of the New York firm, where a large, bearded fellow named Nelson Sizer became Chief Head Examiner.

By the turn of the twentieth century, the first generation of the Fowler clan was dead. With Lorenzo and Lydia's daughter Jessie Fowler in charge, the Fowler family held on until the demise of the American Institute of Phrenology in the 1920s.

END OF THE ROAD

By the 1920s, phrenology had nearly faded from America's consciousness. As the new Freudian theory was accepted as the true science of the mind,

FIVE PRINCIPAL RACES OF MEN

One point of phrenology that was not taken up by its critics was its blatant racism, which no doubt must have fed mainstream America's nineteenth-century belief in manifest destiny. The Fowlers' school required a course called "Ethnology," described as "the races and tribes of men, their peculiarities, and how to judge of nativity of race; especially how to detect infallibly the skulls of the several colored races." During the Mexican War, one phrenologist from Cincinnati who took it upon himself to study Mexican skulls scooped up on the battlefield, argued that they had a "very coarse organization, rather animal than intellectual." The *American Phrenological Journal* ran a full-page essay called the "Five Principal Races of Men," in which it described how the "phrenologist readily detects the mental differences in the races, and can predict with great certainty the destiny of each family of mankind."

phrenology was rejected as a pseudoscience. As scholar Madeline B. Stern, author of *Heads and Headlines,* observes, Jessie Fowler "strove to sell an outmoded product to an increasingly indifferent public."

The *American Phrenological Journal's* final issue appeared in January 1911. Jessie Fowler's firm struggled on, splitting in 1916, with the American Institute of Phrenology under her lead and the publishing and head-analysis arm under her brother-in-law, Michael Piercy. As late as 1925, Stern found "Jessie Fowler, Phrenologist," still listed in the New York City Directory. By the time Jessie died in 1932, Americans were no longer interested in the bumps and grooves of their heads but were, instead, baring their souls to Freudian analysts.

CHAPTER · 9 ·

HYDROPATHY: WASH AND BE HEALED

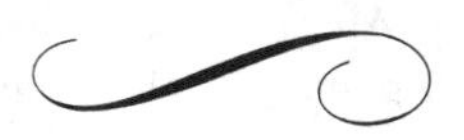

Think! We have treated 600 cases, and our fingers are untainted with the touch of drugs. . . . Nature is our Mistress, and she blesses our household daily, and teaches us how to live.

J.C. Jackson, M.D.
Mrs. L.E. Jackson,
physicians,
Glen Haven Water-Cure

From The Water-Cure Journal, *May 1853*

The Boston-to-Providence train was running late. Dr. Isaac Tabor, a respected Providence physician, waited patiently at the Pawtucket depot. Just as he was about to give up, news of a ''frightful collision'' near Boston reached the depot, followed shortly thereafter by a trainload of the wounded. Along with other doctors present, Tabor boarded the train, examined the sufferers, and tried to comfort them as best he could.

Tabor communicated with all but one of the victims, a ''mangled and bruised'' young man named Stewart Winslow, whose swollen face with blood oozing from his nose and ears and a long gash on the top of his head gave the doctor little hope that the man had long to live.

As, one by one, the other doctors shook their heads and walked away, Tabor patiently waited, holding the victim's hand. As he sat watching the youth's face on that hot August morning in 1853, Tabor decided to try the only method he thought might save Winslow's life.

He quickly removed his patient from the train and laid him on a bed of straw. He then poured a bucket of cold water directly on his head. This seems to have revived the youth, for he ''showed signs of returning animation by struggling and screaming violently,'' much to the shock of the onlookers. On hearing Winslow's screams, the horrified doctors who had given up hope pushed through the crowd with brandy, rum, camphor, and chloroform, all popular cures of the day. Tabor brushed them aside.

Fearing for his life as well as his patient's, Tabor transported Winslow to a makeshift hospital set up for the accident victims. He first wrapped Winslow in a cold, wet sheet and placed an ice pack on the sufferer's head. Within a half hour, Winslow was perspiring freely and appeared to be breathing more easily. After two hours in the sheet, he finally fell asleep.

With the ice pack still on the youth's head, Tabor quietly removed the sheet, washed him in cold water, and placed him in bed. When the youth awoke,

Tabor gently lowered him into a sitz bath, immersing only the lower half of his patient's body, while his legs and feet dangled outside the tub.

For two weeks, day and night, Tabor systematically repeated this treatment. By the time Winslow was strong enough to go home, "not a scar nor discoloration of skin on his body" could be seen.

DISEASE IS THE OPPOSITE OF HEALTH

Although Tabor had been trained as an allopathic (regular) doctor, he had also received training in hydropathy, the cold water-cure therapy that followed the methods of the nineteenth-century Austrian healer Vincenz Priessnitz. Twentieth-century medicine more accurately calls it hydrotherapy (water therapy), since hydropathy actually means "water disease."

In some ways hydropathists shared beliefs with the orthodox doctors of their day, who considered the "water doctors" no more than quacks. Both believed that disease was caused by an imbalance of the body's "vital force." Both believed that the way to restore that balance was to regulate the excretions and secretions of the body by active intervention.

While orthodox medicine's primary way was through the heroic, often life-threatening method of bloodletting, gradually replaced in the mid-nineteenth century by alcohol-based medicines and drugs, hydropathists were vocally anti-drug. They believed that the only way to cure and prevent disease was by both drinking "pure" (as opposed to mineral) water and applying it externally to the body by various methods, such as the wet pack, ice pack, and sitz bath Tabor used to treat Stewart Winslow.

Water-cure theorists placed great emphasis on the skin (the body's "exterior"), whose appearance, they claimed, reflected the condition of the body's "interior" health. If the skin appeared unhealthy (harsh, dry, or discolored), disease was trapped inside. They argued that water cures worked because they opened the pores through stimulation and perspiring, drawing noxious materials to the skin. European theorists called this stage the "crisis." If a patient's skin erupted in boils or perspiration or the patient was overcome by sudden bouts of diarrhea, that meant the cure was working.

Hydropathy in the United States took on a distinctly American wash. American hydropathists eventually disregarded this "crisis" stage. They also used warmer temperatures than were used at the European cures. But most significantly, they incorporated other popular health-reform theories into hydropathy to form what they called the "hygienic system." Along with the water cure, they prescribed a strict regimen of exercise, fresh air, temperance (no alcoholic beverages, coffee, or tea), and a healthy (preferably vegetarian) diet. Their emphasis on pure water and a regimented lifestyle set them apart from the mineral hot springs converts whose numbers grew significantly after the Civil War. The latter "took the waters" at luxurious resorts not for cures, but for rest, recreation, and the fine fare and booze that were offered.

Typical of many antebellum health reformers, American hydropathists blamed their compatriots' illnesses on "artificial habits." Their goal, in fact, went beyond curing sickness. Through hydropathy they wanted to regenerate America.

European hydropathists enjoyed a loyal following on the Continent and England from the 1820s through the early twentieth century. In the United States, hundreds of water-cure establishments dotted the countryside, particularly in the Northeast and Ohio River Valley, from the 1840s to the Civil War, when they were gradually replaced by or turned into the recreational resorts their proprietors had shunned.

HOW TO MEND A BROKEN RIB

Cold-water cures have a long tradition in the history of medicine. Greek physicians used them as early as the fourth century B.C. In the second century A.D.,

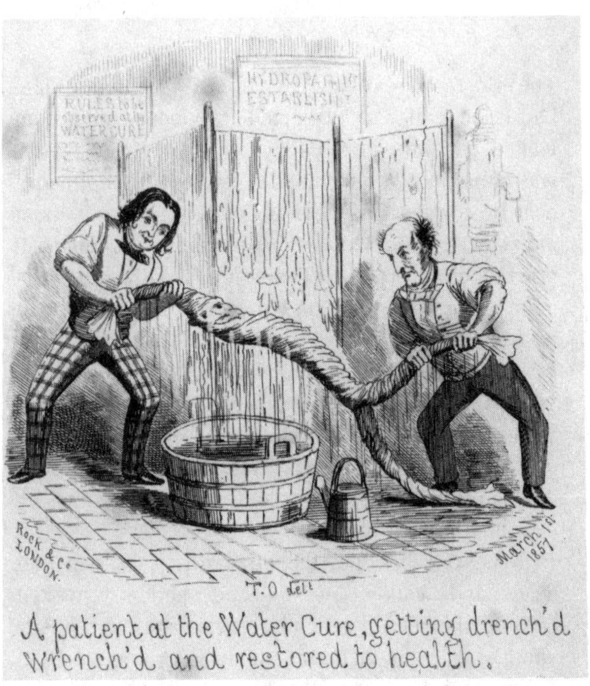
A patient at the Water Cure, getting drench'd wrench'd and restored to health.

34. Thomas Onwhyn. *Pleasures of the Water Cure. London: Rock and Co., 1857. National Library of Medicine.*

the Greco-Roman physician Galen recommended cold water for curing fevers. Healers in ancient China used ice water and wet sheet packs for curing various afflictions.

Hydropathy fell into disuse in medieval Europe, but by the eighteenth century, physicians in Europe and America were recommending hydropathy to cure a variety of illnesses.

Philadelphia physician Dr. Benjamin Rush wrote that cold water would "wash off impurities from the skin, promote perspiration, drive the fluids from the surface to the internal parts of the body, brace the animal fibres, stimulate the nervous system, and prevent the 'diseases of warm weather.' " He recommended cold baths for curing chronic rheumatism, gout, epilepsy, hysteria, palpitation of the heart, rickets, headache, colic, diarrhea, lockjaw, whooping cough, defective hearing, melancholy, and madness.

Vincenz Priessnitz (1799–1851), an Austrian [illegible]-turned-healer from the Silesian village of [illegible] is given credit for hydropathy's revival [illegible]nth century. Priessnitz's conver[illegible]re came purely by accident, [illegible]cident-prone.

[illegible]rative power of [illegible]ge of 13. [illegible] and then [illegible] ually went [illegible]

Three years [illegible] runaway horse-drawn [illegible] three ribs. After the local doc[illegible] wounds and pronounced him incur[illegible] ful teenager tore off the bandages and re[illegible] with wet bandages which he wrapped arou[illegible] chest. He then pressed his abdomen as hard as he could against a chair and swelled his chest by holding his breath. After rewrapping the bandages, he drank a large quantity of cold water, ate lightly, and rested. According to the accounts, Priessnitz was able to move about within 10 days and was back working in the fields in a year.

It didn't take long for Priessnitz's neighbors to hear about his water-cure "miracle." Soon his healing services were in great demand, and he was making house visits throughout the Silesian countryside, asking nothing for his services. When the number of his patients dwindled, he asked his patients to come to his own house and charged a fee. Thereafter, his business took off.

With experience came refinement of his methods. First he discovered that a sponging down, along with wet bandages, was more successful than wet bandages alone. For patients whose diseases were widespread, he used the wet sheet, which he enveloped around the patient's entire body. For local afflictions, Priessnitz used specialized baths—for the head, eye, arm, and foot, and half-baths, sitz baths, and the "douche," a stream of water which he aimed at the afflicted area. For chronically ill patients he also used two or three "sweating" blankets, which, like the wet sheet, he wrapped around the body until the patient perspired freely. This was followed by a sponging down and the "plunge," a quick dunk in a cold bath.

In 1826, Priessnitz opened a water-cure establishment in his home town. The Graefenberg Cure set the stage for the water-cure craze that eventually flooded the United States. His establishment opened with 49 patients. By the 1840s, up to 1,700 patients yearly traveled to Graefenberg. They came with asthma, pleurisy, measles, smallpox, nervous fevers, rheumatism, hernias, gout, syphilis, tumors, and enlarged livers. From all over Europe and America they came, and included barons and baronesses, counts and countesses, artists, civil servants, and physicians.

Elizabeth Blackwell, the first woman to earn a medical degree in the United States, visited Graefenberg in 1850. She described Priessnitz as a white-haired man with a sunburnt and pock-marked face who told her he could cure her eye infection in six weeks. Blackwell's treatment consisted of a daily [illegible]cking, half-bath, plunge, wet bandage, sitz bath, [illegible]ther wet bandage, as well as endless glasses [illegible] throughout the day. Apparently the [illegible]lackwell left before the six weeks [illegible]t her eye.

[illegible] strict regimen for his pa[illegible]g enough, they were encour[illegible]rugs of any kind, gambling, [illegible]ment" were strictly forbidden. Also [illegible]list were "brain work" such as reading and [illegible]g, and flannel or cotton clothing, which Priessnitz claimed weakened the skin.

A heavy, greasy diet was evidently not taboo. In fact, Priessnitz did not appear to be terribly concerned about diet. Unlike American water cures with their vegetarian meals and coarse, butterless Graham bread, Graefenberg offered the heavy Austrian fare popular at the time. According to one account published in the *Boston Medical and Surgical Journal* in 1840, dinner typically consisted of soup, a fried course, beef, mutton, veal, pork, or fowl, and pickled cucumbers. Peas, cabbage, and "sour crout" were the only vegetables served. For dessert there was pastry with fresh butter. Water was the only drink allowed, and patients were told to drink from 20 to 30 glasses each day.

Priessnitz died at his Graefenberg cure in November 1851 at the age of 52 for reasons not described in the literature. Not a single person had been trained to take over Graefenberg at his death, so Europe's first and foremost water cure simply shut down.

Eleven years earlier, the *Boston Medical and Surgical Journal*, precursor to the *New England Journal of Medicine*, had described the "water drinkers" of Europe as an odd lot who "drink no less than five to six gallons daily." The journal warned its readers: "As the water drinkers are beginning to appear in England, they may soon be looked for in the United States, there always being individuals enough among us to copy the absurdities of the old world as fast as they are developed." How right they were. Over the next 20 years, the United States would see its own wave of water-cure heroes and heroines who would attract some of the most famous Americans of the day.

AQUA-MANIA, AMERICAN STYLE

If you happened to be around in the years before the Civil War and were searching for a way to cure a headache or lower back pain without using alcohol-laced drugs, you would probably pick up a copy of *The Water-Cure Journal*, one of the most popular magazines of the nineteenth century.

If you were wealthy enough to afford "the cure" at one of the many water-cure establishments, you would do well to peruse the full page of ads in the back, all of them beckoning you to test the waters—Dr. Sands's Water-Cure Establishment in Lancaster County, Pennsylvania, with its "pure air, pure, soft water, beautiful shady walks on the mountains"; the Wyoming Water-Cure Institute near Buffalo, New York, "treating 400 chronic and acute cases"; or Cleveland, Ohio's Water-Cure Establishment, "entering upon its sixth season, treating diseases peculiar to females." If you thumbed through the rest of the journal, you might also come across an announcement for the opening of Thomas and Mary Gove Nichols's American Hydropathic Institute in New York, the first hydropathic medical school in the United States.

In the 1840s, Russell Trall and Joel Shew opened the first water-cure establishments in America, in New York City. Shew, along with his wife Marie Louise, first treated patients in their home on Bond Street before opening up a cure at Long Island's Oyster Bay. Trall opened his "water-cure house" on Leight Street, and then started the successful New York Hygeio-Therapeutic College that would turn out scores of hydropathists, many of whom went on to found their own cures. Silas and Rachel Gleason ran the Glen Haven Water-Cure with James Caleb Jackson before opening their own Elmira Water-Cure. After selling his shares in Glen Haven, Jackson opened Our Home on the Hillside in nearby Dansville. The Nicholses briefly treated patients at their "elegant residence" at 91 Clinton Place in New York City before turning their home into a hydropathic medical school.

Thomas and Mary Gove Nichols were America's most colorful and controversial water-cure team. Mary was a prolific writer who had fled an unhappy first marriage to lecture and write on the hygienic system, with particular emphasis on women's health. Thomas, trained in regular medicine, adopted hydropathy after the two met, fell in love, and were married. Along with hydropathy, they advocated "free

HOW TO TAKE A BATH

When hydropathy floated across the Atlantic from England in the 1840s, most Americans were not yet ready to take the plunge. The washbowl and pitcher still held reign in most American homes; few had ever taken a bath, except for those who found their way to public bath houses, and these were open only in warm weather. Most believed bathing in the winter would bring on "the chills." Taking a bath was also inconvenient. Bathtubs and piped water in cities did not begin to appear in middle-class households until after the Civil War. Reliable and safe heating devices were not available until World War I.

Aware of these fears and prejudices, hydropathists instructed their readers on the rudiments of bathing. For example, in Marie Louise Shew's 1844 *Water-Cure for Ladies* the author explained: "Let there be a thorough rubbing of the whole body with a coarse wet linen cloth, tolerably well wrung out. Let this be done quickly, and then immediately followed by a dry cloth, or crash towel, until the whole surface is completely dry and warm. . . . No one need, in the least, fear any remote injurious effect. . . . How pleasant and refreshing it is, everyone knows, to wash clean the hands and face of a morning, and how unpleasant, to omit such practice. Precisely so with the whole body, when once accustomed to it."

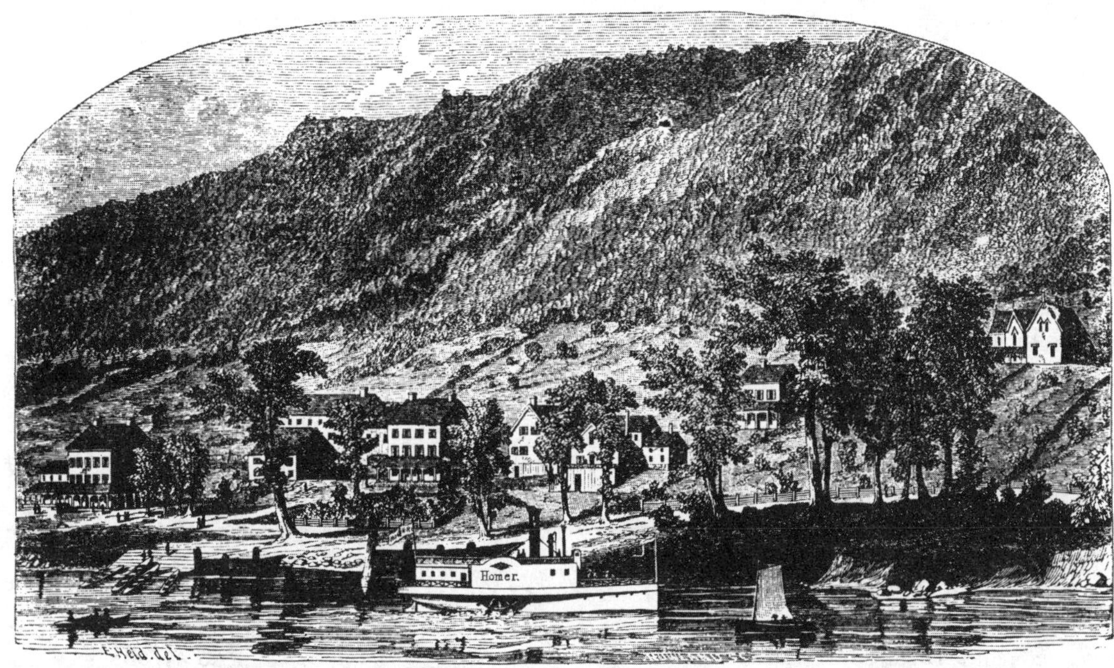

GLEN HAVEN WATER-CURE, HOMER, CORTLAND CO., NEW YORK.

READER:—Our picture describes Glen Haven as it is—lacking its life, which no picture can give. Though called last fall to suffer great loss, yet we have not faltered, and have now a building under contract, every way superior to the old one, which was burned. We mean to make our CURE, before we die, the best in the world. Already are persons seeking homes on our mountain sides, that they may have a residence where *life shall be full of enjoyment*. In a few years, we shall have a hamlet of houses, filled by refined and well-educated Water-Cure families, besides our own family of guests under treatment. And as we are of those who are willing to wait for results till they can grow naturally, so we shall labor on, hopefully and joyfully, in a CAUSE worthy the inspiration and the efforts of all who value health and human redemption.

35. Water cures played up their bucolic settings. *From* The Water-Cure Journal, *June 1855. Countway Library, Boston.*

love,'' arguing that a woman had the right to say ''no'' to lovemaking. Eventually the Nicholses embraced Catholicism, on which they lectured throughout the Mississippi Valley. When the Civil War broke out, they emigrated permanently to England to protest Lincoln's election.

Many hydropathists discovered the cure by way of other popular reforms of the day and imprinted these reforms on hydropathy. Shew was first a temperance reformer and Mary Gove Nichols a follower of dietary reformer Sylvester Graham. Dress reformer Mary Austin popularized the bloomerlike ''American Costume'' at Our Home on the Hillside. As the publishers of *The Water-Cure Journal,* the leaders of American phrenology, Orson and Lorenzo Fowler, mixed their ''bumpology'' with water cures to turn the journal into a slickly designed, widely read magazine that addressed all areas of health reform.

TAKING THE CURE

Americans took to the water cure like ducks to a pond. Four years after Trall and Shew started their New York City cures, 26 more had sprung up, most of them concentrated in New York State. By 1853, *The Water-Cure Journal* listed 41 cures. As many as 200 separate cures came and went by the beginning of the twentieth century, most in operation for only a few years. Almost half were in New York, Pennsylvania, Massachusetts, and New Jersey.

Water-cure proprietors quickly learned that it helped to list staff physicians in their ads. Since it only took three months to receive a degree from most hydropathic colleges in the United States, the problem of an initial shortage of doctors was soon solved. In newspapers and *The Water-Cure Journal,* water-cure ads vied for the sick and exhausted with descriptions of treatments, specialties, facilities, the surrounding countryside, transportation, and increasingly after the Civil War, dining facilities and ''amusements.''

Hydropathists tapped into another consumer need, women's health. Proprietors were aware that many of their prospective clients were, in fact, women who were drawn to hydropathy because of its natural, unobtrusive treatment of pregnancy, childbirth, menstruation, and the ''fallen womb,'' the latter a result of too many tight corsets combined with too much childbearing. Many of the ads assured women that there were separate ''ladies' facilities'' and, most important, specialists in a ''ladies' department.''

American hydropathists paid a lot of attention to and claimed most success with pre- and post-natal care and childbirth. In Mary Gove Nichols's *Experi-*

ence in Water-Cure, for example, a daily regimen for pregnant women is set forth. Nichols also recommended exercise, fresh air, adequate rest, and hydropathic treatments that included a wet-sheet pack, the plunge, two sitz baths, an enema to help prevent constipation, and a vaginal "injection" (douche). This emphasis on health care *during* pregnancy was a radical departure from the relative neglect of prenatal care by the regulars.

Americans found it hard to swallow the full European treatment, so by the 1850s, American hydropathists abandoned the harsher aspects of Priessnitz's cure. Much to the relief of their clients, they raised the water temperature of the baths and cut back on the number of times they wrapped and dunked their patients each day.

Even thus modified, however, taking the cure was still an arduous and demanding experience. Mississippi merchant John Knight, suffering from a "throat and chest affliction," found the regimen at Dr. Wesselhoeft's Brattleboro Water-Cure in Vermont so demanding that he had little time to rest. The Vermont cure was famous for a clientele that included former President Martin Van Buren, historian Francis Parkman, and writer Harriet Beecher Stowe, the mother of five young children, who stayed at the cure for 10 months. (Her husband, Calvin Stowe, followed shortly thereafter. He remained for over a year.)

Knight arrived at Brattleboro early in July 1848 and stayed for one year. He described his experience

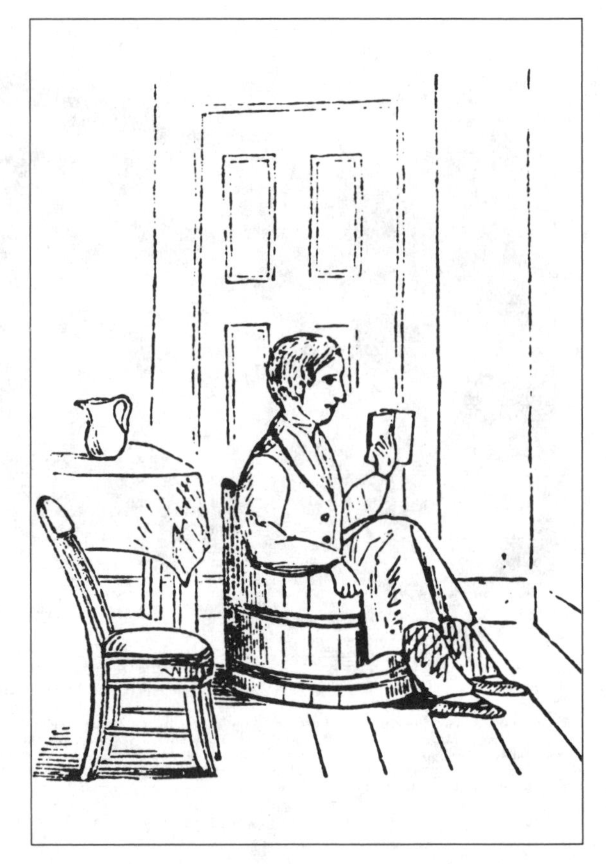

37. The sitz bath got to the seat of the problem. *From* The Water-Cure Journal, *May 1853. Countway Library, Boston.*

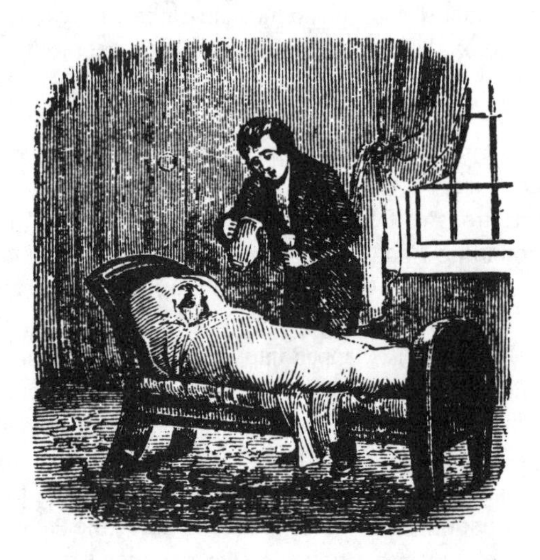

THE WET SHEET PACK—LEINTUCH.

BY JOEL SHEW, M.D.

36. Patients were enveloped in the wet sheet pack for up to three hours. *From* The Water-Cure Journal, *May 1853. Countway Library, Boston.*

at the cure in his letters to his wife, Frances. When he first arrived, every morning at 3 A.M. he was wrapped for three hours in a wet sheet, followed by a plunge, then a half-bath. He then took a three- to four-mile walk. Before and after dinner he sat in a sitz bath. Each evening, he was, again, packed in a wet sheet and took a 15-minute foot bath. Four times each day he gargled with cold water and bathed his chest and throat, using a large bucket of cold water. That was the light treatment. By the end of July, Knight was given the full treatment—13 baths each day, from morning til night. By the time he left Brattleboro in July 1849, his throat problem was gone.

Yet all was not sober at the cures. Recreation was to be found, although carefully regimented. At Our Home on the Hillside, winter patients enjoyed skating on Skaneateles Lake, sleigh rides, concerts, and even dancing. At nearby Glen Haven, the staff and patients enjoyed a Fourth-of-July picnic on a flotilla of boats on the lake, complete with Graham crackers, Graham biscuits, Graham pudding, peas, strawberries, milk, pie, and cold water.

"WASH AND BE HEALED"

The average American could not afford to visit a water-cure establishment; yet in their literature, American hydropathists appeared committed to making hydropathy affordable to anyone who sought the treatment. If you could not scrape together the funds necessary for transportation to a cure and treatment by the pros, treatments that often lasted from several weeks or months to years, hydropathists encouraged you to treat yourself at home. This encouragement of self-doctoring followed a long American tradition of home treatments; it helped make American hydropathy different from the European versions.

Before New York City's Fowlers and Wells took over *The Water-Cure Journal* in 1848, the most widely read self-help hydropathy books available to consumers, in addition to the journal, were Joel Shew's *Water-Cure Manual,* Marie Louise Shew's *Water-Cure for Ladies,* and Russell Trall's *Hydropathic Encyclopedia.* These works were detailed and informative, appealing to an educated audience that could wade through the scholarly style and technical language. They included hydropathic theory, treatments, physiology lessons, and even hydropathic recipes.

Under Joel Shew's editorship, the early issues of *The Water-Cure Journal* followed in the same vein. Shew was a brilliant scholar, but his writing tended to be wordy and dry. In the late 1840s, when Russell Trall took over as editor about the time the journal's offices moved to New York, *The Water-Cure Journal* quickly became the primary source of information for consumers thirsty for the cure without the expense. But what set it apart from other hydropathic literature for the lay person was that Trall targeted an audience that was ready to be entertained as well as educated.

FEMALE DISEASES, OUR SPECIALTY

HIGHLAND HOME WATER-CURE, at Fishkill Landing, Duchess County, New York. O.W. May, M.D., Proprietor.

The pure air and water, beautiful scenery, fine large edifice, an easy access from every direction, combine to render this a desirable place for those who need Hydropathic treatment. This establishment is intended more particularly for the cure of Female diseases; but all other remediable diseases are treated successfully.

The Water-Cure Journal, October 1853

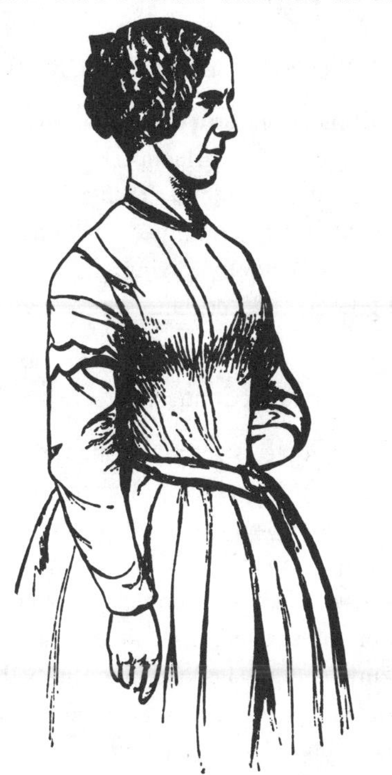

LOOK ON THIS PICTURE:

A WATER-CURE BLOOMER, WHO BELIEVES IN THE EQUAL RIGHTS OF MEN AND WOMEN TO HELP THEMSELVES AND EACH OTHER, AND WHO THINKS IT RESPECTABLE, IF NOT GENTEEL, TO BE WELL!

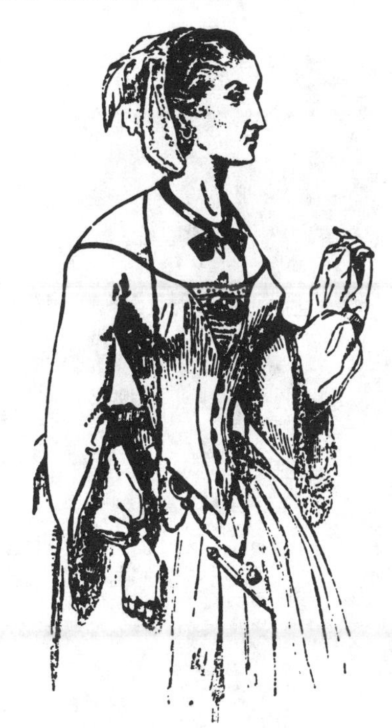

AND THEN ON THIS.

AN ALLOPATHIC LADY, OR A PURE COD LIVER OIL FEMALE, WHO PATRONIZES A FASHIONABLE DOCTOR, AND CONSIDERS IT DECIDEDLY VULGAR TO ENJOY GOOD HEALTH.

38. Dress reform and equal rights were important to water-cure enthusiasts. *From* The Water-Cure Journal, *November 1853. Countway Library, Boston.*

In those years before the Civil War, readers of the journal found not only essays on subjects like "Congestive Fever" and "Water-Cure and the Temperance Movement," but dress-reform stories, vegetarian menus from health-reform conventions, a gossip column, news stories about water cure and animals, a home remedy column in a question-and-answer format, poetry, colorful ads for cures, and even a personals section called "matrimonials."

The Water-Cure Journal lasted until 1913, long after American hydropathy's popularity had faded. Through its long history it underwent changes—in editors, owners, and even its name—to reflect the editors' changing direction away from hydropathy alone and toward health issues in general. When the presses rolled for the last time before the outbreak of World War I, the magazine was simply called *Health.*

QUACKERY AND THE QUACKED

Unlike homeopathy, hydropathy tended to be laughed at or simply ignored by the orthodox doctors and medical writers of the day. For the most part, hydropathy's critics had a heyday poking fun at those who were deluded into thinking that they could be cured by allowing themselves to be wrapped and dunked at the cures and paying for it. The *Comic Annual* for 1846 recommended a free series of hydropathic treatments by simply taking a walk in the rain. You could stand under a spout for a "douche," step into a puddle for a "foot bath," or, if you were clumsy enough to fall into the puddle, you'd get a free "plunge bath" thrown in.

A few came down hard on the water cure, labeling it dangerous. In his 1848 "Hydropathy and Its Evils" published in London's famed medical journal, *The Lancet,* Dr. C.B. Garrett cited the case of a family of children who had been "hydropathed" in which one child died of the treatment. Dr. Stephen Wickes reported on two failed cases of hydropathic treatments that allegedly took place at New Jersey's Orange Mountain Water-Cure in 1852. According to Wickes, a child suffering from "scarlatina" was placed in a tub of cold water and died the following day, and a young woman with epilepsy recovered only after her unsuccessful daily cold wet sheet packs had been abandoned.

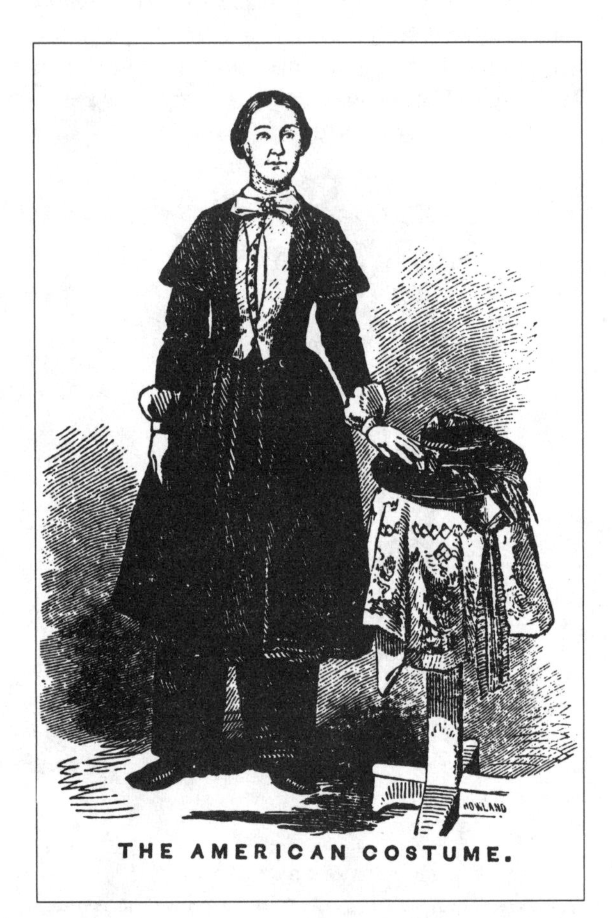

39. This loose-fitting dress-and-pants outfit was a short-lived alternative to corsets and stays. *From* The Water-Cure Journal, *June 1854. Countway Library, Boston.*

A CURE FOR THE OPIUM HABIT

Dr. Trall, please inform a sufferer what is the best antidote against the influence of opium, and the surest way of breaking off taking it? I have tried to quit the habit several times, and when the usual hour comes round for taking it, it seems that I should go crazy if I do not.

A.B.
Norwalk, Connecticut

The antidote is letting it alone. All persons suffer some in breaking off from all habits of taking stimulants and narcotics, and the "craziness" is in proportion to the injury the nervous system has already sustained. If you have not resolution of strength to quit at home, go to a water-cure. Simple diet and plentiful bathing allay much of the suffering. We have cured many such subjects as you represent yourself to be. Hot footbaths and full warm baths are frequently useful.

R. Trall
The Water-Cure Journal, October 1853

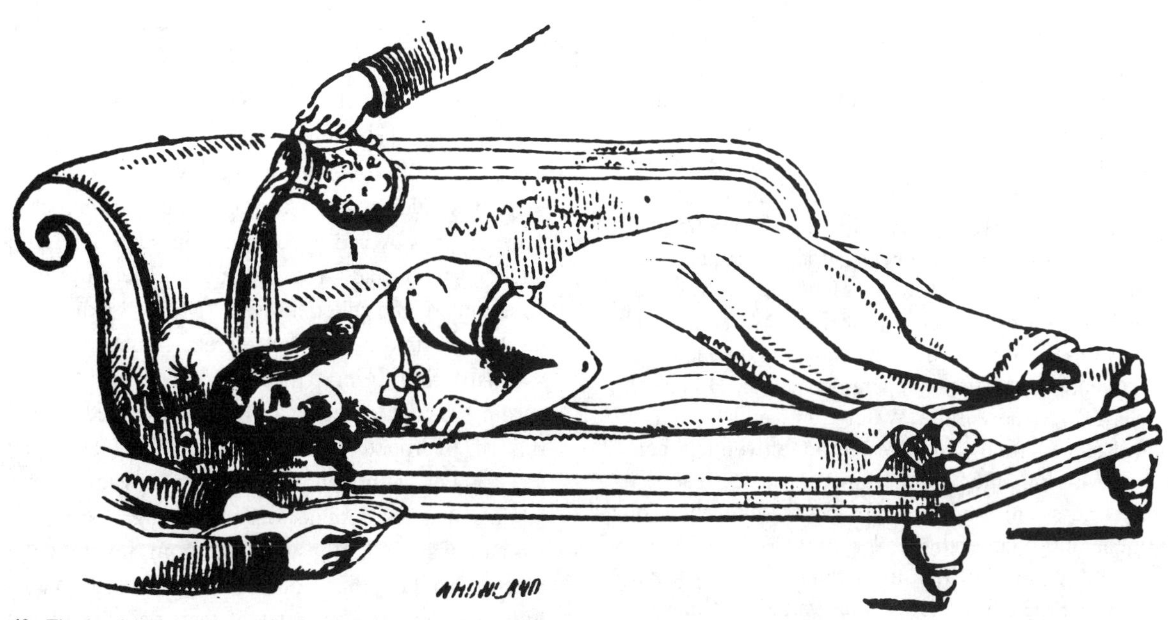

40. The head bath was used for headaches, among other ailments, in the pre-aspirin age. *From* The Water-Cure Journal, *May 1853, Countway Library, Boston.*

Medical writers also criticized what they saw as the inflated prices charged at water cures. In its March 24, 1847 issue, *The Boston Medical and Surgical Journal* described the recently opened Yellow Springs Water-Cure near Philadelphia: "Patients are required to carry with them 'two large woolen blankets; one pair linen, and one pair coarse cotton sheets; long pieces of linen or cotton cloth for bandages, and two comforters.' By taking, in addition, a knife, fork and spoon, an iron pot, and a shin of beef, they might make themselves quite comfortable, on their arrival, independent of the institution. . . . Any person having an obscure farm, difficult of access, in a remote region, may command a price by turning it into a Graefenburg [sic]."

Hydropaths defended themselves against these attacks and, in turn, attacked the regulars in the pages of *The Water-Cure Journal.* One of the most famous is the November 1853 "Water-Cure Bloomer and an Allopathic Lady" drawing, comparing a comfortable, healthy, bloomer-clad water curist with the tightly-laced, corseted woman who took all her prescriptions—including for fashion—from her allopathic doctors.

FROM CURE TO SANITARIUM

American hydropathy reached its peak in the 1850s. After the Civil War, a small number of loyal followers continued to take the waters at the dwindling number of water-cure establishments. But, except for a temporary revival in the 1890s by the German immigrant Father Sebastian Kneipp and his followers, the movement petered out by the end of the nineteenth century. As mainstream medicine began to accept the importance of regular bathing, fresh air, exercise, and diet, all principles of hydropathy's hygienic system, taking the waters appeared less as a cure and more as a way to take a break from one's routine.

HUSBAND WANTED

I am a simple country-girl, daughter of a mechanic, blessed with sound health, a cheerful and contented disposition, a good practical education, with but few of the fashionable accomplishments, and a warm and loving heart. I am a firm believer in the Water-Cure, and an advocate of reforms, but not practically a vegetarian at present. I am, in short, a free child of nature, and an ardent admirer of all her works, and consider a knowledge of the laws of life and health of the utmost importance. As concerns dress, I am neither "Bloomer" nor "anti-Bloomer," but am fearless enough to consult my own taste and convenience, rather than the prevailing fashion.

Now, if I ever marry, I want a husband whom I can look up to and adore. I think I could appreciate true worth, and lose the possessor. What more can I say, except that I am neither old, "ugly," or "rich."

Fanny Freedom
The Water-Cure Journal, March 1854

In an attempt to appeal to the late-nineteenth-century urban American who was less interested in following a strict regimen of diet and exercise than in relaxing and socializing in the country, many cures placed more and more emphasis on their recreational facilities. Others evolved into spas or resorts. As early as the 1850s, descriptions of bowling alleys, gymnasiums, and flower gardening appeared in their ads, welcoming healthy clients as well as patients with serious medical problems. Yet some held on by modifying the treatments, updating them for the twentieth-century temperament. Our Home on the Hillside, the Elmira Water-Cure, and Glen Haven Water-Cure all continued into the twentieth century, evolving into "sanitariums" whose treatment placed less emphasis on the water cure than on hygiene and recuperation.

Today you will find most remnants of hydropathy outside the United States. One variation, "marinotherapy" (seawater therapy), is very popular along Germany's seacoast and in the warmer climes of the Canary and Bahama Islands. The most popular form of water cure still used in the United States is the household ice pack, used for treating swelling.

DEATH AT A WATER-CURE

In August 1874, the newspapers in New York City reported the strange death of a young woman named Isabella Potter, who died while staying in the city's Hydropathic Cure on West 22nd Street. The cure was owned by Charles Christian Shieferdecker, who had studied under Priessnitz at Graefenberg and called himself "M.D.," although he did not hold a medical degree. Isabella Potter was suffering from "rheumatic paralysis," according to Shieferdecker, and he prescribed a series of hydropathic treatments for her. Several weeks later, although the "doctor" assured her parents that his patient was improving, the poor woman was actually suffering from severe neglect. Too late, her concerned parents stormed into the cure, to discover that their daughter was "water-soaked and gangrened." Four weeks after entering the cure, Isabella Potter died. The deputy coroner determined that death was caused by "exhaustion from bedsores." Shieferdecker was charged with criminal neglect. He was never sent to prison and continued to advertise for his West 22nd Street cure, deleting "M.D." from his name.

CHAPTER
· 10 ·

Mineral Water: Cure-All for the New American Nervousness

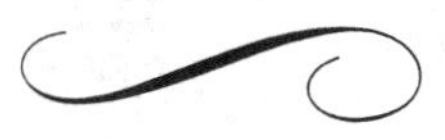

Without civilization there can be no nervousness; there is no race, no climate, no environment that can make nervousness and nervous disease possible and common save when re-enforced by brain work and worry and in-door life.

GEORGE M. BEARD, M.D.
American Nervousness, *1881*

In June of 1871, *The New Republic* newspaper of Camden, New Jersey ran an ad for a bottled mineral water called "Mystic Water from David's Well," drawn near Bristol, Pennsylvania. Touted as "the great diuretic, tonic and alternative remedy of the age," the ad promised that the well water would "purify and enrich the blood, increase the appetite, promote digestion, stimulate the secretions, and vitalize the nervous system." The distributor, D.S. Cadwallander of Philadelphia, offered a box of a dozen bottles for the "low price" of three dollars. For those who preferred to sip directly from the well, a "Healing Institute" nearby was ready to accommodate patients "at all seasons of the year."

Five years after this ad appeared, the institute burned to the ground. No records were kept of the successes or failures of the water from the well, which as of 1960 was still located on the farm where it was first drilled, not far from present-day Levittown.

From the 1870s until January 1, 1907, when the Pure Food and Drug Act went into effect, putting an end to such fraudulently labeled products, thousands of Americans from all walks of life gulped down gallon upon gallon of mineral water for its supposed curative power. A year before the act went into effect, American consumers were drinking bottled water from 589 mineral springs in the United States.

Bottled mineral-water products found their way onto the advertising pages of the popular press in the late nineteenth and early twentieth centuries. They promised to cure their readers' every ache and pain, including constipation, piles, asthma, bronchitis, diseases of the skin, dyspepsia, diabetes, kidney and urinary tract infections, paralysis, and "nervous prostration."

Swilling mineral water was one phase of the mineral water craze that drenched America during the Gilded Age. The other, "taking the waters" at thermal mineral springs, long a tradition in Europe and among Native Americans, had been a regular habit among a small number of wealthy Americans since the late eighteenth century. After the Civil War and until World War I, the spas also attracted a large number of the new urban middle class, products of industrialized America.

The bottled stuff was accessible to millions of Americans. The hot springs were available only to those who could afford to take time away from jobs and families and spend several weeks or months at a spa. Some were graduates of hydropathy treatments, where they had been wrapped, dunked, and doused for days on end. Others, shunning the wet sheet packs and sitz baths of the water cures, were looking for a place in the country to relax. Although the spas drew as many people for the social life, amusements, and food as for the alleged curative minerals in their waters, most patrons sincerely believed that "taking the waters" improved their well-being.

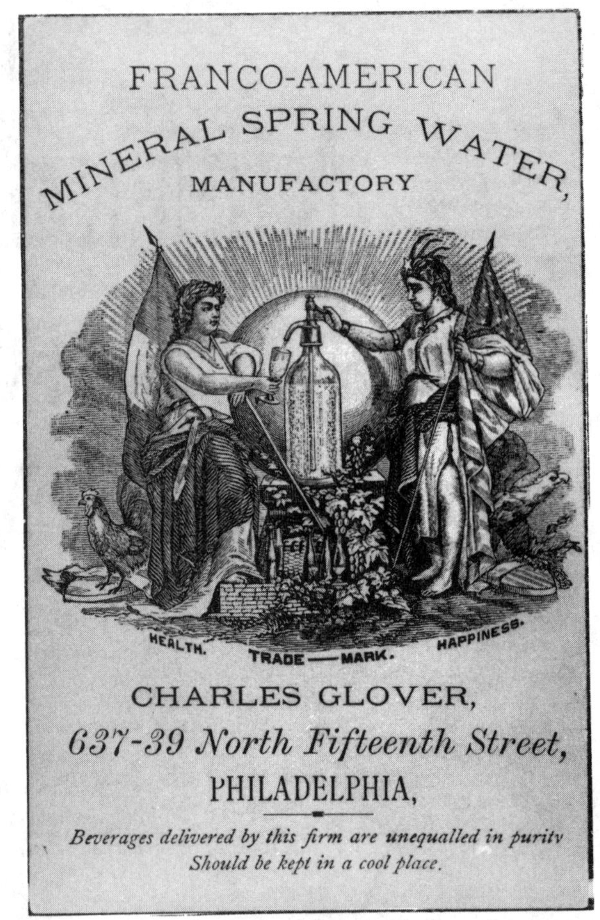

41. Mineral-spring water advertisements, like their modern counterparts, promised health and happiness in a bottle. *Collection of Advertising History, Archives Center, National Museum of American History, Smithsonian Institution.*

"NEURASTHENIA AMERICANA"

Whether swallowing or soaking, mineral-cure advocates in nineteenth-century Europe and America believed that the minerals in the water, absent from public water supplies, could cure a variety of ailments, which at the height of the mineral water craze fell under the general heading of "nervous exhaustion." Today we call it stress.

DRINK AND BE CURED

The United States Dispensatory classes this water with the most renowned of the Alkaline or Carbonated Waters of Europe. Gout, Rheumatism, Neuralgia, Dyspepsia, Gravel, Diabetes, Kidney and Urinary Diseases generally, have all yielded to its influence. It has restored muscular power to the paralytic, cured Abdominal Dropsy and given to the torpid liver healthy action. It has cured Chronic Diarrhoea, Piles, Constipation, Asthma, Catarrh, Bronchitis, Diseases of the Skin, General Debility, and Nervous Prostration from mental and physical excesses. All of these results have been effected by the bottled water away from the spring, and are attested by eminent physicians and medical writers.

Ad for Gettysburg Katalysine Water
by Whitney Brothers, General Agents
Philadelphia, ca. 1870

Nervous exhaustion, or, as it was clinically called, "neurasthenia," "neurasthenia americana," or "americanitis," began to surface in the medical literature just before the Civil War. In 1844, Joel Shew, a medical doctor and leading American hydropathist, argued that the cause of all disease was "an exhausted nervous influence." Other antebellum practitioners expressed alarm about the flood of patients who complained of stress-related ailments. The prime candidates appeared to be "brain workers" —people in business, writing, law, and the professions, who complained of sleeplessness, despondency, anxiety, weariness, debility, and head, back, and groin pains.

After the Civil War, as Harvey Green explains in *Fit For America,* neurasthenia received increasing attention from the medical establishment. In Dr. George Schweig's 1876 article "Cerebral Exhaustion" in the *Medical Record,* for example, the doctor claimed that men, particularly "physicians, lawyers and inventors, were more likely to fall victim to the disease than women." Schweig listed "disinclination for mental labor'' and ''disturbances of the heart'' as his patients' major complaints.

But the most famous ''Mr. Nerves'' was a neurologist from New York, Dr. George M. Beard, whose lectures on nervous disease were published in the *Boston Medical and Surgical Journal* in 1869. In 1881 Beard expanded his theories into a book appropriately called *American Nervousness: Its Causes and Consequences.*

Beard defined ''neurasthenia'' as ''exhaustion of the nervous system,'' a new disease, he argued, that was unique to nineteenth-century Americans. ''Nervousness,'' wrote Beard, ''has developed mainly within the nineteenth century, and is especially frequent and severe in the Northern and Eastern portions of the United States.'' Beard argued that ''the chief and primary cause of the development is 'modern' civilization distinguished by five characteristics: steam power, the periodical press, the telegraph, the sciences and the mental activity of women.''

As causes he listed ''the pressure of bereavement, business and family cares, parturition and abortion, sexual excesses, the abuse of stimulants and narcotics, and sudden retirement from business.'' Nervousness was to be found most frequently among city workers who spent their days sitting at desks, standing at pulpits, or working in counting rooms. Beard listed more than 70 symptoms of nervousness, a list he claimed was not even complete. (One of the more interesting symptoms on this list was ''fear of everything.'') Beard also organized a short list of the primary symptoms into a chart that he called the ''Evolution of Nervousness,'' beginning with ''nervous dyspepsia'' and ending with ''insanity.''

Rather than describe American nervousness in doom-and-gloom terms, Beard celebrated neurasthenia as a reflection of the ''natural superiority'' of American and northern European cultures, and a necessary product of modern civilization. Nervousness, he wrote, was ''part of the compensation for our progress and refinement.''

Healers of all persuasions jumped aboard, each with a cure-all to quiet America's nerves. Some temperance workers pushed the Keeley Gold Cure Treatment, a remedy made of ''chloride of gold.'' Hydropathists running cold-water-cure establishments prominently listed ''treatment of nervous disorders'' in their ads. George Beard himself recommended ''air, sunlight, water, food, rest, diversion, muscular exercise'' and the heroic remedies of phosphorus and arsenic, ''which directly affect the nervous system.'' But the most effective treatment, Beard claimed, was ''general electrization,'' electrical currents using a copper sheet directly applied to the nervous system.

Of all the tonics for neurasthenia, the one that most captured America's imagination after the Civil War was mineral water for both drinking and bathing. For busy urbanities who had grown increasingly distrustful of the quality of their tap water, bottled mineral water was a painless, easy, and relatively inexpensive remedy.

BEFORE NEURASTHENIA THERE WAS GOUT

Mineral-water cures were certainly not discovered by stressed-out nineteenth-century Americans. An age-old remedy with an uninterrupted history since biblical times, mineral water has long been used for its alleged curative powers.

Harry Weiss and Howard R. Kemble describe the history of medicinal mineral-water practices in their informative and entertaining book *They Took to the Waters.* As the authors explain, sulphurous springs flowing into the Dead Sea are described in the Bible. The ancient Greeks built many of their temples near springs for their curative powers. The famed Roman baths, numbering at one time more than 800, were enjoyed by folks from all walks of life, who bathed four or five times a day. When the Romans conquered western Europe, they brought their bathing habit with them, soaking in the mineral waters of Spain, Switzerland, France, Germany, and England; many of their ruins can be seen today. After visiting the newly restored Roman-era baths, visitors to the Pump Room at Bath, England, can sip some of the local water, a warm, sulphurous-tasting drink.

After a lull during the Middle Ages, generations of titled and wealthy Europeans began visiting mineral springs for relief from backaches, rheumatism, and other ailments, particularly gout, the ''prestige'' disease. These springs became famous for treating specific ailments. For example, France's Vichy alkaline waters were supposed to cure gout, liver disease, and diabetes; Germany's Wiesbaden springs were famous for treating rheumatism and gout; France's Aix-la-Chapelle waters, favored by Charlemagne, were supposed to cure chronic rheumatism, metallic poisoning and skin diseases. European springs still draw patrons for treatment of specific diseases.

In North America, native peoples considered mineral springs to be holy water and a gift from the Great Spirit. Long before colonial Americans turned the springs into fashionable watering places in the eighteenth century, warring Native American tribes treated the waters as neutral territory, frequently soaking together while temporarily putting aside their animosities.

In the decades before the American Revolution, propertied American colonials, homesick for the cures of Europe, began soaking in and drinking the natural mineral waters they found along the Eastern seaboard. In addition to immersing themselves in the waters to cure various ailments, many made the trek to get away from the summer heat. As the watering places in America replaced the European spas as *the* place to go in the summer, they attracted the new colonial elite classes—merchants in the North and tobacco and rice planters in the South.

George Washington visited the mineral springs at Bath, Virginia (in present-day West Virginia) in 1748 for relief from rheumatic fever. Bath quickly became a fashionable watering spot for Southern planters. Wealthy New Englanders visited Stafford Springs in Connecticut, known for its power to cure gout, sterility, and something called "pulmonary hysterics." In the middle colonies, the most popular hot spots were New Jersey's Schooley's Mountain Mineral Springs and eastern Pennsylvania's Yellow Springs and Harrowgate, the latter named after the famous spa in England.

IT'S ALL IN THE MINERALS

Mineral-water theorists shared with hydropathists the belief that water, not drugs, would cure disease. But mineral-water advocates have traditionally argued that water would not have its healing properties without the minerals, minerals that the body needs but does not get enough of by simply drinking tap water or taking a bath at home. The major exception to this theory was in the treatment of rheumatism. Mineral-water theorists believed that the heat in thermal waters, rather than the minerals, was the curing ingredient.

One common theme running through mineral-water theory was that specific minerals cure specific diseases, a theme that was greatly expanded during the nineteenth century as modern chemistry came into its own. It is still central to mineral-water theory today, particularly in Europe.

In the eighteenth century, Dr. Benjamin Rush of Philadelphia, the grandfather of American heroic medicine and a temperance crusader, recommended daily doses of "chalybeate" waters (containing salts of iron) found in Philadelphia-area springs as a cure-all for hysteria, palsy, obstinate diarrhea, "female weaknesses," loss of appetite, obstructions of the liver and spleen, and diseases of the kidneys and bladder.

"FOR THE USE OF PERSONS OF CONSTIPATED HABIT"

The Columbian Spring Water is universally acknowledged to be the best *Chalybeate Water Known.* Where the blood requires *Iron,* this water supplies it in the best possible form for use. The assimilation is perfect. *A grain of iron* in this water is in the opinion of a celebrated physician, "*more potent than twenty grains exhibited according to the Pharmacopoeia.*"

FOR SALE BY DRUGGISTS AND HOTELS throughout the country.

Ad for Congress and Empire Springs Waters of Saratoga, New York from Congress and Empire Spring Co., New York City, ca. 1870

TAKING THE WATERS

Doctors recommended that their patients drink or soak in mineral waters only during the inactive phase of the disease. The most common prescription for drinking mineral water was to take from two to four glasses daily, starting with small doses and gradually increasing the amount. Unlike the hydropathists, the mineral-water doctors did not prescribe a strict dietary or lifestyle regimen. However, many believed that the best "water treatment" combined mineral water, exercise, a light diet, and fresh air.

Testimonials of cures in the springs' advertising pamphlets and in newspapers of the day witnessed the miracles of mineral-water therapy.

One such case in the early nineteenth century involved an attorney from New York City who underwent mineral water treatments for pains in his kidneys and lower back. After undergoing the common heroic treatment of bleeding and finding no relief, he visited Schooley's Mountain Springs in New Jersey. There he drank 15 to 20 glasses of the spring's chalybeate water, which acted as a diuretic, as well as a specially prepared carbonated chalybeate. He also took light exercise. To his doctor's delight, the mineral water blackened his patient's urine, and within a few weeks he was "cured."

Before the Civil War, many of the larger mineral-water establishments began to expand their treatments beyond mineral-water soaks and drinks. They promoted, for example, the "electro-thermal bath," combining electrical currents with warm baths. The Russian (steam) and Turkish (hot-air) baths became increasingly popular in bath houses in Boston and New York. At Saratoga Springs after the Civil War, patrons had their pick from a menu of cures that included the Turkish bath, "compressed air baths,"

WHAT AILS YOU? A MID-NINETEENTH-CENTURY GUIDE

AILMENT	*RECOMMENDED MINERAL-WATER CURE*
rheumatism	hot mineral baths
acute gout	alkaline water
chronic gout	saline water
anemia	chalybeate water
hemiplagic paralysis	laxative saline water
hysteria	sulphur and chalybeate water
chronic laryngitis	sulphur and alkaline water
acid dyspepsia	alkaline water
flatulent dyspepsia	saline water
engorgement of the liver	saline, alkaline, and saline–sulphur water
eczema	sulphur water
psoriasis	saline–sulphur water

something called the ''Swedish Movement Cure,'' and ''therapeutical electricity,'' small shocks of electrical current; mineral-engorged hot mud baths became all the rage in the West.

LIFE AT THE SPAS

American mineral-water spas drew two kinds of clients—the sick in search of a cure and worn-out urbanites needing a break from their daily routines. In the decades before the Civil War, many of the former also ''took the cure'' at the highly regimented hydropathic water-cure establishments, where they would sweat enveloped in wet-sheet packs and blanket wraps, plunge in cold baths, and drink 20 to 30 glasses of ''pure'' (*not* mineral) water every day. The latter tended to congregate at the mineral springs. Called ''watering places'' in the eighteenth and early nineteenth centuries, many were renamed ''sanitariums'' in the antebellum years and, finally, ''spas'' by the end of the nineteenth century, as the proprietors placed less emphasis on curing chronic diseases and more emphasis on providing a place for mellowing out in the country. After the Civil War, as Harvey Green explains, the mineral-water cure gradually replaced hydropathy: ''As business ventures, they [the spas] were most successful as therapeutic centers for the wearied neurasthenic businessmen and women who used them as respite from the stress of their lives.'' Not that patrons weren't looking for cures as well. But at the spas they found just enough entertainment and social activity to make the mineral water palatable.

Although the spas of the late eighteenth and early nineteenth centuries were modest affairs compared to their European counterparts or to those in America 75 years later, from the beginning proprietors made it a point to provide necessary comforts and amusements for their well-heeled customers. In Weiss and Kemble's book, for example, the French Captain Ferdinand Marie Bayard described the springs at Bath, Virginia in 1791 as having a troupe of Irish comedians, a dance every week, billiards, and card playing. In 1824, Belmont Hall at Schooley's Mountain Springs, New Jersey, was described as having excellent wines and good, obedient waiters. In 1828, one E. Marsh described Schooley Mountain as providing baths, games, wines, liquors, brown stout, Philadelphia porter and ale, and bottled Saratoga and Congress waters and a chance for guests to meet fashionable company. As an afterthought, he did not forget to praise the mineral water for its medicinal properties.

By the 1850s, patrons of the springs, some of whom had been attracted to the hydropathic cold-water establishments 10 years earlier, began spending summer after summer at the spas. According to Harvey Green, ''for many middle-class Americans, they [the hot springs] were a comfortable compromise with just enough health-related content to assuage any possible guilt about the costs of rising social status.''

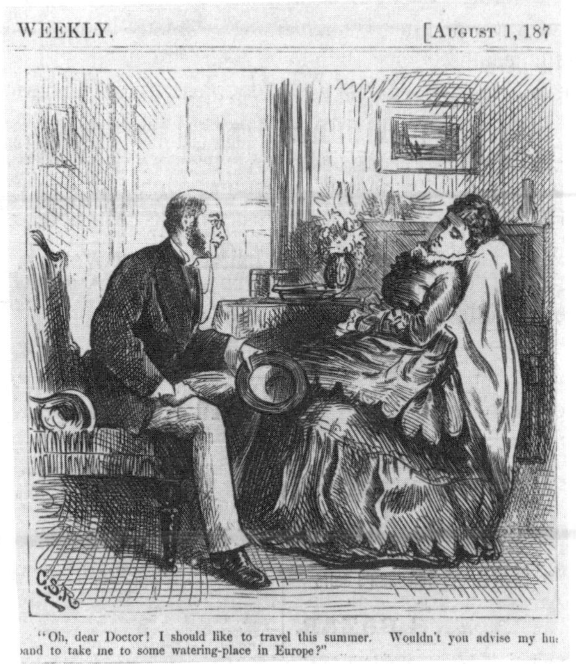
WEEKLY.
[August 1, 187
C.S.R.
"Oh, dear Doctor! I should like to travel this summer. Wouldn't you advise my hu
band to take me to some watering-place in Europe?"

42. *Harper's Weekly* took a jaundiced view of the spa craze. *From* Harper's Weekly, *August 1, 1874. National Library of Medicine.*

A *Macon Telegraph* journalist in the 1920s recalled the scene at Georgia's Indian Springs Hotel before the Civil War:

> They traveled by stage coach or in their carriages, or on horseback, to Indian Springs for a round of dances and gaities. . . . The cotillion, waltz and scottish were danced by the women in brocaded velvet gowns and rustling silks and men in stock collars, the chivalry of the Old South in their looks and manners. . . . Through the throng of beautiful women and courtly men threaded the negro slaves bearing huge silver trays heaped with refreshments for the dancers. Brave days they were in Georgia's history, days of splendor and of plenty.

After the Civil War, Saratoga Springs in New York, with its horse racing and gambling, became one of the most popular vacation spots in the Northeast. In California, the luxurious Paso Robles and Calistoga Hot Springs, named for its founder's promotional malapropism "the Calistoga of Salifornia," drew wealthy patrons from San Francisco. In addition to its hot mineral springs and mud baths, Calistoga Hot Springs provided a direct telegraph line to the San Francisco Stock Exchange for workaholic businessmen who could not leave their jobs behind.

From the beginning, food was a sure way to lure a loyal clientele. For the most part, the menus at the springs ignored the antebellum food reformers' recommendations of lighter meals minus liquor. In eighteenth-century Bath-town near Philadelphia, for example, the clientele enjoyed a breakfast of the best tea, coffee, or chocolate "with plenty of good cream." Before the Civil War, Georgia's Madison Springs, famous for its Southern cooking, served up daily rounds of fried chicken, waffles, biscuits, ham, beef, mutton, veal, and pork. (One exception to the free-flowing liquor atmosphere at the springs was northern California's Wilbur Hot Springs, whose 1890 brochure warned "to obtain the full benefit of the waters, liquor should not be taken during the course of treatment.")

MARKETING THE SPAS

As neurasthenia replaced gout as the prestige disease, the mineral springs habit began to seep into the American urban middle-class lifestyle. Hot spring spas sprouted up all over the United States, particularly in the West, which gradually outshone the East with its promises of ideal climate and dramatic scenery, along with the healing properties of the waters. According to Harvey Green, there were so many spas by 1877 that a special guide to American hot springs was published in a thick volume by D. Appleton and Company, publisher of railroad guides. The railroads, in fact, became a key to many a spa's survival, particularly in the West, since transportation to the springs made all the difference to the pre-automobile generations. The spas, in turn, helped promote the railroads.

The railroads got into the business of marketing the springs through special publications. In 1894, the passenger department of the Union Pacific Railroad published a 166-page book called *Western Resorts for Health and Pleasure Reached via Union Pacific System.* The guide described Idaho's Guyer Hot Springs as a "romantic little mountain resort . . . the accommodations for guests are first-class, and in addition to the hotel, there are bath houses, bowling alleys, croquet and tennis grounds, swings, band stands, and dancing platforms—everything, in short, to make a visit pleasant."

Taking their cues from the railroads' advertising campaigns, proprietors of the Western springs and travel writers drew patrons with promises of romantic settings, ideal (dry) weather year-round, and outdoor sports. Point Arena Hot Springs on the northern California coast described its location in 1903 as "reposing in the midst of a sylvan domain eight miles from the sea." To combat Easterners' image of the wild frontier, the brochure emphasized that "there is no malaria, no snakes or annoying pests." Point Arena welcomed "the nerve-wearied, the mentally-tired teacher, lawyer, artists, and brain workers of all kinds." In his travel guide, *California as a Health Resort,* the English physician Dr. F.C.S. Sanders described central California's famous Paso Robles Hot Springs, which opened in 1888, as having ideal weather for golf throughout the year. "The golf course is property of the springs, and is situated in a park-like country of 115 acres, having natural hazards and gently rolling hills." The doctor assured his readers that " 'Americanitis,' or 'Neurasthenia Americana,' America's new disease, is said to lose its identity by a few weeks' sojourn."

DRINK AND BE DUPED

The mineral water champs were not without their critics. In addition to the hydropathists who sniffed that the spas were nothing more than resorts, after the Civil War the regular medical community began criticizing the bottled-water fad as a bloated and expensive fraud and the spas as nothing more than nice places for a vacation.

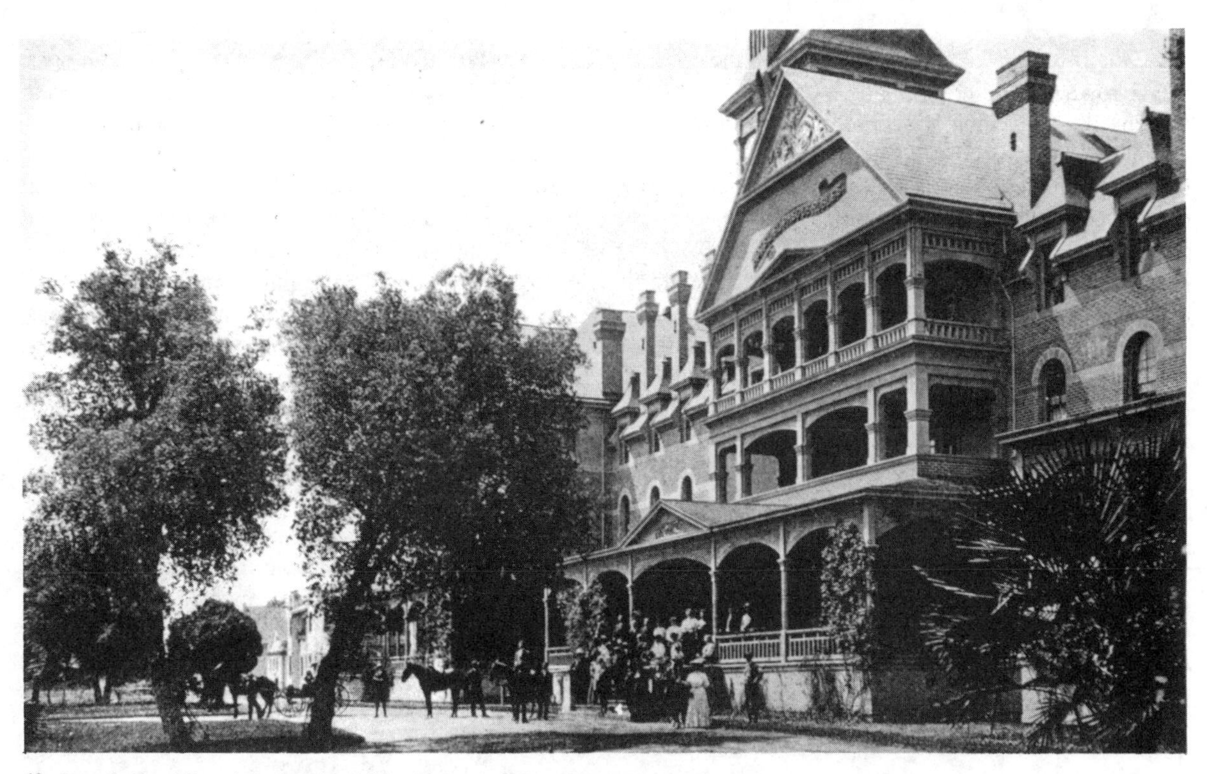

43. Paso Robles Mineral Springs in California was a fashionable destination for ''exhausted'' gentry (1916). *Courtesy, The Bancroft Library.*

In 1868, *The Boston Medical and Surgical Journal* published an article by Dr. Charles E. Buckingham, who came down hard on advertisers who made claims of ''cathartic, alterative, diuretic and antiscrofulous panaceas, which some famous or to-be-famous spring piddles out for the humbugged, who spend money and time for their benefit.'' Buckingham made this recommendation to his readers: ''A quart of pure water, taken a half hour before breakfast will clear out the bowels or wash out the bladders of most men, within an hour after meals, quite as well as the stinking solutions known as mineral waters, whether they are impregnated with Virginia brimstone, or the drainings from some celebrated graveyard in Pennsylvania.'' As for the spas, the writer argued that the change of air, pleasant scenery, and relaxation was what made their clients feel so refreshed. The mineral waters were irrelevant. An 1880 committee of the American Medical Association reporting on the mineral springs claimed that patients at the spas received no supervision and that at many of the spas no supervising doctor was even present.

By the 1890s, bottled mineral water, too, was drowning in criticism, this time from the federal government. In March 1898 a National Pure Food and Drug Congress was organized to fight food adulteration and false advertising, including the claims of bottled mineral-water manufacturers. As Kembell and Weiss explain, the Pure Food and Drug Act of 1906 was a great blow to the mineral-water industry.

In 1918, the American Medical Association published a pamphlet that summed up the medical community's attitude toward the mineral-water craze. ''Mineral waters,'' the AMA argued, ''possess no mysterious or occult virtues in the treatment of disease. No mineral water will be accepted by the medical profession for alleged medicinal properties supported only by testimonials from bucolic statesmen and romantic old ladies.''

NOSE DIVE AND RESURFACING

In the United States, the spas' popularity began to wane by the First World War, particularly in the East, as the automobile provided an easy way to drive to the now-fashionable seaside and mountain resorts.

In the West, the hot springs continued to draw both vacationers in love with the Western landscape and health-seekers in search of the ''climate cure'' well into the 1940s. The Western spas were able to keep their wealthy clientele from Los Angeles and San Francisco, for whom ''taking the cure'' at one of the still-popular European spas involved too many traveling hours in the pre-jet age.

One of the more fashionable spots in the 1930s was Arrowhead Springs in southern California, which advertised the healing properties of its "alkaline, thermal and radio-active" waters and mineral mud baths in a brochure that also advertised the splendor of its accommodations, dining facilities, and golf course. Unlike the advertisements of the pre-World War I era, Arrowhead carefully disclaimed any cure-all properties for its waters. "Arrowhead Springs, while making no claim as a panacea for human ills, is recognized by the medical profession as unique in the variety of treatments which the natural qualities of its radio-active waters permit."

The Arrowhead brochure referred to a special "medical department" at the springs, approved by none other than the American Medical Association. In order not to scare potential vacationers away, the brochure assured its readers that "no guests are received who seek treatment for contagious or communicable diseases or any form of insanity."

By World War II, many of the American spas had closed down. Yet by the 1970s, hot mineral springs began to resurface slowly as one method for dealing with the stresses of American urban life, particularly among the new holistic health-seekers of the West. Gradually, many of the old resorts that had fallen into disrepair were revived, promising once again to provide a respite from the daily grind.

By the 1980s, devotees of mineral-water springs could find both renovated and new spas in all parts of the country. Hot Springs, Arkansas, a hot spot since the early nineteenth century and whose springs are now part of the National Park system, continued to draw visitors for both therapeutic and recreational bathing. But the hot spot for American mineral springs was California, whose spas offered something for everyone. At Murietta Hot Springs in southern California, once used by the Temucula Indians, one could soak in the waters, take tennis seminars, and play golf. Big Sur's world-famous Esalen Institute

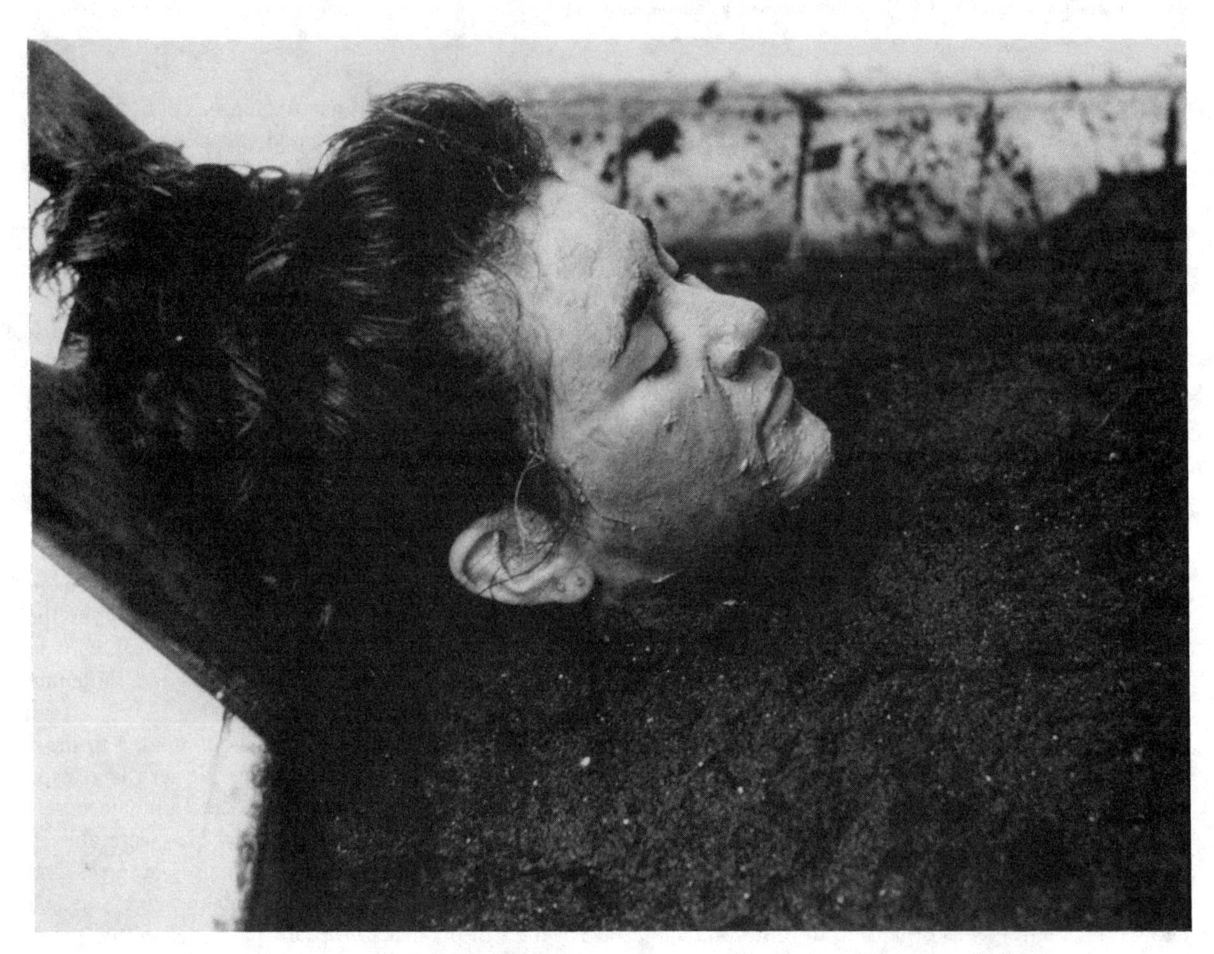

44. Weary urbanites have been recharging in Calistoga, California mud baths for over 100 years. *Photograph by Karen Preuss.*

offered workshops on the latest humanistic psychology techniques, yoga, and aikido, along with hot soaks overlooking the Pacific. Tourists in northern California's wine country could head to the top of the Napa Valley and slip into the hot-springs and mud-bath establishments in Calistoga, where the town's original Calistoga Hot Springs is still in operation under the name Pacheteau. Further north, Wilbur Hot Springs housed guests in its renovated hotel lit only by kerosene lamps. In its 1990 promotional brochure, Wilbur offered its patrons, most of them from the San Francisco Bay Area, an atmosphere reminiscent of the promises of its nineteenth-century predecessors: "Wilbur Hot Springs today is a sanctuary from the tempo of life. No traffic, no electric lights, no pressure; just clean air, incredible starry nights, the rush of Sulphur Creek, wood fires, and the hot baths."

DRINK AND BE HEALTHY

In the 1980s, the bottled-mineral-water fad resurfaced in North America as health-conscious consumers began drinking fewer alcoholic beverages and started worrying about what was in their tap water. Perrier, the top-selling beverage, first swam ashore from France in 1907; by the 1980s it was joined by more than a dozen imported mineral waters and a host of American beverages. With growing competition from locally produced mineral-water companies, by 1986, Perrier had bought Texas's Oasis, Maine's Poland Spring, and Calistoga, California's most popular mineral-water beverage.

Even American breweries began to get into the act. In the mid-1980s, Anheuser-Busch Inc. bought Sante Mineral Water Company, based in Calistoga, and Saratoga Springs Company of Saratoga Springs, New York. To break America's thirst for the most sacred of American beverages, the soft drink, bottled mineral-water companies began offering mineral water flavored with lemon, lime, orange, root beer, cranberry, lemonade, and blackcurrant.

In mid-February 1990, Perrier's domination of the North American market went into a tailspin when Source Perrier voluntarily recalled 72 million bottles after traces of benzene, a toxic chemical, were discovered in several bottles. By the time the little green bottles made their way back to American supermarket shelves and restaurants in April, many consumers had already switched to new, popular bottled spring waters that promised a better taste and purer drink than either tap or mineral water. In a late February 1990 ad in the *San Francisco Examiner* for the prestigious Evian Water of France, which begins its journey "as rain, snow, and ice high atop the northern French Alps, in one of the most pristine places on earth, far from any urban or industrial areas," consumers were promised "effective protection from the outside world of pollutants and organic chemicals."

But even bottling water was no guarantee of purity. In 1991 an FDA survey found that some of the most popular bottled waters in the United States were contaminated by bacteria. Despite the healthful image of bottled water, in some cases consumers would have done as well by turning on their tap.

CHAPTER · 11 ·

SEVENTH-DAY ADVENTISTS: HOLY HEALERS

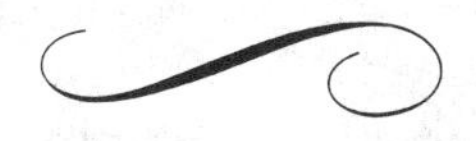

The Lord intends to bring his people back to live upon simple fruits, vegetables and grains . . . .

ELLEN G. WHITE, 1890

She gazed into the middle distance, unblinking. She seemed not to breathe. When she finally spoke, the words "glory, glory, g-l-o-r-y" came from somewhere deep inside her; a companion later described her enraptured voice as "thrilling." Although she was a small woman, only five-feet-two-inches tall, her limbs were unmovable when she was, as she put it, "in vision." She stayed in a trance for about an hour on the evening of June 5, 1863, just outside the farming village of Ostego, Michigan.

The next day, Ellen G. White wrote down what she had seen, filling a 16-page manuscript in her own hand. She and her fellow Seventh-day Adventists were to eat no meat, on God's say-so, part of the message related to her by an angel. Nor were they to down alcoholic drinks, or use tobacco, or pay perfectly good money to physicians. Rather, they were to pray, trust in God, and use His supreme prescriptions: fresh air, clear water, the warm sun, invigorating exercise, and a simple diet of fruit, grains, and nuts to cleanse the corporal temple of the soul. After setting down these rules for living, Sister White, as she was called by fellow Adventists, rested.

It was not the first time that Ellen G. White, a 35-year-old itinerant preacher at the time of her fateful experience, had slipped into vision. Ellen's first glimpse of heavenly health had come in 1848, when she was a young wife of 19. Indeed, health and religion were the intertwined themes that were to preoccupy her for the rest of her life. Variously dismissed by critics as hallucinations, the products of mesmerism, hypnosis, poisoning, or sheer imagination, Sister White's dreams and visions were ac-

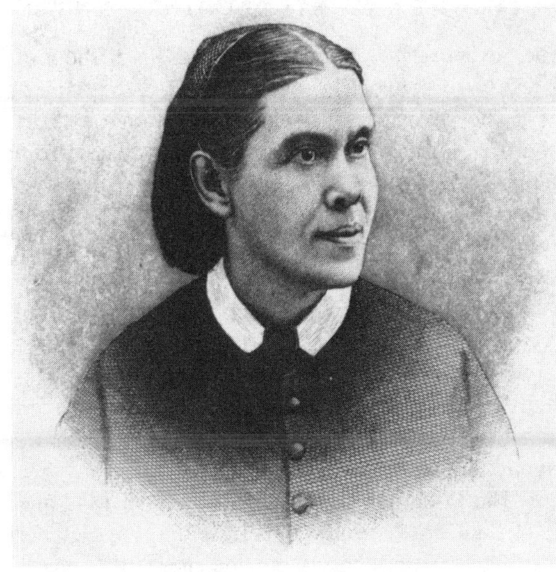

45. Seventh-day Adventist founder Ellen G. White near the beginning of her career. *Photo by Review & Herald Publishing Association. Courtesy, Ellen G. White Estate.*

corded equal status with biblical-era prophesy by believers. They still are.

Like Joseph Smith, founder of the Church of the Latter-Day Saints (popularly known as Mormons), and Mary Baker Eddy, founder of Christian Science, Ellen G. White was a charismatic American mystic. Like them, she was the product of a time when seekers spoke in tongues, divined messages encoded in the scriptures, spoke to God and Christ and the angels—and sometimes grounded their experiences in medical terms.

To White, perhaps even more than her well-known contemporaries, cleanliness was decidedly next to godliness and disease not far removed from sin. Following divinely inspired hygienic principles was essential for right-minded living on Earth and virtually a prerequisite for passing through the Pearly Gates after leaving this vale of tears.

White had many temporal influences, though she was loath to acknowledge them, stoutly maintaining that her precepts were revealed truths shown to her by celestial messengers. Her visions, lasting from a few seconds to several hours, occurred 5 to 10 times a year for 35 years, after which time she continued to receive instructions in dreams.

In a more secular vein, White's followers institutionalized the health reforms of Sylvester Graham, the bran-and-temperance crusader who was one of Sister White's major influences. Although the early Adventists didn't plan it that way, their health regimen led directly to the creation of the modern breakfast cereal industry.

THE GREAT DISAPPOINTMENT

The Seventh-day Adventists started as an offshoot of a nearly forgotten Christian sect called the Millerites, who believed that the Second Coming of Christ (the Advent) was nigh. The sect took its name from William Miller (1782–1849), a Baptist preacher who traversed the country talking about the End of Days, even setting the date, which he calculated from his reading of the Scriptures.

Young Ellen heard Miller speak in 1840, in Portland, Maine. Impressed, the youngster stepped forward when Miller called for soldiers to enlist in Jesus's army. Shortly afterward, she was expelled from her Methodist congregation because of her apocalyptic millennialist beliefs.

The Millerites picked several dates in 1843 and 1844 for Christ's return, finally settling on October 22, 1844. Their faith was emboldened by "signs," natural phenomena such as earthquakes, shooting stars, and a comet that hung in the winter sky over North America in March 1843. There were as many as 50 thousand Millerites, including 500 circuit-riding lecturers who spread the word and urged people to ready themselves for the Advent. As the big day approached, believers gave away their homes, quit their jobs, and waited on hilltops to be swept into paradise by heavenly hosts. When the Savior didn't come for them, many were crushed. Historians refer to the nonevent as "The Great Disappointment."

Ellen was steadfast, however. She contended that something momentous did happen on October 22, 1844. Although Christ did not show himself, she submitted that he moved into his celestial sanctuary that very day, to begin his final judgment of the world. Christ was still coming, although Ellen didn't venture to say when.

Ex-Millerites gathered round the outspoken young "prophetess," as she was called, who had by then started to experience the powerful visions that lent weight to her declarations. Like her, Adventists believed in the imminence of the Second Coming, observed the Sabbath on Saturday (the seventh day), and considered themselves chosen people charged with the duty of spreading the good news.

DAYDREAM BELIEVER

Born in 1827, the daughter of a hatmaker, Ellen Gould Harmon grew up in and around Portland, Maine, a hotbed of temperance reform that, ironically, doubled as a key port for West Indian rum. Like most of New England and New York State, Portland was also a center of fundamentalist religious ferment known as "The Great Awakening."

Young Ellen's life, according to her autobiography, *Life Sketches*, was unremarkable until age nine, when a peevish school chum threw a rock and hit her in the face. The incident left Ellen unconscious. She hovered between life and death for three weeks. Ellen's nose was so badly out of joint that she couldn't breathe through her nostrils for two years.

While recuperating, the girl made hat crowns for her father. Mercury was then in common use among hatmakers and writers have speculated that Ellen's visions, as well as an annoying trembling of the hands that afflicted her after the rock-throwing incident, were the result of mercury poisoning.

Ellen was slow to heal. Her appallingly poor health forced her to drop out of school at age 12, with the equivalent of a third-grade education. The young woman's religious dreams began at 15; her daytime visions, which often took place in the presence of awed witnesses, began at 17.

"My health was so poor that I was in constant bodily suffering," she remembered, "and to all appearance had but a short time to live. I was only 17 years of age, small and frail, unused to society, and naturally so timid and retiring that it was painful for me to meet strangers."

Ellen's transforming early experiences did not center on physical health, but were strictly spiritual. Armed with a unique sense of self, Ellen took to the road to popularize her views. At age 18, in 1846, she married a fellow believer, James White, six years her senior. The Whites spent their early married life traveling from town to town, preaching the gospel and boarding their young children with relatives.

The Whites' travels gradually resulted in a measure of renown for Ellen, whose increasingly forceful personality, absolute belief in herself, and certainty of Christ's return made her a pioneering though unofficial leader of the Adventist movement. James, an editor with more schooling than Ellen, helped her write and publish accounts of her visions, beginning in 1846, the year they were married. He helped launch the periodical *Advent Review and Sabbath Herald* in 1851 and threw its columns open to his wife.

Her first book, *A Sketch of the Christian Experiences and Views of Ellen G. White,* was published in 1851. Showing the intellectual influence of Graham, the book warned against excessive sexual feeling and was especially harsh in its condemnation of masturbation, a term that in that era sometimes also encompassed homosexuality.

Ellen G. White came gradually to her radical views about health. In a vision in 1848, she claimed that the heavens told her to instruct believers to abstain from tobacco, tea, and coffee. In 1854, the heavens advised the consumption of "more coarse food with little grease."

The prophetess's increasingly frequent health messages led to the rapture of 1863. Through it all, the Whites continued their earthly work, often while mired in poor health and poverty. In 1855, they forsook the stony ground of the East for the lush farming country around Battle Creek, Michigan, where a more prosperous life beckoned.

THE NEW CHURCH OF HEALTH

The focus of Adventist activity moved westward with the Whites. In 1860, the still-small fellowship took the name Seventh-day Adventists. In 1863, the

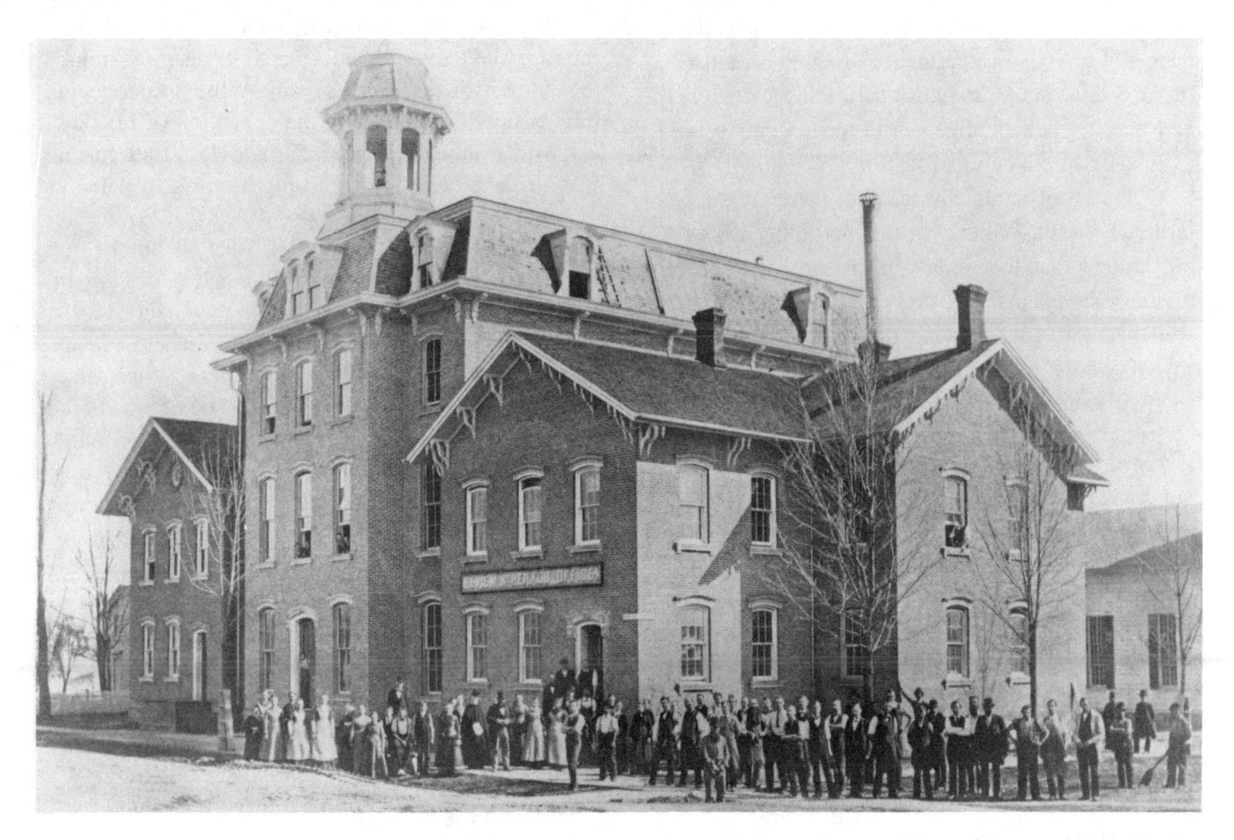

46. The publishing offices of the Adventists' *Review & Herald* in Battle Creek, Michigan. *Courtesy, Historical Society of Battle Creek.*

PROLIX PROPHETESS

In the manner of nineteenth-century health reformers, Ellen G. White was amazingly prolific. The recipient of hundreds of dreams and visions, White recorded her experiences in 37 books published during her lifetime and another 32 posthumous volumes. Her work has been translated into more than 100 languages. All told, White scribbled an estimated 25 million words. Many of her best-known books were about health. They include: *Health: Or, How to Live; Medical Ministry; Counsels on Health; The Ministry of Healing; The Sanctified Life;* and *Temperance.*

During her lifetime, some of White's readers noted close parallels between her work and that of other prominent health writers. In 1976, long after her death, Adventist scholar Ronald L. Numbers published a biography of White that showed strong similarities between her work and books by other authors, especially Dr. Larkin B. Coles, who wrote the 1848 tome *Philosophy of Health.*

Numbers's book, *Prophetess of Health,* caused an uproar. Other modern writers accused White of plagiarism, charging that her visions, and therefore her health rules, were fabricated. The charges triggered a crisis of confidence among Adventists in the 1980s; some, disillusioned, left the church, and one outspoken Michigan dropout went so far as to start a conventional fast-food restaurant.

Church officials allowed that there are similarities between White's writing and other works, but argued that that didn't mean she hadn't had divine visions; instead, they maintained, White, who had not gone beyond the third grade, borrowed words to describe the miraculous things she had seen.

same year that Ellen G. White received her health-minded tablets on the metaphorical mountaintop, the Seventh-day Adventist Church was formally founded. With Sister White's visions showing the way, it soon became a new church of health.

This had an ironic touch, since the church's co-founders were themselves chronically ill. James White suffered from physical and emotional exhaustion and Ellen G. White was scarcely better off. In childhood, she had consumption and frequent fainting spells; as an adult, she was accident-prone, once injuring herself when she fell out of a horse-drawn wagon. She also suffered from bouts of coughing.

Despite her flagging health, Ellen G. White avoided physicians, with their lancets and calomel, in favor of healing prayer sessions. "More deaths have been caused by drug-taking," she wrote, "than from all other causes combined. If there was in the land one physician in place of thousands, a vast amount of premature mortality would be prevented." White also believed in the healing power of the laying on of hands. She claimed to have cured cholera and even her mother's lockjaw with faith.

White placed great faith in hydropathy, especially after she read an 1863 account about the water-cure treatment for diphtheria. The writer of the article was James Caleb Jackson, a medical doctor who ran a spa in Dansville, New York called Our Home on the Hillside. In 1864, the Whites and their children journeyed to Dansville to sit at Jackson's feet.

Ellen G. White was inspired by Jackson's skills, though not by the spa's diversions such as dancing, singing, and card-playing, which Jackson, very much the impresario, believed essential to healing. Jackson's real love, in any case, was hydropathy. "The water revolution," he wrote, "is a great revolution. It touches more interests than any revolution since the days of Jesus Christ."

White was also entranced by Jackson's mastery of phrenology, noting that he conducted expert readings for only five dollars a head. Jackson examined the noggin of the Whites' son Willie, pronouncing him a superior lad, "with the exception of his bowels, which are too large." He was less flattering to Sister White herself, diagnosing her as a hysteric.

Setting their misgivings aside, the Whites returned to Our Home on the Hillside in 1865, after James was struck by a mysterious paralysis. Again, Ellen was impressed by Jackson's therapeutic skills, but put off by the frivolity of the spa, where she and fellow Adventists felt like prim outsiders. When James failed to progress, she took him home to Battle Creek, where he slowly recovered. Ellen G. White began to think that establishing an Adventist retreat true to her fledgling church's principles would not be such a bad idea.

In the meantime, she continued to inform the world of her physical and spiritual precepts. One of her books, modestly titled *Health: Or, How to Live,* sold to the faithful for $1.25 per copy. A bright 12-year-old named John Harvey Kellogg was hired to set type for the tome.

How to Live spelled out Sister White's health principles in black and white. Among them were:

• No sex, or at least precious little of it. With many health reformers of her time, Ellen White believed that sexual energy was easily depleted. Likening erotic energy to a bank account, anti-sex crusaders suggested that every expenditure helped deplete the account. It was evident to White that her neighbors were bouncing checks all over town: "Everywhere I looked . . . I saw imbecility, dwarfed forms, crippled limbs, misshapen heads, and deformity of every description."

In an 1864 book called *An Appeal to Mothers*, White lambasted the solitary vice yet again. Not one to shrink from drawing a radical conclusion, she argued that masturbation induced diseases, cancer being but one.

• No drinking. By this, White meant *no drinking*. One of the first signers of the teetotaler pledge, White was best known outside her small church as a temperance lecturer. A practiced speaker with a big voice, White drew crowds on the anti-alcohol circuit. She once regaled an audience of 20 thousand in Massachusetts without the aid of a public address system, which, of course, hadn't been invented yet. Even given Ellen's rigid anti-alcohol stance, her husband James owned up to using wine occasionally as a medicine, though he stressed it was "domestic" wine, that is, made by church elders who could control its strength and purity.

• No meat. Ellen White believed, with Graham, that animal flesh stirred animal passions in human beings, as did spicy condiments; thus, hot food, hot flesh. White admonished believers to draw nourishment from vegetables, fruits, and unrefined grains, indulging themselves occasionally with tiny, sweetened pieces of Graham bread called Graham gems. Following the Whites' lead, Adventists took but two meals a day: breakfast at 7 A.M. and dinner (lunch) at 1 P.M., with no evening meal. Any more was gluttony.

In 1866, Sister White realized her dream of founding an Adventist retreat by opening the Western Health Reform Institute on an eight-acre spread at the outskirts of Battle Creek. According to a promotional brochure: ". . . no drugs whatever will be administered, but only such means as Nature can best use in her recuperative work. . . ." Typically, the new institution was said to be divinely inspired; on Christmas Eve 1865, Mrs. White had a vision in which she was given sanction to start the spa.

The institute did tolerably well in its first decade, though it was held in far-from-practiced hands. The first medical director, Horatio S. Lay, didn't earn his degree until after he left. The enterprise finally took off in 1876, when the Whites hired the one-time boy typesetter John Harvey Kellogg, now a credentialed medical doctor, as chief physician. Kellogg changed the institution's name to Battle Creek Sanitarium in 1877, and ran the "San," as it came to be known, as a scientific teaching hospital. His younger brother, William Keith Kellogg, served as his assistant.

Although he was at least as dedicated to science as to his hereditary Adventism, Kellogg praised Sister White's health edicts. In 1897, he assured her that ". . . it is impossible for any man who has not made a special study of medicine to appreciate the wonderful character of the instruction that had been received in these writings . . . ."

PRIME TIME FOR PROPHECY

While Dr. Kellogg took care of business on the material plane, Sister White concentrated on serving as a conduit from the celestial realm. The prophetess had her last daytime vision in 1879, at age 52, but continued to take direction in nocturnal dreams from a heavenly creature she identified as an angel and sometimes as "the young man."

She also kept cranking out books, pamphlets, and articles. After James White died in 1881, Ellen White engaged assistants to help with her voluminous writing while she traveled the world as a medical missionary.

One of her preoccupations was women's dress. American women of the nineteenth century wore long skirts that dragged along filthy streets and presented difficulties in going up and down stairs. Moreover, ultra-tight corsets, for that hourglass figure, squeezed the internal organs and left women gasping for breath. Fashionable female regalia could weigh as much as 15 pounds.

"Our feeble women must dispense with heavy skirts and tight waists if they value health," Sister White warned. Accordingly, she developed a modified version of light, baggy bloomers, but the costume never really caught on.

White also worried about the health effects of wigs. "The artificial hair and pads covering the base of the brain heat and excite the spinal nerves centering in the brain," she wrote. "The head should be ever kept cool . . . Many have lost their reason and becoming hopelessly insane by following this deforming fashion."

The prophetess lost that battle, too, as wigs continued to sell briskly. By and large, however, she found the late ninteenth century to be a prime time for prophecy. She disseminated her anti-tobacco and anti-alcohol visions to a growing public and hoisted high the banner of vegetarianism.

Mrs. White found it easier to condemn meat-

A MODERN ADVENTIST SAN

The world's oldest continuously operated Seventh-day Adventist health-care facility sits on a California mountainside with sweeping views of the lovely Napa Valley. Founded in 1878 as the Rural Health Retreat, the St. Helena Hospital and Health Center doubles as a technology-driven acute-care hospital and a detoxification center for victims of the twentieth-century version of "American nervousness."

Founded by Ellen G. White and Dr. Merritt Kellogg (the older brother of Dr. John Harvey and William Keith), the hospital consists of a complex of modern medical buildings and staff housing. The cheery yellow Victorian house where Ellen G. White lived from 1883 to 1891 still stands on the grounds.

Color film footage from 1939 shows the center's own brass band parading through a cluster of vintage buildings, while uniformed nurses twirl American flags, a speaker gives a stem-winder Fourth of July oration, and deer spring by on the tree-covered grounds. The old buildings, along with the band and flag-twirling, are long gone. In their place is a modern, church-owned medical complex where heart transplants and emergency care are highlighted. Hospital meals, however, are still vegetarian unless patients request meat.

The adjoining Health Center, with its nutrition clinics, nondenominational spiritual counseling and psychological coaching, provides a modern restatement of the old Adventist sanitarium concept. Every year, some 700 people enroll in the center's smoking cessation course, alcohol and drug addiction programs, weight-loss clinic, and McDougall program, a vegetarian course in changing one's lifestyle. The center's most famous alumna, syndicated advice columnist Ann Landers, took the no-smoking course in 1974.

Paying patrons live on the premises for up to a month, bunking in well-appointed rooms that—ironically for this teetotaling community—overlook the valley's rich vineyards. Year-round swimming is available, as is a workout room where, on a bright summer day in 1989, the room rocked to a recording of Elvis Presley singing "All Shook Up."

eating than to give it up, however. She scandalized Kellogg and the cooks at the San with her secret vice: juicy fried chicken. White didn't break the finger-licking-good habit until age 66, after an Australian follower convinced her that flesh-eating was cruel to animals and held back the eater's spiritual development.

Convinced that matters were well in hand in her native land, White removed to Australia and New Zealand from 1891 to 1900. While Down Under, she set an example for the church's expanding missionary work, which she linked to its medical vision. She founded health clinics, dispensaries, and sanitaria, describing medical missionary work as "an entering wedge, making way for other truths to reach the heart."

When she returned to America, Sister White discovered, to her dismay, that Dr. Kellogg didn't see things her way. The doctor preferred to operate the church's Battle Creek Sanitarium as a secular business, taking in wealthy boarders such as C.W. Barron, the five-foot-five-inch, 300-pound owner of the *Wall Street Journal*, who died in his room at the San after smuggling in forbidden chocolates. Mean-

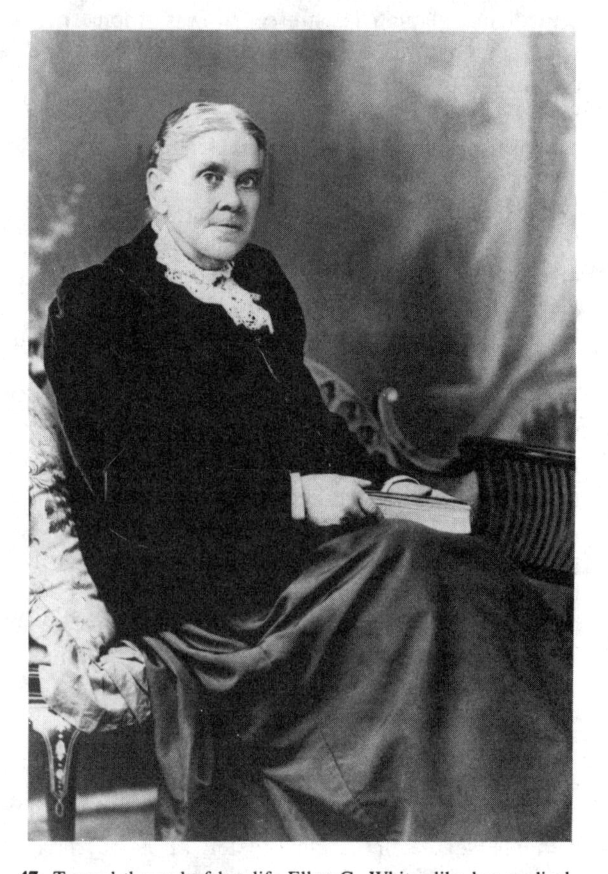

47. Toward the end of her life Ellen G. White, like her medical evangelists, had spread her gospel of health throughout much of the western world. *Courtesy, Ellen G. White Estate.*

while, kid brother William Keith Kellogg was fiddling with new techniques for making cornflakes. He seemed rather more interested in food for the breakfast table than nourishment for the soul.

Sister White met the problem head-on. She "disfellowshipped" the elder Kellogg in 1907. The physician kept control of the San, but again White responded forcefully, promoting a chain of new sanitaria more tightly bound to the church. She scouted locations and raised money herself. She helped to start an Adventist sanitarium in Loma Linda, California in 1905 and added a medical school there, the College of Medical Evangelists, five years later.

Following the tilt of American history and culture to the West, the entrepreneurial White also founded vegetarian restaurants in San Francisco and Los Angeles. The eateries closed, however, when they didn't attract converts along with orders for lentil soup and bran bread.

Ellen G. White never lost her dedication to good health, but her ideas changed over the years. Once fiercely anti-doctor, she came to accept modern medicine when Adventist medical schools began to graduate their own physicians. Her talk in the 1860s about bad "humors" and other ill influences in meat gave way in the 1890s, after the discoveries of Pasteur, to warnings about germs in animal flesh. Comments Ronald L. Numbers, "Mrs. White's intellectual development created a good deal of controversy among those who found the notion of progressive revelation difficult to understand."

White's own health, seldom good, inevitably deteriorated in her surprisingly long old age. She died in 1915 of chronic inflammation of the heart and arteriosclerosis, at age 87.

ELLEN G. WHITE'S HEIRS

The Seventh-day Adventist Church and its distinctive health-reform tradition survived Ellen G. White's passing.

Loma Linda replaced the Battle Creek San as the church's leading teaching hospital and medical school. The church even found a substitute for Dr. Kellogg in Dr. Harry W. Miller, an Adventist medical missionary in China, who developed a soybean-based substitute for milk, treated U.S. Presidents, became friends with General and Madame Chiang Kai-shek and was profiled, admiringly, in *Reader's Digest*. Following the long-lived example of Sister White, Miller died in 1971 at 97.

By the 1920s, the Adventists operated several dozen sanitaria, which they have since converted to high-technology hospitals. In the late 1980s, the Seventh-day Adventists ran the largest Protestant health-care system in the United States, operating 73 hospitals, plus hundreds of dispensaries, clinics, and hospitals abroad. The Adventists also run the world's largest Protestant school system, with a staggering 5,400 colleges, secondary schools, and elementary schools.

Based in Silver Spring, Maryland, the Seventh-day Adventist Church had four billion dollars in assets in 1979, drawn from health-care institutions, schools, supermarkets, publishing houses, retirement homes, and other sources. It was the only church listed in Standard and Poor's index of selected stocks.

Modern Adventists, unlike the Millerites, decline to pick a date for Christ's return, but continue to believe it will be soon. Church members manage to reconcile the apparent contradiction of expecting the end of the world and simultaneously sowing the fertile fields of commerce.

"We have faith, but we go ahead and do things," said communications director James Chase in 1981.

BABY FAE

Loma Linda University School of Medicine, the Seventh-day Adventist showcase 60 miles east of Los Angeles, made headlines in 1984, not for vegetarianism or some other tenet of Adventist health philosophy, but for dramatic and controversial high-tech surgery.

On October 26, 1984, doctors at Loma Linda Medical Center transplanted the heart of a baboon into a 13-day-old girl publicly identified only as Baby Fae. Twenty days later, the infant died when her body reacted badly to a drug used to suppress her immune system.

The surgery touched off an ethical debate. Loma Linda officials defended the transplant as pioneering and medically necessary. Critics disagreed, saying not enough effort had been made to find a human heart donor. In 1985, the *Journal of the American Medical Association* published editorials that stopped short of condemning the surgery but questioned whether Baby Fae's parents had given fully informed consent and concluded that "the overall implication that this particular baboon was 'compatible' with the patient must be rejected."

Right or wrong, it was quite a change for a denomination that had started off as staunchly anti-drug and anti-doctor.

". . . we regard ourselves as being stewards of that which God has given. Christ plainly taught the church to 'occupy until I come.' "

There were 6.2 million Adventists in 1990, some 743 thousand of them in North America. Although the Adventist church is large and rich by the standards of its embattled predecessor, the conservative evangelical group is still distinctive and sometimes embroiled in controversy.

As its chain of hospitals and medical schools grew, the Adventists gradually softened, then dropped, their anti-doctor stance. Church officials explain the transition by noting that Mrs. White availed herself of technology; she was vaccinated for smallpox and had X-ray treatments to remove a spot on her forehead. Nor, they add, was she against all drugs for all time, just the poisonous calomel, opium, and lethal substances prescribed during most of her life.

Modern Adventist communities are close-knit and devout. Adventists don't wear drab, old-fashioned clothing or shun modern conveniences as do, for instance, the Amish, but believers still follow Mrs. White's nineteenth-century dietary laws. They avoid coffee, tea, and alcohol, do not smoke, and go easy on "stimulating" foods like condiments. About half of North America's Adventists are vegetarians. Many rely on processed soybean meat substitutes that are heavily adulterated and texturized, the better to resemble the hot dogs, steaks, and hamburgers they replace.

Residents of a dry Adventist community in Angwin, California—located, ironically, in the heart of California's wine country, where 90 percent of American wine is made—shop at a church-owned supermarket that sells no meat, tobacco, or alcohol and doesn't stock red pepper; mustard was introduced only in the late 1980s. Side-by-side with an extensive bulk-foods section are shelves full of sugary junk foods that would look at home in any supermarket.

Like other conservative Christians such as Mormons and Christian Scientists, Seventh-day Adventists have had trouble holding on to young people in the era of rock music videos and fast-food franchises.

Asked in 1982 about the meatless menu at his school, a 13-year-old Adventist told the *San Francisco Examiner:* "It's lousy. It tastes like barf and it's expensive. Meat tastes better and it's cheaper. This is just a bunch of chemicals and soybeans and it's gross."

Maybe, but it's also evidently healthy. Whether by divine visions, intuition, or some other means, Ellen White anticipated many recommendations of modern nutritionists. Vegetarian Adventists consistently score well in health studies, showing less cancer and heart disease than their meat-eating counterparts.

Although not without problems, Seventh-day Adventists endure on the verge of the twenty-first century, heirs to the reform movements of the nineteenth century and the fratricidal cereal revolution of the early twentieth century.

CHAPTER · 12 ·

THE CEREAL REVOLUTION: THE BROTHERS KELLOGG AND C.W. POST

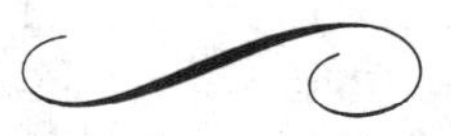

A certain man knew he could do certain things but he could not digest the food necessary to keep him in bodily health and brain power to do the work. So he has perfected the scientific Grape-Nuts, the most scientific food in the world. Get a famous little booklet in each package—The Road to Wellville—*there's a reason. Think it over.*

Post Grape-Nuts ad, 1899

John Harvey Kellogg said the idea came to him in a dream.

An elderly patient at Dr. Kellogg's Battle Creek Sanitarium complained that she broke her false teeth on a hard piece of zwieback, a grainy, twice-baked biscuit, and insisted that Kellogg compensate her or at least serve her food she could chew. Pondering the matter, Kellogg fell asleep. When he awoke, he asked his wife, Ella, to boil some wheat on the kitchen stove. The doctor hand-fed the soft wheat into a hopper, then through rotating rollers which his younger brother William Keith Kellogg scraped with a knife. To the brothers' amazement, the wheat broke off into individual flakes. Baked in an oven, they were crisp, light, and eminently chewable.

The year was 1894. The Kelloggs had invented the world's first precooked, flaked cereal. This seemingly modest accomplishment radically changed the way Americans eat breakfast, changing ideas about nutrition and convenience in the process.

It would be several years before the Kelloggs, chiefly the marketing-minded W.K., realized the significance of what they had done. In the meantime, a driven entrepreneur by the name of Charles William Post became a millionaire by hawking health foods and drinks for the breakfast table, turning the sleepy town of Battle Creek, Michigan into the staging area of the cereal revolution.

Before Post and the Kelloggs, breakfast in America was a salty, greasy, boozy, heavy affair. Salt pork, boiled coffee, potatoes fried in lard, and even shots of whiskey were commonplace. This gut-busting fare served tolerably well when most Americans performed heavy labor on farms. When they moved to towns and cities, clutching their stomachs and complaining of dyspepsia from fatty, 5,000-calories-a-day diets, evangelical businessmen such as Post and the Kelloggs and pioneering health crusaders like Sylvester Graham, whose whole-wheat Graham bread was the precursor of today's Graham cracker, came up with practical alternatives.

Graham, who died in 1851, lived before the age of mass merchandising, but the Kellogg brothers and Post lived to see their innovative ideas accepted, and became rich and famous in the process.

Dr. John Harvey Kellogg parlayed his 62-year association with "the San," as the Battle Creek Sanitarium was known, into international celebrity. Although he took no salary from the San, his many books and public lectures made Dr. Kellogg a millionaire before he was 40. A short, rotund man, he dressed entirely in medical white, right down to the frames of his spectacles, and peddled the short distance from the 20-room Queen Anne mansion he shared with Ella on a white bicycle.

Brother Will, eight years John's junior, was considerably less flamboyant but no less successful. Described by *Time* magazine as "glowering, barrel-chested, bald Will Keith," the younger Kellogg wrested control of what was to become the Kellogg Company from his brother and never looked back. A prominent philanthropist after he earned his fortune, Will was very much the self-made man, jotting down every expenditure, no matter how small, in a little black book and personally attending to details of his food business until he was in his eighties.

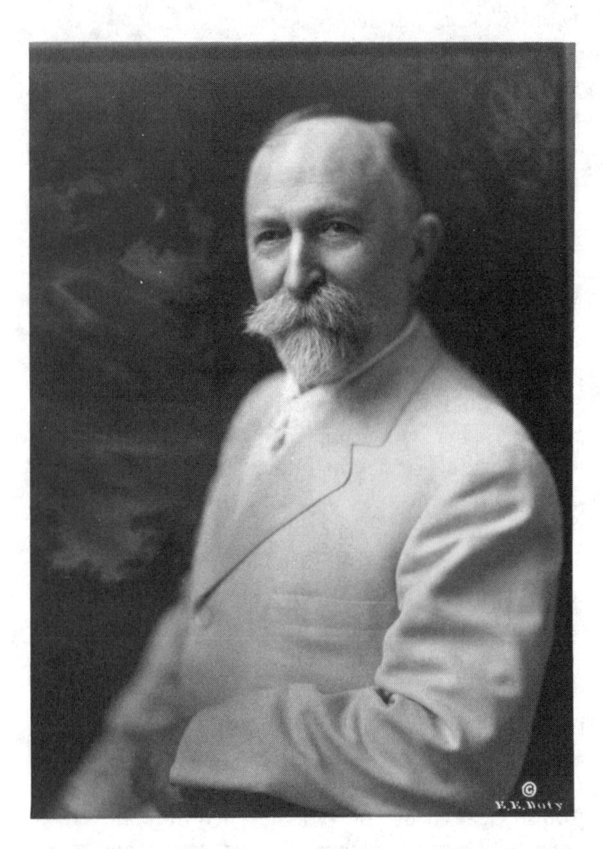

48. Dr. John Harvey Kellogg, physician and author. *Courtesy, Historical Society of Battle Creek.*

C.W. Post, too, was a product of the wide-open capitalism that characterized the turn of the twentieth century. Slender, broad-shouldered, and blunt to the point of brusqueness, Post quickly passed through a variety of careers. He was a real-estate salesman, itinerant farm-equipment peddler, faith healer, and manufacturer of suspenders before finally making it big by becoming an early master of national advertising—some historians say *the* early master—and a confidant of Presidents. About the only thing he didn't do was make rain, though he tried.

Before the barons of Battle Creek came to power, cereal, when it was taken at breakfast, was usually cooked at home and eaten hot. It was the Kelloggs' and Post's genius to change cereal from a hot to a cold food, from uncooked to ready-to-eat and from hearty to light, with standardized products in easy-to-store packages that gave a cachet of modernity to what had been dismissed as "horse food." The new cereals were among North America's first successful convenience foods.

But all that was far from the minds of the Kelloggs as they cooked up the first batch of cereal flakes late one night in the San's basement. They were merely trying to perfect another of the foods—among them peanut butter, a cereal-based coffee substitute, and crunchy granola—invented or adapted for patients at the San, where John Harvey Kellogg had already been medical superintendent for 18 years.

THE MAKING OF A DOCTOR

John Harvey was started on the path to alternative medicine by his Seventh-day Adventist father, John P. Kellogg, who had had horrendous experiences with physicians at a time when becoming a doctor required only a high school diploma and six months of medical school. John P. was given mercury for a wound, and it nearly killed him. His first wife, Mary, on doctor's orders, endured a bleeding "cure" for a cough that had already caused her to lose blood. The treatment, he believed, hastened her death.

A deeply disillusioned John P. Kellogg and his second wife, Ann, mother of John Harvey (born in 1852) and William Keith (born in 1860) and nine other children, became Seventh-day Adventists, subscribing to church leader Ellen G. White's visionary health doctrines. Among them were temperance and vegetarianism, for which she claimed divine inspiration.

When young John Harvey showed promise in school, the church paid for a regulation medical education for him at Bellevue Hospital Medical College in New York City. There, John studied with some of the best medical minds of his day. At night, he returned to a tiny room in a boarding house on the corner of 28th Street and Third Avenue, where he subsisted on a Spartan diet of apples, Graham bread, and one coconut a week, along with Reverend Graham's writings on celibacy and preventive medicine.

Back in Battle Creek, John Harvey was determined to ground Sister White's dietary revelations in newly emerging scientific principles. In 1876, at the ripe age of 24, he became director of the San. The young doctor moved quickly to transform the institution, which Sister White staffed with Adventist volunteers eager to do God's work, into a dynamic combination of a deluxe spa, Chautauqua lecture hall, and state-of-the-art hospital.

Kellogg was a skillful surgeon who attracted distinguished visitors, such as the brothers William and Charles Mayo, namesakes of the Mayo Clinic, who came to admire his techniques. Kellogg himself journeyed frequently to New York and Europe to study with leading medical lights, including Louis Pasteur.

J.H.'s medical acumen was equaled by his promotional flair. Over time, he built the San into a refuge for the well-to-do. A 1957 book, Gerald Carson's *Cornflake Crusade*, reports that "the epileptic, shutter cases, patients with communicable diseases, were refused admittance. The overweight woman and the overworked man were the ideal guests."

By the early 1890s, the San had grown considerably in size and elegance. A chamber orchestra played in the dining room, guests had access to a fully equipped gymnasium, "wheelchair socials" were held on the front lawn, and a brass band invigorated patients with the San's own song, a peppy number dubbed "The Battle Creek Sanitarium March."

According to Carson, "There was nearly a mile of glassed-in halls and wide verandas in a well-maintained setting of lawns, shrubs and landscaping. A tame bear, black squirrels and marmosets, a deer from Indian Territory, helped divert the guests."

Among the 300 thousand patients that passed through the San in its long history were patricians whose surnames have become brand names: Henry Ford, J.C. Penney, Montgomery Ward, R.H. and A. H. Kress, S.S. Kresge, Harvey Firestone, James Buick, and the grape-juice mogul Edgar Welch.

One of the patients in 1891 was a wan unknown in a wheelchair who turned out to be one of the San's most important guests. Although C.W. Post was only 37, he had suffered from nervous exhaustion and chronic appendicitis for years. In despair, he tried the San. He stayed nine months before Dr. Kellogg gave him up as a hopeless case. But Post survived, and he reappeared four years later as the major business rival of the Kelloggs. Their bitter competition continued for 20 years.

RIGHT LIVING AT THE SAN

Most patients at the San fared considerably better than did Post, although some chafed under the Adventist dietary restrictions. The San served no alcohol, no coffee, and no tea. Smoking was forbidden. There was red meat on the menu, but actually ordering it was frowned upon. Those who couldn't abide the San's curious combination of the Spartan and the Sybaritic snuck across the street to the Red Onion, a chops and steak house, or skulked down the way to the firehouse, where a man could enjoy a good cigar in the company of his fellows. Dr. Kellogg's starchy description of this place as "The Sinner's Club" failed to diminish its allure.

But not all of Dr. Kellogg's ideas were punitive or primitive. The menu at the San listed the calorie counts and percentages of fats, carbohydrates, and protein in each dish, long before such ideas were widely circulated. Kellogg is also reported to have made a documentary film on tobacco smoking, which he presciently identified as a major cause of lung cancer—again, years before conventional science caught up with him. And, in an age when established physiologists believed women's respiratory systems were different from those of men, Kellogg attributed the breathing difficulties of nineteenth-century women to the confines of their corsets rather than vagaries of nature.

Within the San's spacious grounds, J.H. Kellogg instructed patients in the principles of "biologic living." Based on Sister White's injunctions, biologic living forbade meat, stimulants and alcohol, and included plenty of fresh vegetables and whole grains, fresh air, and exercise. The San seldom administered drugs, but the doctor frequently performed abdominal surgery, his specialty.

The San was also immersed in hydropathy, the use of water for both prevention and cure of disease. J.H. was especially fond of enemas—he started every day with one himself—and abhorred constipation, which he blamed as the source of "auto-intoxication," or the poisoning of the system. In the

OR YOU COULD EAT A LOT OF APPLE PIE . . .

Dr. J.H. Kellogg considered many of the patients at the Battle Creek Sanitarium to be overweight. This was probably just as well, given what we know about Kellogg's weight-gain regimen for skinny patients. To put on the pounds, Kellogg had patients lie prone after meals with a 20-pound sandbag wedged under each buttock and another sandbag placed directly on the offending abdomen. Kellogg believed this would increase the patient's ability to absorb food and gain weight.

doctor's own words, "Universal constipation is the most destructive blockade that has ever opposed human progress." To help matters along, Kellogg prescribed diets high in roughage, a step that eventually led to the development of Kellogg's whole-grain cereals, and he ordered lubricating paraffin oil to be added to meals. If all that didn't work, he instructed patients to eat 10 to 14 pounds of peeled grapes a day; unpaid Adventist workers did the peeling and pitting.

The San didn't just flood patients' insides with water, it scoured their outsides, too. One patient, describing this rather unnerving experience, remembered: "I stood on a stool and took hold, with my hands, of iron handles in the wall above my head, while my attendant took handfuls of salt, mixed with water until it was like mush, and rubbed me with it from head to foot, until there was a redness all over me."

The patient was then hosed down, subjected to a machine-administered, 15-gallon enema, massaged, and swabbed with body oil.

The vigorous part of the treatment finished, the typical patient ascended to the Grand Dining Room, on the San's top floor, to sup. There, on a 10-foot-long banner on the wall, was another injunction: "Fletcherize!" This was Dr. Kellogg's way of reminding guests to chew their food thoroughly—so thoroughly, in fact, that an automatic "food trap" at the back of the throat would open and trigger the swallowing reflex.

Kellogg coined the verb "Fletcherize" after Horace Fletcher, the millionaire sportsman and world traveler who popularized the technique. A plump self-promoter who gained a wide following with his proselytizing, Fletcher was one of America's great eccentrics. Eventually, Kellogg realized that such thorough chewing liquified roughage, leading inexorably to the dreaded auto-intoxication, and his enthusiasm for Fletcherism waned.

Kellogg's devotion to the health of the colon may seem strangely compulsive to modern-day readers. But he anticipated by nearly a century the popularity of bran, along with the increasing acceptance of low-protein, high-carbohydrate diets.

BROTHER WILL AND HIS HANDY INVENTIONS

Among J.H. Kellogg's many helpers was brother Will, eight years his junior. As children, John made Will shine his shoes and gave him a whack when he thought Will needed it. As adults, the relationship had not changed much. Will Keith worked for 25 years at the San as a bookkeeper, cashier, packing and shipping clerk, and, eventually, de facto business manager. Will's orders came from John, sometimes dictated while the elder brother pedaled his bicycle—a white one, of course. Will jogged alongside and took notes.

This backhanded treatment was to poison the brothers' relationship, making it nearly as bitter as the rivalry each had with C.W. Post. But for a long time Will kept his counsel, running errands and helping John and Ella develop new foods for the San.

One invention, a mixture of oatmeal, wheat, and cornmeal baked and broken up into small pieces, was dubbed Granula. When Dr. Kellogg was sued by James Caleb Jackson, who marketed a related food under the same name, J.H. changed the U in Granula to an O and came up with Granola—then a trade name, although it later became a generic word to describe a dry, crunchy cereal mixed with sugar, raisins, coconut flakes, and nuts. Kellogg's Granola had fewer ingredients than the modern version and was not sweetened, but it was lighter and easier to eat than Jackson's Granula, which was so tough it had to be soaked overnight in milk. Granola was virtually forgotten until the late 1960s, when it appeared in health-food stores and supermarkets as a "new" and healthy food.

Peanut butter was a more consistent success. In a search for nut-based substitutes for meat, Will Kellogg removed the hulls from 10 pounds of peanuts, roasted the kernels in an oven, and put the peanuts through rollers. Voilà! Peanut butter. The new food, sold as Nuttose, was merchandised as a health food for people who couldn't chew nuts and sold mostly to Seventh-day Adventists. "After a while," remembered Will, "the doctor [J.H.] had an idea that toasted peanuts were not wholesome. They were then cooked by steam instead of being roasted, and the little trade that developed was lost.''

The little trade expanded into 700 million dollars in sales for 600 million pounds of peanut butter by the mid-1980s. The Kelloggs, however, made no effort to sell peanut butter on a large scale. Nor did they push Granola—nor, at first, wheat or cornflakes—preferring modest mail-order sales and the few additional dollars they could pick up by selling the foods at the San.

Will Kellogg, his entrepreneurial instincts thwarted, tried to convince John Harvey to mass-market his inventions. He worried that someone else would blitz the cereal market first. He was right.

C.W. POST: ADVERTISING GENIUS

That someone was C.W. Post. Born in Springfield, Illinois in 1854, Post was said to have been blessed by Abraham Lincoln as a boy. When he grew up, Post had the natural salesman's touch, dabbling variously in hardware, farm equipment, real estate, and a product he called Scientific Suspenders. How they differed from unscientific suspenders is unclear, but the relentless work of marketing his ideas exhausted Post by the time he reached his thirties.

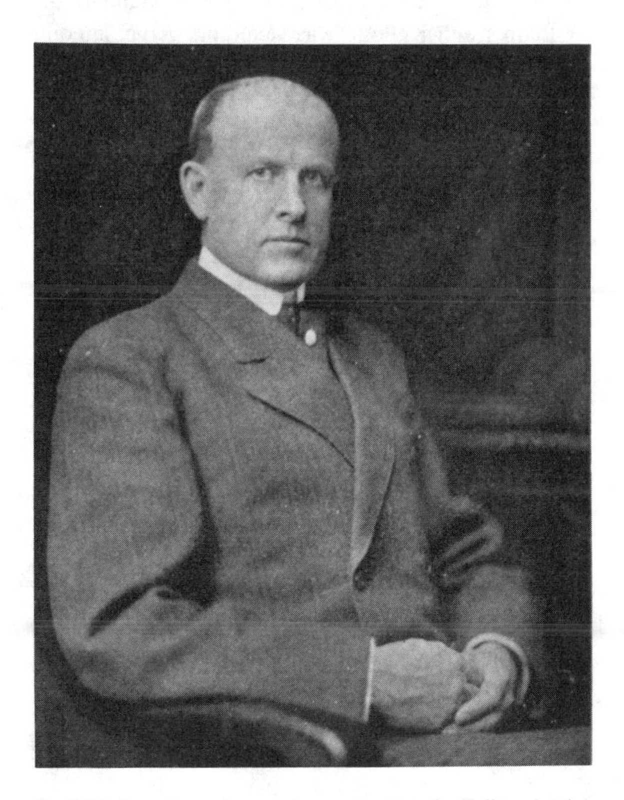

49. C.W. Post, dynamic even in repose, gave the Kellogg brothers stiff competition. *Courtesy, Historical Society of Battle Creek.*

After his unsuccessful treatment at the Battle Creek Sanitarium, Post consulted a medium and a Christian Science practitioner who, he later wrote, helped him cure himself with the power of suggestion. ''I suppose I was a sight,'' he said, ''but the only way I knew how to get well was to be well, however ill I looked, and I began walking around like a man who had business to attend to.''

Post's first order of business was opening a competing sanitarium on the outskirts of Battle Creek, which he dubbed La Vita Inn. The inn featured ''mental'' healing, served hearty portions of meat, and charged less money than the San, frequently taking in the established institution's rejects and overflow. After starting La Vita, Post made Kellogg an offer: he would pray for patients at the San for the modest sum of 50 dollars per week. Dr. Kellogg said no thanks.

Next, Post tried his hand at writing, self-publishing a book entitled *I Am Well!*, based on his experiences and extensive reading of medical and occult literature. ''Seek an easy position where you will not be disturbed,'' the future cereal magnate advised, ''relax every muscle, close your eyes and go into silence where mind is plastic to the breathings of Spirit, where God talks to son.'' Post's advice was later condensed into a booklet called *The Road to Wellville,* which was included in each and every package of his new cereal, Grape-Nuts. Of *I Am Well!*, Post wrote, the book ''possesses the peculiar power of healing the sick while being read.''

In 1895, a year after publishing his book, Post introduced a food that few thought peculiar; it soon surpassed even Scientific Suspenders in sales. Postum Cereal Food, a mixture of bran and molasses that has changed little from its original formulation, was Post's first big success. He made the first batch in a barn, with an initial expenditure of 69 dollars, and peddled it from a handcart on the streets of Battle Creek as a cure for ''coffee heart'' and ''coffee neuralgia.'' One advertisement, which C.W. wrote himself, warned of ''Lost Eyesight Through Coffee Drinking.''

John Harvey Kellogg accused Post of stealing into his experimental kitchen and swiping the formula for the San's Caramel Cereal Coffee to make Postum. Post denied it, and the charge was never proved.

One thing that is certain is that Post was among the first to make use of nationwide mass-market advertising, selling Postum not just as a beverage but as a health aid—this at a time when few foods of any kind were heavily advertised on a national scale. By 1904, nine years after he introduced Postum,

TROUBLE'S BREWING

In his zeal to sell Postum, C.W. Post asked these rhetorical questions of coffee-drinkers: "Is your yellow streak the coffee habit? Does it reduce your working time, kill your energy, push you into the big crowd of mongrels, deaden what thoroughbred blood you may have and neutralize all your efforts to make money and fame?"

Post's corporate successor, General Foods, continued to question coffee drinkers' moral fiber and stamina until 1951, when, by agreement with the Federal Trade Commission, the company altered its advertising so it would not imply that coffee brews ". . . divorces, business failures, factory accidents, juvenile delinquency, traffic accidents, fire or home foreclosures. . . ."

Post was budgeting one million dollars a year for advertising.

Grape-Nuts, introduced in 1898, was Post's second product. Then, as now, Grape-Nuts was a granulated cereal that, despite its name, contained neither grapes nor nuts. The small size of the original package came about, Post ads confided, because the product was "concentrated." Those same ads proclaimed Grape-Nuts "the most scientific food in the world." They also claimed an impressive variety of medicinal powers for the ready-to-eat cereal, among them that it helped combat consumption, malaise, loose teeth, and appendicitis.

In 1906, Post introduced his cornflakes, Elijah's Manna. He changed the name to the more prosaic Post Toasties when consumers in England and the American Bible Belt complained that the name was sacrilegious.

In copy he often wrote himself, Post pioneered the use of epigrammatic, repetitive prose in advertisements, using plain language instead of the flowery phrases then in vogue. Only his medical claims were extravagant. Post Toasties, he wrote, "makes red blood." To potential buyers of Grape-Nuts, he confided "There's a reason." The wily pitchman never said what the reason was.

Post's devotion to advertising brought him trouble in 1911, when *Collier's Weekly,* a leading magazine, attacked the cereal maker for implying that eating Grape-Nuts would make surgery for appendicitis unnecessary. This claim, *Collier's* editorialized, "is lying, and potentially dangerous lying." Post struck back by spending 15 thousand dollars to buy newspaper ads arguing that *Collier's* editors were just angry because he wouldn't buy advertising in their magazine. *Collier's* sued Post for libel. With Condé Nast, namesake of the modern magazine group, who served as *Collier's* ad manager, testifying against Post, the magazine won a 50 thousand-dollar verdict.

Appendicitis would return to pain Post in ways he probably didn't foresee. But for the most part he was riding high. Post netted three million dollars as early as 1900. He built a theater in downtown Battle Creek, named an office block after his daughter Marjorie, planted public gardens, and built Postumville, a housing project for his employees. Living the life of the wealthy grandee, Post maintained homes in Washington, D.C. and Santa Barbara, California, and opened offices in New York and London.

His hard-hitting ads, as well as his products and philanthropy, kept Charles William Post in the public eye. Rare among food manufacturers, he took out ads in favor of the 1906 Pure Food and Drug Act, feeling that his clean factories and healthful foods were things to be proud of. His public policy advertisments made no mention of Post's products, but won their creator plenty of public attention.

CEREAL WARS

Meanwhile, back at the Battle Creek Sanitarium, William Keith Kellogg was steaming. Alone among the Big-Three cereal makers, he was still without wealth, still taking orders. By taking a cue from Post's success, the younger Kellogg argued, he and Dr. John could turn their Sanitas Food Company, long subordinate to the sanitarium, into the tail that wagged the dog. But the older Kellogg, sensing danger to his medical standing by mass-marketing foods, still said no.

"IT'S ALL IN THE SHREDS"

For all their fortune and fame, neither the Kellogg brothers nor C.W. Post invented the first successful pre-cooked cereal. That distinction went to Henry D. Perky, a Denver tinkerer and former Nebraska state legislator who baked—rather than flaked— wheat in 1893 to come up with Shredded Wheat. J.H. Kellogg had a chance to buy the rights to the product, but Perky's asking price, 100,000 dollars, was too high. Shredded Wheat, now made by RJR Nabisco, became a healthy success with Perky's reassuring slogan "It's all in the shreds."

Besides, Dr. Kellogg was doing quite well as he was. As the San grew larger, it also grew away from the precepts, and the control, of the Seventh-day Adventist Church. "The grand display you are making," admonished Sister White, "is not after God's order." Sister White ominously prophesized that "a sword of fire" would descend on the sanitarium. In 1902, one did; in a fire of mysterious origin, the San burned to the ground.

It was rebuilt larger and grander than ever, and control was finally wrested away from the Adventists. In 1907, J.H. Kellogg was expelled from the church, but that was just a formality. The San was his, and when he wasn't holding forth on roughage and hydropathy, he was off in New York and Europe, playing the great man.

It was during one of Dr. Kellogg's journeys to Europe that Will, then 46 and desperate to make his mark, made his move. He added sugar to the cornflakes that he and the doctor had developed a decade before and found consumers liked the taste of a presweetened cereal. Adding sugar was very much against John Harvey's wishes, as was substituting the starchy kernel for the whole corn, but those two changes transformed the original thick, somewhat flavorless Kellogg's cornflakes into the product we know today.

When J.H. returned, he was furious, but it hardly mattered. Will Keith, 46 years in the wilderness, outmaneuvered his brother, snapping up the stock of their Sanitas Food Company. In 1906, he incorporated the Battle Creek Toasted Corn Flake Company, the forerunner of today's Kellogg Company, and began turning out cornflakes in a barn that was soon too small to hold the growing concern.

W.K. Kellogg, emulating Post, plunged into advertising. He sank one-third of his life savings into a single, spectacular full-page ad in the *Ladies' Home Journal*. It was a bold move that paid off. Many more were to follow.

Will's wrinkle was to sell his cornflakes for their taste, not their health-giving properties, to make

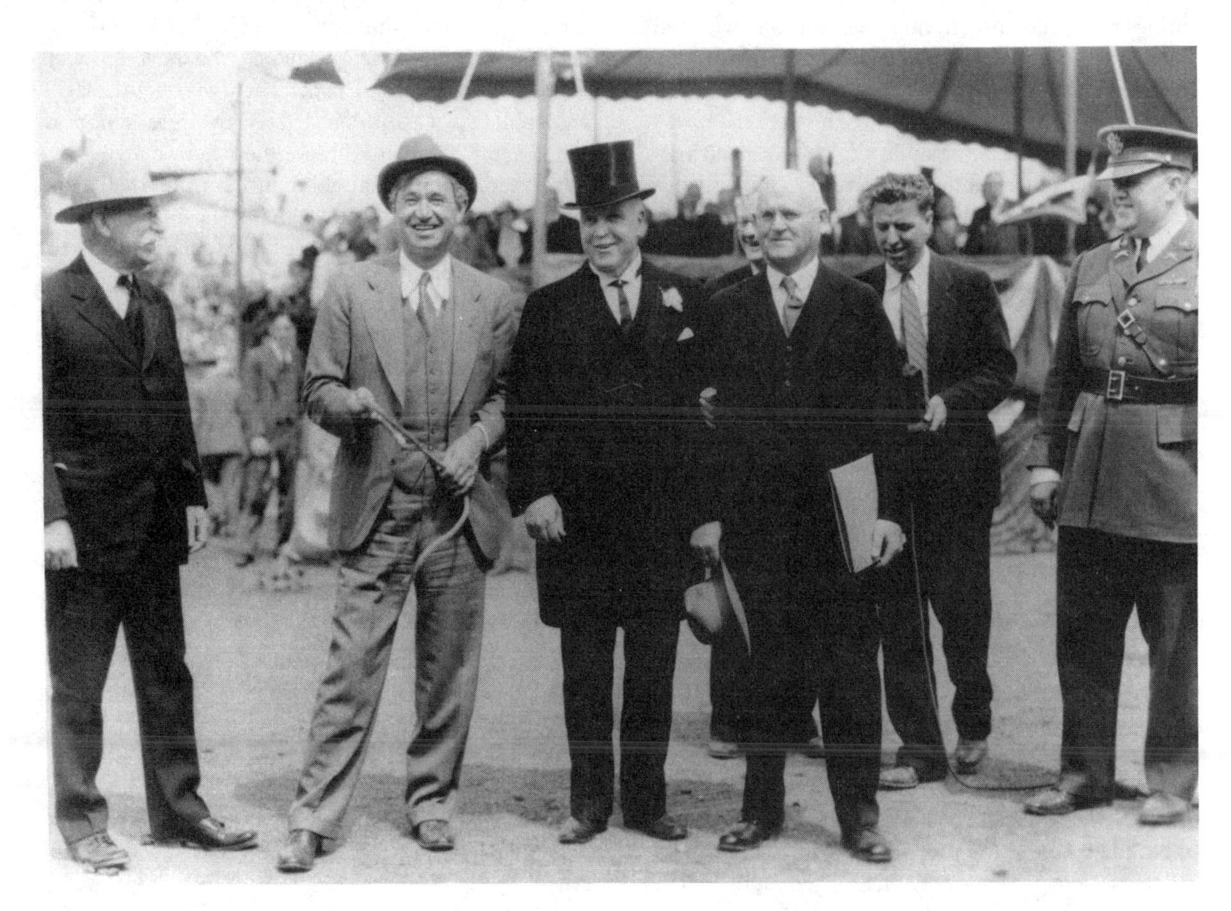

50. A success at last, a bare-headed William Keith Kellogg, fourth from left, hobnobbed with celebrities. Michigan Governor Rolph, in the top hat, is next to humorist Will Rogers. *Courtesy, Historical Society of Battle Creek.*

people want to buy them, not do so out of a sense of duty. That turned the booming health-food industry on its head, and it was just the beginning.

W.K. had his salesmen tramping door-to-door, handing out free samples. He produced appetizing photographs of food in four-color process, commonplace today but revolutionary at the time. He introduced contests and games and photographed a wholesome-looking young woman whom he christened "The Sweetheart of the Corn" to represent the company. He commissioned the world's largest electric sign, in Times Square. According to *Cornflake Crusade,* "the sign showed a small boy's face and the word 'Kellogg's.' When the words 'I want' appeared, tears rolled down the boy's face. Then the spectacular flashed 'I got' and the boy stopped crying."

Eventually, Will Kellogg, too, became a multimillionaire. His belated success engendered resentment from John Harvey, now forced to share the limelight. The older brother sued the younger for control of the company. In 1916, the case was decided in favor of Will, who, while on the witness stand, spoke bitterly of the man who had dominated him during the years of striving and unacknowledged creativity: "I have never claimed any glory, the doctor has claimed that."

But the Kellogg company was his. On the boxes of cereal appeared a facsimile of W.K.'s handwriting. "Beware of imitations," it read. "None genuine without this signature. W.K. Kellogg."

BOOMING BATTLE CREEK

The precaution was essential, for Battle Creek, in the early years of the twentieth century, was a carnival of commerce. The town of 30 thousand was jammed with hustlers trying to cash in on the fame of the cereal kings, Kellogg and Post. Like California's Silicon Valley some 75 years later, Battle Creek was filled with start-up companies, many of them not above industrial spying to steal the state-of-the-art manufacturing technology of established rivals. Eventually, an industry-wide shake-out spared only a few.

But, in 1904, no fewer than 44 firms made cereal in Battle Creek, or claimed to. Some operated from sheds and tents. Some were mainly stock-selling schemes. Some sent salesmen to meet incoming trains, scouring the passengers for investors. And some weren't even located in Battle Creek, but pretended to be, the better to cash in on the town's commercial cachet. Malta-Vita, Maple-Flakes, Food of Eden, and Cero-Fruto are just a few of these long-forgotten trade names.

HEALTH MECCA

Battle Creek became such a health Mecca in the early years of the twentieth century that railroads made all through tickets in Michigan valid for stopovers there, and the telegraph designation for the San was simply "Health." The small southeastern Michigan city remains a popular tourist destination. Some 6.5 million visitors toured the Kellogg's cereal-making plant from 1906 until 1986, when the Kellogg Company, in an echo of the early cereal wars, closed the plant to the public, saying that competitors were taking the tour to steal technological secrets.

Remarked Dr. Kellogg acidly, "The picture of Battle Creek as a health center has made this an attractive place for the operations of various charlatans, and not the least pretentious and predatory of these are the numerous food charlatans . . . posing as experts and discoverers."

In spite of the hyperbole surrounding the new cereals, and the imminent failure of most of their makers, there was real value in the new products pouring out of Battle Creek. They were light, easily prepared, and easily digested. They were simple to store, and—especially before they were heavily presweetened—were admirably nutritious alternatives to the salt-pork and whiskey breakfasts of the past. If they didn't live up to the medicinal claims made for them—and what foods could?—the new cereals set standards of cleanliness and safety unique in the preregulation age.

Their chief manufacturers, the Big Three cereal makers, stood astride the intertwined worlds of health and food. William Keith Kellogg, a success at last, showed the world that he was a businessman to be reckoned with. John Harvey Kellogg still had the San, and it was no small concern.

In the early twentieth century, the sprawling spa was visited by dozens of prominent people, among them President William Howard Taft, tennis star Bill Tilden, Dale Carnegie, Thomas Edison, and George Bernard Shaw. Olympic swimming champion and movie Tarzan Johnny Weismuller dedicated the San's swimming pool, and the famous aviator Amelia Earhart flew Dr. Kellogg over the 27-acre grounds, the facilities for 1,500 guests. A 15-story luxury tower was added some time after the original San burned down.

The most high-profile of the cereal kings was C.W. Post. Vitriolic anti-union broadsides, which he

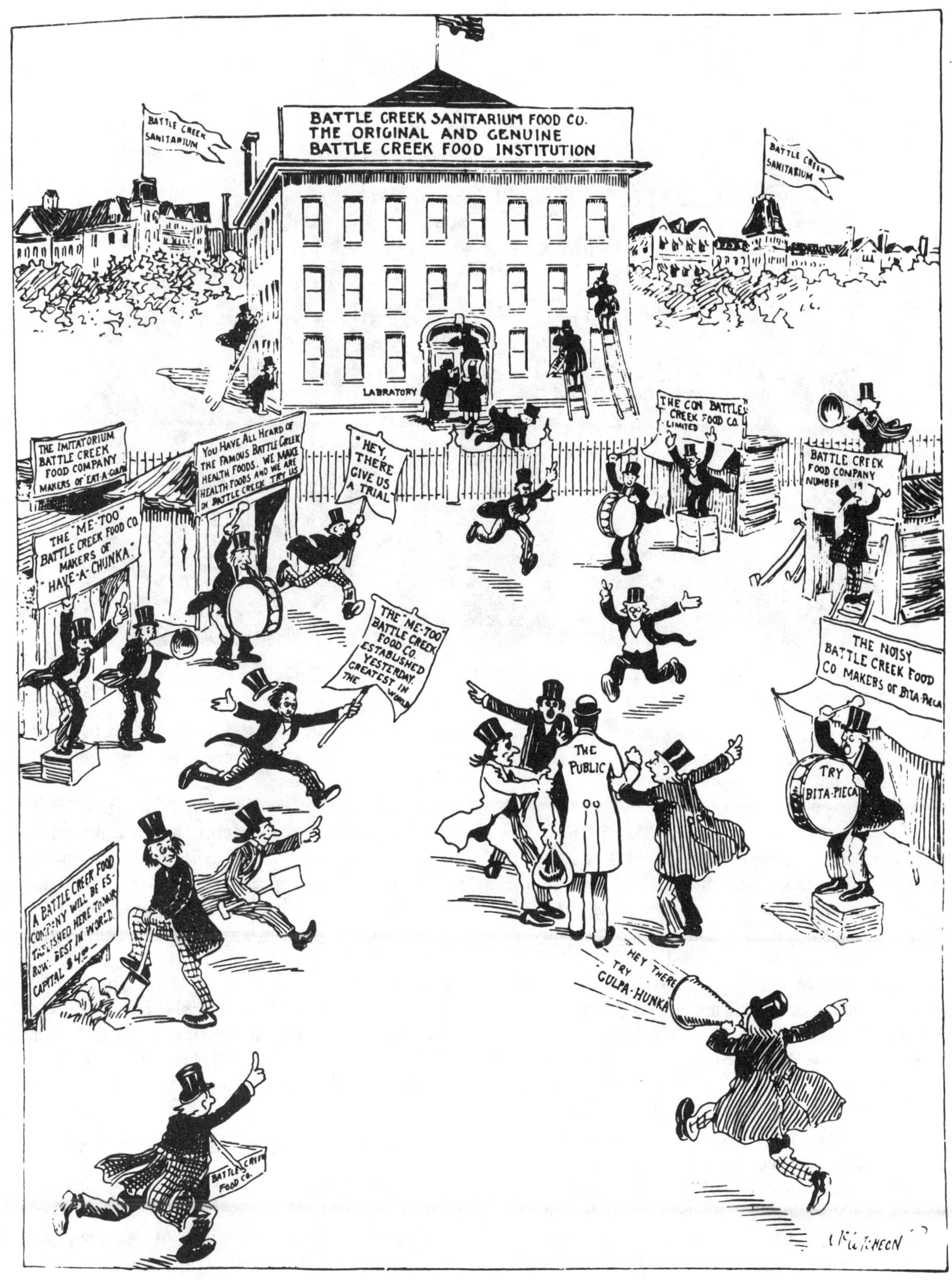
BATTLE CREEK SANITARIUM FOOD CO.
THE ORIGINAL AND GENUINE
BATTLE CREEK FOOD INSTITUTION
BATTLE CREEK SANITARIUM
BATTLE CREEK SANITARIUM
LABRATORY
THE IMITATORIUM BATTLE CREEK FOOD COMPANY MAKERS OF EAT-A-
YOU HAVE ALL HEARD OF THE FAMOUS BATTLE CREEK HEALTH FOODS. WE MAKE HEALTH FOODS AND WE ARE IN BATTLE CREEK TRY US
"HEY, THERE GIVE US A TRIAL"
THE CON BATTLE CREEK FOOD CO. LIMITED
BATTLE CREEK FOOD COMPANY NUMBER 19
THE "ME-TOO" BATTLE CREEK FOOD CO. MAKERS OF "HAVE-A-CHUNKA."
THE "ME-TOO" BATTLE CREEK FOOD CO. ESTABLISHED YESTERDAY. GREATEST IN THE WORLD
THE NOISY BATTLE CREEK FOOD CO MAKERS OF BITA-PIECA
TRY BITA-PIECA
THE PUBLIC
A BATTLE CREEK FOOD COMPANY WILL BE ES- TABLISHED HERE TOMOR- ROW. BEST IN WORLD. CAPITAL $4.00
HEY THERE TRY GULPA-HUNKA
BATTLE CREEK FOOD CO.

51. The *Chicago Tribune* lampooned cerealmania, Battle Creek style. *Drawing by John T. McCutcheon © Chicago Tribune Company, all rights reserved, used with permission.*

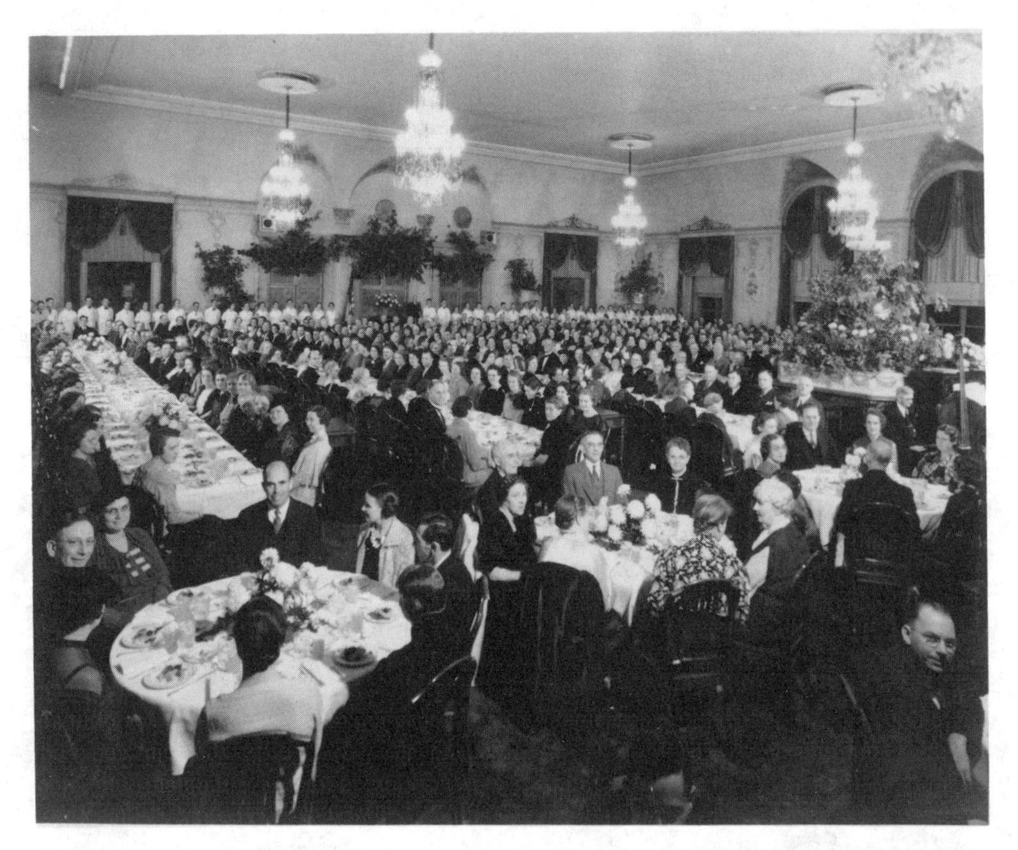

52. Early twentieth-century dining at the San was no spartan affair. *Courtesy, Historical Society of Battle Creek.*

wrote in signed, paid ads in major newspapers, kept him in the public eye, as did his marriage to his secretary, Leila Young, 20 years his junior, in 1904, after Post divorced his first wife.

For the most part, Post had been riding high since his first big success in 1895 with Postum. But in 1914, high drama intervened in the form of his old adversary, appendicitis—the very disease for which Post's ads recommended spoonfuls of Grape-Nuts.

C.W.'s young wife declined to place her faith in cereal. She chartered a special train to rush Post from his Santa Barbara winter home to the Mayo Brothers' Clinic in Rochester, Minnesota. The tracks were cleared for the food magnate's dramatic dash across the continent, a second engine following the train in case the first one failed. The Mayo brothers operated on Post, with apparent success. He returned in the plushly appointed train to Santa Barbara.

However, Post did not fully recover his health, and the melancholia that marked his early life returned. On May 10, 1914, alone in his bedroom, C.W. Post placed the muzzle of a rifle in his mouth and pulled the trigger with his toe. His nurse found the body. He was 59.

The one-time suspenders salesman left an estate of 33 million dollars, most of which went to his daughter, Marjorie. His widow, described in a wire service report as "a very beautiful young woman," settled for a much lesser amount, married the manager of a tavern she owned, and slipped from public view. Marjorie was another story. Married four times, including a union with stockbroker E.F. Hutton, with whom she shared a 54-room New York mansion, Marjorie Merriweather Post became a Palm Springs socialite and owner of a precious collection of art and antiques. When she died at age 86 in 1974, she left a fortune valued at 250 million dollars. Her 118-room Palm Springs palace, Mar-a-Lago, became a showcase possession of billionaire developer Donald Trump, who called it "the most spectacular place anywhere in the world."

THE MODERN-DAY CEREAL KINGS

The Postum Cereal Company survived its star-crossed founder and, in 1925, merged with the Jello-O Company. In 1929, it became part of the mammoth General Foods Corporation.

Post's death left the Battle Creek spotlight to the Kelloggs, both of whom continued their work for a long time. J.H. lived 29 more years and Will Keith another 37.

POST CITY, TEXAS: THE FORGOTTEN DREAM

C.W. Post's quirkiest adventure outside of his cereal business had to be Post City, a godforsaken stretch of prairie in the Texas panhandle that Post purchased for 750 thousand dollars and on which he tried to erect what the *American Mercury* called a "personal city-state." Post took applications from would-be residents of his magic kingdom, screening them for health habits and morals. He built bungalows on the land and even selected the wallpaper himself. He built a hotel, the Post City Hotel.

On tables in the hotel restaurant, near the glass bowls of Grape-Nuts, he placed a card. It read: "The rate in this hotel is $2.50 a day. There are plenty of good boarding houses in town and plenty of room in the mesquite. Four-flushers, kickers and other suspicious characters find board with the sheriff. When in doubt, hit the mesquite."

Then he tried to make rain. Post got the idea from reading accounts of Civil War battles said to be followed by rainstorms. He figured that the heavy artillery called down the deluge, and wanted to do the same in the parched country surrounding Post City. So in 1911 and 1912, he lined up dozens of men to set off large stores of dynamite, some of it donated by the DuPont Company in return for the publicity. In all, he tried 23 times. It rained a few times in the vicinity of the explosions, and Post was quick to claim credit. Once, he even got a congratulatory telegram from his friend President William Howard Taft. Most often, though, the merciless Texas sun kept shining.

His community, now known simply as Post, still stands, though it has long ceased to be a company town. With a population of about 4,000 in the late 1980s, Post is the center of an area rich in fossils up to 225 million years old. It's still as dry as a boneyard.

When he wasn't presiding over the San, John Harvey Kellogg lectured the nation on sex. He was against it. Kellogg admonished parents to catch their children in the act of self-abuse and punish them accordingly. He wrote a 504-page screed, *Plain Facts,* about the dangers of sex. In one passage, Dr. Kellogg described the unchaste response of a young woman dancing the waltz with a young man:

> The mere anticipation fluttered my pulse; and when my partner approached to claim my promised hand for the dance, I felt my cheeks glow a little sometimes, and I could not look him in the eye with the same frank gayety as before.
>
> But the climax of my confusion was reached when, folded in his warm embrace, and giddy with the whirl, a strange, sweet thrill would shake me from head to foot, leaving me weak and almost powerless, and really almost obliged to depend on support upon the arm which encircled me.

John Harvey practiced what he preached. He and Ella kept separate apartments and never consumated their 41-year marriage. They were generous to children, supporting 42 youngsters in need and adopting some of them.

Dr. Kellogg also wrote and lectured widely on the danger of "race suicide," by which he meant the human race. He blamed decline on civilization and its discontents, particularly poor diet. Warning, too, of "that most subtle of all enslaving drugs, cocaine," Kellogg advocted a regimen of "daily cold water and air baths, swimming, work in the gymnasium, wearing of light and porous clothing and frequent changes of underwear."

Dr. Kellogg also established a Race Betterment Foundation, and urged that a registry be created for

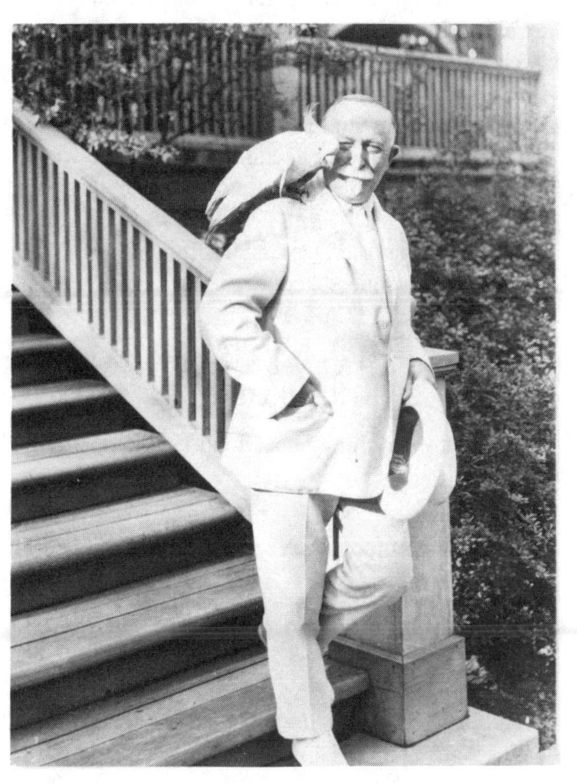

53. John Harvey Kellogg with avian friend—white, to match the doctor's attire. *Courtesy, Battle Creek Adventist Hospital.*

healthy people so that superior marriages and offspring would result. These ideas, which he later dropped, smacked of the discredited pseudoscience of eugenics.

Dr. Kellogg occasionally made news in his last years. In the 1930s, he flew to the bedside of the struggling Dionne quintuplets with soy acidophilus milk for a digestive disorder. At the age of 91, he gave an interview to the Associated Press, attributing his longevity to following the healthy precepts of biologic living. "I have done pretty well for a grass eater," he said. "Man was intended to eat the plants and fruits and not the animals. I haven't touched meat for more than 75 years."

To his last days, John Harvey Kellogg maintained his all-white attire, down to the ever-present white cockatoo he carried on his shoulder. On December 14, 1943, J.H. died of pneumonia. He was 91.

John's brother Will, who survived him, had long since perfected the allied arts of making cereal and making money. In 1915, the younger Kellogg made headlines by driving to the capital of every state in the union in a 37-foot-long automobile constructed for that very purpose. The newspapers described the car as "equipped more modernly than most apartments," and dubbed the huge vehicle Kellogg's "ark."

Will Keith did not indulge himself endlessly, however. In 1930, after a sobering experience in which he had difficulty obtaining medical care for a disabled grandson, W.K. endowed the W.K. Kellogg Foundation with 50 million dollars. Its mission was to bring health care to children around the world. The foundation now has assets of more than one billion dollars.

Even during the Depression of the 1930s, Will, then in his seventies, kept cranking out new products. He built a reputation as a benevolent patriarch by refusing to install machines he said would throw employees out of work, organized four six-hour shifts so that he could employ more people, and actually increased his advertising budget. Yet this hard-charging, complex man, who could be kind to others, had a demanding side, too. In 1938, his grandson, John L. Kellogg, Jr., reportedly under intense pressure to measure up to his famous grandfather, took his own life at age 26.

W.K. survived his brother John by eight years. He lived until October 6, 1951, a flesh-and-blood link to the fierce battles of the cereal revolution. He died of circulatory disease at 91, the same age as John Harvey.

The Kellogg name has, of course, survived the remarkable Kellogg brothers, and even the Battle Creek Sanitarium has survived, after a fashion. Some of the San's historic buildings still stand. Ironically, the San, after passing through many hands, is now a Seventh-day Adventist acute-care hospital, having come full circle with its origins of more than a century ago.

The Kellogg Company is the largest cereal corporation in the world. In 1989, it sold 2.5 billion dollars worth of breakfast cereal in the United States; all told, 38 percent of American cereal sales belong to Kellogg, which sells cereal in 130 countries. The company has continued to follow the path W.K.

THINK WHAT HE COULD HAVE DONE HAD HE HAD MORE TIME

Just about everything about John Harvey Kellogg was prolific.

- He was a physician for 68 of his 91 years, during which time he performed 22 thousand surgical operations.
- His 50 books sold a combined total of one million copies. The longest of his tomes ran to 1,689 pages.
- Kellogg's book *The New Dietetics* made philosopher Will Durant's list of the 100 best books of all time.

BOWLED OVER

The breakfast cereal industry, which started so humbly so long ago in Battle Creek, now coaxes seven billion dollars a year from American consumers. Americans eat an average of 10 pounds of breakfast cereals per year, the most in history. Cereal consumption tops out in Pittsburgh, where the annual average is 13 pounds per person.

The industry is still engaged in health battles. In 1988, Omaha businessman Phil Sokolof made news with a two-million-dollar public relations offensive that convinced the food giants, including Kellogg's, to stop using high-fat tropical oils in their cereals. The next year, the Kellogg Company was embroiled in another controversy when it introduced Heartwise, a cereal with psyllium fiber. Officials in several states pulled the product off the shelves, charging that advertising on the package implied, without proof, that Heartwise could prevent heart disease.

blazed with mass-market advertising. It sponsored popular children's programs such as ''Howdy Doody'' and ''Captain Kangaroo'' on television only a few years after its founder's death and created the popular Tony the Tiger animated character.

In 1985, *Forbes* magazine quoted Kellogg chairman William E. LaMothe, a former cornflakes salesman, as saying the firm planned to hark back to its founders by emphasizing the healthfulness of its products as alternatives to the bacon and eggs on American breakfast tables.

''This is our thing,'' LaMothe told the magazine. ''Dr. Kellogg and Mr. Kellogg were going on either intuition or their basic beliefs coming out of a Seventh-day Adventist background, where they believed that meats were not healthful for the diet.'' In the future, said the chairman, Kellogg's would emphasize ''the whole grain . . . healthy lifestyles . . . avoidance of major disease in the Western world . . . more grains, fruits and vegetables.''

There is still plenty of nonnutritious sugar in Kellogg's cereals, of course, including, very briefly, a product called S.W. Graham, a ready-to-eat cereal named after Sylvester Graham. The heavily sweetened product, promoted as a comforting return to traditional goodness, flopped in the marketplace. But Kellogg's has also come up with a successful line of whole-grain cereals called Nutri-Grain that John H. himself might have approved of. General Foods, Post's corporate descendent, made a similar return to its roots in the mid-1980s with a cereal designed to appeal to the burgeoning health market. Its name: C.W. Post.

CHAPTER · 13 ·

HORACE FLETCHER: THE GREAT MASTICATOR

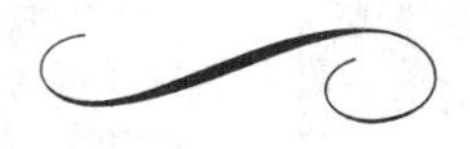

Don't gobble your food, but "Fletcherize"/Each morsel you eat, if you be wise/Don't cause your blood pressure e'er to rise/By prizing your menu by its size.

From the Ladies' Home Journal, *1914*

He was an epicure who once lived entirely on potatoes, a millionaire world traveler who gave up business in middle age to save the world by demonstrating the proper way to chew, and a short, portly man who avoided regular exercise but bested top college athletes in feats of strength. He was the confidant of captains of industry, the author of influential books, the subject of admiring profiles in the popular press and scientific journals, and the food guru for the most illustrious men of his time. His name, said an acolyte, would rival that of Pasteur.

Today, virtually no one remembers him.

Pink-cheeked, cherubic, and apparently always happy, he is barely a footnote in time. Yet historians credit him with proving that healthy people can thrive on only one-third of the protein that conventional wisdom once prescribed. More colorfully, if less significantly, he is also regarded as the man who finally persuaded Americans to drop their generations-old habit of "gobble, gulp and go"—the super-fast bolting of food that created a nation of bewildered dyspeptics and made American table manners the worst since the days of the Visigoths and Vandals.

THE BON VIVANT

Horace Fletcher was born in Lawrence, Massachusetts in 1849, but did not stay around his hometown for long. At 16, eager to see the world, he left for Japan on a whaling ship. Later, he prepped at Andover and attended Dartmouth, but the halls of academe couldn't contain him. As a young man, he lived for six years in Japan, becoming one of the first Westerners to spend an appreciable amount of time there. The experience made him a lifelong Japanophile. When he returned home, he imported Japanese art, toys, and novelties and sold printer's ink for a living. By age 40, he was rich.

A man of virtually limitless energy and eclectic tastes, Fletcher claimed to have circled the world four times by his fortieth birthday, as well as crossed the Pacific 16 times and traversed the North American continent 38 times—all before the age of aviation. He made the Atlantic crossing so many times that he neglected to keep count.

Fletcher claimed to have had 38 occupations, including the directorship of a French opera company and the presidency of the Philharmonic Society of New Orleans. An intensely social being, he was co-founder of the Bohemian Club, whose wealthy members, then as now, gathered yearly under the redwoods on the Russian River 70 miles north of San Francisco to "network" and put on amateur skits. Fletcher became an accomplished amateur painter, marksman, and athlete. He apparently exhibited his characteristic serenity from the beginning;

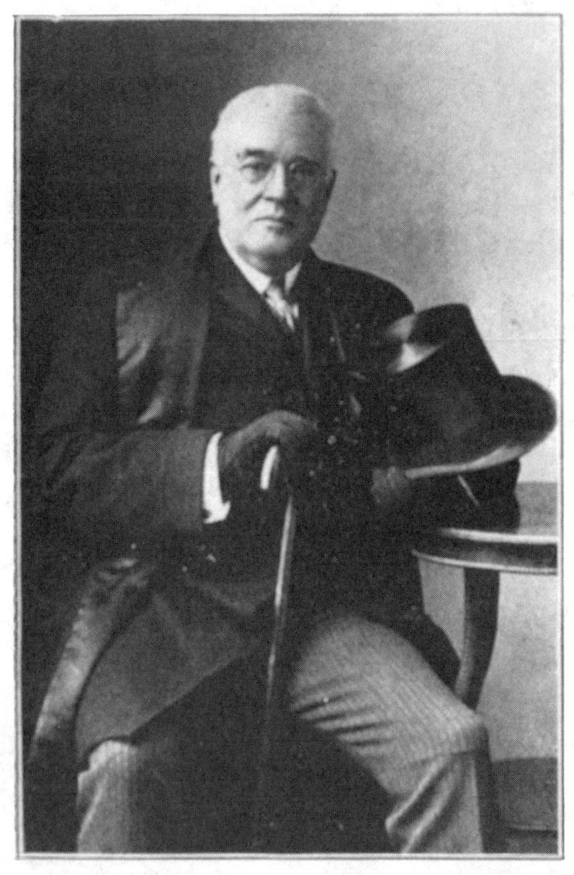

54. Correct chewing was not a hardship for its apostle, the prosperous Horace Fletcher. *From* New England Monthly, July 1906.

his childhood nicknames were Buddha and Old Fletch.

Fletcher's globe-trotting was all the more impressive in an age of glacially slow transportation. "He refers to such remote spots as the Vale of Cashmere as casually as New Yorkers talk of Bronx Park," marveled a magazine writer about his peripatetic subject. When Fletcher married, he settled in a typically exotic locale: a thirteenth-century palace in Venice. Fletcher's abode, wrote a contemporary, "is on the best part of the Grand Canal, and the house is noted for its lavish hospitality."

As befitted a man of his sophistication, Fletcher was an epicure, and by all accounts a charmer. Outgoing but dignified, with white hair and eyeglasses, he was photographed in 1906 for the *New England Monthly* seated at an elegant table and holding a top hat and walking stick. The caption identifies him as an "Apostle of Correct Nutrition."

THE CRISIS

Despite his successes, the excesses of his hedonistic life caught up with Fletcher at an early age. By 40, his hair had turned white and this one-time athlete had gone to fat, packing 217 pounds on his five-foot-seven-inch frame. Noted a contemporary:

> Without ever sinking into dissipation, he enjoyed for several years what is conventionally regarded as a good time. And this existence had precisely the same effect on Mr. Fletcher that it is now having upon thousands of other Americans. It found its outward expression in the protuberant abdomen, the pendant cheeks, the puffy eyes, and the wrinkled neck which seem to have become the stigmata of a prosperous business career.

In short, the good times were killing Fletcher. He hit bottom at age 44, when he applied for a life-insurance policy and was turned down.

The crisis propelled Fletcher in a new direction. Fletcher soon aligned himself with what the philosopher William James, in his classic *The Varieties of Religious Experience,* referred to as "New Thought." In a chapter called "The Religion of Healthy-Mindedness," James quoted Fletcher's early writing and observed that "The leaders in this faith have had an almost intuitive belief in the all-saving power of healthy-mindedness."

The description fit Fletcher to a T. Always an optimist, a doer, and a believer in the cult of efficient management that characterized the Progressive Era, Fletcher became a happy warrior in the battle against ill health. Leaving his business career behind, Fletcher took the first step in his new life, homing in on what a later generation would call stress management.

Fletcher published a book called *Menticulture* in 1895, in which he argued that poor health is the result of poor attitudes. Anger and worry, he wrote, cause disease and constitute a violation of natural law that calls for people to be happy. Wrote Fletcher: "I could no more harbor any of the thievery and depressing influences that once I nursed as a heritage of humanity than a fop would voluntarily wallow in a filthy gutter."

Three years later, in 1898, Fletcher wrote another book. In *Happiness as Found in Forethought Minus Fearthought,* Fletcher—who never had much flair for book titles—submitted that those twin threats, anger and worry, are caused by fear. Do away with fear and you can do away with disease. So confident was Fletcher of his new, can-do philosophy that he advocated mind cures for everything from gout to insanity.

Things were definitely looking up for Horace Fletcher. His biggest discoveries, and the theory for which followers appropriated his name, lay just ahead.

FLETCHERISM AND THE SECRET OF LIFE

Mulling the implications of his mind-cure arguments, Fletcher grounded his philosophy in the physical, specifically in food. Having regained his confidence—while still retaining his extra pounds five years after that fateful insurance exam—Fletcher decided that his "troubles came from too much of many things, among them too much food and too much worry."

As he recalled in his 1903 book, *The A.B.-Z. of Our Own Nutrition,* "We are told that most, if not all, of the diseases which pain, worry and afflict us are caused by indigestion or mal-assimilation of food. . . ." Poor assimilation, Fletcher concluded, came about because people didn't chew their food properly; after all, digestion begins in the mouth. Never one to do things halfway, Fletcher proposed a theory of mastication that he joined to his optimistic outlook.

In Fletcher's reckoning, the presence of saliva—"the watering of the mouth," as he called it—signaled the advent of a true or "earned" appetite. Saliva is needed to mix food in the mouth. One mixes food by chewing but not by chewing just any old way.

Fletcher recommended chewing food until the last hint of flavor disappeared, at which time the Swallowing Impulse (Fletcher capitalized the term) would take over, and the liquified food would automatically slide down the gullet. Any food that was not swallowed in this manner was, perforce, stopped by the Food Filter, an invisible organ at the back of the mouth. The Food Filter was put there by an all-knowing and beneficent Nature to keep her children from swallowing food that the stomach could not digest. Discreetly spitting said food into a napkin would prevent malassimilation and thus forestall disease.

Fletcher's rules for proper nutrition were:

> (1) Never eat except when "good and hungry."
>
> (2) Never eat when worried badly or angry.
>
> (3) Eat only what really tastes good to you.
>
> (4) Exhaust all of the good taste from all food. . . . Don't swallow any food until first it is like a pulp in your mouth and has been fully tasted. When this is so the food will swallow itself.
>
> (5) Leave a little bit of the appetite as a "nest egg" for the next meal.
>
> (6) Eat always somewhat less than what you can; but eat what you do a little more, and so get far better results in the way of both pleasure and nutrition. It isn't how much you eat that does you good, it is how you eat what you do eat.
>
> (7) If you have only five minutes in which to eat, and do not expect to have another chance for a long time, don't hurry. . . . A small amount of food thoroughly masticated is better than much more which is swallowed unmasticated.

That was all there was to it. There was no prescribed number of chews, and there were no restrictions on what enlightened chewers could eat.

Proper chewing—the process came to be known as "Fletcherizing," a term credited to Dr. John Harvey Kellogg—did entail a few additional details. Foods should be held in the mouth for at least 30 seconds after they were liquefied, advised the master masticator, who added: "Industrious munching performs about 100 acts of mastication to the minute, and from 12 to 15 mouthfuls of ordinary food is sufficient to satisfy completely a hearty appetite."

Dining in the prescribed Fletcher manner could be socially disenfranchising, to be sure. Since Fletcher advised eating only when hungry, the true Fletcherite might not take meals when everyone else did. Then, too, chewing food until it was liquefied took time and concentration, which made Fletcherites rather subdued dining companions. Social isolation was a small price to pay, however. Fletcher held in contempt eaters who threw back their food "in the same manner in which a man usually packs a trunk."

In the early stage of his transformation, during the summer of 1898, Fletcher used himself as his own chief guinea pig. Chewing slowly, cheerfully, thoroughly, he found he ate less food and was satisfied with simpler fare than the gourmet treasures he had long been accustomed to; meats and rich sauces no longer appealed to him. From June to October, Fletcher's weight, which had bedeviled him for years, dropped from 205 to 163, a hefty loss of 42 pounds.

As his new regimen took hold, Fletcher discovered that he could easily get by on about 1,600 calories, only one-third the number recommended by

THE LITTLE SHALLOT

Even an expert masticator like Fletcher occasionally had trouble chewing. One stubborn shallot, he reported, required 722 chews before disappearing. "After the tussle, however," Fletcher reported with pride, "the young onion left no odour upon the breath and joined the happy family in the stomach."

medical authorities at the turn of the twentieth century, when 3,500 to 4,500 calories were considered essential.

Although Fletcher devised his approach to improve his own health, he believed it would also improve the health of society in general. Families would spend less money on the simpler foods favored by Fletcherism, and those foods would take less time to prepare.

Most important, if people really began to taste their food and draw all the necessary nutrients from their meals, the human race would be more productive, more efficient. Fletcher lamented that "indigestion and the American plague, dyspepsia, work their evils slowly but surely to cut off our best men and loveliest women in their prime and to rob us of their richest product and their maturest wisdom."

Once determined only to save himself, Fletcher now felt called upon to save the world. "So strong is the conviction of the author that he possess fundamental truth . . . ," wrote Fletcher in *The New Glutton or Epicure,* another of his didactic books, "that where it is seemingly desirable to employ unusual means to attract attention, he feels compelled to do so."

HEAD OF THE CLASS

Fletcher soon found his unusual means of attracting attention. He volunteered for (and often underwrote) batteries of tests at institutions of higher learning, aiming to prove that positive thinking and proper chewing lead to robust health. Fletcher passed the tests with flying colors, amazing his proctors and converting several of them.

Fletcher performed feats of strength and endurance that were astounding, not just for a man his age—he was past 50—but any age. Matched against much younger competitors, the Great Masticator, as Fletcher came to be called, always outclassed them.

Fletcher had performed well before. On the Fourth of July, 1899, while vacationing in France, Fletcher raced 100 miles through the countryside outside Paris on a new contraption called a bicycle, easily outpacing his companion, a 30-year-old American painter who fancied himself in good condition. After making what wheelmen called "a century run" in a day, Fletcher said that he was barely winded. He wasn't even sore the next day. The feat sparked in him "the ambition to see what really could be done . . . ."

The following year, Fletcher interested his personal physician, Dr. Ernest Van Someren, in his radical new ideas. Van Someren, visiting Fletcher's Venice home, tried the regimen himself, felt great, and delivered a fulsome paper in 1901 to the British Medical Association, sparking interest in Fletcher. The British professor of physiology Sir Michael Foster invited Fletcher to Cambridge University for a closer look. Fletcher, full of brio, accepted.

At Cambridge, where Foster and Frederick Gowland Hopkins, a future Nobel Prize winner for vitamin research, observed Fletcher in 1902, several medical staffers took up Fletcherizing. Foster reported "an immediate and very striking effect upon appetite, making this more discriminating, and leading to the choice of a simple dietary, and, in particular, reducing the craving for flesh foods." Foster added that the new regimen, tried for only a few weeks, should be tested by more subjects and at greater length.

Next on Fletcher's itinerary was Yale University, where he was examined in 1903 by Russell H. Chittenden (1856–1943), a distinguished professor of physiological chemistry. Chittenden carried out his work at Yale's Sheffield Scientific School and the Yale gymnasium, where William G. Anderson, a medical doctor and one of the leading lights in American physical culture, supervised the workouts.

Fletcher did the same exercises given to varsity crew members, and handled them with ease. In fact, Fletcher did so well that his performance prompted Chittenden to rethink the minimum daily requirement for protein, regarded as crucial for muscle development. Chittenden began to believe that perhaps Fletcher's 45 daily grams were closer to actual needs than the 118 to 165 grams then generally recommended.

Chittenden designed a study that compared sedentary Yale professors with physically active college athletes. For a group in between those two extremes, he secured the services of 20 U.S. Army men and assigned them to live on a low-protein diet, as Fletcher did. The soldiers were, Chittenden recalled, "at first rather hostile" when they learned that their rations would be cut by two-thirds. Three of the men deserted when they got the bad news; another four were dropped from the study after they availed themselves of free saloon lunches. However, the remaining GIs doubled their strength after up to eight months of Fletcherizing on low-protein diets.

Chittenden, who shared the conventional belief that only high-protein red meat, and plenty of it, built strong muscles, was impressed. The professor slashed his own protein intake. In short order, his painful rheumatic knee improved and his chronic headaches went away. Chittenden went public with his test results in *Popular Science* magazine and his book *Physiological Economy in Nutrition.* These, in turn, attracted press attention. The Fletcher publicity machine, which would not cease until Fletcher died, was plugged in and humming.

In 1907, at age 58, Fletcher returned to Yale for more tests. No one expected him to do as well as he had done four years earlier. Instead he did better, lifting 300-pound weights 350 times in succession using only his calf muscles. The feat more than doubled the Yale student record. Again, scientists and journalists were stunned.

Professors Irving Fisher of Yale and Henry Pickering Bowditch of Harvard joined Chittenden in boosting Fletcher, who was fast becoming a full-blown celebrity. ''To me,'' Chittenden later wrote, ''the chewing business became unimportant.'' Chittenden was primarily impressed by the small amount of food that sustained Fletcher, not the movements of Fletcher's jaw, but the professor did not emphasize his reservations.

Fletcher had his critics, of course. In 1908, New York City's *Medical Record,* noting that Fletcher's disciples came nowhere near equaling their leader's feats of strength no matter how well they chewed, scoffed that mastication had nothing to do with good health. The journal called Fletcher ''a somatic freak,'' concluding that he was simply very strong, for reasons that could not be explained. But these voices went largely unheeded as national and even international enthusiasm for Fletcherism grew.

MUNCHING PARTIES

Aristocratic circles in Edwardian London were much enamored of Fletcher, following the lead of the personal physician to King Edward VII, who expressed keen interest in the American reformer's theories. For a time, in fact, upper-class Englishmen and women took to having ''munching parties.'' At such soirees, reported Fletcher, ''the manager of the ceremony employed a stop watch to time the treatment of the first morsel of food taken by each of the guests.''

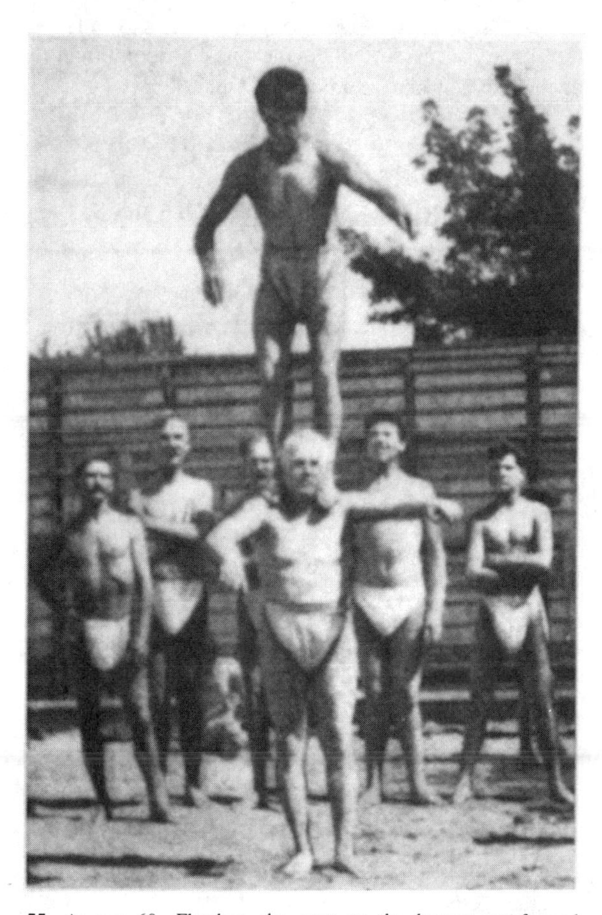

55. At age 60, Fletcher, the gent on the bottom, performed amazing feats of strength. *From* McClure's, *April 1910.*

FAME

Fletcher, derided as ''the chew-chew man'' by skeptics, had no trouble increasing his following. His books went back to press for repeated printings and were translated into Italian, Russian, Polish, and Hungarian. Of his 1913 tome *Fletcherism: What It Is,* the *New York Times* gushed, ''All students of dietetics, indeed, every man and woman who desires to retain a sound, vigorous, healthy body, should read this last book from the pen of the pioneer of Fletcherism.''

The high-rolling philosopher of mastication wrote for leading American magazines; they returned the favor and wrote about him. Serious articles examining his work appeared in the British medical journal *The Lancet* and *Popular Science,* while mass-circulation magazines like the *Ladies' Home Journal* and *Cosmopolitan* became Fletcherite publications.

For a profile of Fletcher in the December 1908 issue of *Cosmopolitan,* the writer remarked that ''most people are human sewers'' who admit indigestible filth into their bodies. Under the heading ''Dietetic Sinners,'' the scribe took matters a step further: ''Cannibals, I am told, always bolt their missionary.'' Then, leaping into the sociological realm, the writer concluded that ''Crime follows malnutrition, as night follows day.''

By 1909, Fletcher was holding forth in the pages of the *Ladies' Home Journal.* Seldom as vociferous as his followers, Fletcher allowed that ''I cannot advise you appropriately what to eat, when to eat and how much to eat, and nobody else can." Fletcher did, however, close his article by offering to answer anyone who wrote to him with questions about nutrition. He also remembered to include the following pronouncement: "Money, leisure and easily accessible cafes are the menace of right nutrition."

Occasionally, Fletcher's critics sounded discordant notes. Fletcherites weren't eating enough food, they said. Their jaws would surely ache from all that chewing. Since no one could equal Fletcher's feats in the gym, he was a special case that no amount of chewing would duplicate.

Although Fletcherism never became a mass movement, its most fervent followers were found among the influential elite who had both the time to wonder about what they ate and the means to eat too much. Fletcher's converts included Thomas Edison, John D. Rockefeller, Upton Sinclair, and Henry James. James invited Fletcher to his home and gave copies of Fletcher's *The New Glutton or Epicure* to neighbors. Henry's brother, William James, wrote of Fletcher in a carefully distanced style in *The Varieties of Religious Experience*. But several years later, William, too, was Fletcherizing. Patients at the Harvard Dentistry School infirmary were issued cards with "Horace Fletcher's Rules for Eating."

At the peak of his fame, Fletcher addressed the New York Academy of Medicine. In 1908, he lectured a convention of home economists at Chautauqua, in upstate New York, where Dr. John Harvey Kellogg shared the rostrum. Kellogg, one of Fletcher's most enthusiastic supporters, estimated that as many as 200 thousand American families Fletcherized in the first decade of the twentieth century. They saved, Kellogg reckoned, a dollar a day in those pre-inflationary times by cutting down on meat and other fancy foods.

"I am sure you deserve to have your name immortalized, as Pasteur's has been," Kellogg wrote in a letter to Fletcher. "I feel myself in the position of an eager disciple sitting at the feet of a master."

In his later years, Fletcher refined his mental and dietary guidelines in a torrent of letters, lectures, articles, and books. The one-time bon vivant affirmed that he had turned against alcohol, tobacco, and meat in his own diet, though he didn't publicly condemn the indulgences in others.

Fletcher retained his sunny disposition and plush lifestyle into his sixties. "The best argument in favor of Fletcherism," observed a journalist, "is Horace Fletcher. People who picture the founder of Fletcherism as a lean ascetic sitting over a plate of prunes or a bowl of breakfast food and solemnly counting his jaw movements would have to make a radical revision of their mental image if they could see the real Horace Fletcher breakfasting at his ease at the Waldorf-Astoria, where he usually stays when he is in New York."

In his final years, Fletcher skipped breakfast, eating only a midday meal, unless he was dining with friends in the evening. Occasionally, he did things that struck even dewy-eyed admirers as a bit odd. He lived, for example, entirely on potatoes for 58 days in 1912. But generally Fletcher was the very model of a well-adjusted soul. Always frighteningly prolific, he arose between 3 A.M. and 5 A.M. and scribbled 7,000 words of correspondence and professional writing before taking his first bite of the day.

"How can I help but work?" he said. "I feel like a man with a life preserver surrounded by thousands of drowning people. I've just got to do what I can to give them the thing that I know will save them."

Fletcher's messianic streak, which grew apace with his success, convinced him that doctors would not be needed if the world would simply chew properly. Physicians would become consultants to hale, hearty people who would need their services only on those rare occasions when the one-two combination of mastication and menticulture failed.

CHEWING STYLES OF THE RICH AND FAMOUS

William James:

In a November 1905 letter to the *Harvard Crimson*, James urged students and faculty to attend an upcoming lecture by Fletcher. His "teaching and example have been of such vital benefit to certain persons whom I know," James wrote. "If his observations on diet, confirmed already on a limited scale, should prove true on a universal scale, it is impossible to overestimate their revolutionary impact."

John D. Rockefeller:

Quoted by Fletcher in the May 1914 *Ladies' Home Journal*: "Don't gobble your food. 'Fletcherize,' or chew very slowly while you eat. Talk on pleasant topics. Don't be in a hurry. Take time to masticate, and cultivate a cheerful attitude while you eat. Thus will the demon indigestion be encompassed round about, and his slaughter complete."

Indeed, the world would be barely recognizable if its inhabitants Fletcherized.

"What, in your opinion, will be the result of perfect alimentary education?" an interviewer asked Fletcher.

"No slums, no degeneracy, no criminals, . . ." the Great Masticator replied. "In a single generation, the whole social problem would be solved."

THE FINAL JOURNEY

When World War I exploded and the German army rolled westward, millions of Belgians were cut off from adequate clothing and food. Fletcher promptly signed on as a food economist with the Commission for Relief in Belgium, a charity headed by Herbert Hoover, a man whose efficiency he admired. Soon after, Fletcher sailed for Europe.

It was an unprecedented opportunity to show what Fletcherism could do. In 1914, the *New York Times* quoted Fletcher as saying: "I have eight million people to work on. Cut off from the world here, we have nothing else to do. Moreover, food is running short, and can be made to last much longer by careful chewing."

"Of course, everybody eats too much," commented a *Times* editorialist. "Belgium ate too much before the Germans took the bread and butter out of its mouth for no fault of its own. Now that there is less to eat, the cult of eating less may spread. Horace Fletcher is its prophet."

History does not record a great triumph for Fletcherism in Belgium, although Fletcher, driven by world-saving zeal, apparently believed he could effect a miracle. In 1916, Fletcher spoke at a tea dance and lace exhibition at the Ritz-Carlton Hotel in New York and assured those in attendance that their charity was being well-spent in war-torn Belgium. No mention was made of his great experiment with mastication.

In January 1919, just months after the conclusion of the Great War, Fletcher journeyed to Copenhagen despite the chronic case of bronchitis that would kill him. On January 12, he died in that city at age 69, possibly exhausted by wartime service and ceaseless travel.

Fletcher clearly hoped that his philosophy would outlive him. With a nod to professors William James and Henry Pickering Bowditch, he bequeathed part of his estate to Harvard and endowed a prize for a thesis on this mouthful: "Special Uses of Circumvaliate Papilli and the Saliva of the Mouth in Regulating Physiological Economy in Nutrition."

Fletcher's Harvard prize and the reams of publicity he received during his lifetime weren't enough to secure his memory in the ever-fickle public mind. Without his considerable energy and gift for self-promotion, the world forgot him in the pell-mell hedonism of the Roaring Twenties.

Nevertheless, Fletcher's legacy endures, if not under his name. "Horace Fletcher taught the world to chew," declared one of his obituaries, and there's some truth to the statement. Americans finally slowed down at mealtime, with happy consequences for the nation's table manners. Gluttony was no longer celebrated; slenderness began to gain some of the chic it would have among later generations.

With reduced calories came reduced intake of protein. Today's standards—56 grams a day for 70-kilogram men and 44 grams a day for 55-kilogram women—are nearly identical to the recommendations that emerged from the Chittenden experiments at Yale. The Swallowing Impulse and the invisible Food Filter are, of course, forgotten. Fletcher wouldn't be happy about that, but, in ways he couldn't foresee, the gourmand-turned-dietary-crusader has left his mark.

"ECONOMIC ASH"

One of Fletcher's most idiosyncratic touches was his detailed interest in excrement, to which he attached the scientific-sounding term "economic ash." The term reflected his belief that human waste was merely the inoffensive residue of proper digestion.

Even Fletcher produced waste, but—and he was very proud of this—only in small amounts that did not offend the senses. Fletcher was so eager for one and all to notice his accomplishment that he took to sending samples to scientists in sealed packages via the first-class mails.

All people, Fletcher figured, should produce such stools, if they had to produce any. In a chapter in *The New Glutton or Epicure* entitled "Tell-Tale Excreta," Fletcher decreed that human stools should be "in pillular shape," adding that "There is no stench, no evidence of putrid bacterial decomposition, only the odour of warmth, like warm earth or 'hot biscuit.' "

CHAPTER · 14 ·

CHRISTIAN SCIENCE: "HEAL THE SICK, RAISE THE DEAD"

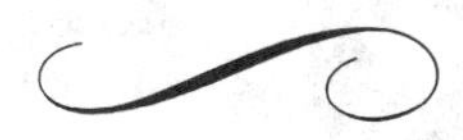

To the Christian Science healer, sickness is a dream from which the patient needs to be awakened.

MARY BAKER EDDY

Mary Baker Eddy was not the most likely nineteenth-century American to become rich and famous. At a time when careers for women were severely restricted, Eddy had the additional handicaps of poverty, sickness, lack of education, and advancing age. She was 54 years old, unknown, and recently removed from penury when her first and most important book, *Science and Health With Key to the Scriptures*, was published in 1875. She was 58 when her Christian Science Church was founded. Riches finally found her when she was in her seventies.

Yet Eddy became the most important American woman of her era. She fused health and spirituality, founding a "religion of healthy-mindedness" (to use William James's phrase) that endures on the verge of the twenty-first century. The white, colonnaded Christian Science churches and quiet reading rooms that are fixtures in many towns—not to mention the serious, highly regarded *Christian Science Monitor* newspaper—seem the epitome of pious respectability. Yet Christian Science, founded in the wake of the mind-cure movement that swept America from the mid-nineteenth to the early twentieth century, is anchored in profound radicalism.

Christian Scientists are understandably loath to be linked to the sometimes-outlandish alternative health movements of the past (and, for that matter, the present). Commented a modern-day church lecturer: ". . . Of course Christian Science isn't some form of alternative health care . . . [Christian Science] includes healing as a natural part of Christian life, but its most basic aim is to truly have God as God."

Clearly Christian Science is a religion. Yet, just as clearly, history shows that the church developed in a time of great ferment in American medicine and that its founder was deeply immersed in a variety of alternative health-care movements even before she started her church, which had a distinctive medical mission. Indeed, the formative years of Christian Science are virtually synonymous with the life of Mary Baker Eddy.

IN THE BEGINNING

Mary Baker was born on July 16, 1821 in the farming village of Bow, near Concord, New Hampshire. The pampered youngest of six children, she was a frail girl, subject to chronic dyspepsia, nervousness, and depression, as well as seizures that a

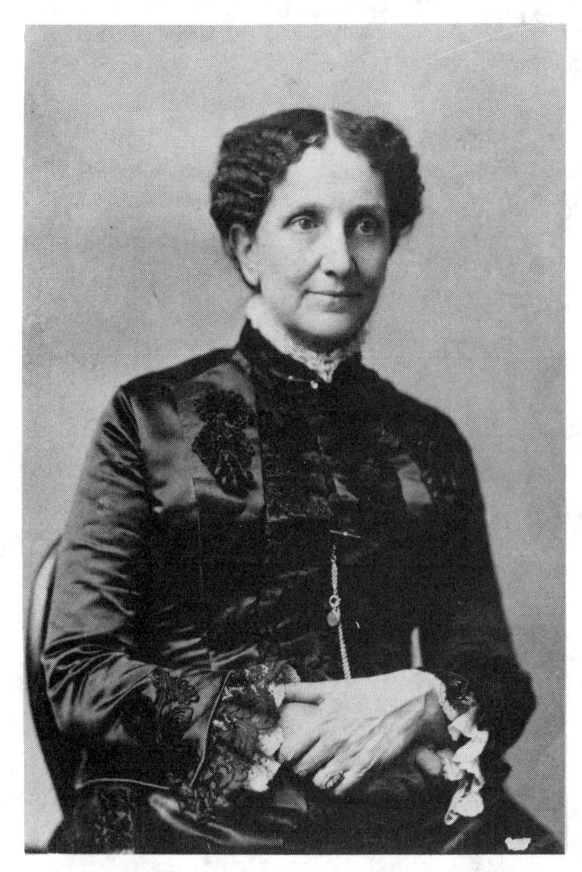

56. Mary Baker Eddy, the dynamic and disciplined founder of Christian Science, held that disease is a false belief (1886). *Courtesy of the Library of Congress.*

local physician called hysteric. She was also given to fainting spells, especially during the tantrums that she threw during arguments with her strong-willed father.

Young Mary frequently had theological disputes with her father, a Congregationalist who subscribed to the Calvinist doctrine of predestination. Rejecting his hellfire sentiments, Mary—foreshadowing the optimistic theology of Christian Science—insisted that God was good, not cruel. Early on, she showed an unusual physiological trait: She had no sense of smell and, therefore, virtually no sense of taste. This was a kind of a foreshadowing, too, perhaps explaining the grown woman's detachment from the life of the senses and her exaltation of the mind.

In 1843, Mary Baker married businessman George Washington Glover at age 22 and moved with him to Charleston, South Carolina. At 23, she was a widow and mother. Glover died only six months after their marriage, evidently of yellow fever. A son, George Glover, was born soon after his father's death. Young Mrs. Glover moved back north with her infant son.

When she returned north, Mary Glover was broken in body and spirit. Childbirth had been difficult, and Mary was for some time thereafter considered an "invalid," though she was only in her mid-twenties. To dull the pain—she complained of a spinal inflammation, and could barely walk—she used morphine. This was not an uncommon solution to pain in that era and no social stigma was attached to it.

In this latest spasm of ill health, Mary Glover began investigating alternatives to the bleed-and-purge "regular" doctors of the 1840s. She subscribed for a while to the whole-grain-and-water dietary regimen of Sylvester Graham, and indulged her curiosity about the Great Beyond by dabbling in spiritualism, then all the rage in New England.

She also read up on homeopathy, finding it a most satisfactory alternative to standard medicine, with its often-toxic *materia medica.* Mrs. Glover decided that the highly diluted medicines of homeopathy were really more akin to ideas about medicine than actual drugs, seeing in the science of Samuel Hahnemann a bridge between the material and spiritual. (Homeopaths disagree, considering their drugs to be material medicines, not ideas.) Mrs. Glover also immersed herself in the water cure, visiting Dr. Vail's Hydropathic Institute in Hill, New Hampshire to ease her pain.

In 1853, Mary Glover became Mary Patterson after marrying her second husband. Dr. Daniel Patterson was an itinerant dentist who used homeopathy in his practice. Wandering from town to town in New England, the couple eked out a living. The new Mrs. Patterson was still not well, so Dr. Patterson dispatched letters to a highly regarded healer in Portland, Maine, entreating the man, a mind-cure doctor, to heal his wife.

PHINEAS P. QUIMBY, MIND HEALER

Phineas Parkhurst Quimby (1802–1866) had the perfect nineteenth-century name. It combined, in about equal parts, dignity and silliness. The name suited Quimby, who combined seriousness and silliness in his medical practice as well.

A pragmatic man with an inventive mind, Quimby made and repaired clocks and took daguerreotypes during the early years of photography. Quimby, who considered himself a semi-invalid, became interested in healing after he treated himself with hypnotism. His instructor was Charles Poyen, a touring French lecturer on mesmerism, as hypnotism was then known. After Quimby's 1837 meeting with Poyen, he began treating others with mesmerism and appended "doc-

THE NAME GAME

Thrice-married, the founder of Christian Science had four names in all. They were:

Mary Baker, 1821–42.

Mary Baker Glover, 1842–55.

Mary Baker Patterson, 1855–73. Note: She unofficially reverted to the surname Glover several years before her divorce from Daniel Patterson was granted.

Mary Baker Eddy, 1873–1910.

tor" to his name. The title was self-conferred; Quimby's formal schooling totaled six weeks.

Quimby didn't let his lack of formal education—which was, in any case, not unusual in early nineteenth-century America—stop him. He joined forces with a 17-year-old assistant, Lucius Burkmar, whom he put into hypnotic trances. Burkmar then diagnosed and prescribed for paying members of the public. Often, the sick felt better after these sessions. Quimby and Burkmar worked together for three or four years.

Over time, however, Quimby came to think that it was the sufferers' belief in the medicine that Burkmar prescribed—with scant knowledge of what the drugs actually did—that cured. So Quimby fired Burkmar and went into business by himself, using positive thinking and the power of suggestion in place of medication. "Whatever we believe," Quimby said, "that we create."

Quimby retained some mesmerist's tricks, such as wetting his hands and rubbing patients' heads, because it seemed to comfort them. But he no longer hypnotized the sick who came to see him; rather, he asked where it hurt and counseled them. He believed that the healer imparted vital electricity to the patient and, in return, took on the sufferer's own aches and pains, acting like a medical lightening rod. Once the vital connection was made, Quimby believed, healer and patient could communicate from afar and needn't be present together in the same room or even the same town.

Quimby called his technique by several names, one of which was "Christian Science." He did not, however, consider it a religion, although he was a religious man. He regarded himself as simply a healer.

In 1859, Quimby opened a medical office in Portland, charging little money and treating poor patients for free. Three years later, a sick woman named Mary Baker Patterson came to see him. Witnesses remember her as a pale, emaciated woman who barely made it up the stairs to Quimby's office, although she was not yet 40.

Quimby temporarily but dramatically cured Mrs. Patterson of her spinal pain. Soon, she was walking unaided. She was so grateful, and so curious about Quimby's methods, that she stayed for three weeks. On a return visit, Mrs. Patterson stayed in Portland for two months.

Quimby's visitor proved herself to be an apt and eager pupil. She poured over his unpublished manuscript, "Questions and Answers," and sat in on his healing sessions, closely observing his work. When they weren't together, she believed that Quimby attended to her in spirit through what she called his "angel visits."

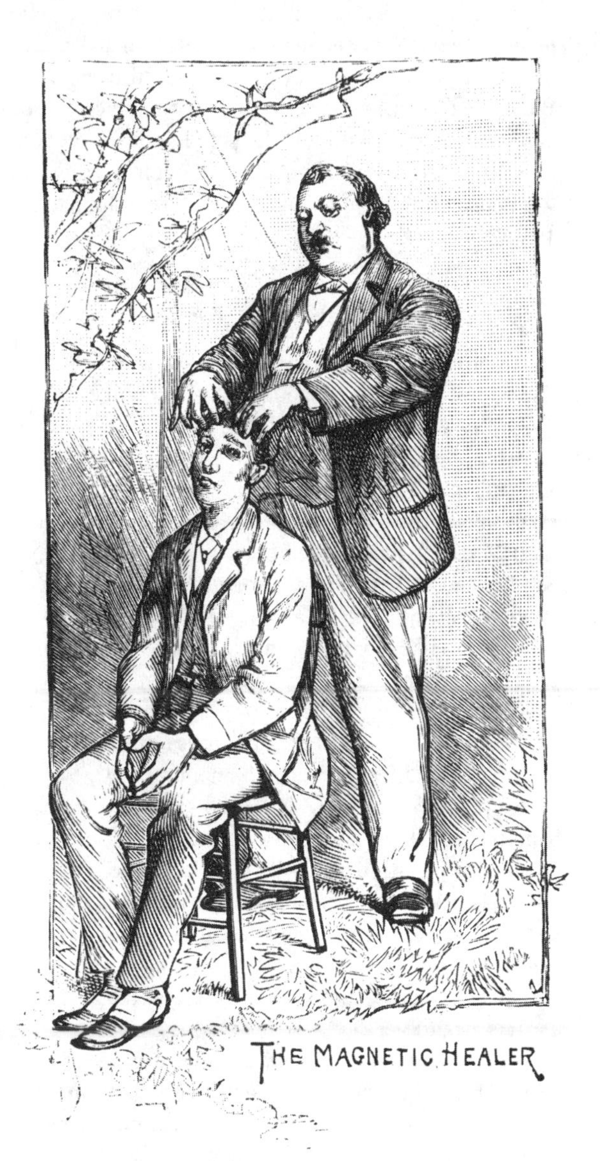

57. Although she fashioned her own distinctive philosophy of health, the young Mary Baker Eddy was influenced by magnetic healers. *Culver Pictures.*

Mrs. Patterson could not say enough about the marvelous Dr. Quimby. In one of her many missives to the newspapers, she observed: "P.P. Quimby rolls away the stone from the sepulchre of error and health is the resurrection." Scoffed another paper in its editorial columns: "P.P. Quimby compared to Jesus Christ! What next!"

In 1863, Mrs. Patterson gave her first treatments, using the Quimby method of suggestion and head-rubbing in place of outright hypnotism, surgery, or drugs. She began to think of herself as a healer, too, although she allowed that she was merely in her "pupilage."

Only three years later, Mrs. Patterson's world turned upside-down. On January 16, 1866, Quimby died from an abdominal tumor. His family, who never believed in his theories, called in a homeopathic physician, to no avail. A grief-stricken Mary Baker Patterson memorialized Quimby in verse. She continued to use his method, including head-rubbing "manipulation," for six years, although Quimbyism without Quimby was about to undergo a momentous change.

AFTER THE FALL

On February 1, 1866, only two weeks after Quimby died, Mrs. Patterson, negotiating the icy winter streets of Lynn, Massachusetts, slipped and suffered a concussion. Suffering from spinal pain, she later said she fell into a condition "pronounced by the physicians incurable" and was near death. On the third day, Mrs. Patterson called for her Bible. While reading the sacred text, she was healed—simultaneously discovering the basic principle of Christian Science, which she likened to the healing powers of Christ and his disciples. Her fall and recovery came to be regarded as the mystic birth of Christian Science.

Mrs. Patterson's contemporaries remembered the event rather differently. In a monumental, 14-part series published in 1907 and 1908, *McClure's* magazine tracked down the physician who had treated the stricken woman 40 years before. In a sworn affidavit, Dr. Alvin H. Cushing, a homeopath, attested that Mrs. Patterson was never incurable or near death, adding that he treated her for a nagging cough some months after she claimed to have found the secret of perfect health.

Mrs. Patterson insisted that the fall and recovery transpired exactly as she described them, making hers a dramatic break not only from orthodox medicine but also from Quimby since, as she put it, her discovery came about through divine revelation. Plunging into the writing of the book later published as *Science and Health,* Mrs. Patterson devoted the rest of her life to the religion of health that she called Christian Science. Meanwhile, Dr. Patterson left his single-minded wife in 1866; in 1873 they were divorced. He became a recluse, dying in poverty in 1896, by which time his former wife was a worldwide celebrity.

The decade between the demise of Quimby and the publication of *Science and Health* were Mary's years in the wilderness. Reverting to her first married name, Glover, she stayed in private homes, usually moving in with spiritualists and sharing with them her still-enthusiastic opinion of the late Dr. Quimby.

Mrs. Glover was a demanding guest. On at least one occasion, she implored the woman of the house to leave her husband and become a full-time teacher of the Quimby method. Once, Mrs. Glover so incensed her host that she was put out of the house in a rainstorm in the middle of the night.

Life began to brighten for Mary—now in midlife, widowed, divorced, and without her mentor—when she shifted from healing to teaching. She formed a partnership with a young man named Richard Kennedy. In 1870, she and Kennedy opened shared offices, Dr. Kennedy curing by the Quimby method and Mrs. Glover teaching metaphysical healing. The partnership lasted only two years, but it launched her on a career path at last.

Mrs. Glover now considered herself a creative theoretician and teacher. Her teaching reached its apogee in 1881, when she opened the Massachusetts Metaphysical College, which she operated under state license until 1889, when medical licensing laws were tightened. The college faculty consisted of one person—Mary herself—and was quartered in her home.

The college mission statement promised that the institution would show "how to improve the moral and physical condition of men, to eradicate in children hereditary traits, to enlarge the intellect a hundred per cent, to restore and strengthen the memory, to cure constipation, rheumatism, deafness, blindness and every ill the race is heir to."

Some 4,000 students matriculated at the Massachusetts Metaphysical College during its eight-year existence. Most were women. Healing was one of the few fields in which women could make money, especially in the long years when mainstream medicine shunned women. Indeed, women long regarded Mary as what their descendants would term a "role-model." There were five times as many female Christian Science healers as male healers in the 1890s; by the early 1970s, the ratio had widened to eight-to-one.

"MORTAL MIND" AND MATTER

However much she owed to Quimby, Mrs. Glover had ideas of her own. It was not the patient's limited "mortal mind" that cured, she decided, but the "divine mind" of the Deity, channeled through a practitioner or healer. Quimby had formulated a primitive concept of the unconscious, holding that what he called "spiritual matter" contained beliefs, ideas, images, and memories that could be called forth. Mrs. Glover rejected the idea of an unconscious, maintaining that healing takes place when there is a direct line to God.

Other elements marked Christian Science as distinctly different from mind cures. Quimby had allowed for the reality of the physical world even while asserting that it could be controlled by the mind. Mrs. Glover, by way of contrast, held that matter is not real, and only divine mind—"All-in-all," as she put it—really exists. People just believe that matter is real. Consequently, she dispensed with Quimbyisms, such as head-rubbing and hand-wetting, as merely reinforcing belief in matter.

In her radically revamped theology, nearly as far removed from the mainstream of Christian thought as Christian Science healing is from mainstream medicine, she also denied that sin is real. Evil, which causes sin, is merely a collective, cumulative belief. Disease, a manifestation of evil, is error. If thought is reformed, evil is exposed as a fraud. In modern terms, through thought reform the student can reprogram himself to vanquish disease.

Mrs. Glover and her growing number of student–practitioners claimed to cure people, and in some cases they may have done so. Psychosomatic diseases seem especially responsive to suggestion, and given the primitive state of medicine in late nineteenth-century America, Christian Science practitioners may have done as well, or better, than medical doctors.

As Christian Science medical practice grew, the movement created its own vocabulary. One was not sick; one had a "belief" that one was sick. A testimonial in the founder's book *Miscellaneous Writings* refers to "an ulcerated tooth belief." When one cured sickness, one "demonstrated" the truth of Christian Science.

From the beginning, Christian Science theory was ambitious and was applied literally. *Miscellaneous Writings* also contains a passage on contagious disease that reads:

> People believe in infections and contagious diseases, and that anyone is liable to have them under certain predisposing or exciting causes. This mental state prepares one to have any disease whenever there appear the circumstances which he believes produce it. If he believed as sincerely that health is catching when exposed to contact with healthy people, he would catch this state of feeling quite as surely, and with better effect . . . .

With her emphatic belief in mind, Mrs. Glover discarded all other health systems. She no longer followed a Graham diet, or put stock in the water cure, or believed it necessary to learn physiology,

M.A.M.

Mary Baker Eddy's strong belief in mind and spirit convinced her that evil can be projected mentally just as easily as can good. She attributed evil thoughts to "malicious animal magnetism," or M.A.M. Mrs. Eddy believed that M.A.M. was the prime ingredient in "mental malpractice," a charge she frequently leveled at her enemies.

In 1878 she brought a suit against Daniel Spofford, a former associate, on behalf of one Lucretia L.S. Brown, a student of Christian Science who endured severe spinal pain. The charge was witchcraft. The case went to court, appropriately enough, in Salem, Massachusetts, the site of the infamous witch trials of 1692–94. But times had changed. The judge ruled that the workings of Spofford's mind were beyond the jurisdiction of the court and dismissed the charges.

The decision did nothing to allay the late-night anxiety attacks that Mrs. Eddy attributed to M.A.M. To preempt the attacks, she formed a PM ("private meeting") group to direct mental energy at the presumed offenders.

Convinced of the pervasive power of M.A.M., Mrs. Eddy's personal life took on comic overtones. Defective household appliances, missing buttons on dresses—nearly any problems, really—were attributed to M.A.M. Many of her lectures were devoted to M.A.M. and how to combat it.

Indeed, Mrs. Eddy took no chances when it came to M.A.M. She convened a group of supporters to give positive "absent treatment" to the pressmen and binders working on the 1891 edition of *Science and Health*, just to make sure everything went well. The book still includes a seven-page chapter entitled "Animal Magnetism Unmasked."

even to attend childbirth. They were all illusions, like the body itself.

Her increasingly bold claims did not go unnoticed. One disaffected former student publicly challenged her to make good on her claim to bring eyesight to the blind, and backed up his challenge with 2,000 dollars. Mrs. Glover disdained the wager. "I performed more difficult tasks 15 years ago," she retorted. "At present, I am in another department of Christian work."

In 1875, after a decade of laborious writing, Mary Baker Glover published her magnum opus, *Science and Healing With Key to the Scriptures*. An author at last, Mrs. Glover expounded on Christian Science theory, blasted malicious animal magnetism, and promoted her own interpretation of the Bible, grounding her healing techniques—which she believed to be her own rediscovery of Christ and the Apostles' methods—in biblical authority.

As for *Science and Health,* she claimed it was prompted by divine revelation. "No human pen or tongue taught me the Science contained in this book," she wrote in the revised 1898 edition. She urged followers to read no books on metaphysics or healing save the Bible and *Science and Health.* "Centuries will intervene before the statement of the inexhaustible topics of that book become sufficiently understood to be absolutely demonstrated," she intoned.

Evidently, her followers agreed. Referring to *Science and Health,* a believer wrote, "When we think we are advanced far enough to let that book alone, then we are in trouble." Some Christian Scientists believed they were cured merely by reading *Science and Health.*

Two years after the publication of *Science and Health,* Mary Glover married her third husband, Asa Gilbert Eddy, and became Mary Baker Eddy. A student of hers, he was 10 years her junior. The union was brief. In 1882, after only five years of marriage, Mr. Eddy died of heart disease. He expired under a physician's care after Christian Science treatments failed to arrest his decline.

Mrs. Eddy rejected the autopsy findings out of hand, insisting that Asa Eddy died of "mesmeric poison." Although she didn't save her husband, she said that she could have cured him. "I have cured worse cases before," she assured her shaken followers, "but I took hold of them in time."

UPON THIS ROCK

In addition to her revolutionary ideas about healing, Mary Baker Eddy showed formidable organizational skills and a flair for public relations. Gradually, she transformed her flock from a small, radical health-reform sect with strong religious overtones into an established church with a unique approach to health.

Mrs. Eddy's followers were drawn largely from the ranks of health reformers. Spiritualists, astrologers, water-cure fans, Grahamites, and phrenologists all flocked to the new movement. The Christian Science Church was founded in 1879 ". . . to reinstate primitive Christianity and its lost element of healing." Commented *McClure's*: "Mrs. Eddy's teachings brought the promise of material benefits to a practical people, and the appeal of seeming newness to a people whose mental recreation was a feverish pursuit of novelty." Like any new church, Christian Science had its power struggles and schisms.

One of Eddy's brightest followers, Josephine Woodbury, who had attracted a flock of her own with a romantic, nature-loving version of Christian Science, gave birth to a son by a man not her husband after announcing that she and her spouse had stopped having sexual relations in favor of a higher form of congress. Mrs. Woodbury, who claimed that she didn't know she was pregnant, attributed the changes in her body to "some fungoid formation." She suggested that her son, whom she called Prince (after the "Prince of Peace"), was the product of immaculate conception. She was expelled from the church.

The church grew throughout the 1880s and 1890s. Mrs. Eddy built her main church, the Mother Church, in Boston in 1895, but Christian Science soon outgrew those cramped quarters. In 1906, the much larger Excelsior Extension was opened next to the Mother Church; 20 thousand worshippers crowded into six dedication services. That same year, church membership was estimated to be between 55 thousand and 85 thousand.

Mrs. Eddy's star never shone brighter than at the dawn of the twentieth century. Although she never received the title "reverend" through benefit of clergy, she took the title Pastor Emeritus to preside over what was (and is) formally known as the First Church of Christ, Scientist. Many in her flock referred to her reverently as "Mother."

THE MATRIARCH

The once-sickly girl had become a formidable, rich old woman known in most of the Western world. "No other American woman has made a greater fortune by her efforts," observed *McClure's.* ". . . None other is so famous; none other has half the power."

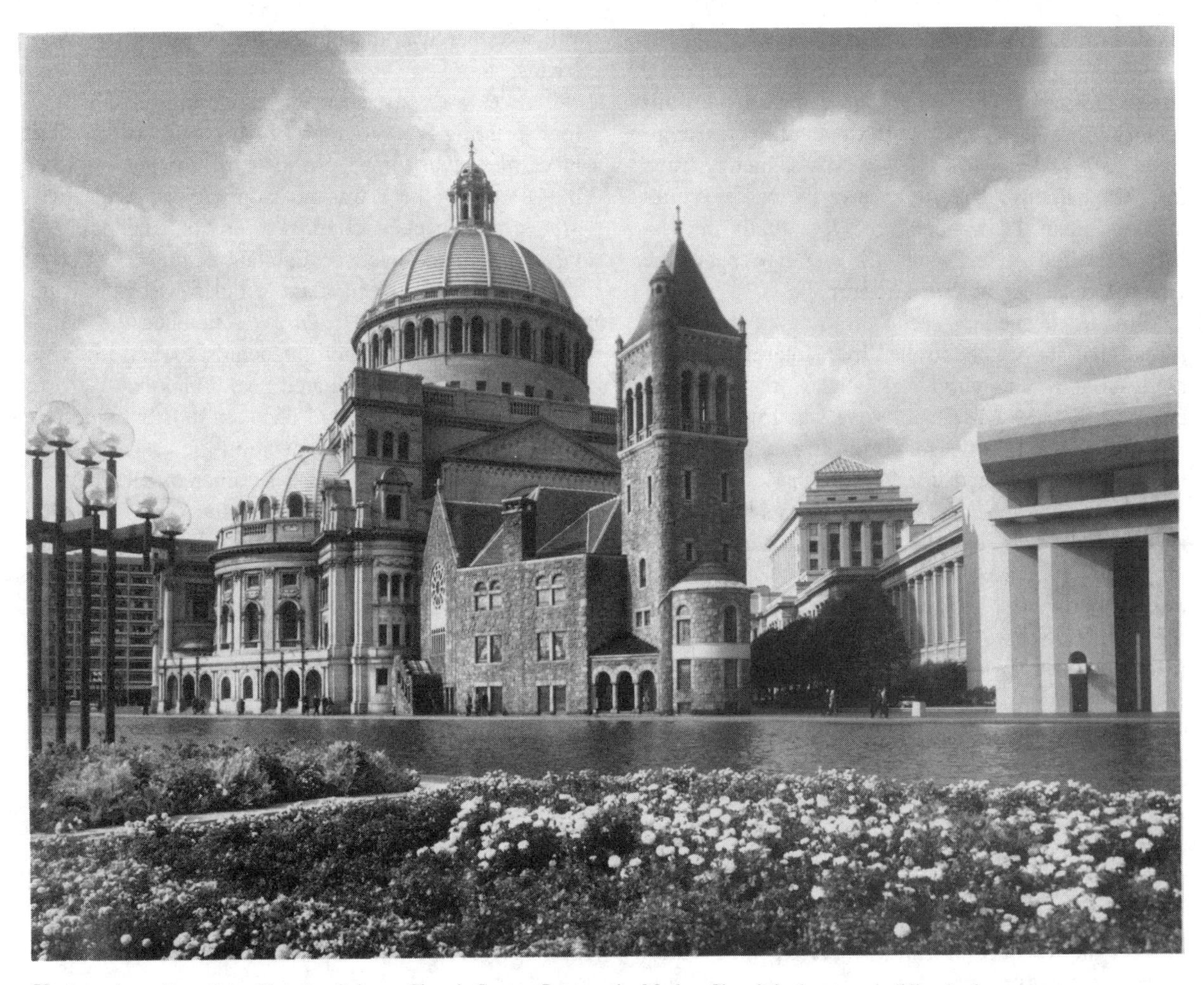

58. A modern view of the Christian Science Church Center, Boston; the Mother Church is the stone building in the center.

The magazine did not exaggerate. Mrs. Eddy was compared to Christ, and not unfavorably. As Jesus was said to represent the masculine principle of godliness on Earth, Mary Baker Eddy was said by Scientists (as church members called themselves) to embody the feminine—the more refined, spiritual principle.

Mrs. Eddy's control over the temporal organization she had made was virtually total. In 1894, she abolished clergy in Christian Science churches and replaced them with lay "readers," devout members who read aloud from the Bible and *Science and Health* during services and were enjoined from commenting on the passages.

Science and Health, meanwhile, went through a series of revisions. Mrs. Eddy's idiosyncratic style was cleaned up, courtesy of the Reverend Henry Wiggin, a Unitarian who served for several years as her literary advisor and is considered by some scholars to have extensively rewritten the text.

At about the same time, Mrs. Eddy ordered Christian Science dispensaries, which offered low-cost health care to the poor, to exchange their healing couches for bookshelves. This was the origin of the now-familiar reading rooms stocked with Christian Science literature.

Mrs. Eddy amassed a fortune in royalties from her books and the sale of merchandise. In the Boston Mother Church, hard by the "Mother Room" dedicated to her, an array of mementos was available: cufflinks, photographs of Mrs. Eddy, and teaspoons such as the "Mother Spoon," a silver spoon that bore Mrs. Eddy's likeness and sold for five dollars.

The matriarch wrote the bylaws of the church. Her followers were required to journey to her home and render unto her one year of service if she so desired. Church services were periodically to feature hymns written by her. Mrs. Eddy hired and fired the board of directors. Church members, stipulated the bylaws, "shall not patronize a publishing house or bookstore that has for sale obnoxious books.''

As she grew old, Mrs. Eddy reduced her public appearances. For several years, thousands of pilgrims journeyed to her home in Concord, New Hampshire, to hear her speak a few words or merely wave from the balcony. The presence of the petite, white-haired woman thrilled believers. Eventually the visits were ended. ''Her isolation is now like that of the Grand Lama,'' commented a journal.

In her deepening seclusion, rumors inevitably spread that she was controlled by a coterie of household servants and church associates, that she was crazy or that she was dead. None was true; she was just old. In the first decade of the twentieth century, her son George joined in a lawsuit charging that his mother was not in her right mind. She was found to be as sharp as a tack, and the suit went nowhere.

Mrs. Eddy's power and isolation fueled public interest, however, and not all the attention—from the nation's most famous author and a leading magazine—was favorable.

BLOWBACK

In the first decade of the twentieth century, Mark Twain and *McClure's* magazine weighed in with highly critical looks at Christian Science.

In a 1907 book entitled simply *Christian Science,* Twain expanded on themes he had sounded in articles for the *North American Review.* Opening with a characteristically satirical sketch, Twain told mischievously of his supposed misadventures with a Christian Science practitioner, a devout woman who tried to heal his broken bones with prayer, assuring him the pain was imaginary. ''I gave her an imaginary check, and now she is suing me for substantial dollars,'' wrote Twain. ''It looks inconsistent.''

More seriously, Twain worried that Mrs. Eddy's fast-growing church, with what he saw as its vainglorious leader and disturbing, cultlike tendencies, would soon be a worldwide power and its octogenarian leader an all-powerful pope.

Twain's critical attention was not helpful to Christian Science, and the *McClure's* series was another blow. *McClure's* was the home of leading investigative reporters, popularly known as muckrakers, such as Lincoln Steffens and Ida Tarbell, and it had considerable prestige.

A young Rochester, New York writer, Georgine Milmine, devoted what an editor's note described as ''nearly two years of close research'' to the series, double- and triple-checking Mrs. Eddy's path through life as attested to in her autobiographical writings. Soon-to-be-eminent *McClure's* staffers helped out. Willa Cather was the chief editor, assisted by Will Irwin.

McClure's started off by shooting itself in the foot, printing a photograph of Mrs. Eddy in the first installment that turned out to be of another woman, but after that there was no stopping the magazine. *McClure's* checked court records, obtained affidavits, and interviewed acquaintances of Mrs. Eddy. The cumulative effect of the articles was powerful. The all-star team at *McClure's* concluded that Mrs. Eddy had fudged important details of her life and made largely unsubstantiated health claims.

Christian Science had received mostly favorable press coverage as the organization grew. This was a significant departure. In the summer of 1907, Mrs. Eddy gave interviews to the *Boston Globe* and the Hearst newspaper chain, offsetting some of the bad publicity from *McClure's* and Twain.

In 1908, she founded the *Christian Science Monitor*. The internationally circulated daily newspaper was started to publish generally uplifting news and promote a more positive image of Christian Science. Perhaps surprisingly, it was a serious and good paper from the start, not a simple propaganda organ. The *Monitor*, now augmented by church-owned television, radio, and magazine enterprises, remains respected.

Mary Baker Eddy's life was nearly over. She was approaching 90, and, biographer as Julius Silberger, Jr. writes, ''repeatedly promised her house-

MR. CLEMENS AND MRS. EDDY

Mark Twain (Samuel L. Clemens) could get downright vituperative about Mary Baker Eddy and her church. In his book *Christian Science,* Twain took aim at nearly everything about the new religion of health.

On Mary Baker Eddy's literary style: ''She has a perfectly astonishing talent for putting words together in such a way as to make successful inquiry into their intention impossible.''

On the origin of Christian Science healing: ''Her enemies charge that she surreptitiously took from Quimby a peculiar system of healing. . . . Whether she took it or invented it, it was—materially—a sawdust mine when she got it, and she has turned it into a Klondike. . . .''

On Mary Baker Eddy herself: ''In several ways she is the most interesting woman that ever lived, and the most extraordinary.''

hold that her ultimate demonstration would be against Death himself."

Ironically, for someone who spent her life issuing pronouncements on health, Mrs. Eddy's own health was seldom good. She was plagued by nightmares and chronic pain from kidney stones and renal colic. When Christian Science "treating"—both self-administered and guided by her disciples—failed to end her pain, she took injections of morphine. At first, physicians (one of them Mrs. Eddy's cousin) were summoned, but this proved embarrassing. Later on, Mrs. Eddy's staff, who had often been called to attend to her late-night attacks, gave her the shots.

Mrs. Eddy had, of course, been dead-set against drugs, but in 1905 she revised *Science and Health* and added this line: "If from an injury or any cause, a Christian Scientist were seized with pain so violent that he could not treat himself mentally . . . the sufferer could call a surgeon, who would give him a hypodermic injection . . ."

In her last days, Mrs. Eddy grew increasingly eccentric. She berated her church's Benevolent Committee for failing to produce "scientific" weather to comfort her, and confided to friends that she didn't expect to die, but if, perchance, she did, it would be because the mesmerists had gotten to her with their mental poisoning at last.

On December 3, 1910, in the 34-room stone mansion in Chestnut Hill, Massachusetts where she had lived for the last three years, Mary Baker Eddy died. The cause of death was pneumonia. She was 89. She left an estate valued at 2.5 million dollars. Her body was attended day and night in a room equipped with a device that church leaders thought she might need in case the mesmerists' foulest work was foiled: a telephone.

MODERN CHRISTIAN SCIENCE

Christian Science has survived its founder by nearly a century, maintaining its tradition in the age of high-technology medicine. The church still uses Mrs. Eddy's *Science and Health*— with its chapters on malicious animal magnetism and practical instruction on how to use the divine mind to heal—as its sacred text. Elected lay readers still read aloud from *Science and Health* and the Bible during Sunday services. On Wednesdays, at evening testimonial meetings, church members speak about personal experiences with Christian Science healing.

Although membership is believed to have declined in the late twentieth century, there may be more Christian Scientists today than in Mrs. Eddy's era, in some 60 countries. Church leaders don't release membership figures; outside estimates vary widely, putting the number of Christian Scientists at between 100 thousand and 400 thousand.

A spring 1989 visit to the church's Boston headquarters revealed a phalanx of modern and older buildings constructed around the 1895 Mother Church. Drought had drained the reflecting pool of its sparkle, but the spacious headquarters were impressive. This is a prosperous institution, composed largely of well-educated, middle-class, middle-aged and elderly people. The church's sober-sided image does little to attract young members.

There is nothing about the massive buildings to remind a visitor of the organization's dramatic history or still-radical healing theories. Yet the Christian Science past is often manifest in the church's present.

Nowadays, when Christian Science makes news, it is seldom due to spectacular successes in medicine but because of supposed failures. Christian Science was put on trial in the late 1980s when children of members died while under the care of church practitioners who refused to allow treatment by medical doctors. In a 15-month stretch in 1989 and 1990, five sets of Christian Science parents in four states were convicted of crimes, including third-degree murder, felony child abuse, and involuntary manslaughter. None of the parents was imprisoned.

Christian Scientists defend the right of parents to bypass orthodox medical care on freedom-of-religion grounds and are supported by civil libertarians. Medical authorities usually oppose the church. By the late 1980s, 44 states had amended child-abuse statutes to permit spiritual healing of youngsters—the result of lobbying by Christian Scientists, Jehovah's Witnesses, and others—but unfavorable court rulings threatened to neutralize that protection.

Christian Science practitioners and nurses licensed by church authorities are reimbursed by most private and public insurance plans, prompting a church critic to declare, "When it comes to getting money, they qualify as a health-care system. When it comes to taking responsibility for death, they say they are a religion."

Nathan A. Talbot, a church spokesman, countered that ". . . .There does exist an impressive cumulative record of Christian Science healing over more than a century—including the healing of diseases medically diagnosed as incurable or terminal. At the same time, serious concerns are being voiced about the unfulfilled expectations raised by popular medical hype."

The church says it has published more than 50 thousand personal testimonials on the efficacy of

Christian Science healing. But medical authorities, citing a lack of specificity and medical oversight, dismiss the testimonials as mere anecdotes.

Christian Science has modified its traditional opposition to material medicine, even as Mary Baker Eddy modified her views to accept morphine. Christian Scientists submit to drugs to kill pain and see physicians for broken bones. They accept blood transfusions and will wear hearing aids and eyeglasses. But devout Christian Scientists do not regularly frequent physicians or psychiatrists, although they are free to do so.

In the late 1980s, the Mother Church in Boston listed 3,000 health practitioners and 500 nurses in the United States. A licensed practitioner in California told the *San Francisco Chronicle* that his practice consists mainly of prayer tailored to the individuals he treats. ''Over the years [a healer] gets filled with wonderful ideas and when people call me to pray for them, it usually isn't very difficult at all to listen to some angel thought from God.''

Nurses help practitioners by keeping the patient's body clean and providing a low-key, pleasant environment so he or she can concentrate on thinking pure thoughts. Nurses also help ''hold thoughts'' by focusing on uplift. The church operates sanitaria and convalescent homes as alternatives to hospitals.

Christian Scientists don't attribute cures to miracles from a personal God who hears their prayers and decides to reward them; they believe they have tapped into a divine principle that allows healing power to flow, rather like throwing a cosmic switch. Devout Christian Scientists believe that absent treatments work; practitioners sometimes talk to patients on the phone and direct positive thoughts from afar.

Church leaders reject outsiders' contentions that Christian Science uses faith healing, will power, or suggestion. It is the always-present divine mind that heals, they contend. Nor is healing really the point; religion is the point. ''The change in physical condition or personal circumstance,'' reads one church publication, ''is only the outward and visible evidence of an inward and spiritual grace. . . .''

Mrs. Eddy's spiritual descendants haven't fared well in comparative studies, even though most don't smoke or drink (not chiefly for nutritional reasons but because they believe tobacco and alcohol cloud the mind).

In 1989, in a study published in the *Journal of the American Medical Association,* 5,000 Christian Scientists were compared to 30 thousand non-Christian Scientists. Christian Scientist women were found to die four years earlier on average than did female nonbelievers; Christian Scientist men died two years earlier than male nonbelievers.

Present-day physicians have come to value the mind, even if they stop well short of endorsing exclusively spiritual care. Christian Scientists, with their long institutional history and high public profile, have surely contributed to this growing appreciation of the powers of mind and spirit.

CHAPTER
· 15 ·

OSTEOPATHY: THE "LIGHTNING BONESETTERS"

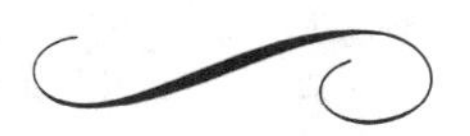

The rule of the artery must be absolute, universal, and unobstructed, or disease will be the result.

ANDREW TAYLOR STILL, 1897

The year was 1864, and times were hard. Over much of America, the Civil War was raging. In Missouri, a recently mustered-out Union veteran named Andrew Taylor Still was waging another kind of war, making a hardscrabble living as a traveling country doctor. At this time, Still's own children were desperately ill with spinal meningitis. Still did everything he could to save them, but one of his children died. Then a second child expired. Then a third. Neither Still nor his fellow physicians who were called in to minister to the stricken family could arrest the course of the dreaded inflammatory disease.

Years later, writing in his autobiography, Still was generous to the doctors but heartbroken over their failure: "It was when I stood gazing upon three members of my family—two of my own children and one adopted child—all dead from the disease spinal meningitis, that I propounded to myself the serious question: 'In sickness, has not God left man in a world of guessing? Guess what is the matter? What to give and guess the result?' "

Still's lament soon gave way to a practical course. Like Columbus, he wrote, "I trimmed my sail and launched my craft as an explorer." When, years after his children's deaths, he finally put ashore, it was in a new world of health, with a system he claimed as his own invention.

Unlike Samuel Hahnemann, who found his truth in biochemistry, the Reverend Sylvester Graham, who preached on diet, or Still's contemporaries, Ellen G. White, who revered faith, and Mary Baker Eddy, who exalted the divine mind, Still brought his attention to bear on the structure on the human body.

Still decided that the spinal column—with its tangle of nerves and arteries sending nourishing blood to the organs—held the key to good health. He called this principle the "rule of the artery." Should any of the spine's vertebrae be out of place, however, disease would result. But Still had an answer to disease: He would put the vertebrae right again with mechanical adjustments by using his own hands—he was literally a "hands-on" doctor. Still called his new system "osteopathy," a word he coined by combining the Greek words for "bone" and "suffering."

When Still developed his technique in the 1870s and 1880s, he made a radical break with mainstream medicine and his own recent past as a "regular" doctor who used *materia medica*, or pharmaceutical drugs, to effect cures. "All the drugs man needed were put in him by Nature's Quartermaster," declared Still, a religious man. So Still set off to lead a medical revolution, guided, as he believed, by the heavens.

THE HEADACHE CURE: A BOY'S OWN STORY

Andrew Taylor Still was born on August 6, 1828, the third of nine children, in backwoods Virginia. When he was a boy, Andrew's family, headed by his father Abraham Still, a circuit-riding Methodist preacher and doctor, moved to Tennessee. Later they moved to Missouri, where Andrew lived most of his adult life.

At age ten, Andrew had an experience that he later counted as momentous. Suffering from a headache and upset stomach, he improvised his own therapy by throwing a rope over a tree branch, putting a blanket over the rope, and laying his head on the makeshift swing. The tactic allowed him to stretch and relax. Andrew fell into a deep sleep. When he awoke, his headache and stomach sickness were gone.

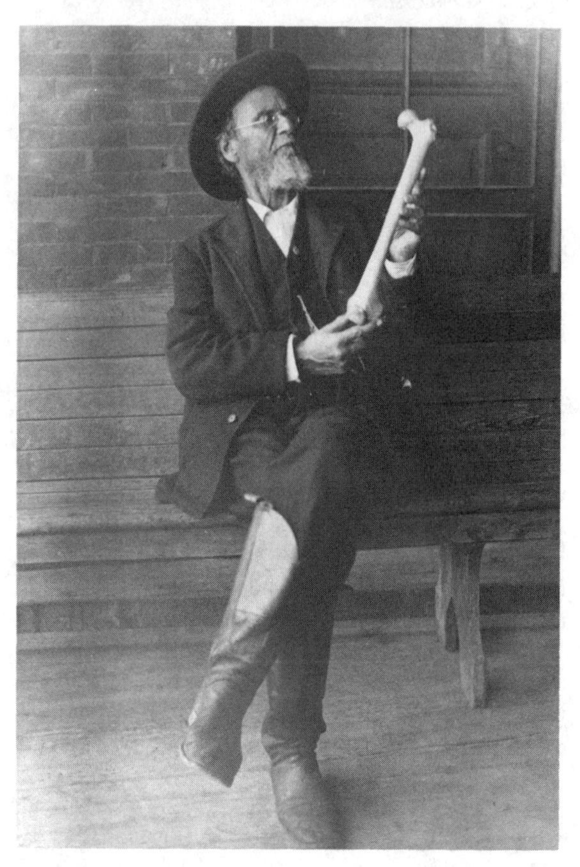

59. Still life with femur: Osteopathy's founder, Andrew Taylor Still. *Courtesy, Kirksville College of Osteopathic Medicine.*

"I followed that treatment for twenty years," he recalled, reckoning that "I had suspended the action of the great occipital nerves, and given harmony to the flow of the arterial blood. . . ." Still considered the boyhood experience his "first lesson in osteopathy."

As a young man, Still followed his father into medicine, accompanying him to revival meetings where healing sessions took place. Andrew became a doctor in 1854, at age 26. There is no firm evidence that he attended medical school, but that was not unusual. In the West, in those days, people were known by what they did, not what they studied in school; therefore a doctor was a person who practiced medicine.

Although he eventually rejected other systems of alternative medicine along with mainstream doctoring, Still was touched by several reform movements before he codified osteopathy.

One of his influences was mesmerism, the "magnetic healing" that enjoyed a vogue in mid-nineteenth-century America. Mesmerists believed that a free flow of "universal magnetic fluid" was a necessary component of health, and Still decided that blood was that fluid.

Still also lived at a time when bonesetters were popular. Bonesetters were working-class people who showed a gift for setting dislocated bones; some also manipulated joints and muscles by hand, working until a click or pop convinced both bonesetter and patient that something had just been put right.

According to Norman Gevitz, whose book *The D.O.'s: Osteopathic Medicine in America* is the prime scholarly work on Still and his professional heirs, Still ". . . put together some of the major theoretical components of magnetic healing and bonesetting in one unified doctrine; the effects of disease, as the magnetic healers said, were due to obstruction or imbalance of the fluids, but this condition itself was caused by misplaced bones, particularly of the spinal column. At this point, Still had given birth to his own distinctive system."

YOUNG DOCTOR STILL

Still's system did not spring full-blown, as from the head of Zeus. As a young doctor, he used an eclectic mixture of techniques, setting a bone here, pressing hard on a spine there, giving a drug to this patient, performing surgery on that one. He moved through the countryside in the Midwest, using his young sons who had survived the meningitis attacks or been born afterward as assistants. A bearded, unkempt-looking man, Still became known as an eccentric who carried a sackful of bones to demonstrate his powers.

As Still moved about, he attracted students, including a young man who was attempting to cure piles with a medicated ointment and another whom Still described as "a lightning-rod peddler." With his sons, his students, and his sackful of bones, Still must have been quite a sight:

> Children gave me all the road, because I said I did not believe God was a whiskey and opium-drug doctor; that I believed when He made man that He had put as many legs, noses, tongues, and qualities as he needed for any purpose in life for remedies and comfort. For such arguments I was called an infidel, crank, crazy, and God was advised by such theological hooting owls to kill me and save the lambs.

The tart-tongued Doctor Still was not without rhetorical defenses of his own, however, as he showed by characterizing one of his critics as "some old gimlet-eyed blatherskite."

By the 1880s, Still was advertising himself as a "lightning bonesetter," a description that could be applied just as well to his growing number of followers. He had by then weaned himself from attachment to orthodox medicine, claiming that his evolving system of osteopathy was a sovereign remedy not just for backaches and other chronic complaints, but all diseases, including contagions.

Still's bold citations of cures were legion. He claimed to have cured his brother, E.C. Still, of a morphine habit that took him through 75 bottles of the narcotic per year. An "Irish lady with asthma" he made well by adjusting her spine and a few ribs; "for asthma," he wrote, "Osteopathy is king." Rheumatism, heart disease, lumbago, and Still's old adversary, headache, all yielded to osteopathic treatment. He claimed to have developed "painless obstetrics" and to have banished "flux," an infectious form of diarrhea that killed children; flux was common on

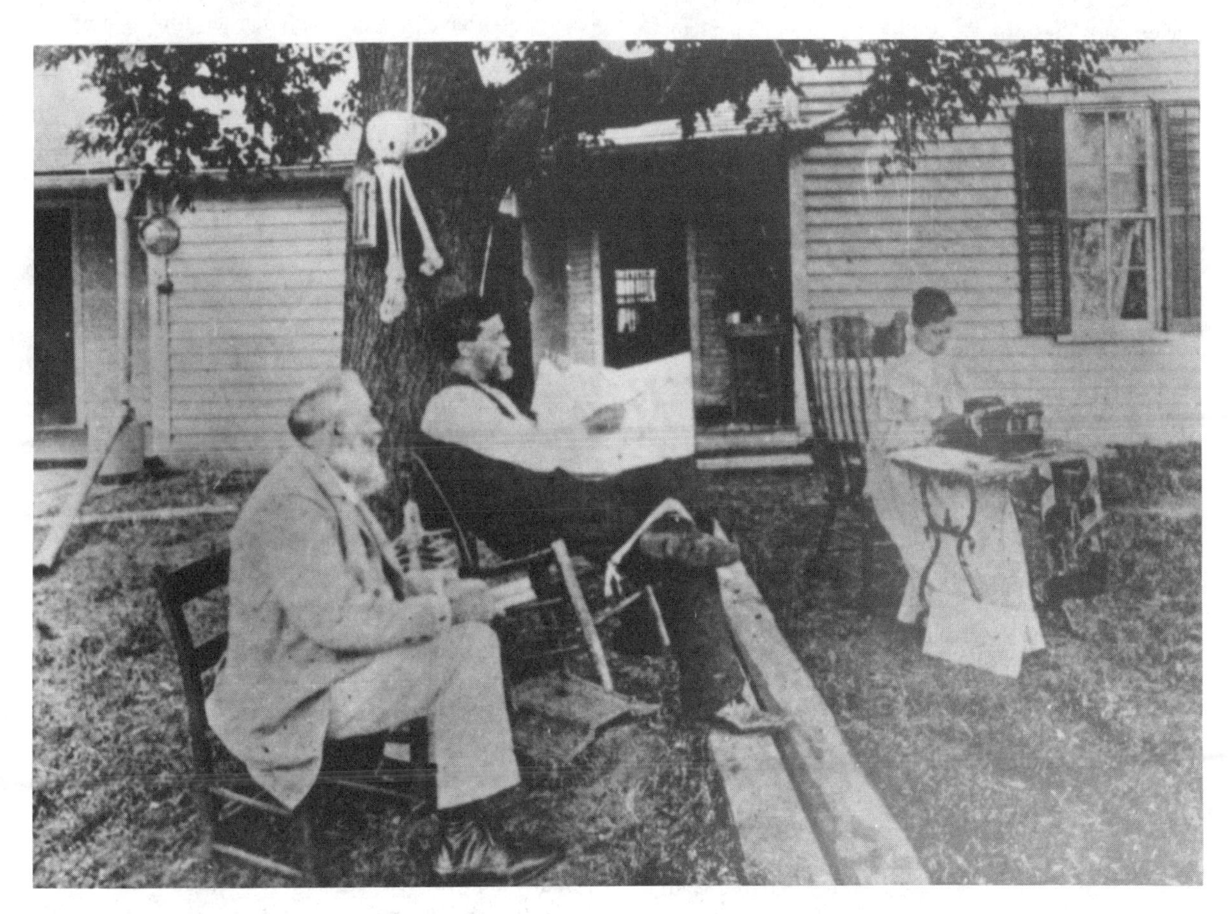

60. Still, seated center, was never too far from his favorite skeleton (on the tree trunk), which he used for teaching. *Courtesy, Kirksville College of Osteopathic Medicine.*

the frontier. He also said he cured through manipulation 75 percent of the appendicitis cases brought to him.

Although Still's assertions sound extravagant and improbable, he had enough satisfied patients to expand his practice. In the late 1880s, he helped the invalid daughter of a minister in the northeastern Missouri town of Kirksville to walk again. Pleased with the high regard in which he was subsequently held in Kirksville, Still and his family settled there in 1887. His sons followed in his footsteps, becoming osteopathic doctors. Still's autobiography includes a photograph of him resting comfortably in his grassy backyard; nearby, part of a human skeleton is laid against a sturdy old tree. The lightning bonesetter didn't like to get too far away from his bones.

THE RULE OF THE ARTERY

Healthy arteries pumping blood throughout the body were essential to Still's vision of health; but arteries could be constricted by spinal displacements, thus disturbing the circulation and inducing disease.

Still and his followers came to call such displacements "lesions." By this they meant mechanical lesions, made visible (or at least palpable) by a spine that was out of alignment. A primary lesion originated on the spine; a secondary lesion originated elsewhere and carried irregularities to the spine. Still taught his students to locate osteopathic lesions by feeling their protrusions or by noting temperature changes in the spinal column by palpation.

The examining osteopath looked for "stiffness, tension, contractures and other changes in the ligaments and musculature of the spine." Once found, the dislocations were repaired by hand, as "the bones could be used as levers to relieve pressure on nerves, veins, and arteries."

With such skills, who needed drugs? "The body itself contains within itself all the chemicals, all the medicines, necessary for the cure of disease," assured osteopath M.A. Lane, a professor in the college that Still established in Kirksville. Unleashing the body's defenses, Lane and other osteopaths asserted, granted "general immunity against all diseases." Their eventual rivals, the chiropractors, had similar views.

Osteopaths, busy setting up their fledgling practices, took care to differentiate their approach from mere massage, bonesetting, and other physical therapies, which they regarded as imprecise if not downright useless. "On the whole," sniffed one osteopath, "those manual systems compare with osteopathy as does the shotgun with the rifle."

". . . an osteopath . . . treats disease by manipulating . . . the tissues of the body, especially the tissues that constitute and support the backbone and

BONE-CRACKING COMPETITION

Osteopathic doctors got their first new competitors after 1895, the year Daniel David Palmer (1845–1913) cracked the vertebrae of a deaf janitor and ostensibly restored the man's hearing. Palmer, who founded a school in Davenport, Iowa, to teach his method, had invented chiropractic.

Osteopaths looked down their noses at chiropractors, considering them johnny-come-latelies who were imitating their method, cranking out graduates of diploma mills, and cutting into their business. Chiropractors did have a shorter course of study, but mail-order schools sold diplomas in both chiropractic and osteopathy, cheapening both degrees.

Although chiropractors—who, unlike osteopaths, cannot legally prescribe drugs or perform surgery—have had a much harder time gaining acceptance from the medical establishment, they have maintained their distinctive appeal, unlike most osteopaths, and become familiar figures in the medical landscape.

Osteopaths and chiropractors maintain that they use very different techniques to manipulate the spine. The theories behind their techniques also differ in emphasis. While both schools believed in the body's innate ability to heal itself, chiropractors concentrated on enhancing the health of the nerves, while classic osteopaths focused on freeing up the flow of blood.

Writes Norman Gevitz:

> Osteopathic manipulations were based on the lever principle, namely, the application of pressure on one part of the body to overcome resistance in motion elsewhere. This meant twisting the patient's torso in certain directions while maintaining a steady hold upon the point in structure to be influenced.

By contrast, "The most common chiropractic procedure had the client lying prone with little, if any, support below the spine. The operator would then place both hands directly over the subluxated [dislocated] segment and administer a quick thrust downward with all possible force."

the nerves that issue between the vertebrae," wrote Lane. "This manipulation, however, is no hard and fast system, but can and does vary from a single movement by which 'sub-luxations' great or small, or any other unusual stress, tension, or deflection may be removed, to a general treatment, in which the entire vertebral column and its anatomical clothes are thoroughly relaxed and readjusted."

Still's disciples were nothing if not confident. Wrote Lane in 1918: "Today, in the great center and mother institution of osteopathy at Kirksville, a city made world-renowned by Dr. Still and the system of therapy he founded, there are young osteopaths, yet in the student stage of their career, who with entire confidence in their own powers and the science under it, treat all kinds of infectious disease with a courage, or rather an entire want of fear, that reminds one of the primitive Christians."

SCHOOL DAYS WITH "THE OLD DOCTOR"

Kirksville, which hosted the first osteopathic dispensary in 1889, was also home to the world's first osteopathic school of medicine, established in 1892. The American School of Osteopathy granted Diplomates in Osteopathy, the D.O. degree that was Still's answer to the M.D. Unusual for its time, the school was open to black students and women; indeed, in the years just before 1900, one in five osteopathic graduates was a woman.

Still, who was 64 when the American School of Osteopathy opened its doors, was affectionately known by his students as "the old doctor." Still lectured frequently, sailing off into improvised dialogues and long, discursive stories; but osteopathy was a practical system, and his hands-on demonstrations of technique were highly valued.

According to a former student, "We would hold the patients in position while Dr. Still . . . worked upon them. . . . He would tell us what it would mean to the nerves from that particular region if nerves were 'tied-up' or a bone was out of line." To make a diagnosis, Still said "that we should place the patient on his side and then pass our hands carefully over the spinal column from the base of the spine, noting temperature changes as we went along. Should there be a lesion along the spine . . . it would easily be detected through an abnormal coldness or hotness of the tissue at that point."

Still concentrated on teaching anatomy, diagnosis, and osteopathic manipulative technique—the OMT. Later, as Missouri state regulation of medical schools tightened, he added courses in surgery and

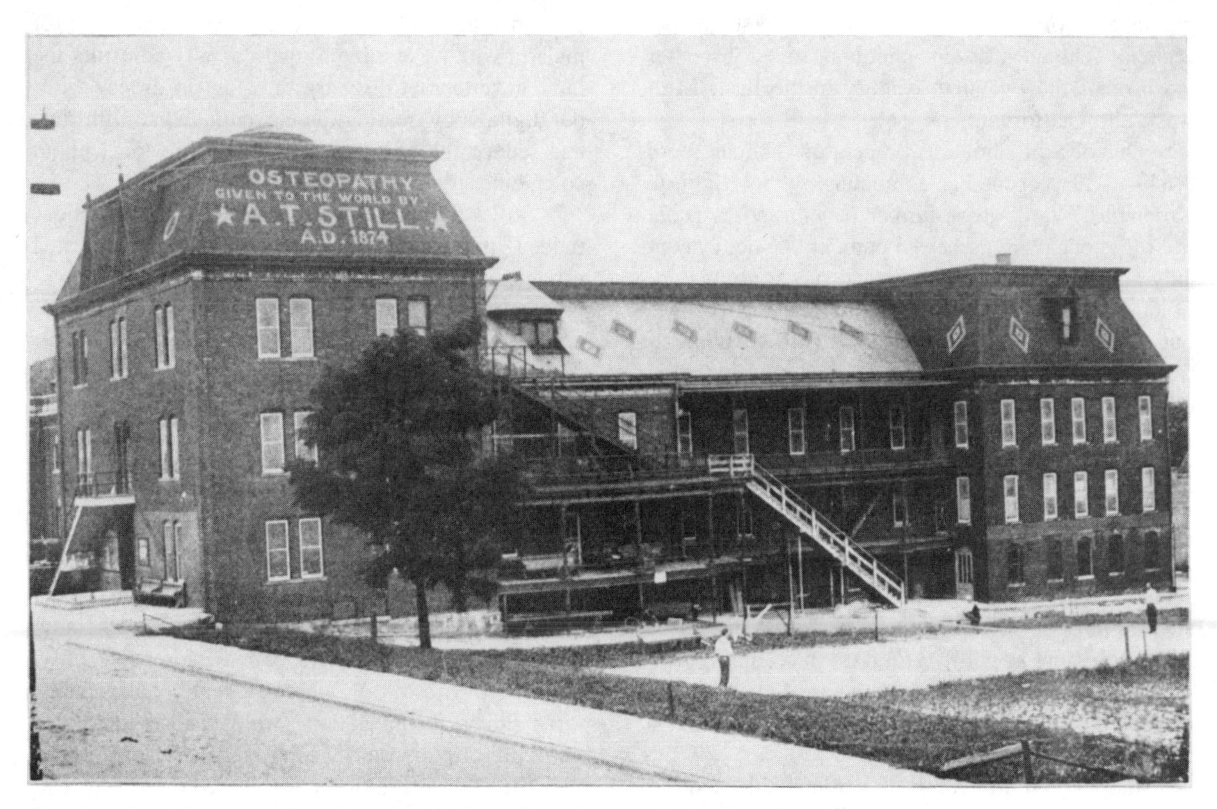
OSTEOPATHY
GIVEN TO THE WORLD BY
★A.T. STILL★
A.D. 1874

61. A late nineteenth-century view of osteopathy's first college. *Courtesy, Kirksville College of Osteopathic Medicine.*

chemistry and lengthened the course of study. In 1897, the state granted Still and his followers a big victory by legalizing osteopathy, much to the displeasure of medical doctors, who derided osteopathy as quackery.

Given official sanction and boosted by widespread testimonials, the Kirksville school and dispensary flourished. Patients came to cure headaches, nagging backaches, and flux. They came to combat rheumatism, and even for infectious diseases, even though the public was beginning to understand that contagions were caused by microorganisms and differed considerably from the chronic structural and muscular conditions that lent themselves directly to OMT.

Other privately owned, for-profit schools opened to compete with Kirksville. Advertisements for a new osteopathic school in Des Moines, Iowa derided the small-town atmosphere of Kirksville. But Kirksville was acquiring a trendy reputation similiar to that of Battle Creek, Michigan, where the cereal kings and their sanitaria were flourishing at about the same time. Hotels and boarding houses cropped up around town, and railroads initiated reduced rates to the "Missouri mecca."

Despite the growth of Kirksville and its school, competitive proprietary schools continued to open. By 1904, half of the 4,000 American D.O.s had graduated from schools that competed with Still's academy. About a dozen schools operated just after the turn of the twentieth century in the East, Midwest, and California.

One of Still's boldest competitors, Marcus Ward (1849–1929), opened a competing school right in Kirksville. Ward was a former patient and assistant of Still's; but Ward eschewed pure, or classic, osteopathy and added pharmacology and surgery to his use of OMT. Ward's school later merged with Still's, but other osteopaths, chafing under Still's manipulation-only dogma, heeded Ward's restless declaration of independence. In the long term, osteopathy would follow Ward's lead, although it would be years before Still's charismatic authority was superseded.

Fundamental changes in osteopathic education—and thus in osteopathic practice—were given a boost by publication of the Flexner Report in 1910. Flexner scolded osteopathic schools for providing little bedside training or basic laboratory work and dismissed their professors as poorly grounded in scientific principles. As with other medical schools of every stripe, osteopathic schools were devastated by the criticism and the public scrutiny it brought.

In the coming years, the osteopathic schools that survived the post-Flexner scrutiny tightened their entrance requirements and added courses to try to keep up with the on-rushing changes in mainstream medical science. By 1940, they all required at least two years of college for admission; by 1954, at least three years. And, as the schools spent ever more time teaching surgery and once-forbidden pharmacology, they spent ever less time on OMT, the technique that defined A.T. Still's therapeutics and made them unique.

MAINSTREAMING

From the profession's early days, free-thinking D.O.s, impressed though they may have been with Still's method, questioned his dogmatic assertion that OMT cured everything. Even Still himself, whose belief in his creation was quasi-religious, made some allowances for advances in scientific knowledge.

"I believe but very little of the germ theory," osteopathy's founder scoffed in 1901, "and care much less." In practical terms, however, Still modified his therapeutic approach, accepting what he termed "adjuncts" to OMT. He conceded that surgery could be performed as a last resort and endorsed antiseptics for wounds, surgical anesthetics, and chemical antidotes for poisoning.

Despite such concessions, Still's faith in basic OMT did not waver. Observes Gevitz: "Still claimed . . . that he could prevent the chills and fever of malaria without quinine by periodically adjusting the lumbar vertebrae; dispense the fluid in dropsy without digitalis by treating the eleventh and twelfth ribs; and reduce the swelling of a gouty big toe without colchicine by manipulating the foot."

Still's faith was rooted in religious conviction. Indeed, this son of a preacher very nearly elevated osteopathy to the status of a religion, even as he was proclaming it to be a science. Osteopathy, he said, was "the only exact method of healing." It represented "the most significant progress in the history of scientific research."

Some of the founder's followers shared his faith, or at least adhered to his technique. Known as "lesion" osteopaths, they also called themselves "ten-fingered" osteopaths, 10 fingers being the number necessary to perform hands-on OMT. Their eclectic brethren who embraced drugs, surgery, and other therapies, such as hydrotherapy and electrotherapy, were called "broad" osteopaths. More colorfully, they were known as "three-fingered" osteopaths, three fingers being all that were needed to scratch out a prescription on a writing pad.

Still's criticism of three-fingered osteopaths was scathing: "Medicine and osteopathy as therapeutic agencies have nothing in common either theoretically or practically, and only an inconsistent physician will attempt to practice both," he declared. In 1915, at a national convention, the 87-year-old patriarch, sensing that the vandals were inside the gates of his shining city on a hill, made an impassioned appeal for broad osteopaths to return to the straight and narrow, but it was too late. Changes in the profession, while incomplete and uneven, were irreversible in the face of scientific advances and competition from M.D.s. Two years later, on December 12, 1917, Still passed away. He died of unspecified causes, at age 89, a visionary whose life spanned the age of Conestoga wagons and airplanes, calomel and X-rays.

After the passing of osteopathy's founder, the revisionist three-fingered osteopaths won the struggle for power hands down. Their cause did sustain a temporary setback during the great influenza epidemic of 1918–19. The grippe, as influenza was called, killed more people than all the combat deaths in World War I. Some 650 thousand people died in the United States, 41 million worldwide. In a two-week period, 5,100 flu victims expired in Philadelphia.

Medical authorities were helpless. There was no recognized cure for the flu, and no vaccine had been developed to prevent it. Osteopaths claimed great success against the epidemic by applying general OMT to the necks and spines of sufferers who, in their frustration, turned to alternative medicine, but M.D.s disputed the osteopaths' statistics and rejected their claims of cures.

Osteopaths submitted that OMT fought contagious diseases by helping the blood form antibodies, thereby boosting the immune system. M.A. Lane, in a book published in 1918 at the height of the epidemic, wrote that OMT "proceeds actively to assist nature, first by adjusting any existing anatomical abnormalities in the spine . . . and . . . by stimulating the spinal nerves and thus energizing cells that in all probability are doing all they can to manufacture the anti-poisons . . . in the patient's blood." Conversely, dislocations predisposed the body to infection.

In spite of their best efforts to defend Still's nineteenth-century theories in a rapidly modernizing world, traditional osteopaths found that fighting scientific research was like trying to sweep back the ocean with a broom. In 1929, the American Osteopathic Association okayed "supplementary therapeutics" to go with OMT, giving belated official recognition to a process that had long been underway.

OMT was falling into disrepute and disuse. Modern osteopaths declared themselves too busy to use the technique, especially when they could get faster results from drugs. Sometimes OMT was used in pre- and postoperative periods. George A. Still, the founder's grandnephew, who held both D.O. and M.D. degrees, used OMT in obstetrics after surgery to build the body's defenses, and claimed a sharp decline in postoperative pneumonia. In the long run, however, it was easier for osteopaths to use three fingers to write a prescription, and most did just that.

WAR AND (ALMOST) PEACE

Relations between osteopaths and medical doctors had seldom been good. M.D.s quite logically saw the standard-bearers for this new theory of the spine as competitors and, by their lights, scurrilous ones at that.

In 1893, Charles Still (1865–1955), A.T.'s son, was sued by an M.D. for practicing medicine without a license when he treated diphtheria-stricken children in Red Wing, Minnesota. The younger Still claimed to have lost but one of his 70 patients, an impressive cure rate if true. Public opinion rallied to the beleaguered osteopath's support, and the doctor who brought the charges dropped his lawsuit.

Overall, things were slow to change, however. In 1897, the same year that Missouri decided to legalize and regulate osteopathy, the *Journal of the American Medical Association* denounced A.T. Still's followers as "degenerates who constitute most of the devotees of and the practice of quackery." M.D.s further upped the ante by arguing that there were no such things as osteopathic lesions and that students in schools of osteopathy were there only because they couldn't get into real, that is, conventional, medical schools.

Concluding, as had many before them, that the best defense is a good offense, osteopaths formed the American Osteopathic Association in 1901. The AOA started a magazine, the monthly *Journal of the American Osteopathic Association,* modeled on the *Journal of the American Medical Association,* and began AMA-style lobbying to liberalize licensing laws.

Over the span of decades they were spectacularly successful. In 1973, Mississippi became the last state to legalize osteopathy. California, which stopped licensing new osteopaths in 1962, started again in 1974, completing a sweep of all 50 states.

OSTEOPATHY TODAY

Osteopathy's bid for acceptance was much closer to success in the early 1990s than it had ever been before. All 50 states gave D.O.s the same rights accorded to M.D.s. By 1990, Americans paid 25 million office visits to osteopaths every year. Even so, many consumers are not quite sure what osteopaths do, often confusing them with a wide range of physical therapists, specialists in sports medicine, orthopedic surgeons (M.D.s who treat the bones, muscles, and joints but do not practice OMT), and especially chiropractors, who still adjust the spine but are not legally allowed to prescribe drugs or perform surgery.

D.O.s, who can do all three, prefer to compare themselves to M.D.s, although they are careful to spell out their differences. D.O.s still study osteopathic manipulation in college (though many do not use it) and feel that their knowledge of this nondrug technique makes them more holistically inclined than orthodox doctors.

In 1990, there were nearly 200 osteopathic hospitals and close to 30 thousand D.O.s in the United States. Moreover, there were 15 American osteopathic medical schools, including Still's original school, renamed the Kirksville College of Osteopathic Medicine.

Osteopathic colleges offer courses in OMT, Still's most enduring legacy. A 1974 study showed, however, that only 17 percent of patients at osteopathic hospitals received any OMT. The figure may have climbed since then, as hospitals that still use OMT report that their patients, happy to have a noninvasive alternative to drugs and surgery, say they like the technique.

Does traditional osteopathic manipulation work? The question is difficult to answer. Even conventional physicians acknowledge that OMT is effective for chronic backaches, joint pain, and muscle aches; but many D.O.s have abandoned claims that OMT is

''THE LITTLE M.D.S''

Perhaps the most unusual turn in the long and generally unfriendly relationship between medical doctors and osteopaths came in California. In 1962, 2,000 of the state's 2,300 osteopaths accepted M.D. degrees in return for giving up their separate status as osteopaths. The merger was mutually beneficial to M.D.s—led by the state branch of the American Medical Association, which adopted an ''if you can't beat 'em, absorb 'em'' strategy—and D.O.s, who craved the status that came with their new degrees.

The degrees, derided by the national American Osteopathic Association as ''the little m.d.s,'' were only good for practicing medicine in California. To snare the new degrees, California osteopaths agreed not to license any new D.O.s and osteopathic medical schools synchronized their curricula with mainstream schools.

The merger removed the most dynamic and free-thinking osteopaths in the country as a competitive force. California osteopaths had spearheaded modern ''broad'' osteopathy and long topped the nation's schools in academic requirements.

Dramatic as it was, the merger did not remain intact. In 1974, the state supreme court struck down part of the deal, again permitting the licensing of new osteopaths. Even so, osteopathy has never fully recovered in the nation's most populous state. The Yellow Pages of the 1990 San Francisco telephone directory listed only 10 osteopathic physicians, while medical doctors took up 25 pages in the same directory. Chiropractors covered another 13 pages.

THE ''MISSOURI MECCA''

Kirksville may not be the fashionable destination it used to be, but the Missouri town is still a major center of osteopathic education and historical lore.

When one of the authors visited the Kirksville College of Osteopathic Medicine in the summer of 1990, the world's first osteopathic college was gearing up for its 1992 centennial. Home to 500 students on a 50-acre campus shared by a modern medical center, the college honors A.T. Still's backcountry roots by dispatching apprentice D.O.s to rural clinics. The college also emphasizes traditional OMT, requiring 267 hours of osteopathic theory and practice, well above the 120 to 150 hours offered in most of its sister schools.

The Still National Osteopathic Museum is also located on campus, right near the log cabin where Still was born, which was relocated from his Virginia home. The museum, founded in 1978 and open to the public, displays writings in Still's hand, orginal drawings from his autobiography, and the skeleton that Still used in his first classes. Just a few blocks away, Kirksville has erected a statue of ''The Old Doctor,'' right in front of the town courthouse.

an effective general treatment for disease, as Still insisted it was.

Although, as noted, many patients report feeling better after receiving OMT, there are few hard data to verify their feelings, which some observers attribute to the soothing power of touch and suggestion. Studies in the 1930s and 1940s suggested that Still's osteopathic lesions might be real, but not enough subsequent research has been done to convince a skeptical medical profession.

Brian Inglis, professor of psychological medicine at the University of Edinburgh, asserts that osteopathy and its rival, chiropractic, are more closely linked than devotees of either discipline care to acknowledge, and may work in much the same way. Of Still's "rule of the artery" and Daniel David Palmer's "rule of the nerve," Inglis writes:

"Both 'rules' are really rationalizations designed to give a plausible explanation of why spinal manipulation works. Both may be right (for blood and nerves can both be the beneficiaries); and both could be wrong without necessarily discrediting manipulative therapy—for whose results some other explanation might eventually be found."

Authorities can debate how, and if, spinal manipulation works, but there is no debating American osteopathy's growth. Ironically, much of this growth has come about at the expense of osteopathy's identity. Indeed, many D.O.s are now virtually indistinguishable from M.D.s and some practitioners hold both degrees.

CHAPTER · 16 ·

CHIROPRACTIC: THE SPINE ADJUSTORS

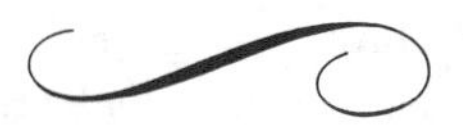

A Subluxed vertebra is the cause of 95 percent of all diseases.

DANIEL DAVID PALMER, 1910

Harvey Lillard never dreamed that the man with the long flowing beard would ever cure him of his deafness. Seventeen years earlier, the Davenport, Iowa janitor had suddenly lost his hearing when he felt something snap in his back while he was bending over. As he watched the man who called himself a ''magnetic healer'' adjust the examining table that September day in 1895, Lillard had no idea that he was about to help make medical history.

Fifteen years later, the healer, whose name was Daniel David Palmer, described that historic session in his autobiography. After convincing Lillard to let him try his hand at a cure, he asked the janitor to lie face down on the examining couch. Running his hand over his patient's back, Palmer discovered an abnormal protrusion and concluded that the snapping sound must have been a misplaced vertebra. ''If the vertebra was replaced,'' he reasoned, ''the man's hearing should be restored.'' With that in mind, Palmer first placed his hands on Lillard's spine, and then quickly moved the vertebra back into place. The janitor's hearing, recalled Palmer, was ''instantly restored.''

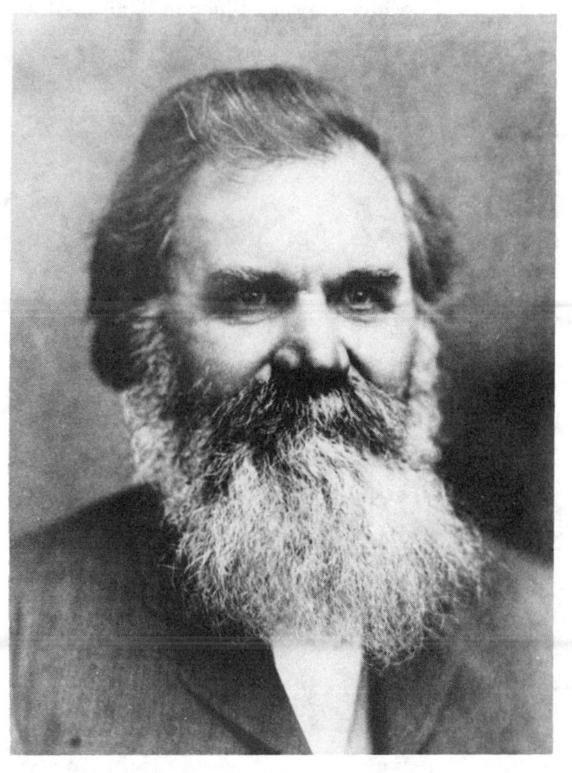

62. ''Old Dad Chiro'' (D.D. Palmer), founder of chiropractic. *Photo courtesy of the Archives, David D. Palmer Health Sciences Library, Palmer College of Chiropractic.*

The skeptics questioned Palmer's curative powers, pointing out that Lillard must have been able to hear in the first place since he had carried on a conversation with the healer before the adjustment. The skeptics notwithstanding, Lillard's treatment would become known as the first chiropractic adjustment, and "D.D.," as Palmer was called, the "discoverer" of chiropractic. The term *chiropractic,* from the Greek "to work by hand," was invented a year later by D.D.'s friend, fellow Iowan Reverend Samuel Weed.

The principles of chiropractic as described by D.D. and others at the end of the nineteenth and beginning of the twentieth centuries, are, as D.D. himself readily admitted, "as old as the vertebrata." (He claimed that it was his *method* of spinal adjustment that was original, "replacing displaced vertebrae by using the spinous and transverse processes as levers.") These principles are still the core of chiropractic theory today.

Simply put, chiropractors believe that the key to health is the condition of the nervous system, through which every part of the body is related to the spinal column. These nerve "highways" can function properly only when the spine and bones of the vertebrae are in proper alignment. A misaligned vertebra such as Lillard's, known as "vertebral subluxation," puts pressure on the nerves, which lowers the body's resistance to disease. Wrote D.D. in his 1914 *The Chiropractor,* "by restoring them [the vertebrae] to their normal position, normal function is restored."

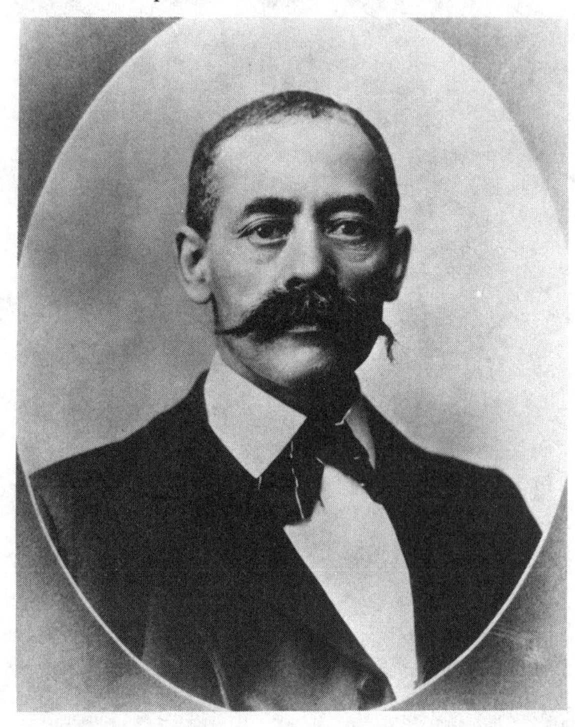

63. Harvey Lillard, the Davenport, Iowa janitor who said D.D. Palmer cured his deafness, was the first chiropractic patient. *Photo courtesy of the Archives, David D. Palmer Health Sciences Library, Palmer College of Chiropractic.*

Opposed to both drugs and surgery, chiropractors correct misaligned vertebrae by "adjusting" (also called "manipulating") parts of the body, in particular, the spine. The spinal adjustment is meant to strengthen the body's natural healing ability (called the "Innate Intelligence"). And while many chiropractors also use other forms of treatment, such as massage, homeopathy, diet, or vitamin therapy, the chiropractic adjustment has been the principal method of treatment ever since Lillard stepped out of D.D. Palmer's magnetic healing studio.

Vertebral subluxation, according to chiropractic textbook author A.E. Homewood, may be caused by a whole host of factors—badly designed furniture, stress, fatigue, bad posture, automobile accidents, strains from lifting, falls, heredity, changes in environment, such as temperature, and even body type. Drugs, walking on cement, poor shoe design, working at a computer, and, for newborns, forceps at birth may also damage the spine.

Through much of its history, chiropractic has been maligned by its critics as quackery, and chiropractors stereotyped as "bonecrackers." Back in the 1930s, when a good number of chiropractic schools were forced to shut their doors for financial reasons, the critics happily predicted that the "dangerous cult" would soon disappear. Yet today chiropractic is very much alive and well, thanks not only to successful political lobbying and major legal victories, but also to the army of loyal patients who consider their chiropractors nothing less than miracle workers.

"LOOK WELL TO THE SPINE FOR THE CAUSE OF DISEASE"

Manipulation is, indeed, "as old as the vertebrata." As medical sociologist Walter I. Wardwell describes, as early as 2700 B.C., the Chinese practiced a form of spinal manipulation, while the pre-Hippocratic Greek mythological god of healing Aesculapius was believed to have used spinal manipulation as a healing method. Hippocrates, the father of Western medicine, referred to spinal manipulation in his writings and the spine "as the cause of disease." Many of the Native Americans of North, Central, and South America regularly used manipulation for healing purposes. European settlers in the New World reported seeing Native American children walk on the sore backs of their elders.

By the Middle Ages, spines were manipulated not for health reasons, but for form. "The most important requirement was that the spine be straight."

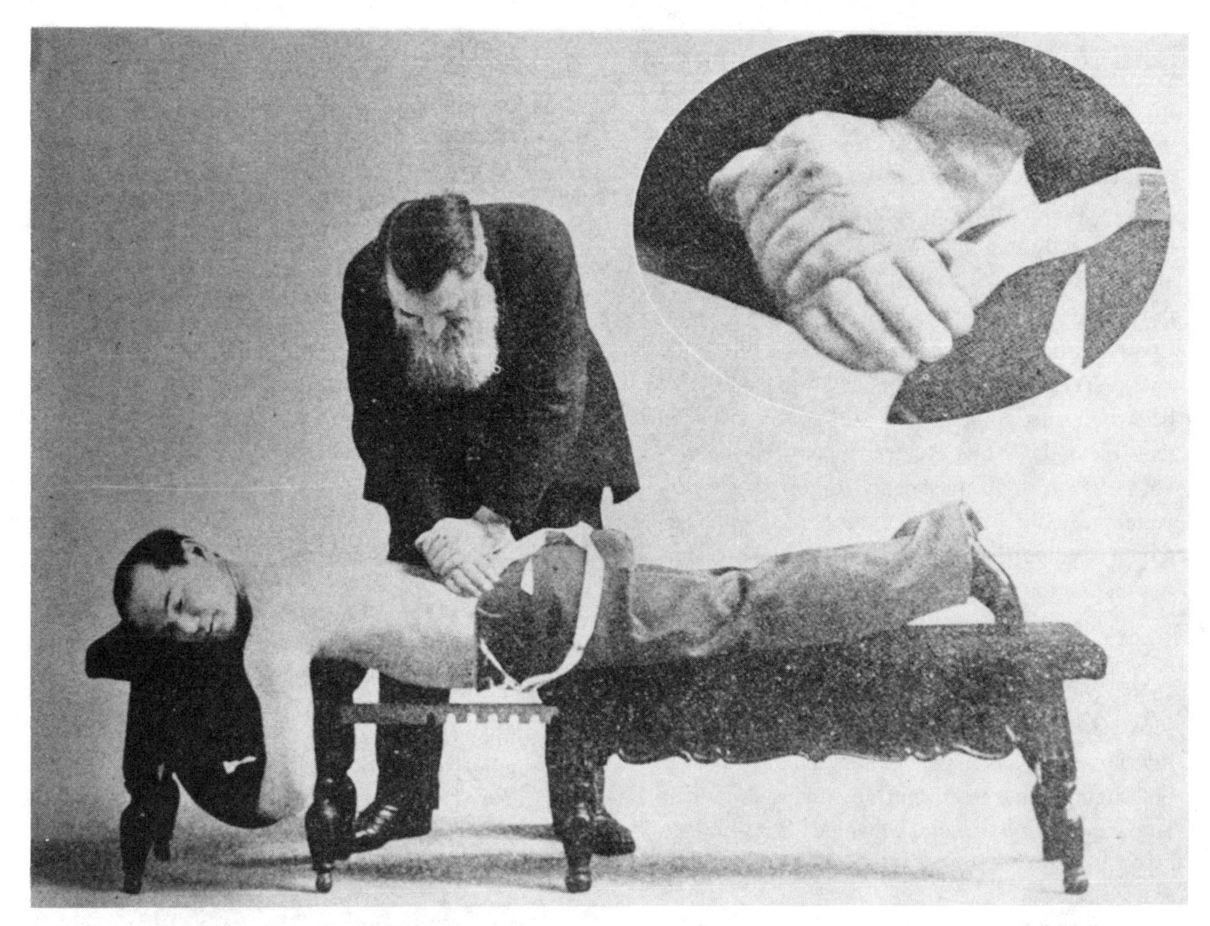

64. A patient gets an adjustment from the hands of the master (D.D. Palmer). *Photo courtesy of the Archives, David D. Palmer Health Sciences Library, Palmer College of Chiropractic.*

Healers known as "bonesetters," precursors of chiropractors, first made their appearance in seventeenth-century Europe, and bonesetting rapidly turned into a folk healing art in England, France, Germany, and Spain. From its beginnings bonesetters were labeled as "peasant healers" by the regulars, who refused to allow bonesetters access to their hospitals. By the nineteenth century, bonesetting had made its way to the United States. There, as in Europe, the art of bonesetting was a family affair, handed down from father to son or from mother to daughter. Although on both sides of the Atlantic bonesetting was derided by allopathic physicians as quackery, some regulars evidently manipulated many a spine in the course of their healing.

According to Wardwell, the most famous nineteenth-century bonesetter in England was Sir Herbert Barker, who by 1906 was calling himself an osteopath. Across the Atlantic, "Bonesetter Reese" practiced his art in western Pennsylvania and Ohio, while the Sweet family manipulated spines throughout Rhode Island, Massachusetts, Connecticut, and New York, even receiving referrals from orthodox physicians. As late as 1917, a Sweet family member was known to have practiced bonesetting in Rhode Island.

Like many folk-healing practices, bonesetting had strong ties to spiritual healing traditions. European bonesetters were seen as having a special gift for healing. In the United States, Mormon leader Joseph Smith (1805–1844) employed bonesetting as part of the laying on of hands, a process described by one witness as sounding like "the crushing of an old basket."

Like bonesetters, magnetic healers also employed the "special healing power" of the hands; their method was to rub the spinal column vigorously to infuse a "life-giving force" into all of the organs of the body. Palmer writes that he practiced magnetic healing for nine years before discovering chiropractic.

D.D. PALMER AND "THE BIG IDEA"

Daniel David Palmer was born in 1845 in the small town of Port Perry, Ontario, Canada, east of Toronto. As the American Civil War was ending, he and a brother took off for the United States for the

CHIROPRACTIC VS. OSTEOPATHY

In the early days of chiropractic, debunkers charged that chiropractic was just another version of osteopathy, invented by the Kirksville, Missouri healer Andrew Taylor Still. Chiropractic's champions said it was exactly the other way around.

Both systems shunned drugs and surgery in the nineteenth century. According to Still's son, Charles, Still and Palmer met in Kirksville in the 1890s. Yet both chiropractors and osteopaths have been quick to point out the differences between their methods: While Palmer emphasized the nervous system and adjustments to correct specific vertebrae, Still believed in the "rule of the artery," arguing that the blood circulation system, not the nervous system, determined one's health.

Today, many regulars continue to relegate both chiropractic and osteopathy to second class status. Chiropractic has reponded by continuing to separate itself from orthodox medicine. Osteopathy, however, has moved closer to the regulars in both training and treatment, employing drug therapy and surgery as well as manipulation.

greater financial opportunities postwar America appeared to offer. While his brother ended up in Oklahoma, D.D. settled in the Mississippi River town of New Boston, Illinois via Buffalo, Detroit, and Davenport, Iowa. Soon after arriving in New Boston, he met and married Lavina McGee, widow of a Confederate soldier. In 1881 Lavina gave birth to their only child, Bartlett Joshua ("B.J."), who would sell his father's "big idea" to twentieth-century America.

When B.J. was only three, Lavina died, and the young widower purchased a grocery store. Figuring that his landlocked neighbors could use a good fish market, D.D. specialized in selling fish. Debunkers of chiropractic would later use his early career choice as an excuse to call him "nothing more than a fish peddler."

Besides fresh fish, D.D. also became interested in magnetic healing after consuming books on magnetism, Chinese philosophy, and thought reading. In the mid-1880s he moved across and up the Mississippi to Davenport, Iowa, where he hung out his shingle on the fourth floor of the Ryan Building at Second and Brady streets. According to his grandson, David Daniel ("Dave") Palmer, by the time D.D. adjusted Harvey Lillard's back in his Brady Street studio, D.D. already had a substantial practice in the laying on of hands. His method, wrote Dave Palmer, was "to draw his hands over the area of the pain and with a sweeping motion stand aside, shaking his hands and fingers vigorously."

One can only imagine the impression D.D. must have made on his patients, for he was, according to his grandson, "a rare type standing out from the common herd." He was "rather short and of heavy stature, usually wearing a broad-brimmed black sombrero of the type known in Western days. He wore a heavy beard, trimmed in full fashion."

The year after he discovered chiropractic, D.D. incorporated a school in Davenport to teach "the big idea," calling it Palmer's School of Magnetic Cure. Records show that there were three students in 1899, two in 1900, five in 1901, and four in 1902, one of whom was his 21-year-old son B.J.

In 1903, the founder of chiropractic, along with his son, was arrested for practicing medicine without a license. With a legal cloud trailing behind him, D.D. left Davenport and headed west, where he introduced chiropractic in Oklahoma, Oregon, and California. He left behind a 2,000-dollar debt and a disgruntled son who ran the school in his father's

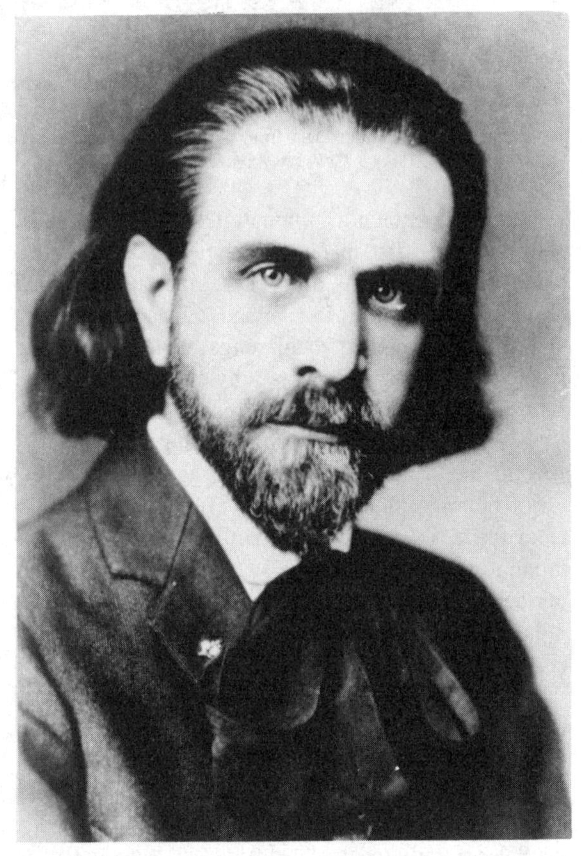

65. The charismatic and eccentric B.J. Palmer, D.D.'s son, popularized chiropractic. *Photo courtesy of the Archives, David D. Palmer Health Sciences Library, Palmer College of Chiropractic.*

absence. Three years later D.D. was brought to trial and convicted, the first chiropractic martyr. Sentenced to a term of 105 days in the Scott County Jail, D.D. was released after serving 23 days and paying a 350-dollar fine. Somehow B.J. was able to avoid the same fate.

Apparently there was no love lost between D.D. and his son, who was 13 years old when "Old Dad Chiro" discovered chiropractic. From the beginning of their professional relationship, these two strong-willed men never saw eye-to-eye on a thing. Unlike his cautious father, who was not eager to spread chiropractic beyond a select circle because it would not be "properly interpreted," the precocious B.J. envisioned chiropractic as the next wave.

The first explosion between the two came when B.J. upstaged his father by publishing the first book on chiropractic, *The Science of Chiropractic: Its Principles and Adjustments,* in 1906. Dedicating his book to his father, he wryly wrote, "With my kindest regards, I present you with the No. 1 of the 1st issue of the first book ever published on chiropractic. From B.J. Palmer, D.C., to father Dr. D.D. Palmer." Four years later, D.D. would follow with his own book, *The Chiropractor's Adjustor,* in which he publicly aired his irritation with his son. "I objected to its [B.J.'s book] being published at that time, because I thought and now know that the science had not been sufficiently developed. But in spite of my objections, the book was printed."

D.D. returned to Iowa in 1906, and soon thereafter B.J. purchased the struggling school from his father, incorporating it as the Palmer School and Infirmary of Chiropractic (PSC). According to Dave Palmer, the name "Infirmary" was added because chiropractic patients lived on the top floor next to the classrooms. After paying 500 dollars, students took a six-month course in the new science and earned a diploma. This diploma was soon replaced by the degree of "Doctor of Chiropractic" (D.C.), a title that raised the ears and wrath of the regulars. By 1908, 130 students were enrolled at the school. By 1910 it offered a 12-month course with classes in anatomy, physiology, dissection, analysis, hygiene, chiropractic orthopedy, nerve tracing, histology, gynecology, obstetrics, theory, philosophy, and chiropractic practice.

The final break between D.D. and B.J. came in the summer of 1913, when D.D. tried to lead on foot an alumni homecoming parade through downtown Davenport. What happened next is not entirely clear. Apparently B.J., who was riding in a faculty car, did not want to be upstaged by his father. One version has B.J. begging his father to join him in his automobile. When D.D. refused, B.J. had him escorted to the sidewalk. Another version has B.J., in a fit of rage, deliberately plowing the car into his father. When D.D. died only three months later in Los Angeles, his executors blamed B.J. for his father's death. They claimed that D.D.'s health rapidly failed after the car incident and sought 50 thousand dollars in damages. Although the district attorney sought a murder indictment, a grand jury refused to indict B.J. In his final days, "Old Dad Chiro" left instructions that his son be barred from his funeral.

B.J. PALMER: "THE DEVELOPER"

Ever since he was expelled from the seventh grade, rebelliousness and eccentricity were a way of life for Bartlett Joshua Palmer, who, writes his only child Dave, "in his whole life didn't conform to any pattern of life."

Dave's earliest memory of his father was waking at daybreak to the sounds of B.J.'s typewriter echoing through their Davenport mansion. B.J.'s habit of retiring at 9 P.M. and rising at 5 A.M. to work never varied; if dinner guests were present, he simply excused himself promptly at 9 and went to bed.

In his memoirs Dave Palmer described how B.J. liked to wear a shoestring around his head to hold his long hair in place, which he washed only once a year, apparently so as not to lose its natural oil. No matter the season, B.J. evidently wore suits made only of homespun material made in Asheville, North Carolina. He always slept with his head toward the North Pole and his feet toward the South Pole—he would rearrange the bed to suit his needs whenever he was on the road. Wrote one reporter in the Davenport *Times Democrat,* "He was a striking figure. He was an image—and that is exactly what B.J. wanted—to portray a distinct personality."

A compulsive collector, B.J. gathered into his home everything from swords and walking sticks to pigeons and alligators. The third floor of his mansion housed a world-famous collection of spines, while on the grounds stood a three-story greenhouse filled with lush tropical plants and rare statues made of bronze and marble imported from Italy. Always up on the newest technological breakthroughs, he was the first in Davenport to own an automobile. On many an early morning, the townsfolk would see him whiz by in his chauffeur-driven car on his way to an adjustment appointment at a wealthy client's home.

His wife, the former Mabel Heath, whom he married in 1904, seems to have tolerated his odd habits with good humor. A chiropractic graduate

The World's Greatest Chiropractor
A Fascinating Lecturer and Crayon Artist
"The man who is to medicine what Tolstoy is to Russia." Press Comment
"Lincoln saved a race, Palmer is saving the Entire Human race." Nutting
- - A Rare Opportunity To Hear - -
B. J. Palmer, D. C., Ph. C.
Don't Miss It
Pres. The Palmer School of Chiropractic, Davenport, Iowa, U. S. A. the School conducting the largest open Clinic in the World.
WHO WILL DELIVER A
FREE ILLUSTRATED LECTURE
Setting forth the principals and demonstrating the science of

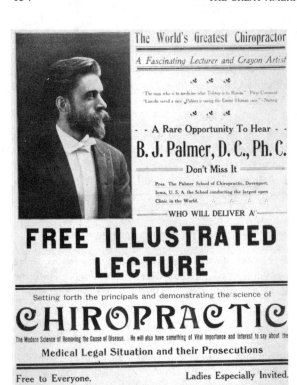

The Modern Science of Removing the Cause of Disease. He will also have something of Vital Importance and Interest to say about the
Medical Legal Situation and their Prosecutions
Free to Everyone.
Ladies Especially Invited.
Patterson's Opera House Mt. Carroll. Illinois
SATURDAY, AUG. 27, 1910, 8 P. M.

66. *Photo courtesy of the Archives, David D. Palmer Health Sciences Library, Palmer College of Chiropractic.*

herself, Mabel, known as the "Sweetheart of Chiropractic," wrote a textbook on anatomy and taught at the Palmer school for 35 years before her death in 1949. She often acted as referee between young Dave and B.J., who, like his own father, bore down hard on his son. When the college-age Dave insisted on leaving Davenport to study business at the University of Pennsylvania's Wharton School and "break loose from parental tyranny," B.J. promised he would never allow him in the house again. Mabel must have intervened, for Dave spent his first Christmas break in Davenport with his parents.

"EARLY TO BED, EARLY TO RISE, WORK LIKE HELL AND ADVERTISE"

His father may have discovered "the big idea," but B.J., called "the Developer of Chiropractic," was responsible for introducing chiropractic to the American public. He did so with aggressive marketing—through broadsides, advertisements, books, pamphlets, newspaper articles, an alumni newsletter, a journal, a speaker's bureau, and, at PSC's annual lyceum, a conference, reunion, and in-service training workshop held in Davenport every August from 1913 until 1960.

To manage his own campaign, B.J. created the PSC Printery, a combination printing press and public relations/advertising bureau. Festooned with plants and fine works of art, the printery was known as the "prettiest printing plant in America." (Son Dave, who did not share his father's taste in interior design, simplified the decor when he took over the school after B.J.'s death in 1961.)

B.J. was a prolific writer, pouring out thousands of words on a typewriter made with an extra-long carriage. His 1926 book, *Selling Yourself,* cajoled his audiences to get out there and sell chiropractic. It listed 58 topics and epigrams, such as "Only the mints can make money without advertising," and "Early to bed, early to rise, work like hell, and advertise," which is, today, painted in bold letters on the porch of the PSC student union. His weekly alumni newsletter, "The Fountainhead," reminded his graduates that they would always be members of a large chiropractic family. His monthly journal, *The Chiropractor and Clinical Journal,* begun by his father in 1904 and lasting until 1961, kept his growing chiropractic family, many of them isolated in rural areas and small towns, informed of major legal and technical updates and entertained with poetry and cartoons. B.J. made no bones about its purpose, which was stated under the masthead: "A national magazine devoted to the Promotion and Perpetuation of Straight Chiropractic."

B.J.'s pride and joy was PSC, which by 1920 was the largest chiropractic college in the United States, spreading out over three square blocks, educating 2,000 students and treating 3,000 patients in

RADIO DAYS

Chiropractic was not B.J.'s only obsession. In 1921 he purchased a 100-watt "radiophone" station from a man in nearby Rock Island, Illinois, which was assigned the letters WOC (that some people joked stood for "Wonders of Chiropractic"). From the fourth floor of the college's administration building, WOC beamed weather reports, stock market conditions, farm information, and live piano and pipe organ music across the Midwest. When it made its debut in 1922, it was only 1 of 10 stations on the air in the United States. Today WOC, along with WOC-TV, the first television station in Iowa, is still on the air at its modern headquarters across the street from Palmer College in Davenport, Iowa.

its clinic. B.J.'s "organizational and merchandising skills," writes Wardwell, "led to remarkable success in recruiting staff and students and in retaining the support of PSC graduates."

B.J.'s finest moments were at the annual PSC lyceums, during which time chiropractors and their families and patients, as well as sightseers from all over the world, gathered under the hot Davenport sun. The lyceums, lasting as long as a week, featured picnic lunches held on the banks of the Mississippi River, speedboat rides, demonstration clinics, sessions on new techniques, and introductions to new technological breakthroughs, in addition to speeches by visiting guests and, of course, B.J.

Writer Marcus Bach describes the lyceum he attended in the early 1940s:

> The atmosphere had the high pitch of a world series, the fervor of an old-time revival, the passion of a circus, even to a tent, an enormous tent pitched in the midst of the pretentious ivy halls of a big and booming chiropractic school. . . . But the impression that came to me out of the mood of the milling men and women streaming into the big top was that here was a pioneering, evangelizing crowd with the overtones of a crusade. Whatever these people had found, they believed in it; whatever they believed in, they were proud of it, proud to a point of zealotry.

The most popular feature of every lyceum was B.J. himself. At the lyceum Bach attended, B.J. spoke for an hour-and-a-half in a sweltering tent, packed with thousands of his followers. "Though in his sixtieth year," writes Bach, "he was as vital and sharp as an executive of thirty-five. Though not very tall, say five-feet eight, he seemed to tower over taller men. Not always correct in his views, he gave the impression of infallibility, and not always original in the cryptic, graphic, axiomatic things he said, he spoke as though everything he uttered was straight out of the unexpurgated gospel according to B.J."

The introduction of new chiropractic methods was always a high point of the Davenport lyceum, so when B.J. introduced something called the Neurocalometer, or NCM, at the 1924 gathering, it was nothing out of the ordinary. Yet his speech, aptly named "The hour has struck," caused such ripples through the profession that many of his colleagues left both the lyceum and B.J.'s beloved college.

B.J. introduced the NCM as the first instrument that could locate subluxations directly, whether or not the patient had symptoms, which won points for the "straights" and further alienated the "mixers."

"STRAIGHTS" AND "MIXERS"

Not all chiropractors agreed with B.J.'s gospel. From the beginning, two major splits have existed within the profession, divided along both philosophic and therapeutic lines.

B.J.'s "pure, straight and unadulterated" (shortened to "straight") followers have focused on subluxations, whether or not symptoms (like back pain or stiff neck) are present. They believe that the chiropractor's main job is to locate and remove subluxations, with the goal of bringing total health to their patients.

"Mixers," who have criticized "straights" for being too narrow, place more emphasis on removing symptoms by combining a variety of drugless therapies with spinal adjustments. These have included water, heat, ice, and massage therapies, food supplements, and herbal and homeopathic remedies. Some mixer schools have also taught minor surgery and applied obstetrics. St. Louis's Logan College had a birthing cottage on its campus until 1946, while Carver College in Oklahoma City required obstetrics as a prerequisite to graduation into the early 1960s.

Today, the majority of chiropractors are "mixers" and combine drugless therapies, particularly physical therapy, with spinal manipulations.

According to his adversaries, B.J. then predicted that no chiropractor would be able to remain in business without using the NCM.

He managed to make even more enemies when word got out that PSC had bought patents on the NCM and that it would be available only to PSC graduates at a cost of 2,200 dollars. Although B.J. denied any profit motive, the news sent three-quarters of the PSC staff packing, including some of his most loyal followers.

For many already alienated by B.J.'s domination of chiropractic and his straight approach to healing, the 1924 lyceum was the last straw. Scholar Kathleen A. Crisp writes "B.J.'s 1924 lyceum speech was like gasoline thrown on this fire smoldering in the profession."

The 1924 lyceum, attended by 8,000, was the beginning of the end of PSC's domination of American chiropractic. Two years later, attendance at the annual lyceum had dropped to 700; attendance at the college matched this decline. Former staff members and graduates went on to found their own schools.

Yet not even the mass desertions of his colleagues discouraged the stubborn B.J. In his later years, although he suffered from painful ulcers, the developer continued to sell the big idea both at the annual lyceums and on the road at the same pace and with the same optimism he had had all his life. Although son Dave dropped the Davenport lyceum after his father's death, South Carolina's Sherman College and the Pennsylvania Straight College, considered the most extreme "super-straight" colleges in the United States, revived the lyceum format in honor of their mentor. As of 1991, Sherman College continued to hold an annual lyceum each May.

THE "DANGEROUS CULT"

While B.J. was holding forth in Davenport, some members of the regular medical profession were shaking their heads at the presence of yet another healing "cult" claiming to do their job. From 1912, when the first antichiropractic article appeared in the *Journal of the American Medical Association,* to 1987, when chiropractors won a historic antitrust lawsuit against the American Medical Association, the battle lines were clearly drawn.

Before World War I, chiropractic colleges, which like many medical schools of the era were nothing more than diploma mills, became an easy target for a growing and increasingly confident AMA that was finally winning the public's trust. During this same period, the AMA created its Department of Investigation, which, according to scholar Cooper, concentrated most of its efforts on chiropractic colleges in a "long-term war."

Although the Flexner Report of 1910, *Medical Education in the United States and Canada,* sponsored by the Carnegie Foundation for the Advancement of Teaching, shut down a good number of chiropractic colleges because of their lack of emphasis on "scientific education," surviving chiropractic colleges continued to thrive until the Depression.

And they continued to come under AMA fire. In one study by the AMA's Committee on the Costs of Medical Care, called *The Healing Cult,* the author clearly stated his goal: "the containment, if not the elimination of chiropractic."

Although B.J. and his followers deliberately set themselves apart from regular medicine, the orthodox medical world cringed whenever they heard chiropractors call themselves "doctor." Mixers were particularly offensive, since they claimed to be able to cure many of the same disabilities as the regulars. In 1947, the AMA asserted that "there is no pathological basis whatsoever for the theory of chiropractic and it is silly to allude to it as a science." When the AMA created a Committee on Quackery in 1962, lasting until 1975, chiropractic continued to be its chief target.

By the early 1960s, medical writers were joining the battle. Chiropractors were harshly criticized in a book called *Bonesetting, Chiropractic, and Cultism* written by Samuel Homola in 1963, which can still be found in medical libraries. Dedicating his book to his wife, "and to the progress of medical science in its eradication of cultism and quackery in the healing arts," Homola accused chiropractors of everything from treating "imaginary subluxations" and making patients dependent on long-term care involving endless office visits to "diluting the high quality of modern medical care—making it difficult for the public to distinguish between low-grade and high-grade medical practice."

Debunkers of chiropractic made their way into the mass media, in particular in comic strips from the 1930s to 1960s. For example, "bone crunching back doctors" appeared regularly in Canadian-born artist J.R. Williams's strip, "Out Our Way," which ran in papers throughout North America in the 1930s and 1940s.

LEGAL PAINS AND VICTORIES

From the time D.D. Palmer was arrested and jailed in 1906 for practicing medicine without a license, chiropractors have had their fill of courtrooms and jails. Walter I. Wardwell reports that the Universal Chiropractic Association handled 3,300 legal battles by 1927 and that during the first 30 years of chiropractic's existence, more than 15 thousand prosecutions were brought to trial; one-fifth ended in convictions.

A HAZARD TO RATIONAL HEALTH

It is the position of the medical profession that chiropractic is an unscientific cult whose practitioners lack the necessary training and background to treat human disease. Chiropractic constitutes a hazard to rational health care in the United States because of the substandard and unscientific education of its practitioners and their rigid adherence to an irrational, unscientific approach to disease causation.

American Medical Association
House of Delegates Statement, 1966

GO TO JAIL FOR CHIROPRACTIC

In 1917, the Alameda County (California) Chiropractors Association adopted the slogan "Go To Jail for Chiropractic." The Association required its members to go to jail instead of paying a fine, and 450 did so in one year alone. These bone-cracking jailbirds then proceeded to set up their examining tables and adjust patients who showed up to support them, right in jail. Their tactic must have worked, because in 1923 California Governor Friend William Richardson pardoned all chiropractors then in jail.

Chiropractors' first major legal victory came in 1913, when Kansas granted them their first state licensing law. Although the AMA continued to argue against licenses for chiropractors because "the public health must be protected from an unproved therapy that could be harmful to its patients," by 1931, 30 states gave professional recognition to chiropractors. By 1974, chiropractic was legal in all 50 states. (The last states to legalize it were New York in 1963, Massachusetts in 1966, Mississippi in 1973, and Louisiana in 1974.) Chiropractors are licensed in all the Canadian provinces as well as in other countries around the world.

By the mid-1970s, chiropractors were turning the guns against the regulars, helped by the fact that a record number of Americans, about eight million, were visiting chiropractors, then numbering 23 thousand. In 1976, five Illinois chiropractors took the profession's most aggressive legal stand to date when they filed an antitrust suit against the American Medical Association and nine other medical organizations. Similar suits followed in New York and Pennsylvania. Soon thereafter, the AMA stepped back from its public criticism of chiropractors, and even revised its consultation clause to read "a physician shall, in the provision of appropriate patient care, except in emergencies, be free to choose whom to serve, with whom to associate, and the environment in which to provide medical services."

The Illinois lawsuit would not be settled for another 11 years, but it was a sweet victory for the spine manipulators. In 1987, a U.S. district judge in Chicago found that the AMA had engaged in a conspiracy "to contain and eliminate the chiropractic profession." The judge barred the AMA from "restricting, regulating or impeding" its members or hospitals where its members worked from associating with chiropractors.

"OH, MY ACHING BACK"

The same year chiropractors won their lawsuit against the AMA, the media reported a rise in the number of backaches in the United States. *Prevention* magazine estimated that about seven million Americans were being treated for back pain, "considered the most prevalent single medical ailment in the United States." The following year, the Associated Press reported that back injuries were costing employers more than 20 billion dollars annually because of absenteeism, and that back pain was "the second leading cause of lost work in the United States after the common cold, according to the National Insurance Council."

Where did many of those sufferers go for relief? In 1985, *Newsweek* reported that more than 10 million Americans sought relief in a chiropractor's office. The following year *Prevention* reported that 85 percent of those visits were for back and neck pains.

Since the mid-1970s, chiropractors have enjoyed a kind of second "golden age" that would have tickled B.J. Palmer's backbone. In 1990, 45 thousand chiropractors practiced in the United States, according to the Foundation for the Advancement of Chiropractic Tenets and Science. Worldwide, in the early 1990s chiropractors had the right to practice in 26 countries, either through licensure or under common law, as in England, Ireland, and Israel. The United States led in the number of chiropractors, followed by Canada and Australia.

In 1983, Lindell Hospital in St. Louis became the first American hospital to establish a chiropractic program, including 40 staff chiropractors who worked with other specialists. "About 300 patients each year were admitted under the program after consulting an M.D. first," reported Russell Forbes, who coordinated the chiropractic program. (In 1987, the hospital shut down for financial reasons.)

Other hospitals in Arizona, Virginia, Michigan, Washington, and Rhode Island followed Lindell's example, although not without some controversy. When Rhode Island's Cranston General Hospital–Osteopathic became the first New England hospital to welcome chiropractors, Dr. Stephen Barrett of the National Council Against Health Fraud grumbled, "Any hospital that is willing to make an uncritical acceptance of chiropractors probably has something seriously wrong with its management."

Sports medicine has also opened doors for chiropractors. In 1988, Jan Corwin, an Oakland, California, chiropractor and sports-medicine specialist, joined the U.S. Olympic medical team in Seoul, South Korea, winning one of six spots picked from hundreds of applicants. His inclusion was urged by the track and field members, who wanted a chiropractor on hand for last-minute "tune-ups."

Alone among unorthodox healers in the United States, chiropractors have managed to survive professionally and gain legal recognition while remaining outside orthodox medicine. Yet American chiropractors have a long way to go. With the trend in health insurance bending toward health maintenance organizations, most of which do not include chiropractors on their staffs or lists of practitioners, more chiropractic patients are having to pay for all of their care themselves. And American chiropractors have yet to gain the kind of government recognition that their colleagues have in New Zealand. In that country, a government-authorized commission in 1979 urged closer cooperation between doctors and chiropractors, stating that "it has become plain that much medical criticism of chiropractors is based on simple ignorance of what they do."

CHAPTER · 17 ·

PATENT MEDICINES: "IT WILL CURE YOU AT HOME WITHOUT PAIN, PLASTER OR OPERATION"

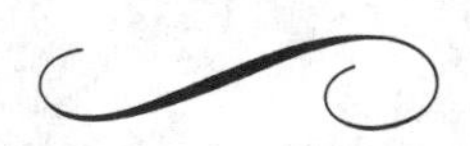

Gullible America will spend this year some seventy-five millions of dollars in the purchase of patent medicines. . . . It will swallow huge quantities of alcohol, an appalling amount of opiates and narcotics, a wide assortment of varied drugs ranging from powerful and dangerous heart depressants to insidious liver stimulants; and, far in excess of all other ingredients, undiluted fraud.

SAMUEL HOPKINS ADAMS
"The Great American Fraud"
Collier's Weekly, *October 7, 1905*

Back in 1715, Pennsylvanians Thomas and Sybilla Masters applied for a patent from the English king on a device for refining corn. As recipients of the first patent ever granted to American subjects by the mother country, the Masters had more in mind than pounding maize to feed their neighbors. For as their petition read, "the said Corn so refined is also an Excellent Medicine in Consumptions & other Distempers." Known as Tuscarora Rice, the Masters' ground maize holds the distinction of being America's first patent medicine.

Today we may look back in disgust at the odd-tasting potions in strange-looking bottles that promised to cure our ancestors' consumption, liver and bladder ailments, dyspepsia, and "female diseases." Yet during patent medicine's heyday—from the 1870s to 1930s—remedies like Lydia E. Pinkham's Vegetable Compound, Hostetter's Celebrated Stomach Bitters, Microbe Killer, and Kickapoo Indian Sagwa were as much a part of the American household medicine cabinet as aspirin is today.

Unlike Tuscarora Rice, most American patent medicines were not actually patented, a term held over from the days when European royalty granted patents to their favorite medicine makers. If they had been patented, medicine makers would have had to

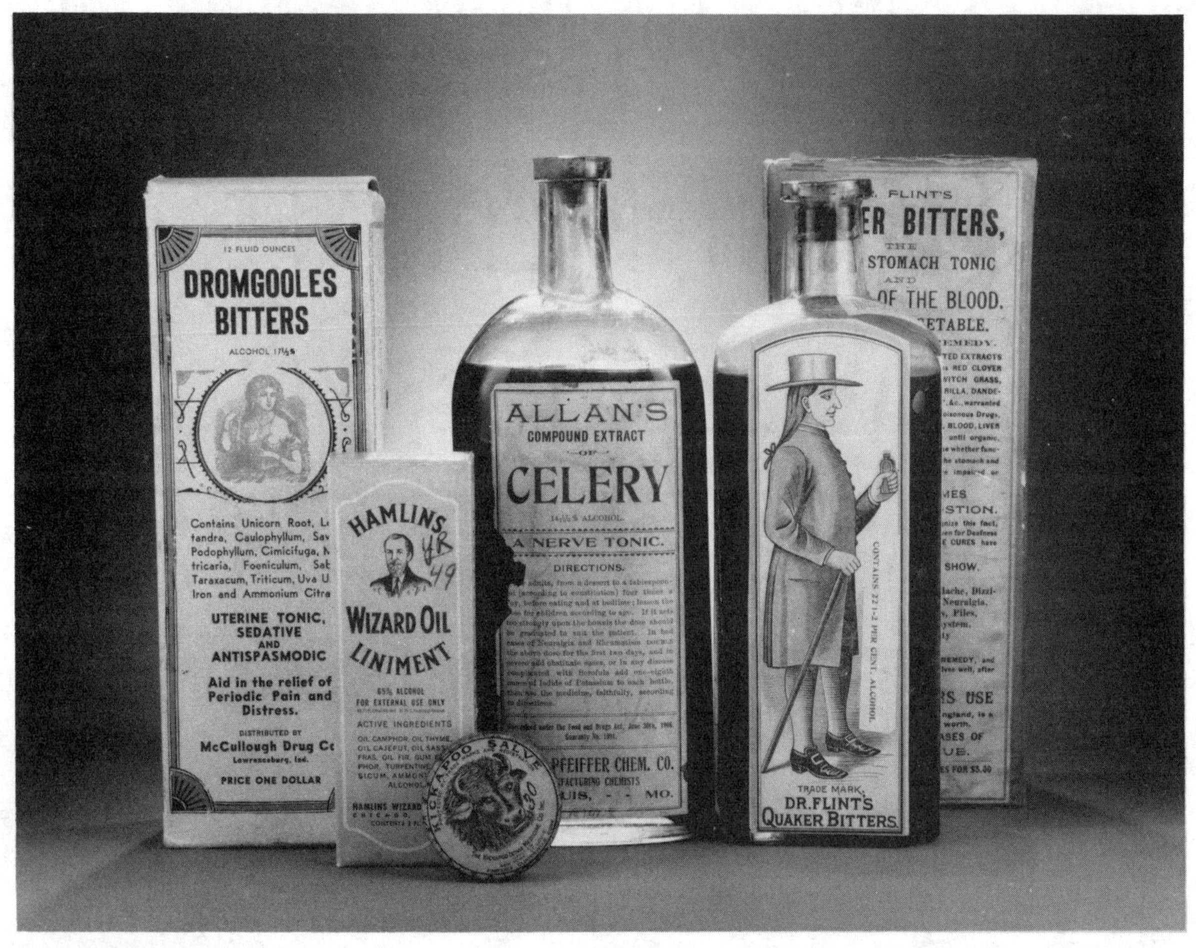

67. A patent medicine sampler: Hamlin's Wizard Oil and Kickapoo Salve (small tin, foreground) were especially popular. *Medical Sciences Department, National Museum of American History, Smithsonian Institution.*

disclose their secret formulas, which often changed. More important, a patent would have expired after seventeen years, after which time the product's formula and name would have been up for grabs.

Legally, ''patent'' medicines were in fact ''proprietary'' drugs. For the medicine men and women were far more interested in protecting, through copyright, their trademarks—the unique shapes and colors of the bottles, along with the label designs and printed matter—than their formulas. In the nineteenth century, the Pinkham family proudly published the recipe for its popular Lydia E. Pinkham's Vegetable Compound; but the name and trademark, with Mrs. Pinkham's smiling visage, has never been copied. As scholar James Harvey Young points out in *The Toadstool Millionaires,* the most comprehensive book on the history of American patent medicines, ''That the names of medicines, year after year, were printed in the same distinctive type induced a feeling of familiarity. Pictorial symbols served the same function. The trademark, indeed, was a fixed star in the universe.''

Through most of their history, patent medicines enjoyed a free-flowing existence. No government agency required that medicine makers prove their tonics were effective or even safe. No law stopped them from listing on the labels or in advertisements whatever ''cures'' happened to be in fashion at the time, or required a list of ingredients or warnings on the labels.

Some of the most popular medicines of the nineteenth and early twentieth centuries were brimming with alcohol, opium, and cocaine, which, no doubt, convinced many an unknowing consumer that the medicine ''worked'' very well indeed. Cocaine was a major ingredient in many popular medications, such as Rogers's Cocaine Pile Remedy, made in Moundsville, West Virginia; Coca Beef Tonic, from New York City; and Lloyd's Cocaine Toothache Drops, from Albany, New York. Some patent-medicine makers assured consumers that their tonics contained no addictive drugs, when the opposite was true. Yet patent-medicine defenders always argued that their brews were far safer than the heroic alter-

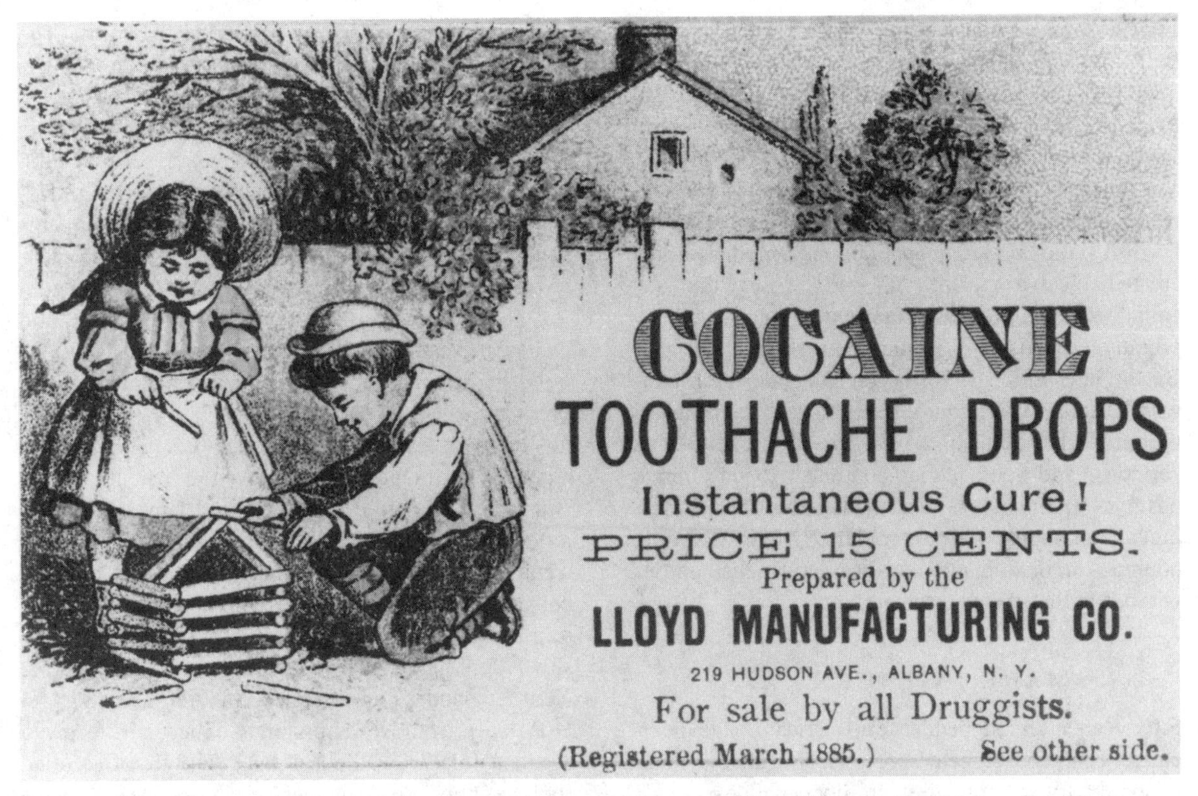

68. Cocaine was a common ingredient in many patent medicines, including those given to children. *National Library of Medicine.*

natives of the day—bleeding, calomel, prescription drugs, and surgery.

THE BRITISH INVASION

Seventeenth-century colonial Americans picked up the patent-medicine habit from their English cousins. Britons had their pick from a host of cures, such as Dr. Bateman's Pectoral Drops (created not by a doctor but by a businessman) and John Hooper's Female Pills, and Americans gulped down these remedies with gusto. By the eighteenth century, the fashion in medicine was to dump as many ingredients as possible into the brews. A remedy called Venice Treacle contained more than 60 ingredients, including the flesh of a viper.

English patent medicines sailed over with the first settlers to North America and dominated the American market until the revolutionary era. Some settlers brought English patents with them, giving them the right to make and sell medicine in America. Self-medication for every ill, including dysentery, malaria, smallpox, yellow fever, and consumption, was a way of life that few people questioned. Going along with the dictum that disease must be driven from the body by a cure at least as awful as the disease itself, the colonials, like the English, believed that the worse a medicine tasted, the more effective the cure. Cotton Mather was known to have recommended the medicinal properties of one remedy that was essentially cow urine and dung.

The first English patent medicine to be advertised in America, according to Young, was Daffy's Elixir Salutis, for "colic and griping," in the October 4, 1708 *Boston News-Letter*. The *Boston News-Letter,* America's first regularly published newspaper, was partly supported by ads from patent-medicine makers, a foreshadowing of the special relationship the nostrum makers would develop with the press a century later. As early as 1692, the *Boston Almanac* advertised something called "Aqua anti torminales," a cure for "the Griping of the Guts, and the Wind

THE TASTE THAT REFRESHES

The original Coca-Cola, created in 1886 by Atlanta pharmacist Dr. John Pemberton, contained a small amount of cocaine. It was advertised as a "brain tonic and intellectual beverage" that was also supposed to ease menstrual distress. By 1903 the narcotic was removed from the popular beverage. Today, the world's hottest-selling soft drink is flavored with a nonnarcotic extract of coca, the plant from which cocaine is made.

Cholick'' and ''that woeful Distemper of the Dry Belly Ach.'' It was sold by Benjamin Harris at Boston's London Coffee House. Harris published America's first newspaper, *Publick Occurances,* in 1690, although it lasted but one issue.

Just before the American Revolution, American-made remedies were vying for attention with the English potions. Benjamin Franklin's mother-in-law created a salve for the itch and for lice that she called Widow Read's Ointment. Her son-in-law proudly advertised it in the *Pennsylvania Gazette.* But as late as the 1770s, even after the trade bans with Britain went into effect, most colonials still preferred the English brands to the home-brewed varieties, and apothecaries continued to do a brisk business in English bottled medicines. The increasingly short supply was no problem. Druggists simply poured American-made remedies into English bottles without telling their customers.

MADE IN THE U.S.A.

Fifty years after independence, American-made medicines began to compete successfully with the time-honored British nostrums. In honor of America's independence, some of the earliest American-made potions had names like Dr. John Hill's American

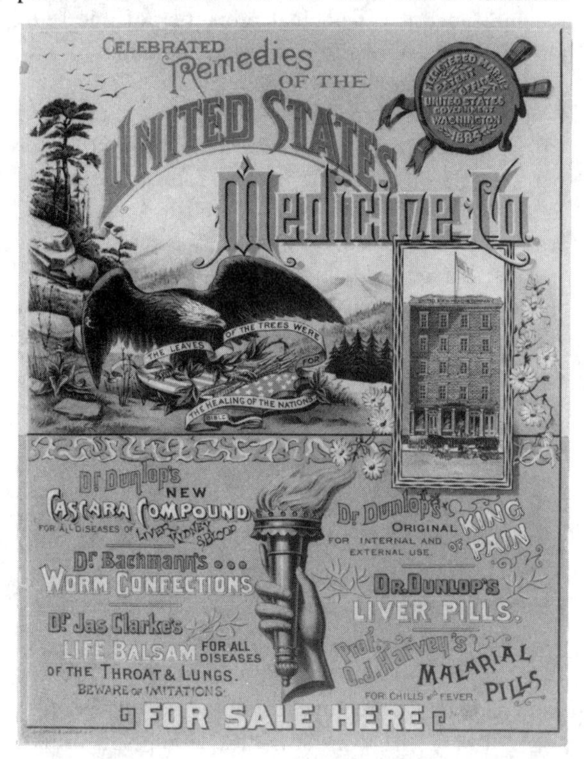

69. This nineteenth-century patent medicine advertisement played on consumers' patriotic feelings. *Collection of Advertising History, Archives Center, National Museum of American History, Smithsonian Institution.*

Balsam, proudly made from American herbs. The balsam was supposed to cure whooping cough, hypochondria, and a host of other illnesses.

Before independence, patent-medicine vendors in America enjoyed a seller's market. Competition was low-key and newspaper ads were straightforward if not dull. By the late eighteenth century this situation changed, as more would-be American medicine makers grabbed their mixing pots and fought for the market. The battle of the brews was on, and one of the earliest battles fought was with ''bilious pills,'' a popular cure for liver ailments and various other ailments.

First on the scene was Samuel Lee, Jr. of Windham, Connecticut, who received a patent for his Bilious Pills to fight yellow fever, jaundice, dysentery, dropsy, worms, and ''female complaints.'' As a marketing tool, Lee emphasized that his nostrum contained no mercury-laden calomel, a popular heroic medication of the day which often ''cured'' by slowly killing its victim. Three years later another New Englander, also named Samuel Lee (Samuel H.P. Lee), from New London, Connecticut, received a patent for *his* ''Bilious Pills.'' The first Lee cried foul, pointing out that the New Londoner used the hateful calomel in his remedy. Calomel or no, both pills sold quite well throughout the young country.

America's appetite for bilious pills was clearly insatiable, for by the early nineteenth century two other Lees, Michael of Baltimore and Richard of Baltimore and New York, each sold his own brand.

By the antebellum era, American medicine shelves were brimming with American-made elixirs, setting the stage for patent medicine's ''golden age'' a half-century later. Drugstores, many of them owned by physicians, and general stores had special patent medicine departments, often located alongside remedies for barnyard animals and horses. (One skeptical druggist in Topeka, Kansas displayed a sign that read, ''We sell patent medicines but do not recommend them.'') Everywhere one looked, newspapers, almanacs, magazines, billboards, barn displays, posters, and trade cards bombarded an increasingly literate consumer with messages to try one medicine or another, such as Swaim's Panacea, America's first sugar-coated pill; David Jayne's Vermifuge, a tapeworm medicine for children; Thomas W. Dyott's Infallible Worm Destroying Lozenges; and Radway's Ready Relief.

If the tonics didn't deliver to the consumer all that they promised, they did deliver fortunes to many a would-be Horatio Alger. Such was the case with America's first ''king of nostrum makers,'' a Philadelphian named Thomas W. Dyott.

THE MAYOR OF DYOTTVILLE

Thomas Dyott was the first patent-medicine maker to break into the national market. And he did so with the single-minded ambition many others would repeat 50 years later.

Thomas Dyott was making his living polishing shoes in Philadelphia when he first developed his line of "family remedies" in the 1810s. Most of these medications, as, for example, his Robertson's Infallible Worm Destroying Lozenges, were named for a "Dr. Robertson," who Dyott claimed was his grandfather, a distinguished Edinburgh physician. Even after a Philadelphia physician reported that no Dr. Robertson had practiced in Edinburgh for at least two centuries, Dyott continued to sell his tonics, helped by agents in Cincinnati and New York. When he took on the self-conferred title of "Doctor of Medicine," his line of medicines sold even better.

Soon Dyott figured that it would be smarter to manufacture his own medicine bottles than depend on the imported English glassware still favored by American medicine makers. With this end in mind, he bought the Kensington Glass Works on the Delaware River, not far from Philadelphia.

Two decades before the Civil War, Thomas Dyott was making 25 thousand dollars a year and claimed a personal estate worth 250 thousand dollars. Envisioning himself as a humanitarian sort of fellow, Dyott sold his remedies at half price to the poor. He also turned his glass works into a model village, which he called Dyottville, for his 450 employees. No swearing, gambling, or liquor was allowed (no matter how much alcohol may have been poured into his nostrums), and workers had to bathe and attend Sunday school. Infractions were translated into deductions from paychecks.

Dyott's dream community didn't last. After branching out yet again, this time to start his own bank for his workers, the bank went under in the 1837 panic. After he distributed his stock among his relatives and filed for bankruptcy, he was convicted of fraudulent insolvency and sentenced to one to seven years in prison. Released early, Dyott was soon back on his feet again and managed to make a small fortune before he died in 1861.

PATENT-MEDICINE FEVER

Dyott would have been in good company after the Civil War, for most American patent medicines did not reach a national audience until the late nineteenth century, when many a fortune was to be made in the potion business. Thanks to the new transcontinental railroad, lower postal rates, an expanded popular daily press, and the punch of professionally written advertising copy, patent-medicine makers were able to reach a market that spilled across a continent.

Most patent-medicine makers were not as successful as Dyott. But everyone looked for some sort of gimmick that would grab the consumer's attention. The most colorful and successful (before print advertising) was the traveling medicine show, a colorful blend of circus-style entertainment and sales pitch that remained popular in rural America up to the 1940s.

To reach a national audience by the end of the nineteenth century, however, most nostrum makers turned to print advertising in all its forms—trade cards and brochures to be left on drugstore counters, posters for shop windows, paintings on barns and rocks, and ads in almanacs, religious and country weeklies, daily newspapers, and on the back pages of popular novels.

C.F. Richards & Co., a San Francisco drugstore, advertised its own patent-medicine line in its special *Domestic Receipt Book*. In its 1872 edition, readers found medicine ads for Richards's Bronchial Pellets and Richards's Oriental Invigorator, as well as Trapper's Indian Oil and Armstrong's Pulmonary Syrup, on the same pages as recipes for muffins, tea cakes, and pickles.

In books, brochures, and full-page ads, patent-medicine makers fed their messages into America's consciousness. In the mid-1880s, the Kickapoo Indian Medicine Company published an illustrated 170-page book called *Life and Scenes Among the Kickapoo Indians: Their Manners, Habits and Customs*. The book included colorful stories on such topics as "Kickapoo Indian Life in a Kickapoo Village" and "the Scalp Dance." Every page was festooned with ads for the company's "family line" of medicines—Kickapoo Indian Oil, Indian Salve, Indian Worm Killer, Indian Cough Cure, and Sagwa, the firm's panacea.

As the costs of advertising rose dramatically, only those with big bucks to spend survived. Many a patent-medicine firm was bought out, sometimes by advertising agencies. Beginning copywriters often showed off their talents by first writing patent-medicine copy. Some moved on to more glamorous enterprises, among them P.T. Barnum, who got his start writing ad copy for a baldness cure, during which time he may have coined his famous phrase, "There's a sucker born every minute."

"IT CURES WHERE OTHERS FAIL"

One of the most successful advertising campaigns was for the long-surviving Lydia E. Pinkham's Veg-

None Genuine without our Stamp over the neck of each Bottle.

KICKAPOO INDIAN MEDICINES.

First in order comes **KICKAPOO INDIAN SAGWA,** a vegetable Remedy composed of roots, herbs, barks and leaves. Sagwa acts directly upon the Stomach and Liver, and will cure all the various symptoms of Dyspepsia, including Neuralgia, Headache, Constipation, Kidney Diseases, &c. $1.00 per bottle.

KICKAPOO INDIAN OIL is a very valuable remedy, affording effectual and speedy relief in all nervous and inflammatory diseases. As a Pain Killer it is *magical.* The Oil may be taken internally or applied externally, according to the printed directions. For children it is excellent. 25 cents per bottle.

KICKAPOO INDIAN WORM KILLER is prepared by the Kickapoos from their native formula of roots and herbs. It is a positive specific for the removal of Stomach, Seat or Pin Worms, whether in adults or children. It is a pleasant, safe, prompt and effective remedy, and requires no physic. 25 cents per box.

KICKAPOO INDIAN SALVE is made by the Kickapoo Indians from the best Buffalo Tallow (not hog's lard). It is a specific for Skin Diseases, soothing and excellent for Erysipelas, Eczema, Boils, Piles, Burns. 25 cents per box.

KICKAPOO INDIAN COUGH CURE is an invaluable Indian Remedy for Coughs, Colds, Asthma, Throat and Lung Diseases. It is purely vegetable and pleasant to take. Its action is specific. 50 cents per bottle.

SOLD BY ALL WHOLESALE AND RETAIL DRUGGISTS IN THE UNITED STATES.

NONE GENUINE WITHOUT THE SIGNATURE OF

Healy & Bigelow.

COPYRIGHT 1887. HEALY & BIGELOW NEW HAVEN, CONN.

70. So-called Indian remedies always sold well. *Collection of Advertising History, Archives Center, National Museum of American History, Smithsonian Institution.*

etable Compound, which hit the market out of Lynn, Massachusetts in the mid-1870s. Lydia Pinkham's story reads like a fairy tale, but in many ways she was a product of her times.

Lydia Estes (1819–1883) grew up in a middle-class Quaker household in Lynn, in a family whose parents were involved in the abolitionist, feminist, and temperance movements of the day. Through them, Lydia was introduced to both Frederick Douglass and the abolitionist Grimké sisters of South Carolina. Early on, the young Lydia was drawn to alternative medical theories and read the works of Sylvester Graham and the Eclectics. In the process, she learned how to make homemade remedies for various ills. By the time she was married to Charles Pinkham and raising three sons and a daughter, she was busily concocting brews for her neighbors. One of these was her vegetable compound for "female complaints and weaknesses."

Perhaps if Lydia had been married to a successful businessman—Charles had big dreams of striking it rich, but never managed to support his family for any length of time—or the panic of 1873 hadn't hit just about the time the Pinkhams were teetering on the edge of poverty, the vegetable compound might never have gone commercial. As the story goes, the family was sitting in the kitchen trying to decide what to do next, when two strangers from Salem came to the door wanting to buy "a vegetable compound." As Lydia Pinkham's major biographer Jean Burton writes, "The only detail marking the transaction as in any way extraordinary was that these visitors were not only willing but anxious to pay." It was the first time Lydia had received any money for her brew. "Why not," the family asked, "sell it in the stores?"

Through most of its history, Lydia E. Pinkham's Vegetable Compound remained true to its roots, a family enterprise. Son Dan left the family nest to distribute pamphlets in Brooklyn and Manhattan while Lydia and the rest of the family brewed the remedy back home. (Ever tuned in to marketing trends, at one point Dan suggested that they expand the list of cures to include "kidney complaints" because it was a popular malady at the time. The family back in Lynn rejected this idea, however.)

The Pinkhams realized that their most important decision was the trademark design. At first Dan came up with the idea of a little New England cottage and the likeness of a striking young woman, emphasizing the remedy's New England roots. But he soon gave up that idea for another, his mother's own face. When the children asked Lydia what she thought of the idea, she replied with a smile, "Do as you please, boys." That smile helped turn the compound into one of the most popular patent remedies in America.

Their next smart move was committing a large portion of their budget to advertising that face. It all began when son Will, on a whim, walked into the offices of the daily *Boston Herald* and asked how much it would cost to print one of the Pinkhams' four-page pamphlets on the front page of the paper. Having just sold 84 dollars' worth of remedies to a wholesaler, Will decided to hand over the 60 dollars it cost for the ad. His mother's smile so startled the *Herald's* readers that sales picked up immediately. Subsequent ads were so successful that the family moved their brewing operations out of the basement into the building next door.

The Pinkhams showed their marketing savvy by playing up the fact that they were a family-run business and that the compound was "home-brewed." They conducted tours of the plant and happily published the recipe of the tonic which, like many remedies of the day, also contained a stiff dose of alcohol (about 18 percent at the time) "used only as a solvent and preservative."

Lydia herself wrote most of the ads, in collaboration with her sons and her daughter, Aroline. (Her son Charles and Aroline took over the business after their parents' deaths. Both Dan and Will died of consumption during the company's growing years.) Lydia's straightforward style, with messages such as "LYDIA E. PINKHAM'S VEGETABLE COMPOUND is a positive Cure for all those Painful Complaints and Weaknesses so common to our best female population" and "REJOICE THAT A PAINLESS REMEDY IS FOUND," appealed to her readers, for whom Lydia had become a kind of surrogate grandmother. Believing that it was important to reach her readers personally, Lydia also wrote a "Guide for Women," a 62-page booklet that was eventually translated into five languages.

But the Pinkhams' most clever marketing tool was "Write to Mrs. Pinkham," Lydia's invitation to her readers to write to her for advice, medical and otherwise. Until her death in 1883, Lydia insisted on answering all of the correspondence herself. After her death, the *Ladies' Home Journal* reported that duped readers were still writing to "Mrs. Pinkham." The Pinkhams argued that there still *was* a "Mrs. Pinkham," namely son Charlie's wife.

At the time of her death in 1883, Lydia Pinkham's face was said to be the best-known female face in America. The compound was bringing in about 300 thousand dollars a year, with over half spent on advertising. After her death the family hired ad man James T. Wetherald to take over the advertising campaign. He successfully brought the compound into the twentieth century.

In 1925, sales of the product were up to three million dollars. By the 1940s, Lydia E. Pinkham's Vegetable Compound was marketed in 33 countries. The company remained a family-run operation until 1968, when Mrs. Pinkham's heirs sold it to a pharmaceutical firm. In 1972, the operations were moved to Puerto Rico, and as of the late 1980s the compound was still being made there.

OPEN UP AND SWALLOW

Much like the words "natural" and "preservative-free" have helped to sell products in the late twentieth century, certain key words were fashionable during

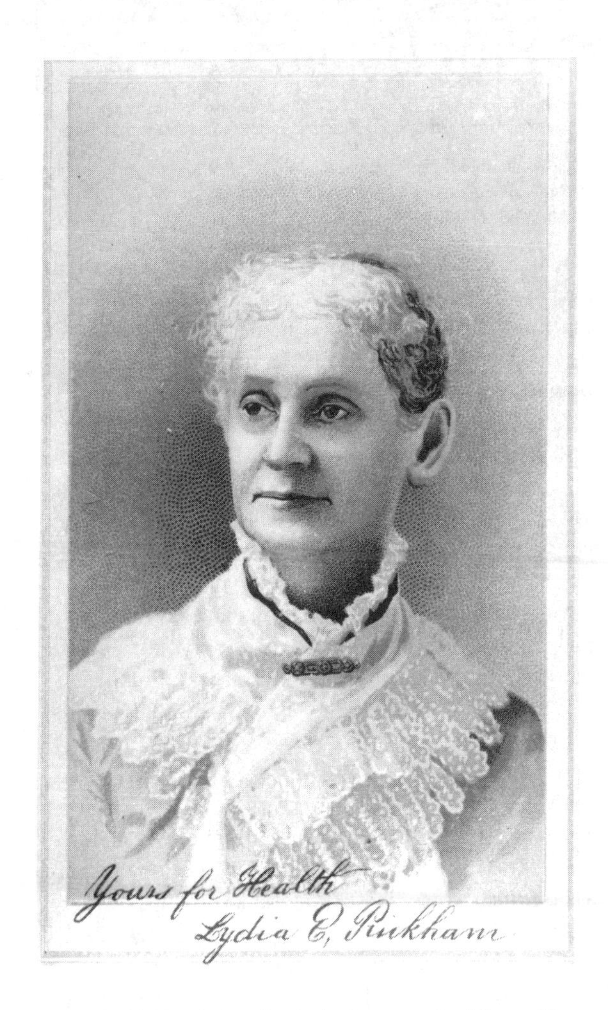

71. Lydia Pinkham's grandmotherly face graced millions of bottles of the best-selling Vegetable Compound. *Collection of Advertising History, Archives Center, National Museum of American History, Smithsonian Institution.*

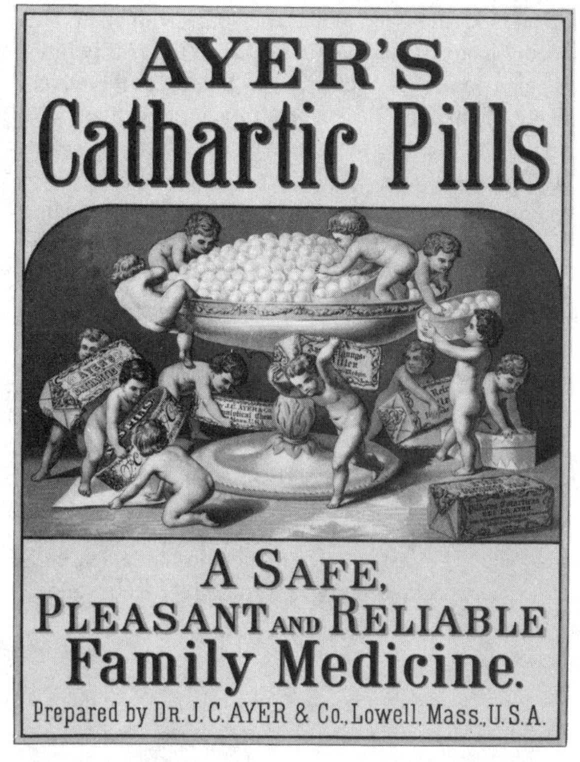

72. Would these cherubs lie to you? *Collection of Advertising History, Archives Center, National Museum of American History, Smithsonian Institution.*

patent medicine's heyday. They changed with whatever names and "cures" happened to be in style at the time. "Vegetable" and names of vegetables always helped. Lydia E. Pinkham's Vegetable Compound sounded simple, homemade, and unadulterated. Purely Vegetable Taraxacum (Dandelion) Bitters was also a big hit, as was Paine's Celery Compound, a "nerve tonic" that hit the market in 1872. By the 1890s, celery remedies were so much in demand that consumers were drowning in Celery Bitters, Celery Crackers, and a tonic called Celery-Cola. Sears, Roebuck, one of the biggest producers and distributors of patent medicines, got in on the act by coming out with its own celery remedy called Celery Malt Compound.

Customers wanted their medicine safe and fast-acting, so names like Dr. Sweet's Infallible Liniment and Warner's Safe Cure were popular. Anything with the word "Indian" was a sure winner, as was Kickapoo Indian Sagwa, which its creators claimed was "at all times under the Indians' personal supervision, they alone possessing the secret of its combination." So were remedies with the name "Quaker." C.F. Richards & Co.'s *Domestic Receipt Book* for 1872 advertised something called Golden Bitters, the *Quaker tonic* "prepared from select Shaker roots and herbs, according to the old Quaker recipe." Anything that sounded foreign or exotic also did well, as, for example, Dr. Drake's Canton Chinese Hair Cream, Persian Balm, Westphalia Stomach Bitters, and Redding's Russian Salve.

Nineteenth-century Americans were obsessed with kidney, bladder, liver, and heart afflictions and consumption, one of the most dreaded diseases before World War II. Texans claimed that their cowboys always carried Simmons Liver Regulator with them, "washed down with a little water." Out of Binghamton, New York, the Kilmer brothers brewed a whole line of "family remedies" whose names promised to appeal to every consumer's fancy: Indian Cough Cure, Autumn Leaf Extracts for Females, Ocean Weed Heart Remedy, Prompt Parilla Liver Pills, and the hot-selling Swamp Root. William Swaim, whose origins are a little fuzzy (he was from either New York or Philadelphia), came up with the best name of all: Panacea, a "cure" for cancer, scrofula, rheumatism, gout, hepatitis, and the early stages of syphilis.

Medicine makers needed only to convince the consumer that their remedies actually worked. A little hyperbole mixed in with a bit of downright lying usually did the trick.

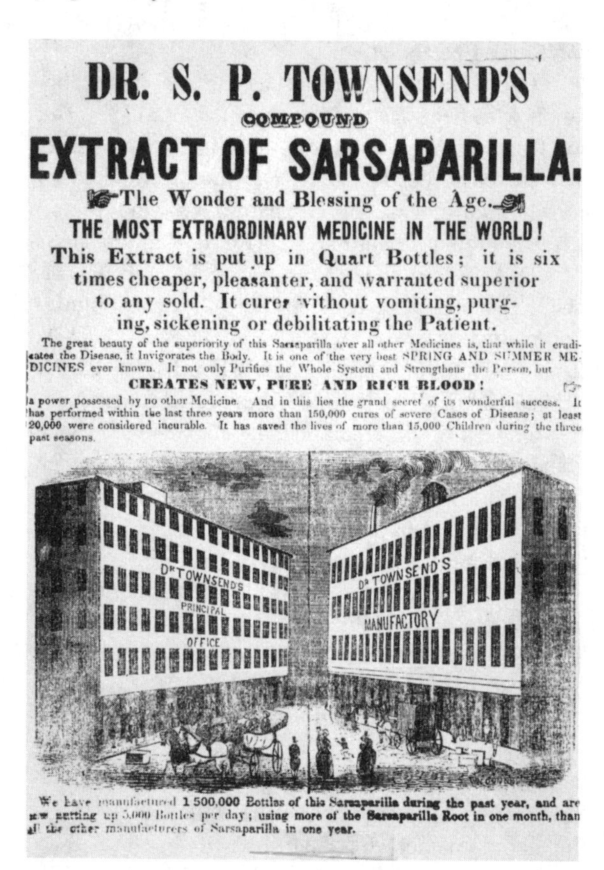

73. No hyperbole was too far-fetched in patent medicine advertising. *Collection of Advertising History, Archives Center, National Museum of American History, Smithsonian Institution.*

Ad copy often played on consumers' fears of the heroic medical treatments of the day or of doctors in general. One ad in the 1880s for Kickapoo Indian Sagwa had the headline "Poisoned by Calomel—Cured by Sagwa." The copy described a Pullman train conductor who claimed he had tried calomel for his chronic diarrhea, "which nearly poisoned me." After taking Sagwa, he was "perfectly well." A 1906 ad in the *San Francisco Examiner* for Lydia E. Pinkham's Vegetable Compound read: "Few Women confide fully in a physician. They simply will not tell him all. That's why many doctors fail to cure female diseases."

Just as first-hand accounts are used in modern-day ads for reducing aids, testimonials were used in patent-medicine ads as late as the 1930s. Sometimes they backfired. The May 27, 1935, Allentown, Pennsylvania *Call Chronicle* printed an ad for something called Natex, in which a satisfied consumer described how she had suffered from indigestion, headaches, and dizzy spells before taking the remedy. "Natex seemed to go to the root of my trouble," she claimed. "I'm still enjoying good health." Four columns over on the same page was the woman's death notice. She had apparently died just two days earlier.

Patent-medicine sellers used scientific breakthroughs to legitimize their potions. According to James Harvey Young, the germ theory of disease was popularized by a patent medicine called Microbe Killer, the creation of Prussian-born William Radem, who emigrated to Texas. Microbe Killer was soon followed into the market by a flood of allegedly germ-eradicating nostrums.

PATENT-MEDICINE TRIVIA CORNER

- The United Society of Believers in Christ's Second Appearing (Shakers) were once the largest producers of patent medicines in America.
- One of the hottest nineteenth-century American patent medicines was Dr. Miles's Compound Extract of Tomato, today known as catsup.
- Moxie, a New England-based soft drink once as popular as Coca-Cola, was originally a patent medicine. Known as Beverage Moxie Nerve Food, its label promised to cure "brain and nervous exhaustion, loss of manhood, imbecility and helplessness, softening of the brain, locomotor ataxia, and insanity."
- The Giant Oxie Company of Augusta, Maine produced a hot-selling remedy called Oxien, billed as an "improved Moxie nerve food." Its founder was William H. Gannett, whose fortune from the remedy helped son Guy start his chain of newspaper and radio stations. Today the Gannett Company publishes *USA Today*.

"UNCONSCIOUS DRUNKENNESS"

Not everyone was enamored of patent medicines. By the turn of the twentieth century, regular doctors, helped by a strengthened American Medical Association and a growing pharmaceutical industry in "ethical" (prescription) drugs, teamed up with muckraking journalists and a handful of politicians to investigate the patent-medicine industry and publicize the "truth" about these dangerous potions.

They pointed a finger at the high alcohol content of many of the medicines, arguing that duped customers were unknowingly becoming medicine junkies. When Samuel Hopkins Adams wrote "The Great American Fraud," a multi-part investigation of the patent-medicine industry, for *Collier's Weekly* from 1905 to 1907, the author compared the alcohol content of whiskey and several popular patent medicines: Paine's Celery Compound had 21 percent and Hostetter's Stomach Bitters contained a whopping 44.3 percent, not much lower than the alcohol content of whiskey, at 50 percent. "While the 'doses' prescribed by the patent-medicine manufacturers are only one to two teaspoonfuls several times a day, the opportunity to take more exists, and even small doses of alcohol, taken regularly, cause that craving which is the first step in the making of a drunkard or drug fiend."

Adams argued that some of the country's driest states, like Maine and Kansas, were doing a thriving business in patent medicines. James Harvey Young points out that, as the American temperance movement gained strength in the 1870s, thirsty customers sought relief in patent medicines. "For those deprived, one legal and almost respectable recourse was open: the steady pursuit of health through high-proof bitters."

In its *Nostrums and Quackery,* a three-volume exposé published in 1912, 1921, and 1936, the AMA presented examples of the "evils" of patent medicines. One story from the 1912 volume described a remedy called Marjorie Hamilton's Obesity Cure that included Healthtone-Obesity Bath Powder. It was supposed to dissolve fat while the patient soaked in a bath twice a day. In the same volume the authors reprinted an ad for Toxo-Absorbent, touted as "the great drugless treatment" that promised to cure 38 different ailments.

Collier's

THE NATIONAL WEEKLY

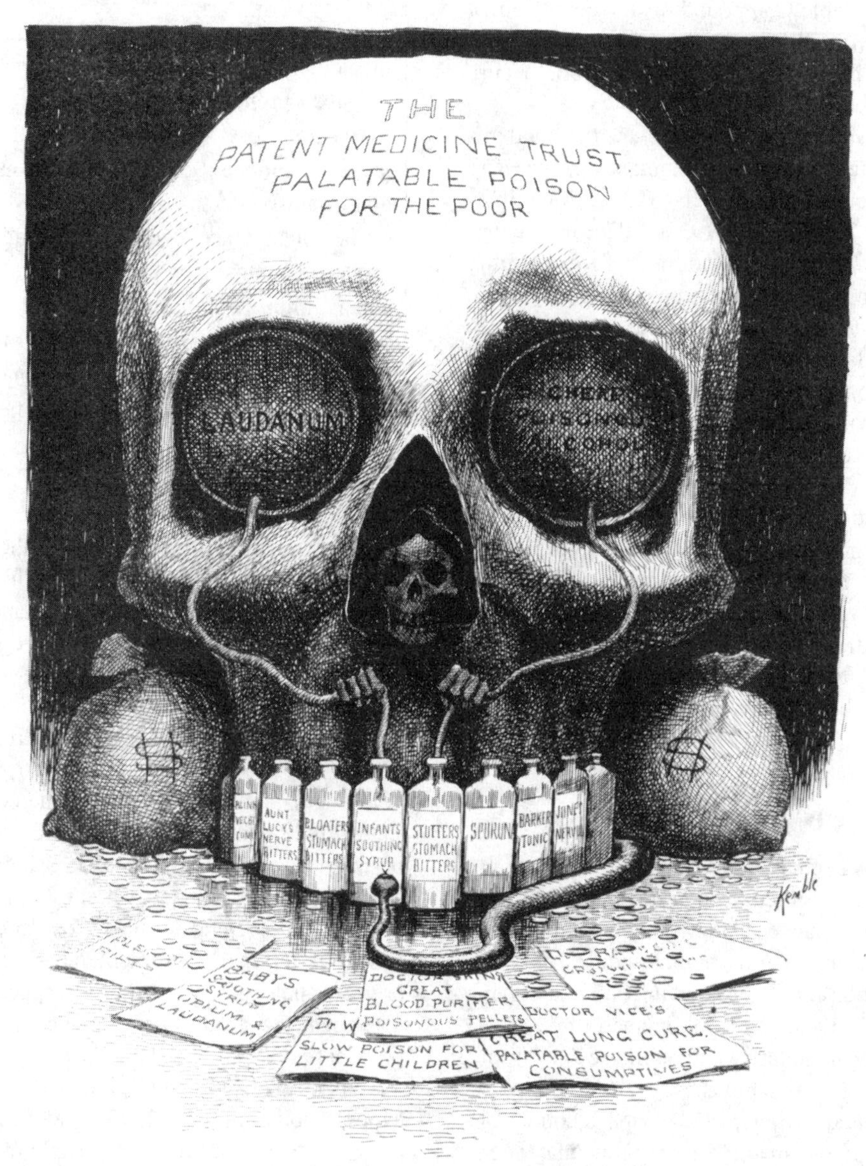

DEATH'S LABORATORY

Patent medicines are poisoning people throughout America to-day. Babies who cry are fed laudanum under the name of syrup. Women are led to injure themselves for life by reading in the papers about the meaning of backache. Young men and boys are robbed and contaminated by vicious criminals who lure them to their dens through seductive advertisement

DRAWN BY E. W. KEMBLE

74. *Collier's* powerful investigative series on patent medicines spurred badly needed reform (1905). *Courtesy of the Library of Congress.*

Critics such as Adams blamed the press for supporting the patent-medicine industry through its dependence on huge advertising revenue. Quoting a Dr. Humphreys, a leader in the powerful Proprietary Association of America—the medicine makers' major lobbying arm formed in 1881, which in the late twentieth century represented over-the-counter drug manufacturers—Adams wrote, "The twenty thousand newspapers of the United States make more money from advertising the proprietary medicines than do the proprietors of the medicines themselves." The AMA blamed the press for giving too much publicity to patent medicines: "Printer's ink is the very life blood of quackery." To illustrate how much clout the medicine makers had over the press, Adams reprinted an example of a typical newspaper-advertising contract, this one from the Cheney Medicine Company, makers of Hall's Catarrh Cure, that included the so-called "muzzle clause." It explicitly stated that the contract would be void "if any law is enacted by your State restricting or prohibiting the manufacture or sale of proprietary medicines."

FEDERAL LEGISLATION—NO PANACEA

In spite of the strong lobbying muscle of the proprietary-medicine makers and their powerful muzzle clauses, by 1895 about half the states had passed food and drug laws. But the laws were inconsistent from state to state and could easily be ignored once a remedy crossed the state line.

The Pure Food and Drug Act of 1906, the first federal food and drug law, was introduced by Dr. Harvey Wiley, chief chemist for the Department of Agriculture. Although its final, watered-down version was nothing more than a labeling law, most proponents agreed it was a step in the right direction. For the first time, manufacturers engaged in interstate sales could not make false statements on the label. They also had to list on the label the presence and amount of specific narcotic drugs as well as alcohol.

From 1906 to 1938, when the more powerful Food, Drug and Cosmetic Act was passed by Congress, the 1906 law became known for what it did not do. As Gerald Carson explains in his article "Who Put the Borax in Dr. Wiley's Butter?", at first many patent-medicine makers considered the act a joke. "In time the manufacturers . . . learned the

A CANCER CURE FROM THE SHOW ME STATE

One of the most fascinating stories in Samuel Hopkins Adams's 1905–07 investigative series for *Collier's Weekly* was that of "Rupert Wells, M.D." of St. Louis, maker of an alleged radioactive (or miracle) cancer and consumption cure called Radol. Wells, whose real name was Dennis Dupuis, conveniently created an M.D. for himself by inventing the "Postgraduate College of Electrotherapeutics of St. Louis" and appointing himself "chair of Radiotherapy." To gather clients, Wells heavily advertised in newspapers throughout the country, inviting readers to write to him for free information and promising, "I can cure cancer at home without pain, plaster or operation." If a sufferer answered, Wells urged the correspondent to purchase his treatment immediately for 15 dollars a month. By the time the Post Office Department caught up with him and issued a fraud order, Wells was doing a lively business, sending out an average of 25 treatments a day. A chemical analysis by the Department of Agriculture revealed that Radol was a watery solution containing about 10 percent glycerin and a small amount of inorganic salts.

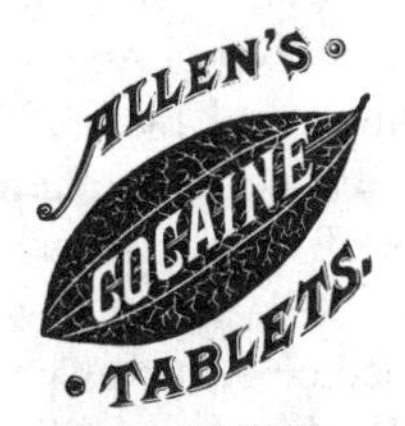
ALLEN'S
COCAINE
TABLETS.
For Colds, Sore Throat, Nervousness, Neuralgia, Headache, Sleeplessness, Dyspepsia, Indigestion, Heartburn, and Flatulency.
USED BY ELOCUTIONISTS, VOCALISTS, AND ACTORS.
NASAL TABLOIDS.
For Catarrh, Asthma, Hay Fever, Cold in the Head.
COCAINE OINTMENT.
For Burns, Scalds, Sunburn, Prickly Heat, Eczema, Hives, Itching Skin Eruptions, Mosquito Bites.
PRICE LIST.
TABLETS, - - - - - - - $4.00 PER DOZEN.
OINTMENT, - - - - - - 4.00 " "
NASAL TABLOIDS, - - - - 8.00 " "
For Sale by Wholesale Druggists and
ALLEN COCAINE MFG. CO.,
1254 BROADWAY, NEW YORK.

75. In the absence of drug laws, over-the-counter narcotics were perfectly legal (1885). *National Library of Medicine.*

hard way that they were living dangerously when they ignored the precept 'Thou shalt not lie on the label.' "

Medicine makers could still dump narcotics into their remedies; they simply had to list them on the label. Ironically, the law did not require that poisons like arsenic, found in some patent medicines, be listed on the label. Also frustrating to the law's champions, it did not cover cosmetics; nor did it regulate advertising copy. Although in 1912 the law was amended to include fraudulent claims of cures, claimants had to prove manufacturers *intended* to make false claims.

What difference did the label law make on the patent-medicine industry? Not much, according to critics. In fact, many medicine makers embraced the Pure Food and Drug Act as their own, using it to legitimize themselves. Included along with several other examples in the AMA's 1912 volume of *Nostrums and Quackery* was the label for Dr. Kilmer's Cough Remedy (formerly Dr. Kilmer's Indian Cough Cure), then still sold under its old label in Britain. The old label read "has a wonderful effect on those suffering with coughs, colds, croup, hoarseness, congestion, inflammation, tightness across the chest, catarrh, bronchial catarrh, asthma, bronchitis, consumption, and all diseases of the chest, throat and lungs." The new, more conservative American label read "is intended for coughs, hoarseness, colds, tickling in the throat, croup, congestion, inflammation, tightness across the chest, catarrh, bronchial catarrh, and bronchitis." True to the law, the label stated "10 percent of pure grain alcohol." And to sweeten its appeal, prominently displayed in boldface was the message "Guaranteed by Dr. Kilmer & Co. under the Food and Drug Act, June 30, 1906."

By the 1920s and 1930s, the fashionable ailments were no longer consumption and cancer, but acid indigestion, body odor, bad breath, irritability, fatigue, and obesity. In an ad for Lydia E. Pinkham's Vegetable Compound from the *San Francisco Examiner* on April 4, 1935, the reader was asked "Does Your Husband Call You Grouchy? If he knew how good Lydia E. Pinkham's Vegetable Compound was, he'd go straight to the nearest drug store and buy you a bottle." While the ads were more subtle, patent medicines were still far from safe, as attested by the militant consumer's group Consumers' Research, whose best-selling *100,000,000 Guinea Pigs* reminded the American public that danger still lurked inside many a tonic bottle.

Patent medicines still did a brisk trade in the Depression years. In their book, *Border Radio*, Gene Fowler and Bill Crawford describe the advertisements for questionable doctoring that reached thousands of radio listeners in the 1930s, such as Dr. John Romulus Brinkley's goat-gland transplants, guaranteed to cure male impotence, and Norman G. Baker's cures for cancer and tumors "without operations, radium or X rays." In its 1936 volume of *Nostrums and Quackery,* the AMA detailed the dangers of certain cosmetics, including popular freckle removers that contained mercury and face makeups with arsenic. One "obesity cure" called Jad Salts had been misbranded while being touted as a kidney cure and was doing quite well on the market as a diet remedy.

Alcohol-laced medicines, along with bitters, were hot sellers during the Prohibition years. Peruna, given a new boost from radio advertising, contained a hefty 18 percent alcohol in the 1920s.

Safety was still an issue. Harold Hopkins, former editor of the magazine *FDA Consumer,* described how his father lost mobility of his legs in the late 1920s after taking a popular alcohol-based remedy called Jamaica Ginger that was spiked with a toxic substance. An estimated 35 to 50 thousand Americans suffered severe reactions to proprietary medicines in the same era.

In the late 1930s, it took another mass-scale tragedy to get a new federal drug law passed. Ironically, one of the arguments against a new law was its possible power to stop new miracle drugs from reaching the market, drugs to battle pneumonia, blood poisoning, and meningitis. One of these miracle drugs was called Sulfanilamide, not a patent medicine, but one of the first-generation sulfa drugs to fight infections. As a tablet it was hard to swallow; as a liquid medicine, it was palatable, or so the experts thought. By October 1937, the first poisoning reports came in from doctors in Tulsa, Oklahoma. The solvent used in the drug was actually a poison similar to antifreeze. By the time the drug was tracked down, 107 people had died, most of them children.

Too late for Sulfanilamide victims, the Food, Drug and Cosmetic Act of 1938, engineered by New Deal brain truster Rexford Tugwell, required that a product had to be proven safe *before* it reached the market. For the first time, the Food and Drug Administration could also regulate cosmetics and diet aids. (Under the 1906 law, diet aids were not considered drugs because obesity was not considered a disease.) Drug labels had to include directions for use and warnings against misuse. Drugs were considered "misbranded" if they were dangerous to health when used in the manner prescribed on the label.

Even so, some patent medicines survived. By the 1950s, according to James Harvey Young, five giant companies controlled nearly half of latter-day American patent medicines. The hottest sellers were analgesics, laxatives, vitamins, cold and cough preparations, antacids and stomach remedies, antiseptics, liniments, and tonics.

In 1962, the Food, Drug and Cosmetic Act was revised to require that all new drugs or old drugs claiming new uses had to show that they were not only safe but also effective. Ten years later the FDA officially organized an Over-the-Counter Drug Review, which as of the late 1980s was still in progress. Certain ingredients found in popular over-the-counter medicines were removed because they were found to be unsafe, as, for example, hexachlorophene, once found in soaps, underarm deodorants, baby powders, and toothpaste.

Advertising, that thorn in the side of patent medicine's most vocal critics, still hovers in the gray area. While the Federal Trade Commission is in charge of preventing false or misleading claims in advertisements, the wheels of justice move ever so slowly. It took the FTC 16 years to take the "liver" out of Carter's Little Liver Pills and nearly that long to take the "tired blood" out of Geritol ads, two of the most widely advertised over-the-counter drugs on television in the 1950s.

THE "NEW" PATENT MEDICINES

Self-medication is as popular as it ever was, and the over-the-counter medicine industry offers the consumer a larger smorgasbord of products than ever before. Now bound tightly in their tamper-resistant seals, modern over-the-counter drugs attest to the new "in" ailments, like wrinkles, but for the most part promise us relief from the same old standbys—headaches, coughs, menstrual cramps, back pain, insomnia, stress, and allergies.

Anti-aging nostrums were big business in the early 1990s. In March 1990, *Newsweek* reported that Americans spent two billion dollars each year on fountain-of-youth products. Skin products came increasingly under fire. Two years earlier the FDA had sent out letters to 22 cosmetic firms with the warning that they had to stop any anti-aging claims or risk seizure of their products.

Health-food stores may be the biggest marketplace for the new medicines, drawing the consumer with assurances that their 100-percent "natural," "organic" remedies contain no alcohol or toxic substances. Some echo the old patent-medicine names—Liver Guard, Brain III Formula, Perfect 7 Intestinal Cleanser, and Male Factors. One product found in a San Francisco store in the late 1980s called Urban Air Defense promised relief from a very modern problem—smog.

Many of the old patent medicines continued to sell to loyal customers in drugstores throughout the country: Sloan's Liniment for "the temporary relief of minor rheumatic and arthritic pains"; Dr. Kilmer's Swamp Root; Doan's Pills; Father John's Medicine, a bitter-tasting "cough suppressant for coughs due to colds," that, according to its label, "contains NO ALCOHOL nor HABIT FORMING INGREDIENTS."

In 1990, on a bottom shelf in a Walgreen's Pharmacy in a quiet, middle-class San Francisco neighborhood, the authors found a bottle of Lydia E. Pinkham's Tablets. According to the label, the compound was to be taken "to help relieve hot flashes and certain other discomforts of 'Change of Life' (Menopause) and Monthly Periods (painful Menstruation) and that 'Too Tired' feeling due to simple iron deficiency anemia." On the package was the smiling face of none other than Lydia E. Pinkham.

OH, THAT NAGGING COUGH

Some things don't ever change. According to an Associated Press report in 1985, many over-the-counter medications still contain large doses of alcohol: "Some of the popular cold medications range from 10 percent to 25 percent alcohol. There are cough syrups with up to 38 percent alcohol, and many popular mouthwashes range from 6 percent to nearly 27 percent."

CHAPTER
· 18 ·

MEDICINE SHOWS: PITCH DOCTORS TAKE TO THE ROAD

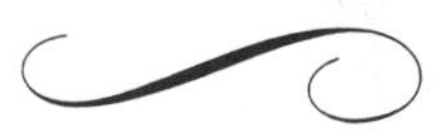

My friends, before your very eyes I will demonstrate these remedies. . . . Come closer! Let me help you!

''DR. LAMEREUX,'' circa 1880

In the colorful, wide-open decades near the turn of the twentieth century, the big-top barnstormers from Barnum and Bailey and the Ringling Brothers had a barely legitimate yet immensely popular rival for the title of Greatest Show on Earth. These were the years of the traveling medicine show. Lured by the romance of the road, and the chance to earn big money by peddling patent medicines to gullible consumers, self-appointed ''doctors'' set off across North America, cobbling together a form of theater that ''combined the mystery of magic with all the delights of a circus, the romance of savagery and the ecstasy of religion.''

The pitch doctor—characteristically a white man of middle or advanced years wearing a top hat and frock coat—who delivered the sales talk (the ''pitch'') had a lot of help. He was surrounded by performers drawn from the circus, traveling theater troupes, minstrel shows, Wild West extravaganzas, and vaudeville. As he traveled from town to town, he worked from temporary wooden stages with canvas backdrops flanked by flickering gasoline torches or electric lights.

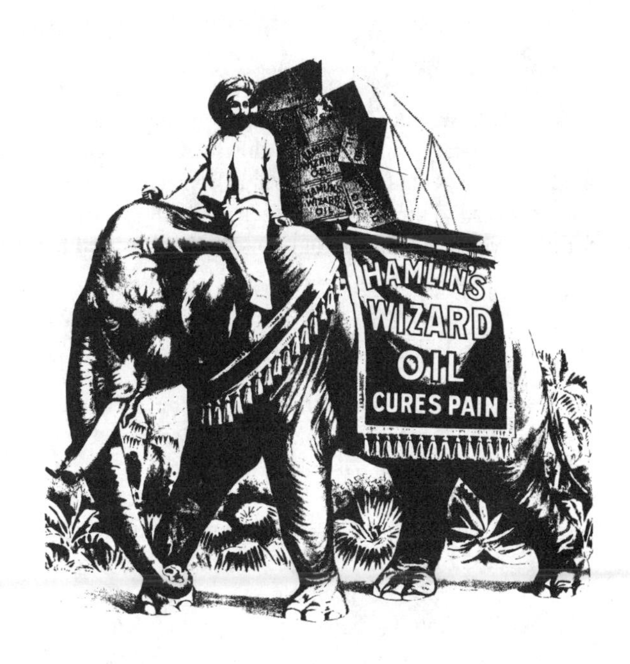

76. Traveling medicine showmen didn't hesitate to think big. *Collection of Advertising History, Archives Center, National Museum of American History, Smithsonian Institution.*

Eventually consumers caught on to the hucksters' game, making the very words "snake oil" virtual synonyms for fraud.

It took decades, however, for traveling medicine shows to run out of gas. From roughly 1870 to 1920, medicine shows were leading forms of entertainment and providers of health care, however questionable, especially in the hinterlands. They found their most appreciative audiences among poorly educated country people, credulous folks whose love of tall tales fed the medicine show doctors' grand claims.

"The medicine show was the one breath of romance, the one touch of lands across the seas that invaded the isolation of our remote little town," recalled a writer for the *American Mercury* magazine. "The light from its torches was reflected from eyes that were only too seldom opened wide in interest and pleasure. It was a splash of color and strange movement against a dull and drab background."

REHEARSAL: THE MOUNTEBANKS

The medicine shows that once crisscrossed North America originated with the antics of Europe's mountebanks, traveling quack doctors who sold assorted notions and cures, pulled teeth, and performed magic and comedy to draw and hold a crowd. Working from small, temporary stages, mountebanks often employed assistants to help with treatments, sales pitches, and entertainment, such as singing and juggling, to attract attention.

The mountebanks' deceptions were, of course, eventually discredited. Today the word mountebank means charlatan or crank. The clowns that accompanied the mountebank, called "zanni" in Italian, gave another word to the English language: "zany," transformed over time from a noun to an adjective used to describe a madcap character.

The mountebanks and zanni who toured Italy, France, and England had counterparts in colonial America by the early eighteenth century. So numerous and irritating to the authorities did they become, in fact, that Connecticut passed a law against the sale of "any Physick, Drugs or Medicines" by "any Mountebank," since "the Practice of Mountebanks in dealing out and administering Physick and Medicine, of unknown composition . . . has a practice to destroy the Health, Constitution and Lives of those who receive such Medicines." The colony's legislature also voted to bar medicine shows themselves, declaring that said performances induced "Corruption of Manners, promotion of Idleness, and the detriment of good Order and Religion. . . ."

Such laws did little, however, to slow down the bandwagoning medicine shows, which continued to flourish on both sides of the Atlantic. In 1866, nearly a century after the Connecticut law was passed, P.T. Barnum, who liked a good show and knew one when he saw it, wrote about an Italian who served as a "model for our quack doctors." Known as Christoforo, he worked Florence's "grand piazza before the Ducal Palace" in the 1840s and 1850s. According to the American impresario, Christoforo hawked potions for a patent-medicine manufacturer, and then sold his own panacea during breaks in his well-attended magic act. Observed Barnum in his delightful 1866 book *The Humbugs of the World*:

> It was to me a strange and suggestive scene—the bald, beak-nosed, coal-eyed charlatan, standing in the marketplace . . . peering through his gold spectacles at the upturned faces before him while the bony skeleton at his side swayed in the wind, and the grinning skulls below made grotesque faces, as if laughing at the gullibility of the people.

Barnum's shrewd reading of the trickster's appeal explains why laws alone could not suppress the medicine shows, either at home or abroad. Of Christoforo, Barnum wrote: "He understood human nature . . . its superstitions, tastes, changefulness, and love of display and excitement. He has done no harm, and given as much amusement as he has been paid for. . . . I dare say his death . . . will cause more sensation and evoke more tears than that of any better physician in Tuscany."

SMALL-TIME OPERATORS: THE PITCHMEN

In the mid-nineteenth century, American cousins of the great Christoforo were everywhere: in the rude mining camps, rough frontier towns, bursting cities, sleepy villages, and especially in isolated farming communities, where the love of display and excitement could not be indulged enough.

Like the sensation of Florence, American pitch doctors worked alone or with a few assistants. They were forerunners and counterparts of the more elaborate traveling medicine shows, with their dozens of performers, that came to life late in the nineteenth century.

Pitchmen accompanied by animal acts, singers, and acrobats worked on street corners and vacant lots hawking their medications. Some sold from the back of a wagon or stage (a "high pitch"); others contented themselves with selling samples out of a satchel mounted on a tripod (a "low pitch"). In later years, pitchmen traded in their buggies and wagons for cars and trucks, sometimes living in the cramped vehicles. Theirs was a nomadic, no-frills existence.

Regardless of their reduced circumstances, pitchmen generally affected a high moral tone for their medical lectures, which they illustrated with brightly colored anatomical charts or skeletons. Top hats, brocaded vests, and frock coats lent an air of dignity to the occasion, and every occasion led sooner or later to the pitch.

A "proof" or demonstration of the world's greatest pills accompanied the pitch and was carried out with the aid of a shill (a confederate who bought the first bottle and pretended to be cured) or a gullible-looking person in the crowd who would be too embarrassed to admit in front of his fellows that the cure made available at such a low, low price from the distinguished doctor—the title was nearly always self-conferred—wasn't for him.

TRICKS OF THE TRADE

Since proofs and demonstrations were used by medicine men to validate their products, showmen worked up tricks of the trade that they played on their unsuspecting marks. Here are a few of them.

• *Arthritis and rheumatism*: Patients were "cured" by vigorously rubbing liniment on the afflicted area—say, the elbow—which was also then pressed hard against the back of a chair. The rubbing and pressing dulled the pain just long enough to make the patient feel better.

• *Deafness*: Difficulty in hearing (not deafness caused by nerve damage) can be caused by impacted earwax. Knowing this, showmen rubbed the area outside the ears, dribbled in several drops of oil, inserted their fingertips in the patient's ears and quickly withdrew them, to make the ear "pop."

• *Tapeworms*: Pills to expel tapeworms contained string with an outside layer that dissolved in the stomach. Only the suspicious-looking strings exited from the body.

• *Liver disease*: Liver pads carried a spot of red pepper and glue. When placed on the patient's body above the liver, body heat melted the glue, producing a comforting warmth.

The etymology of the word *pitch* was explained by Dr. N.T. Oliver, a 70-year-old ex-medicine-show star who published his memoirs in the *Saturday Evening Post* in 1929. Wrote Oliver: "The word 'pitch' and its derivative, 'pitchman,' come either from the pitch-pine torch under which he once worked by night, before the coming of the gasoline flame and the electric light, or from the verb, as 'to pitch a tent.' "

Most pitchmen are long forgotten. But at least one solo pitchman is remembered today, more for his family's famous name than anything he did on the road. He is William Avery Rockefeller (1810–1906), known as "Doc" Rockefeller, who traveled the Midwest after the Civil War.

Rockefeller peddled packaged herbs and billed himself as "the Celebrated Cancer Specialist." He sold his cancer cure for the then-stupendous sum of 25 dollars and was known as a good storyteller who played a mean banjo. Leaving his wife and soon-to-be-famous son, John D. Rockefeller, behind, Doc lived in a bigamous marriage in South Dakota as Dr. William Levingston. Although relations between father and son were understandably strained, John D. never entirely rejected the influence of Doctor Bill. Indeed, the petroleum mogul took patent medicines for his health long after the family business changed from snake oil to Standard Oil.

Violet McNeal, a relatively rare pitchwoman, recalled in her memoirs that she mixed her medications herself in a disinfected bathtub before bottling and labeling the goods. Vital Sparks, her medicinal boost to male virility, were pieces of rock candy rolled in powdered aloes. Tiger Fat, a salve with supposedly exotic ingredients, was composed of items purchased wholesale from a mainstream druggist and suspended in a Vaseline base.

The pitchman's supposed panaceas were far cries from what they were alleged to be; but unless they contained high concentrations of alcohol or narcotics (most often opium), they usually caused no direct harm.

In any event, the number of people who shelled out good money for such remedies from solo or small-group pitchmen was fairly small. Not so the multitudes that flocked to the full-blown, full-tilt medicine shows of the 1880s and 1890s.

THE BIG TIME: "ANOTHER SOLD, PROFESSOR!"

"Advertising," wrote Barnum in his droll book about humbuggery, "is to a genuine article what manure is to land—it largely increases the product." The big traveling medicine shows were conceived as advertising vehicles by patent-medicine manufacturers, who coveted national markets. True, they already used magazines, posters, and handbills, and even graffiti painted on rocks and the sides of barns, to ballyhoo their products. Patent-medicine sellers also bought a considerable amount of space in newspapers, whose phenomenal growth was fueled in part by ads for cure-alls in a bottle. Still, patent-medicine makers liked the idea of using the touring extravaganzas as three-dimensional billboards, ads that sprung to life before the very eyes of awed consumers.

The biggest manufacturers mounted their own touring companies. One of the best-known medicine shows sold Hamlin's Wizard Oil, a liniment bottled by John A. Hamlin, a magician with his eye on the main chance. Hamlin's ads proclaimed Wizard Oil "the great medical conqueror. There is no sore it will not heal, no pain it will not subdue." In the 1870s, Hamlin's troupe took to the road to sell his Wizard Oil. Hamlin, who opened an opera house in Chicago, considered his show to be what later generations would call a class act. Frock coats, vests, silk hats, spats, and wing collars were *de rigueur* for his performers, who dropped in to sing with church choirs and maintained a strict sense of public decorum.

Stalwarts such as Doc MacBride, the Great King of Pain; Silk Hat Harry; and Big Foot Wallace followed on the heels of the Hamlin troupe. Such performers, especially in the late nineteenth century, when medicine shows peaked, fell into three broad categories.

Among them were Quakers—not actual members of the Society of Friends, but pretenders who cashed in on the Friends' reputation for honesty. Of the medicine-show Quakers, Violet McNeal recalled, "They called each other 'thee' and 'thou' and 'brother.' They dressed in fawn-colored clothing and wore wide-brimmed, low-crowned hats." One such Quaker, Brother John, toured in a horse-drawn chariot and demonstrated his versatility by pulling teeth in public.

Another popular guise was that of "Oriental" healer. To most Americans, the Far East signified everything mysterious and exotic; facts could dispel this aura of mystery only with difficulty. McNeal, a white American, performed for a time as Lotus Blossom, Oriental healer. Other medicine-show troupers

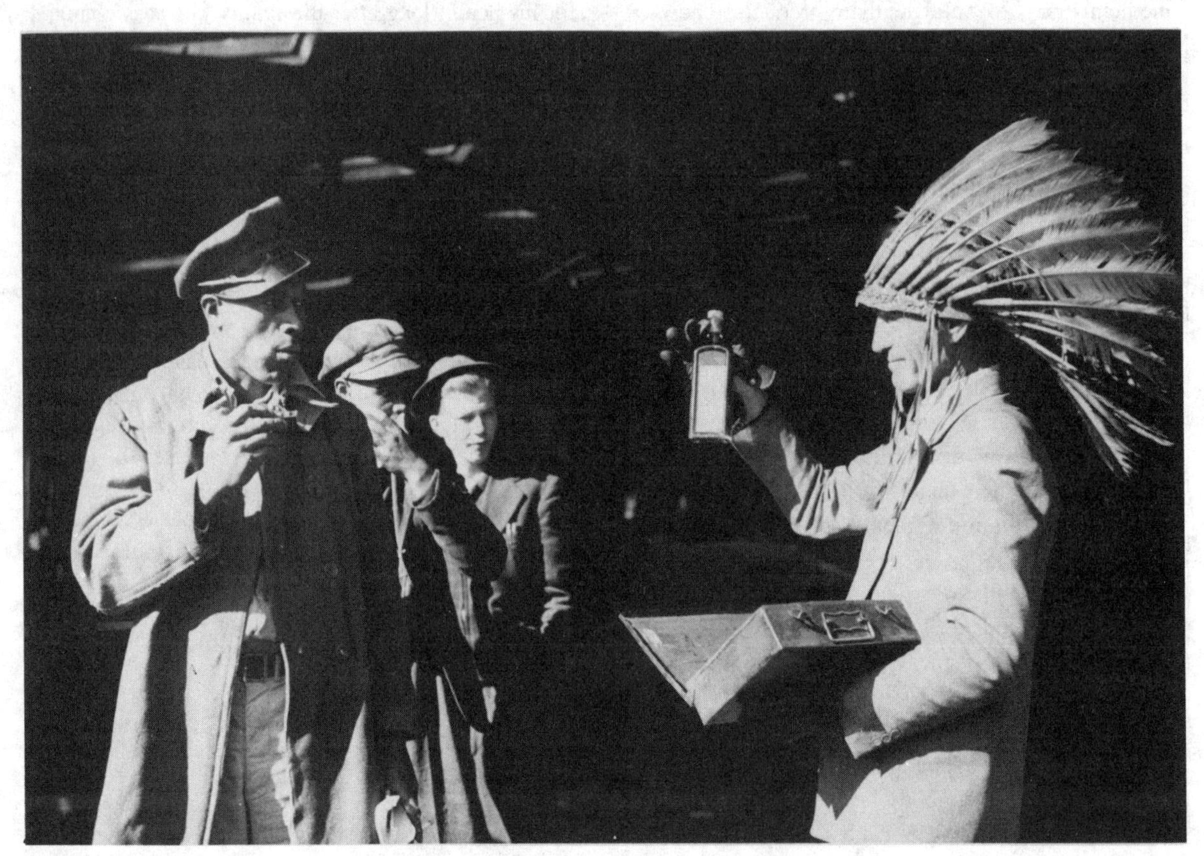

77. This "Indian" low pitchman peddled his tonics on the street. *The Bettmann Archive.*

TERMS OF THE TRADE

Like other show people, medicine-show veterans spoke in tangy slang that described their job and the restless, driven life that went with it. Below is a sampler.

Chopped grass: herbal medicine
Flea powder: powered herbs
Keister: satchel that opened into a display case, mounted on a tripod
Bally act: added attraction, like dancing girls, acrobats, or strongmen
Lot lice: show patrons who hung on without buying anything
Alagazam: the pitchman's hello
Velvet: profit

From *Step Right Up,* by Brooks McNamara

claimed to have escaped from China or Tibet, where they learned the wisdom of the East, now available for a small fee.

Probably the most crowd-pleasing acts of all were those of "Indian" medicine men. Although most nonnatives considered Native Americans to be bloodthirsty savages, they were also believed to be clever children of nature. Exploiting this idealized notion, medicine-show impresarios featured costumed, befeathered Native Americans (some were actual Native Americans, and some weren't) and borrowed features of the Wild West shows such as trick shooting to embellish their pitches.

Medicine-show performers used horse-drawn wagons, trains, and, later, trucks to get around. They slept in the cramped confines of their vehicles, pitched tents, or stayed in hotels that would accept disreputable show-folk, hostelries with walls "so thin, you could hear the fellow in the next room making up his mind," as one veteran of the road wryly recalled. Small operations disbanded during the winter or stayed in warm-weather climes; southern California and Florida were popular choices. The bigger shows toured year-round, moving indoors when the snowflakes flew.

Advance men publicized the shows with handbills, posters, and newspaper ads. Noisy rallies were held in front of drugstores and special displays of the show's medicines graced the windows of pharmacists who might otherwise resent the competition from the peripatetic entertainers. Major shows were heralded by parades down Main Street. If the troupe had a band, the musicians played in the parade and again on stage that night. If it had "Indians," they rode into town astride "genuine Indian ponies" or walked single-file in full regalia—war bonnets and war paint—past awed spectators.

Touring medicine shows played parks, fairgrounds, vacant lots, Grange halls, and bandbox "opera houses" hardly worthy of the name before audiences ranging from several dozen to the houses of 12 thousand fans claimed by Dr. Thomas Kelley, a Canadian medicine-show star who toured the United States and Canada. "Fixes," or payoffs to local officials, were made to secure the necessary permits to set up for business.

There was no rigid format for medicine shows, which borrowed freely from each other and other forms of entertainment. In general, however, a big touring company was apt to offer a variety show that ran for about two hours.

On the bill could be displays of marksmanship, broad ethnic comedy steeped in rough stereotypes, magic, stunts and acrobatics, dancing, or perhaps a strongman. Entertainment would make up about two-thirds of the show. The performers worked on a stage with a runway into the crowd and a canvas backdrop with painted scenes of nature and life among the Native Americans. On the lip of the stage might be glass jars with repulsive-looking tapeworms suspended in clear liquid. The huge worms, said to be removed from prominent local citizens, were actually purchased from stockyards. Tapeworm expellers—need it be said?—were big sellers.

The essentials of the pitch were the same in large medicine shows and solo pitch acts. Having charmed the audience into paying attention, medicine-show doctors were not beyond frightening spectators to part them from their money.

As Thomas Kelley reminded his listeners:

> You are all dying, every man, woman, and child is dying; from the instant you are born you begin to die and the calendar is your executioner. That, no man can hope to change. . . . Ponder well my words, then ask yourselves the question: Is there a logical course to pursue? Is there some way you can delay, and perhaps for years, that final moment before your name is written down by a bony hand in the cold diary of death? Of course, there is, ladies and gentlemen, and that is why I am here.

Having built up intolerable tension, the medicine-show doctor shrewdly released it by holding up a bottle or jar of the miracle-working medicine that he just happened to have with him. Shills made the first purchase, as the medicine-man's assistants walked through the audience with samples. Each sale was followed by cries of "Another sold, professor!" and finally "All sold out, doctor!"

The medicines fell somewhat short of the miraculous. According to Brooks McNamara, whose 1976 book *Step Right Up* is probably the major scholarly work on medicine shows, "the staples . . . generally included an herb compound with some tonic or cathartic properties, a liniment or oil, a salve, a catarrh cure, a corn remedy, and some sort of medicated soap." The popular Hamlin's Wizard Oil, according to McNamara, included "camphor, ammonia, chloroform, sassafras, cloves and turpentine." It also contained more than 50 percent alcohol. Ka-Ton-Ka, a mainstay of the Oregon Indian Medicine Company (actually headquartered in Pennsylvania) contained mundane ingredients: sugar, baking soda, aloe, and alcohol.

Although they could not deliver on their claims, medicine shows had to take care that their medications didn't directly harm anyone. They wanted to play the same towns the next year. As well known in their day as medicines advertised on television are now, Hamlin Wizard Oil, the Oregon Indian Medicine Company, and, most notably, the Kickapoo Indian Medicine Company were trusted and familiar names.

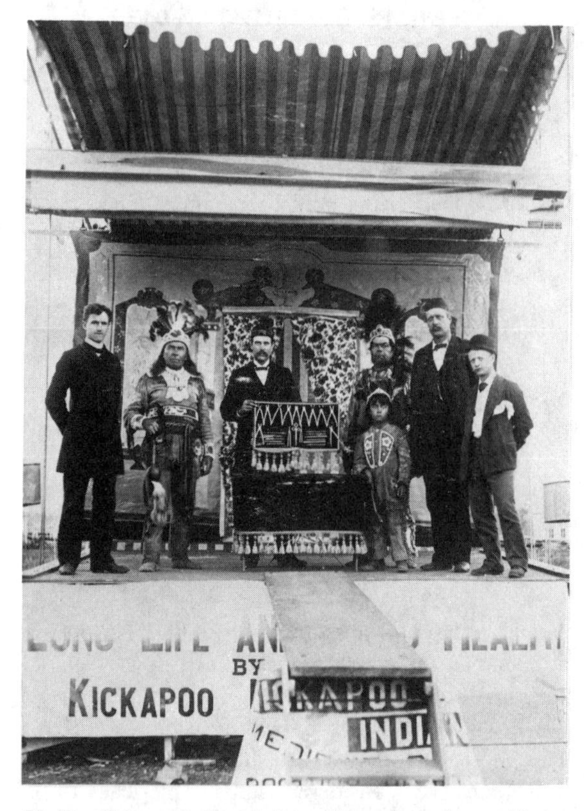

78. The Kickapoo Indian Medicine Show, shown here at Marine, Minnesota, circa 1890, was exotic and entrancing to small-town audiences. *Minnesota Historical Society.*

THE KICKAPOO INDIAN MEDICINE COMPANY

The Connecticut-based Kickapoo company sent out the biggest, most famous, and, according to contemporaries, the best of the touring medicine shows. The enterprise—named after the Kickapoo nation, resident in Indian Territory (Oklahoma) with which the firm was in no way connected—was founded in 1881 by two Caucasians, New Haven's John E. "Doc" Healy, a veteran salesman of King of Pain liniment, and Charles "Texas Charlie" Bigelow, of Beeville, Texas, a glamorous hombre who wore shoulder-length hair and a sombrero.

There were, to be sure, Native American employees at the Kickapoo Indian Medicine Company, headquartered near New Haven in Clintonville, although none were Kickapoos. Dubbed the Principal Wigwam, the headquarters served as a dormitory, factory, museum, and curio shop for tourists.

The attraction of the Kickapoo line was based on the notion of Native Americans as wise, mystical healers with magical knowledge of botanical medicine. The "mystical" Kickapoo goods included Kickapoo Cough Syrup (made from rum and molasses), Kickapoo Indian Oil (braced with a big dose of camphor), and Kickapoo Worm Expeller. By far the best-known product was a medication called Kickapoo Indian Sagwa.

Sagwa—Healy and Bigelow made up the word—was advertised as a cure for dyspepsia and rheumatism, among other things, although its chief actual value was as a laxative. Sagwa was said by Healy and Bigelow to be made by elders of the Kickapoo tribe who shipped the makings to Connecticut for finishing, bottling, and labeling. Sagwa supposedly contained a secret ingredient that defied laboratory analysis. In fact, Sagwa was a mixture of herbs, buffalo tallow, roots, bark, leaves, gum, and alcohol. The ingredients were purchased from a standard pharmaceutical firm.

According to legend (carefully nurtured by Healy and Bigelow), Sagwa was discovered by Texas Charlie when, nearly dead from a prairie fever, he was nursed back to health by a Native American family who told him of the powerful brew. A real-life legend of the frontier, Buffalo Bill Cody, was enlisted to endorse the product. Cody was quoted in Kickapoo ads as saying, "An Indian would as soon be without his horse, gun or blanket as without Sagwa." The entrepreneurial Kickapoo owners even

SNAKE OIL

Snake oil, or something that passed for it, was taken very seriously indeed by patrons of nineteenth-century medicine shows. Any kind of snake oil lent mystery and magic to a medicine, but rattlesnake oil was especially prized, given that rattlers presumably didn't happily donate the oil. Actually, rattlesnake oil didn't come from slithering reptiles, but rather from drug laboratories. White gasoline and wintergreen oil was a popular ''snake oil'' mixture.

came up with a fabricated symbol of Indian healing—Little Bright Eye, a princess, no less—whose sayings adorned the company's promotional magazines along with idealized illustrations of ''Life and Scenes'' among the Kickapoos at home on the range.

The first Kickapoo touring shows appeared in Boston, Providence, and New York City, but found their real home in secondary cities and towns and in the sensation-starved countryside. The shows were managed by seasoned white ''scouts'' and ''Indian fighters.'' Sites of the shows were ''Indian villages.'' In the late 1880s and early 1890s, some 100 Kickapoo companies, with as many as 100 Native American and non-Native American performers, took to the road, some ranging as far as Europe. At the peak of their success, Healy and Bigelow claimed to have 800 Native American employees. Like their rivals the Hamlin troupes, the Kickapoo showmen made a point of being well-behaved, staying in each town at least a week to dispel the medicine-show business's fly-by-night image.

Healy bailed out of the original Kickapoo company in the 1890s, heading off to Australia. By 1912, even Texas Charlie grew tired of the charade, selling the company to a buyer who ended the tours in 1914. Imitators continued to motor along America's highways as late as the 1930s, and the Healy and Bigelow medicines were obliquely recalled in Al Capp's popular ''Li'l Abner'' newspaper comic strip, which featured an elixir called Kickapoo Joy Juice.

HEADLINERS

Running away to join the circus once symbolized freedom to children; so did running off to join the circus's jaded cousin, the traveling medicine show. One young man who did just that, James Whitcomb Riley (1849–1913), worked for Dr. C.M. Townsend, selling the doctor's Cholera Balm and King of Cough medicine as he beat a bass drum, sang, played the violin, and recited doggerel. ''Why let pain your pleasure spoil/for want of Townsend's Magic Oil?'' Riley rhymed.

Riley made his name after his apprenticeship to Townsend, but several others became stars on the medicine-show circuit. Among them were Nevada Ned and Painless Parker.

Nevada Ned, the stage-name of Dr. N.T. Oliver, took his Western-flavored moniker for promotional purposes, ''though I had not, as yet, been within 2,000 miles of Nevada,'' as he later admitted. Oliver ran shows for both Healy and Bigelow and John A. Hamlin in the 1880s and 1890s. When he wasn't doing trick shooting in medicine shows, Ned cranked out crime novels. Originally from Philadelphia, Oliver dropped out of Yale to follow the same wanderlust that gripped Riley; unlike the poet, he made a life's work of it.

Oliver acted the tough ''Indian scout'' before audiences, but he was bright enough to understand the less-than-uplifting reason for the success of ''In-

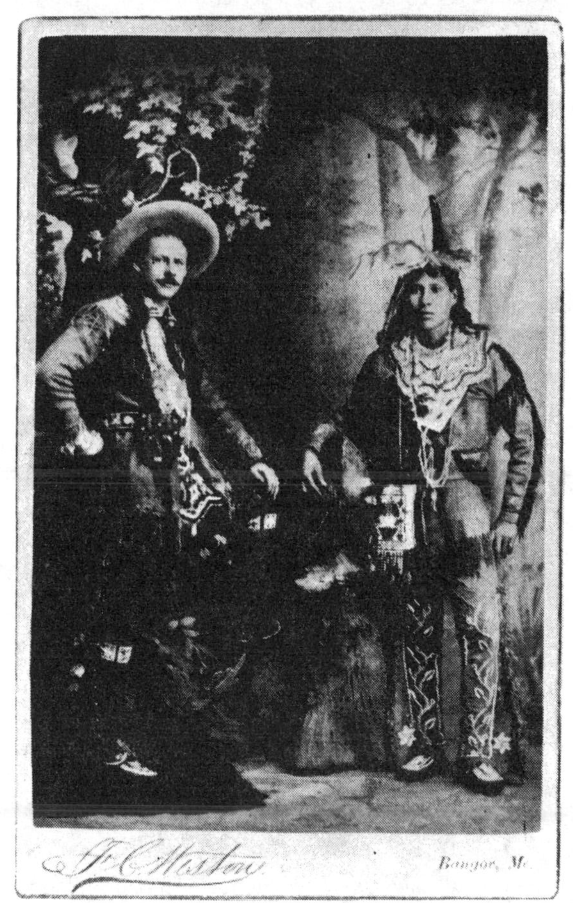

Nevada Ned in Kickapoo Regalia, and Spotted Wolf, Member of His Company

79. *From* Saturday Evening Post, *October 19, 1929.*

dian'' medicine shows. ''Now that the redskin no longer stood in the white man's way,'' he wrote in 1929, ''he became a figure of romance. Fiction discovered him anew, added the cowboy, the gold camp and the desert, and the stage was set for the showmen.''

Oliver was also honest enough to laugh at himself. As the manager (''Indian Agent'') of a Kickapoo show, Oliver was supposed to translate the speeches, given in various Native American languages, of the ''Kickapoos'' on stage. But, as he later wrote, ''What the brave actually said, I never knew, but I had reason to fear that it was not the noble discourse of my translation, for even the poker faces of his fellow savages sometimes were convulsed.''

Occasionally taking out his own shows, Oliver once hit the road with two Syrians berobed to look like Hindu priests, and threw an elephant into the bargain. It was at the head of a Kickapoo show in Chicago that Oliver (or Nevada Ned) oversaw what, at 110-members strong, may have been the biggest medicine show ever mounted. It was the only time, he recalled, that a big-city daily newspaper dispatched a critic to review a medicine show.

Wherever he went, Oliver made sure he was noticed. ''In 1886,'' he wrote, ''I had added ten-dollar gold pieces as buttons on my velvet and corduroy jacket, five-dollar gold coins as buttons on my fancy vests, three-dollar gold pieces as cufflinks. Around my neck, I wore 3,000 dollars' worth of real diamonds and two gold-mounted mother-of-pearl .44s. My moustache was long and prettily waxed to points, my clothes foppish in the extreme. In such fashion I liked to stroll up Broadway or through the markets in Washington and Fulton streets, followed by bootblacks, newsboys and messengers, who could not decide whether to hoot or cheer.''

Scarcely less flamboyant was Dr. Painless Parker, who billed himself as ''the greatest all-around dentist in this world or the next.'' Unlike most medicine-show stars, whose degrees were self-conferred, Parker was a licensed dentist, practicing a common sideline in the traveling extravaganzas—tooth-pulling. In rural areas, dentists were scarce. People who needed a diseased tooth filled or capped, or, more than likely after a delay, pulled, waited until a visiting dentist showed up. Extractions took place in public, in the street or on stage, as a form of entertainment.

Born Edgar Randolph Parker in the Maritime region of Canada in 1872, Parker attended Philadelphia Dental College (later incorporated into Temple University). The future ''molar mogul,'' as one wag described him, began practicing at age 21, bouncing in a buckboard wagon through the backwoods of Canada. When customers were slow to materialize, he took to working outside and blowing a cornet to attract attention. Parker kept on with his theatrical dentistry for the next 59 years. He pulled teeth on city streets, worked in traveling medicine shows, ran a circus, and started a lucrative chain of dental parlors staffed by dentists who worked for him.

Some of what Parker did was serious dentistry. He promoted preventive tooth care at a time when few consumers gave much thought to saving their teeth. He also helped to pioneer the use of local anesthetics when dentists put their patients to sleep with ether. Parker injected his patients with hydrocain, a predecessor to novocaine, which he considered more convenient than ether.

Near the turn of the twentieth century, the young Canadian moved to Brooklyn, New York, where he opened an office on Flatbush Avenue. On the advice of a press agent, Parker mounted signs all around the second floor of his building: ''Painless Parker. I am positively IT in painless dentistry! Yes, me!'' The IT was four stories high. Tightrope walkers angled between Parker's office and buildings across the street, singing the doctor's praises. The crowd-pleasing dentist often left his office to pull teeth in the street, to the accompaniment of a small brass band. The band drowned out the cries of the afflicted whom hydrocain apparently didn't help.

Parker's Brooklyn business was a success, but he sold it and moved to Los Angeles to start a new life with his wife, Frances. The old itch came back, however, and Parker returned to show-biz in a big way. He bought a circus, which he took up and

MEDICINE-SHOW GRADUATES

As Nevada Ned diplomatically put it in 1929: ''The actors, famous in legitimate pictures and vaudeville who have, in their time, passed out the Indian Prairie Flower and the Buffalo Salve are many more than the records show. Few have chosen to mention it to interviewers.'' Among the famous names: Harry Houdini, James Whitcomb Riley, George Burns and Gracie Allen, George M. Cohan, Minnie Pearl, Chico Marx, Carmen Miranda, Roy Acuff, and Lester Flatt (on a radio show that pitched patent medicine). Hank Williams's medicine show turn was re-created in his 1964 film biography *Your Cheatin' Heart*, starring George Hamilton as the country music great.

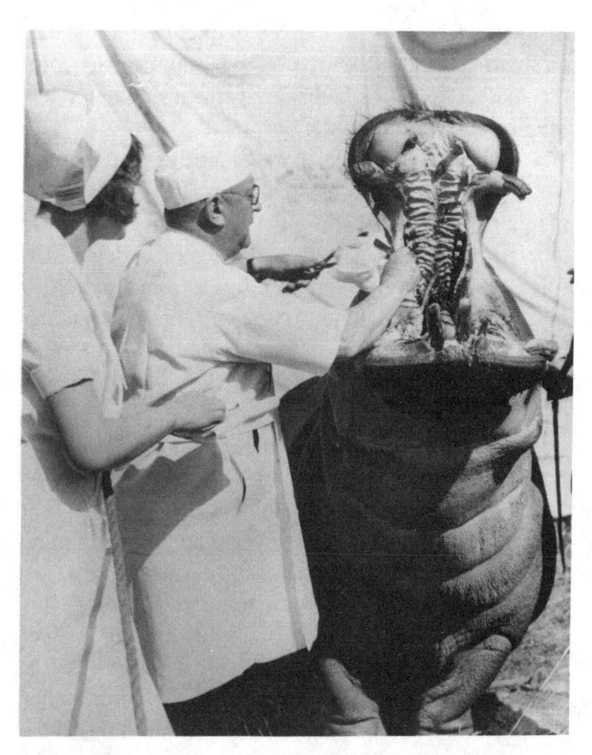

80. No tooth problem was too tough for medicine-show dentist Painless Parker. *San Francisco Public Library.*

down the West Coast, stopping to open branches of his dental office. (He had started a second chain.)

"The Parker Dental Circus was a little queer as the big shows went," observed the writers of a magazine feature on Parker, "but that did not seem to bother the crowds that stormed it nightly. Draped all around the main tent was a 20-by-200-foot banner sign proclaiming: 'Dr. Painless Parker. I am positively IT in painless dentistry!' Inside were placards, and more banners, all bearing the Parker crest—a giant facsimile of a molar tooth with the doctor's handsome portrait superimposed on it. The bandstand was built in imitation of a gaping set of uppers and lowers so that the red-coated bandsmen seemed to be sitting in a gigantic, open mouth, in instant peril of mastication.

"Outside, between the tattooed lady and the living skeleton, the doctor had set up a large tent labeled 'Painless Parker Dental and Medical Clinic,' and staffed it with four dentists, four doctors, four oculists and a dozen white-frocked nurses." Back under the big top rode Parker, ". . . smiling and bowing and tossing showers of small coins to the natives from the back of a genuine, 100 percent East Indian pachyderm."

Parker sold the circus and settled in a 14-room mansion on a 300-acre spread near Saratoga, 50 miles south of San Francisco in the Santa Clara Valley—now covered by high-technology industry but then abloom with orchards. But Parker went back to street dentistry, not because he needed the money, but because he missed the crowds and the fun of showing off. Blowing his cornet and yanking teeth at the San Francisco cable car turnaround at Powell and Market streets, Parker was in his element. He opened more offices and continued to prosper. He bought a yacht, the biggest on San Francisco Bay, and joined the Roundtable, an exclusive luncheon club that set places for muckraker extraordinaire Lincoln Steffens and the great lawyer Clarence Darrow. A.P. Giannini, founder of the Bank of America, became Parker's pal.

Despite his affluence and growing social status, the doctor's later years were marked by legal battles with officials who rejected his claims to painless dentistry, worried about the lack of sanitation in his street dentistry, and objected to his growing chain of clinics. California authorities suspended his dental license from 1930 to 1935, but Giannini intervened with the governor to have it restored. When authorities moved to tone down his ads, Parker outwitted them by legally changing his first name to Painless, so that even a simple telephone-directory listing would be an ad. In 1935, California outlawed sidewalk dentistry, but by then Parker had moved most of his operations inside. Ten years later, when his wife died, Parker sold his mansion and land and moved into cramped, cluttered rooms above his Market Street headquarters. Clearly this was a man who lived for business.

As an old man, Parker was tolerated if not exactly clasped to the bosom of establishment dentistry and was considered a legendary survivor of a bygone era of medicine. In 1952, just before he died at age 80 of a heart ailment, the national magazine *Collier's* printed an affectionate three-part series on Parker, still busy operating 28 dental offices on the West Coast. Describing him as "a stocky, white-coated old gentleman with silvery hair and moustache, a pointed Vandyke beard and an expression of restrained glee," *Collier's* photographed Parker in an old top hat. Around his neck was a necklace of 357 teeth. Parker had pulled them all in one wild day in 1905, near Poughkeepsie, New York.

RUNNING ON EMPTY

Painless Parker's long golden age was unique. The great tide of medicine shows—of road-wise pitchmen, doctors and dentists, "Indians" and frontiersmen got up in buckskin—began to ebb even before World War I. The causes were many: The growth of cities

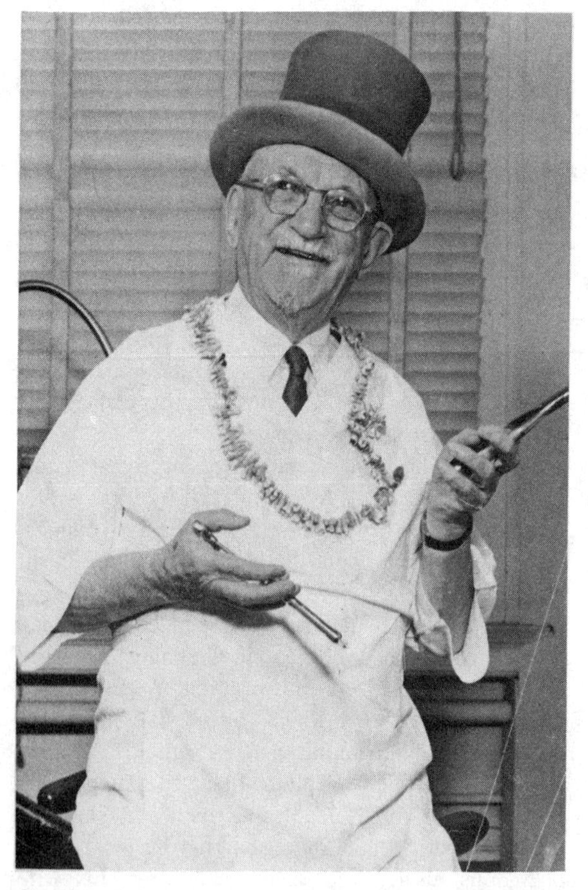

81. Tools of the trade: Painless Parker with impresario's hat and necklace of 357 human teeth. *From* Collier's, *January 5, 1952.*

reduced the market of country people who flocked to medicine shows; the inroads of radio and motion pictures made even the farmers who stayed on the land more worldly; and new laws forced the medicine shows that tried to tough it out in the new age to tone down their health claims.

Thomas Kelley, who toured Canada and 37 American states with his Shamrock Medicine Show (earning, he said, two million dollars), saw the end coming long before it arrived. ". . . Progress is on the march to shatter the rural customs of yesterday," Kelley wrote. "The natives are wiser now, here, there, and everywhere in North America. Soon there will be no such thing as a rube. . . ."

Kelley also recognized the unbeatable competition from movies: ". . . What chance has a med-man with big expenses, tons of equipment and seven-to-nine performers, against a fellow who comes along carrying his entire show in a tin can?" The first flickering, silent, black-and-white films were shown in makeshift cinemas and even in medicine shows as novelties. By the late 1920s, however, movies had taken over so completely that they turned to medicine shows as sources of picturesque characters and settings. Like the Native Americans, whom the medicine shows had once patronized, the shows themselves were considered quaint.

Moreover, once-lax laws were being tightened. The 1906 Pure Food and Drug Act required patent-medicine manufacturers to list ingredients on product labels. Health claims had to be watered down. Before 1906, Kickapoo Indian Oil was promoted as "a quick cure for all kinds of pain. Good for man or beast." After 1906, it was sold only for "the relief of aches and pains."

State medical authorities also pressed medicine shows to carry licensed physicians, although this did not immediately curb abuses. Indeed, some shows already carried a doctor, usually referred to as "The Boozer." Many were heavy drinkers who couldn't maintain a respectable practice. Medicine shows set up "consultation rooms" on the showgrounds, funneling anxious patients to the doctors for private sessions. Receptionists engaged patients in seemingly casual conversation and encoded cards which enabled the doctors to make miraculous (and time-saving) diagnoses. In the new era of regulation, such practices were frowned upon.

In 1938, the Food, Drug and Cosmetics Act stiffened penalties for lawbreakers. By the 1940s, federal agents were sitting in on medicine shows to check health claims. But by then there were few medicine shows left to regulate. The Depression had already taken money from the pockets of working people and World War II gasoline rationing had the motorized shows running on empty.

In 1950–51, a Louisiana Cajun by the name of Dudley J. Le Blanc pushed the pedal to the floor one more time. Concocting a medicated tonic he called Hadacol, Le Blanc mixed B-vitamins, honey, and alcohol. According to Brooks McNamara, "The first batches were stirred up in vats behind Le Blanc's barn by local girls equipped with boat oars."

The new product found a ready market as a dietary supplement. Le Blanc, already splurging on advertising, decided to augment his ads with a traveling medicine show. So the Hadacol Caravan, with the gregarious Le Blanc as master of ceremonies, made its way across the South in 1950, winding up with a month-long stay in Los Angeles. Le Blanc did not sell Hadacol at the shows, although the product name was plastered everywhere. Rather, he collected box tops from Hadacol packages as admission.

The Hadacol Caravan had star power. Performers such as Carmen Miranda, Mickey Rooney, George Burns and Gracie Allen, Minnie Pearl, Roy Acuff, and Chico Marx entertained. In Los Angeles, Groucho

Marx and Judy Garland dropped by. In 1951, with Cesar Romero acting as master of ceremonies, country-music great Hank Williams singing, and former heavy-weight boxing champion Jack Dempsey plugging Hadacol on stage, the caravan went forth again, traveling in chartered railroad cars. That same year, however, Le Blanc, who had political ambitions, sold the business and the Caravan rolled no more.

A few medicine shows sputtered into the 1950s, the last one leaving the road in 1964. Their erstwhile customers, already sated with movies and radio and protected by laws that didn't exist in the heyday of the medicine show, were further distracted by glowing electronic boxes made by RCA, Zenith, and Philco. Fading into folklore, the great cure-all caravans were well and truly gone.

CURTAIN CALLS

Even the most elaborate traditional shows were considered beneath the notice of documentarians. Besides, their popularity peaked before portable film-making and sound equipment were cheap and widely available. Consequently, film libraries and archives of recorded sound hold only scraps of actuality from this once-omnipresent form of theater. Even feature films with medicine-show settings are hard to come by, especially on home video, even though the fictional re-creations feature stars such as W.C. Fields, Jack Benny, George M. Cohan, Harold Lloyd, and Jimmy Durante. Other physical traces of the old hucksters are equally hard to uncover. A writer in search of the Kickapoo headquarters in New Haven found a vacant lot, with no sign that the company had ever been there. In San Francisco, the flatiron building that served as Painless Parker's headquarters was demolished and replaced by a modern bank branch.

Traditional medicine shows are not likely to reappear. But some observers, especially gimlet-eyed federal agents, believe they have seen their descendents at the "New Age" fairs and expositions that began multiplying in the 1970s.

In makeshift booths, along with samples of health foods, audio tapes that teach relaxation techniques, video tapes that illustrate exercise routines, demonstrations of massage, and artfully arranged displays of "healing" crystals, are vitamin-rich dietary supplements and bottles of glandular extracts. These medications, Food and Drug Administration officials believe, are marketed by manufacturers who make unsupported if not outright fraudulent health claims.

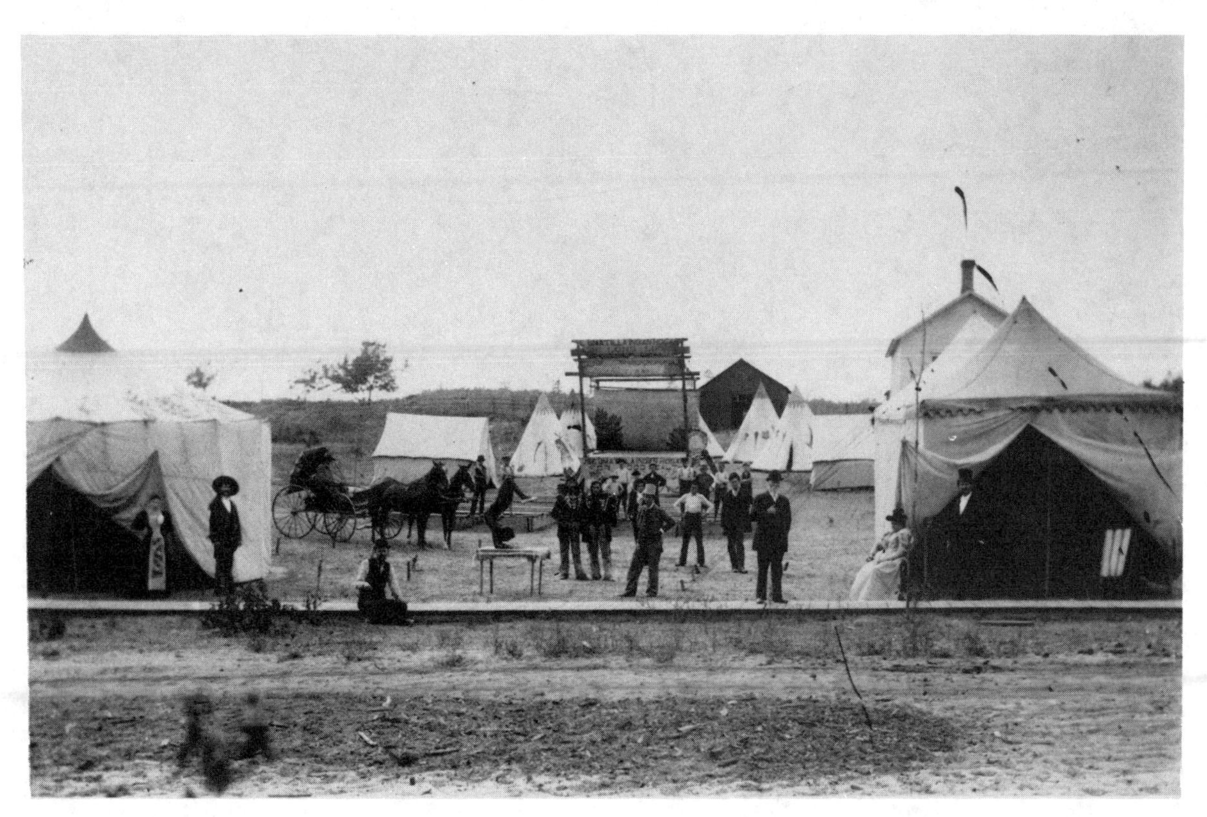

82. A traveling medicine show ready for business near Black River Falls, Wisconsin (circa 1902). Photo by Charles Van Schaick. Van Schaick Collection, State Historical Society of Wisconsin.

In a 1985 Associated Press dispatch, FDA officials were quoted as saying that extravagant verbal pitches were common. According to the AP story, "Two exhibitors at a health fair in the Northwest 'sold simple hydrogen peroxide, an antiseptic and bleaching agent, with claims the chemical would cure cancer, kidney stones, multiple sclerosis, inflamatory illness, viral infections and bacterial organisms,' said agency spokesman Bill Griss." The report continued: " 'Years ago, fraudulent health products were promoted by snake oil peddlers who traveled the country,' said Griss. . . . He said that in recent years, operators have banded together to rent large exposition halls for a short period . . . made a hard-sell pitch to prospective buyers and then skipped town."

Although they no longer travel with large companies of compatriots, a handful of medicine men still work at county and state fairs, swap meets, flea markets, and other gatherings. Akin to the solo pitch doctors of old, modern pitchmen are occasionally sighted in press accounts, like members of an endangered species of migratory birds.

In 1984, the *Los Angeles Times* ran a feature story on Michael Roe, a 38-year-old man who toured southern California in a 1950 Dodge cattle truck that served as his office, transportation, and home. Roe, who compounded bottled medications from 70 to 80 herbs that he said he gathered himself, made pitches for his Survival Magic Show while dressed in a top hat and vest. "Many people take me very seriously," Roe told the *Times*. "They can't afford a doctor, and they know that herbs can heal, and here I am. And I hear wonderful success stories from people who use these herbs."

Roe, who cautioned that he neither diagnosed nor prescribed for individuals, said he learned about herbs chiefly from "Old Indians and Mexicans. . . . People are over-entertained these days," Roe complained, 70 years after the Kickapoo Indian Medicine Company gave up its road shows. "You really need to get their attention before they'll listen to you. It's not easy being a medicine man anymore."

CHAPTER
· 19 ·

THE BODY ELECTRIC: FUTURE SHOCKS

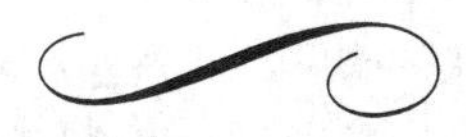

Electricity is the greatest power on earth. It puts life and force into whatever it touches; gives relief to rheumatism, backache, kidney, liver and bladder troubles, early decay, night losses, lack of nerve and vigor, nervous debility, constipation, dyspepsia, undevelopment and lost vitality, and all female complications.

Ad for Addison's Galvanic Electric Belt
Quoted in Journal of the American Medical Association, *1915*

Ever since people first saw evidence of electricity—and long before they knew what it was—this mysterious, unseen force has captivated the imagination. Brilliant stabs of lightning, the pale dance of St. Elmo's Fire, and the crackle of brushed hair were signs of invisible magic. Were such magic to be tamed, there would be no limit to what it might do: light the night sky, power mighty engines, or even heal the sick.

Today, applied electricity is a fact of life, and nowhere is it more useful than in medicine. Electric pacemakers regulate human heartbeats. Sensitive instruments record the brain's faint electrical charge. Powerful jolts even rewire the brain in controversial treatments for clinical depression.

While mainstream scientists struggled to capture lightning in a bottle, their rivals on the fringes of medicine put the new technologies to work. Electric belts, electric baths, and other gadgets appeared in the nineteenth century, touted as cures for everything from cancer and cholera to writer's cramp and upset stomach.

Best of all, from the sellers' standpoint, debunking the new machines was difficult, even for eminent physicians. In the early days, not even top doctors were quite sure what electricity was. (For the record, *Webster's New World Dictionary* defines electricity as "a property of certain fundamental particles of all matter, as electrons [negative charges] and protons or positrons [positive charges] that have a force field associated with them and that can be separated by the expenditure of energy: electrical charge can be generated by friction, induction, or chemical charge . . . .")

LODESTONES AND TWITCHING MUSCLES

The ancients were, of course, well aware of electricity's effects. They noted that amber, when rubbed, attracts hair, straw, and other light objects. They observed the halos on ships' rigging and the tips of spears, which they considered to be messages from the gods.

Magnetic lodestone, which attracts pieces of iron and steel, was considered the philosopher's stone. Paracelsus (1493–1541), a Zurich-born healer and teacher who championed mineral medicines, alchemy, and astrology, ascribed occult powers to lodestone and used it to treat epilepsy.

Several generations after Paracelsus, the physician William Gilbert (1544–1603), who attended England's Queen Elizabeth I, wrote about the principles of magnets and the difference between magnetic attraction and electricity. In his 1600 book *De Magnete,* Gilbert named what we now know as electricity, calling it "electrica," a word he derived from *elektron*, the Greek word for amber.

Knowledge about electricity accelerated in the eighteenth century. In 1752, Benjamin Franklin (1706–1790) sent his famous kite into the stormy sky over Philadelphia, showing that lightning was electricity (and inventing the lightning rod). Toward the end of the century, Luigi Galvani (1737–1798), an anatomy professor in Bologna, induced violent contractions in the muscles of frogs with electrical discharges. At about the same time, the Italian physicist Alessandro Volta (1745–1827) developed a crude battery.

While Franklin, Galvani, and Volta were making their discoveries, a contemporary, Christian A. Kratzenstein (1723–1795), was pioneering medical uses of electricity. Giving electrical charges to his patients, Kratzenstein "observed an increase in the pulse beat and acceleration of the blood circulation and contractile effect on the muscles," writes historian Bern Dibner. "He then began to administer electrical charges in cases of such congestive ailments as rheumatism, malignant fever and the plague . . . . Other experimenters turned to applying electrifying charges and sparks to alleviate human suffering."

Still other experimenters turned to bizarrely colorful applications of electricity and its cousin, magnetism, even as their true properties were only beginning to be understood.

THOSE ELECTRIFYING PHOSPHENE PARTIES

Benjamin Franklin has long been remembered for the risky business of putting a metal key on a kite during a thunderstorm. That, however, wasn't his most enjoyable experience with electricity. When he was in a more playful mood, Franklin took part in phosphene parties.

"At these parties," according to one modern account, "groups of people would join hands in a circle and receive a high-voltage shock from an electrostatic generator. Somehow, the completion or breaking of this people-circuit created an electrical stimulus to their brains that unleashed colorful phosphene light shows." Adds the report: "You can also generate these images at will by rubbing closed eyes or pressing against the lids with fingertips."

MESMERISM

Franz Anton Mesmer (1734–1815) was practicing medicine in Vienna in the 1770s when he came under the sway of a Jesuit priest with the unlikely name of Father Hell. Herr Hell, it turns out, was more than a priest; he was a healer who applied magnetized metal plates to the naked bodies of sick people to effect cures. The priest/healer was a big influence on Mesmer, an impressionable young man who wrote his dissertation at the University of Vienna on the influence of the planets on the human body.

Mesmer believed that an imbalance of an invisible electrical universal fluid was the cause of all disease. Later, he decided the fluid was really magnetic in nature.

In 1778, Mesmer left Vienna for Paris. The ambitious physician caused a sensation in the French capital, where his theories became all the rage, especially among well-to-do women.

Charles Mackay, in his compelling 1843 book *Memoirs of Extraordinary Popular Delusions and the Madness of Crowds,* quotes Mesmer's explanation of his theory in a letter to a friend. Wrote Mesmer:

> I have observed that the magnetic is almost the same thing as the electric fluid, and that it may be propagated in the same manner, by means of intermediate bodies . . . . I have rendered paper, bread, wool, silk, stones, leather, glass, wood, men and dogs—in short, everything I touched—magnetic to such a degree that these substances produced the same effects as the loadstone on diseased persons. I have charged jars with magnetic matter in the same way as is done with electricity.

Mesmer characterized his mysterious power as animal magnetism, but awed acolytes referred to the magic by the name of their magus, calling it Mesmerism.

Mackay, a British doctor of law with a keen eye for the absurd, describes Mesmer's treatments thusly:

> In the centre of the saloon was placed an oval vessel, about four feet in its longest diameter, and one foot deep. In this were laid a number of wine bottles, filled with magnetised water, well-corked-up, and disposed in radii, with their necks outwards. Water was then poured into the vessel so as just to cover the bottles, and filings of iron were thrown in occasionally to heighten the magnetic effect. The vessel was then covered with an iron cover, pierced through with many holes, and was called the baquet. From each hole issued a long movable rod of iron, which the patients were to apply to such parts of their bodies as were afflicted. Around this baquet the patients were directed to sit, holding each other by the hand, and pressing their knees together as closely as possible, to facilitate the passage of the magnetic fluid from one to the other.
>
> Then came the assistant magnetisers, generally strong, handsome young men, to pour into the patient from their fingertips fresh streams of the wonderous [sic] fluid. They embraced the patients between the knees, rubbed them gently down the spine and the course of the nerves, using gentle pressure upon the breasts of the ladies, and staring them out of countenance to magnetise them by the eye. All this time the most rigorous silence was maintained, with the exception of a few wild notes on the harmonica or the piano-forte, or the melodious voice of a hidden opera-singer swelling softly at long intervals. Gradually the cheeks of the ladies began to glow, their imaginations to become inflamed; and off they went, one after the other, in convulsive fits. Some of them sobbed and tore their hair, others laughed till the tears ran from the eyes, while others shrieked and screamed and yelled till they became insensible altogether.
>
> This was the crisis of their delirium. In the midst of it, the chief actor [Mesmer] made his appearance, waving his wand, like Prospero, to

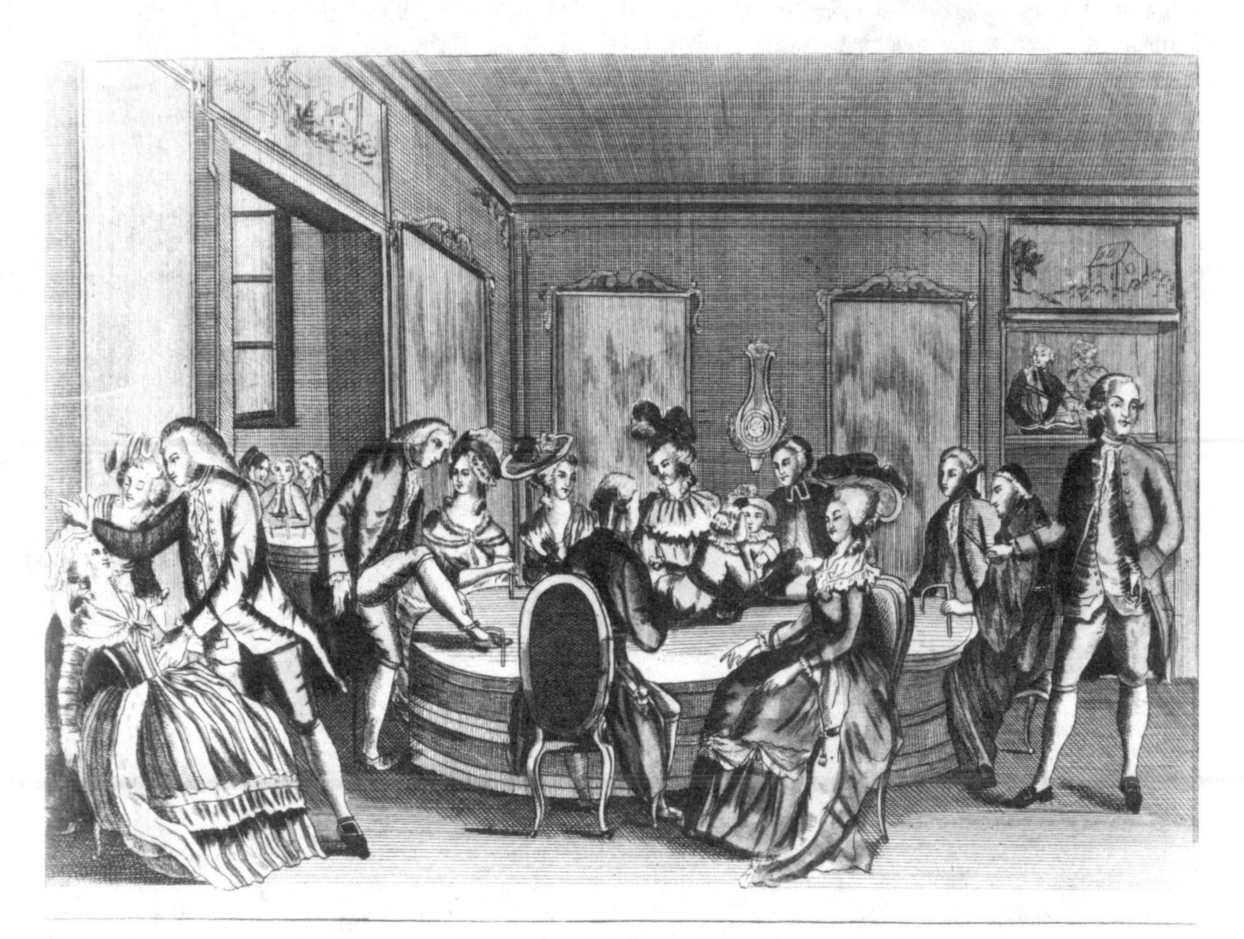

83. Late eighteenth-century Mesmerism was equal parts therapy and theater. *National Library of Medicine.*

> work new wonders. Dressed in a long robe of lilac-coloured silk richly embroidered with gold flowers, bearing in his hand a white magnetic rod, and with a look of dignity which would have sat well on an eastern caliph, he marched with solemn strides into the room. He awed the still-sensible by his eye, and the violence of their symptoms diminished. He stroked the insensible with his hands upon the eyebrows and down the spine; traced fingers upon their breast and abdomen with his long white wand, and they were restored to consciousness. They became calm, acknowledged his power, and said they felt streams of colour or burning vapour passing through their frames, according as he waved his wand or his fingers before them.

Mesmer's thrilling theatricality attracted much attention, not all of it as uncritical as the shrieks and swoons of his patients. In 1784, the French Academy of Sciences conducted a study of Mesmerism. One of the investigators was Benjamin Franklin, then residing in Paris. The academy concluded that there was no such thing as magnetic fluid, and that the humid results of Mesmer's elaborate demonstrations could be obtained without any touching. Mesmer, they concluded, had tapped the well of imagination; he worked his miracles by suggestion.

The report damaged Mesmer's reputation. He left Paris, eventually abandoning France altogether, and dying years later at age 81. Today, Mesmer is recognized as a pioneer of hypnosis (a word he didn't use) who, however unwittingly, paved the way for Sigmund Freud and other explorers of the psyche. In the process, Mesmer bequeathed his name to the English language: to mesmerize is to cast a spell; to be mesmerized is to be enthralled.

Although Mesmer's scientific pretentions were punctured, his ideas did not immediately disappear. His followers continued to hold sessions without the master and were denounced in respectable circles as depraved voluptuaries. Indeed, the French Academy of Sciences expressed concern that women under the spell of Mesmerism would compromise their virtue for rakes posing as healers.

Stripped of its sensual elements, Mesmerism was transplanted to America, where it proved influential in surprisingly changed fashion. In 1836–37, the Frenchman Charles Poyen lectured in the United States, where Phineas P. Quimby, a health practitioner in Portland, Maine, heard him speak and was sorely impressed. Quimby, who used touch and suggestion in his practice as a magnetic healer, was a major influence on Mary Baker Eddy, the founder of Christian Science, who railed into her old age against "malicious animal magnetism" beamed at her by her enemies.

Mesmerism was so popular that a disgusted New York physician, David Meredith Reese, was moved to write: "That this and kindred delusions should have prevailed in the dark ages, need not be a source of wonder; but that it should receive countenance in the nineteenth century, demonstrates the present to be indeed the age of humbug."

Reese wrote in 1838, just a year after Poyen popularized Mesmerism in America. By the early 1840s, professional Mesmerists were thick upon the ground. An 1843 advertisement in the *Boston Courier* proclaimed:

> Mrs. W. FERGUS begs to state that she has secured the assistance of a superior Somnambulist and Clairvoyant, and is now prepared for the highest order of Mesmeric experiments, as well as examination for disease. References can be given to some of the most intellectual and influential individuals in the city. Terms made known at her residence, No. 4 Winter Place. Physicians are invited to call.

Popular as it became, Mesmerism, with its pseudo-scientific baggage and scandalous origins, was never accepted by mainstream science. In 1889, a century after Mesmer shocked Paris, the *Electrical World,* a trade journal devoted to news about Thomas Edison's wondrous inventions and the role of electricity in industrial engineering, reported:

> Dr. Pinel, of Paris, has succeeded in hypnotising several subjects by means of the phonograph . . . . The conclusion deduced by Dr. Pinel is that the theory of magnetic current passing from the operator to the subject is entirely baseless, and that the real cause of the phenomena of hypnotism is nervous derangement on the part of the subjects . . . .

Indeed, by the late nineteenth century, a new age—not of suggestion, but of humming, sparking, and shocking devices, often used without a physician's supervision—had arrived.

THE SHOCK OF THE NEW

Reduced to essentials, the role of the new electronic contraptions was to put "good" electricity into the bodies of sufferers or draw off "bad" electricity. Electric devices had powerful appeal. In addition to their novelty, they required no drugs or surgery and promised relief from even chronic pain without causing harm.

CURE OF DISEASE WITHOUT DRUGS OR MEDICINES.

An Air-Tight Dry Cell Pocket Battery which furnishes 4000 Electro-Magnetic Vibrations Per Minute.

(Patented in U. S. and Foreign Countries A.D. 1888–89.)

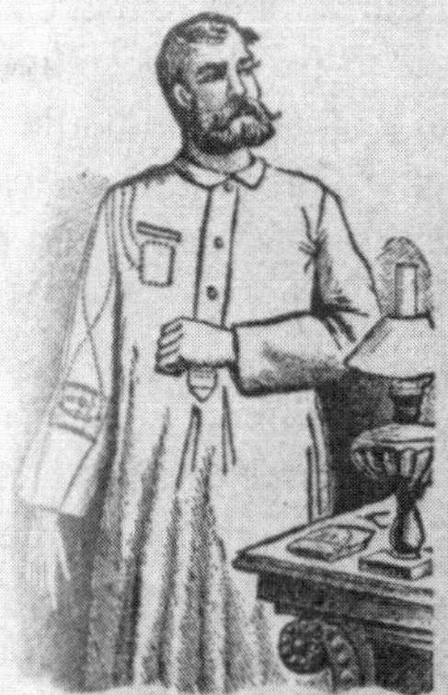

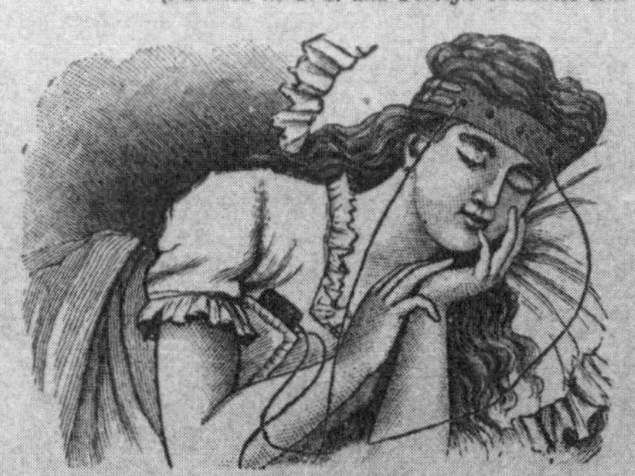

Battery in Pocket with conducting cables; Armature and Electrodes attached for use in all cases of Nervous or Sick Headache, Neuralgia, Dizziness, Insomnia, or Sleeplessness.

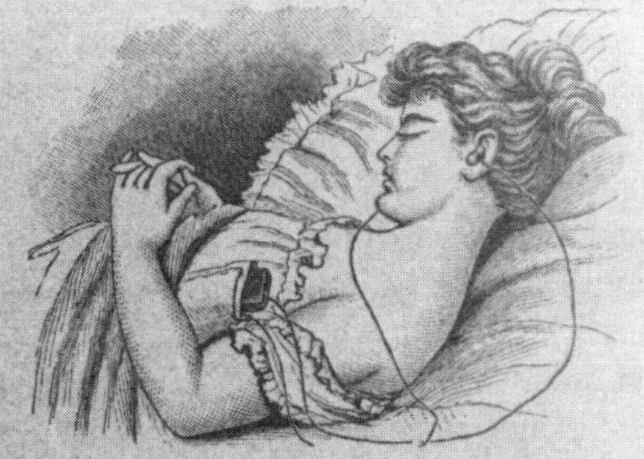

Battery in Pocket with conducting cables and Adjustable Ear Nasal Electrodes, for use day or night, in all cases of Deafness, Catarrh, and Catarrhal Deafness.

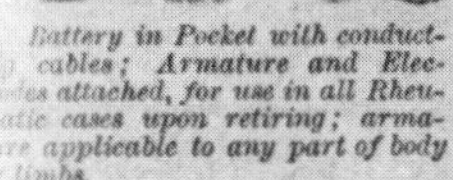

Battery in Pocket with conducting cables; Armature and Electrodes attached, for use in all Rheumatic cases upon retiring; armature applicable to any part of body or limbs.

ARE you afflicted with either Partial or Total Deafness, or Catarrh, or Catarrhal Deafness, Rheumatism, Neuralgia, Lumbago, Gout, Nervous Debility, or any other Disease, from any cause or of any Length or Standing?

If so, send your name and full Post-Office address for Illustrated Book containing **sworn statement** showing the positively permanent cures that have been effected **in cases pronounced incurable,** by means of **mild, pleasant, continuous currents of Electricity of Low Intensity and Long Duration** directly applied to the seat of the disease by any sufferer, allaying all inflammation, soothing the nerve centres, and producing healthy secretions by means of the **DR. HUBER ELECTRO-MAGNETIC DRY CELL POCKET MEDICAL BATTERY SUPPLIED WITH CONDUCTING CABLES. ARMATURES TO FIT ANY PART OF BODY OR LIMBS, AND ADJUSTABLE EAR AND NASAL ELECTRODES.** They can be worn in pocket day or night, but chiefly at night upon retiring, without the least inconvenience. Invariably produces sound, refreshing sleep. Duplicate cells always ready and sent prepaid by mail. No waste. No acids or disagreeable odors. Always ready for immediate use. A child can perfectly operate one. **The Battery and different Appliances can be used by all the members of an entire family for various ailments.** Their success has been so thoroughly established that perfect satisfaction is guaranteed in all cases. **Price, $7.50 to $13.50, according to Appliances needed.** Sent C. O. D. with privilege of full examination. Charges prepaid. **Trial of Batteries and Appliances and Electrodes in Office, FREE! In the Ladies' Department** of our business a thoroughly competent and experienced woman is always present to give instructions for use of all appliances.

Address THE DR. HUBER DRY CELL POCKET MEDICAL BATTERY CO.

(Please mention this paper.) **No. 88 Fifth Avenue** (3d door above 14th St.), New York City.

84. *National Library of Medicine.*

Some of the gadgets were, indeed, harmless. In *Medicine: An Illustrated History,* Albert S. Lyons and R. Joseph Petrocelli note that electromagnetic generators in hand-held cylindrical electrodes were "widely used . . . for relieving pain." Many devices, however, were unlikely to do more than relieve buyers of extra cash.

Around the turn of the twentieth century, Heracles Sanche ("The Discoverer of the Laws of Spontaneous Cure of Disease") marketed an invention he called the Electropoise. According to one of Sanche's ads, "The Electropoise supplies the needed electrical force to the system, and by its thermal action places the body in condition to absorb oxygen from the lungs." Sanche, who advertised this gizmo in *Cosmopolitan* magazine, charged 10 dollars for it.

According to the second volume of the American Medical Association book *Nostrums and Quackery,* published in 1921:

> The Electropoise was a metal cylinder . . . three and one half inches long and weighing about five ounces. The cylinder was sealed at both ends and to one end there was attached an uninsulated cord. At the free end . . . there was a small disc, which, by means of an elastic band and buckle could be fastened to the wrist and ankle. The Electropoise cylinder, when broken into, was found to be hollow and empty.

An enterprising self-promoter, Sanche sold another device called the Oxydonor, which he claimed "forced oxygen into the system." The Oxydonor looked impressive, exuding ozone and exhibiting a blue glow in a glass container. Powered by a small high-voltage generator, it was said to be beneficial for no fewer than 86 diseases. Declared worthless by the AMA, the invention sold for 35 dollars.

To the credulous, there was nothing an electrical spark at the right time and place couldn't do. Testimonials in the *Electro-Clinical Record* claimed that electricity cured writer's cramp, hay fever, cholera, and constipation—the latter yielding after a patient's third immersion in an electric bath.

Electric baths used very low currents to zap patients nearly submerged in water while they held electrodes attached to a battery; other electrodes connected the battery to the inside of a metal-plated bathtub. Even regular physicians made some use of electric baths as the nineteenth century gave way to the twentieth.

Most uses of electricity were employed by fringe doctors or nondoctors and could be used directly by the patient. Many were sold by mail order and were advertised as quick fixes and miracle cures. An AMA author in the first volume of *Nostrums and Quackery,* published in 1912, sneered, "The comparative ease with which the medical faker is able, by the most preposterous claims, to separate the trusting from their money indicates the enormous potentialities in advertising."

Would-be electronic wizards sought to turn that potential into kinetic profit. The makers of Addison's Galvanic Electric Belt—pieces of copper and zinc separated by blotting paper to generate a current and worn around the waist—marketed their product as "Nature's Vitalizer."

Handy electric belts that could be discreetly worn under coats, vests, and dresses were fast-moving items in the last years of the nineteenth century. Their popularity occasionally angered not only medical authorities but also rival health reformers such as Bernarr Macfadden, who pointed out that "purveyors of these belts usually charge you from 5 to 20 times the cost of their manufacture." Other critics made an even more telling point: Some of the so-called electric devices used no electricity.

Nolan's Famous Catarrh Cure, for example, consisted of what were purported to be electric pills—"50,000 volts of electricity in a two drachm bottle." The Galvano Necklace, used to treat goiter, was tested by the U.S. Post Office in 1930 and found to have no electrical current. It was banned from the mails that same year.

Still, the parade of products continued, outpacing authorities' attempts to keep up. These products followed a technological progression from hand-turned dynamos to wet batteries to dry cells and finally to plugs for wall sockets. Or, rather, those that generated actual electricity did.

AT THE PINNACLE WITH PULVERMACHER

Makers and marketers of electric gimcrackery for medical purposes came and went. Most were little-noticed, even in their own day. Pulvermacher's Galvanic Company was an exception. The Cadillac, as it were, of late nineteenth-century electric devices, Pulvermacher's sold products under the slogan "Electricity is Life." The corporate logo showed a globe,

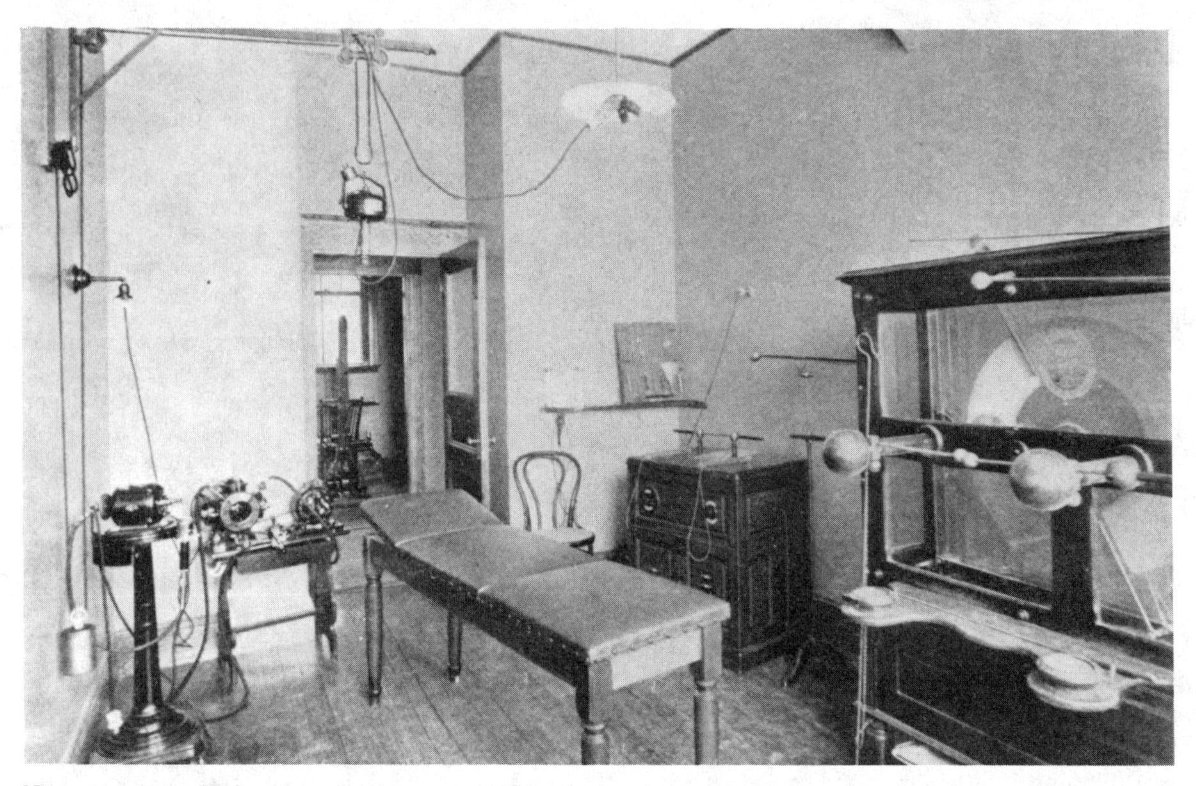

85. Awaiting the next patient in the electric room of the Adams Nervine Asylum, Boston (1904). *From* Twenty-seventh Annual Report of the Managers of the Adams Nervine Asylum, *Boston, 1904. National Library of Medicine.*

complete with flashes of electricity streaking toward a presumably grateful planet. Company promotional literature said that the firm operated in Great Britain, France, Prussia, Austria, Belgium, Canada, and the United States.

Pulvermacher's bore the name of a Professor J.L. Pulvermacher, who, as company literature had it, invented Electro-Galvanic Chains, which were made into belts and bands, in 1846. Pulvermacher was said to reside in London while the firm sold products described as "self-applicable for the cure of chronic diseases without medicine."

In the fashion of the day, Pulvermacher's did not hesitate to occupy the pinnacles of science, health, and marketing simultaneously. Declaring electricity to be "Nature's Chief Restorer," the company sniffed that "little reliance can be placed in medicine . . . it is generally of no avail." Electricity, on the other hand, was invaluable, "so near does it approach a panacea for the numerous Nervous and Chronic diseases to which mankind is liable."

Pulvermacher's broad belts and narrow bands provided "mild, continuous currents" that were said to be less of a shock to the system than brief, powerful jolts. Adjustable metallic devices that were worn on the outside of the body for 8 to 12 hours a day, the contraptions were immersed in a vinegar solution to generate a weak current. They buckled in front, like regular nonelectric belts; unlike regular belts, Pulvermacher's cost 20 dollars each.

The costly gadgets were supposedly effective for nearly everything. Dyspepsia was a snap to cure, since Pulvermacher's calmed the nerves of the stomach by regulating "abnormal electrical conditions." Kidney ailments, lumbago, deafness, and morphine habits were not a problem with Pulvermacher's. Neither were female complaints, given that the marvelous belts were, withal, "the greatest blessing ever vouchsafed to womankind."

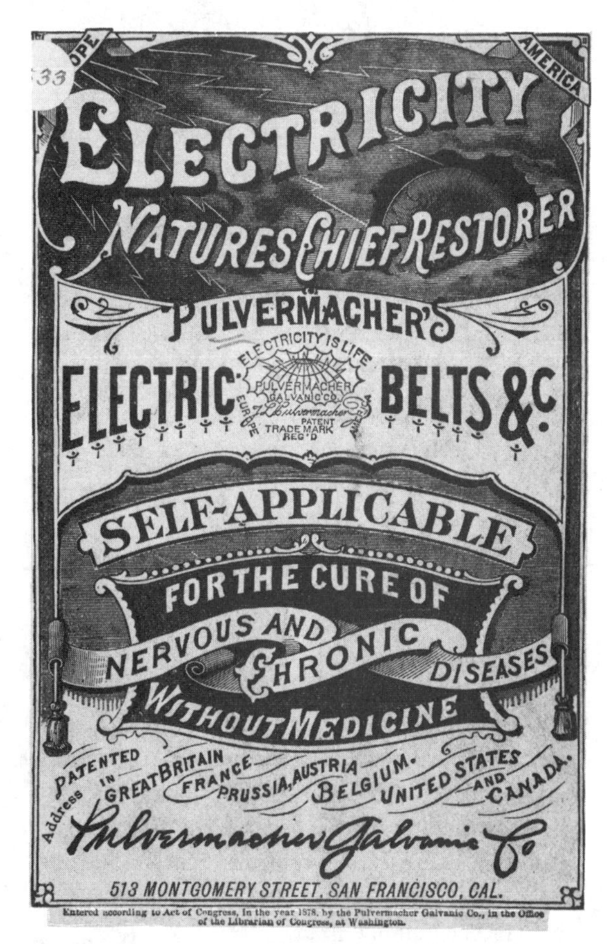

86. Late nineteenth-century Americans plugged into Pulvermacher's electric cures. *Courtesy, The Bancroft Library.*

To spread the good news, the firm mailed out free copies of its publication, the *Electric Review*. The curious were invited to come on down to "our Galvanic Establishment" at 513 Montgomery Street, San Francisco and see for themselves.

Although Pulvermacher's pushed the self-application of electricity, it was not loath to claim the endorsements of physicians and other mainstream authorities. Company literature quoted *Popular Science* as noting that Pulvermacher's belts produced "action so tender that a baby would not wince at it." The firm even cited *The Lancet*, Britain's leading medical journal, which wrote, "In these days of medico-galvanic quackery, it is a relief to observe the very plain and straightforward manner in which Pulvermacher's apparatus is recommended to the profession."

"THE SWITCHED-ON P.M."

Although one might think that novelties like electric baths went down the drain years ago, they haven't quite done so. The racy British tabloid newspapers had a field day in 1989 with a report that then Prime Minister Margaret Thatcher took electrically charged baths as part of a health and beauty regimen that also included mud baths and herbs. The baths were said to be charged with 0.3 amps of electricity.

"The Switched-On Prime Minister's Amazing Secret" and "Shock Revelation on the Source of Mrs. T's Vigor" were two headlines on news reports of the buzzing baths, broken as a scooplet in *Vanity Fair* magazine. Thatcher declined to comment.

"THE DEAN OF TWENTIETH CENTURY CHARLATANS"

While their versatility and efficacy were certainly oversold, Pulvermacher's products were probably not directly harmful. (Indirectly, they may have been, by encouraging the sick to avoid medical attention.) For sheer audacity, though, Pulvermacher's was surpassed by Albert Abrams, an American physician who might have given even the flamboyant Franz Mesmer a run for his money.

Born in San Francisco in 1863, Abrams took his medical degree at Germany's respected University of Heidelberg in 1882 at age 19. He earned another degree at Cooper Medical College (later absorbed by Stanford University Medical School), where he became a professor of pathology. Abrams was elected vice president of the California Medical Society. He also authored well-received medical textbooks and won a reputation as a gentleman of letters. His 1900 memoir, *Scattered Leaves of a Physician's Diary,* includes a photograph of Abrams, a handsome, bearded man of 37, and brief sketches such as "My First Patient."

The literature on Abrams does not establish why the successful physician gave up his quiet professional life to break with standard medicine; a midlife crisis is the best explanation anyone has come up with about Abrams, who was twice a widower. In any case, break with standard medicine he certainly did.

His 1909 book *Spinal Therapeutics* placed the cause (and cure) of disease in the spine, a thesis that won Abrams a following among struggling osteopaths and chiropractors. In 1910, in his next book, *Spondylotherapy,* Abrams argued that stimulating centers of the spine with percussive touch was the key to good health. Abrams wrote: "Every organ has governing nerve centers in the spinal cord which when stimulated by manipulation of the vertebrae can be made to contract or dilate."

Abrams's winding road took a hairpin turn into electronic medicine a few years later when he invented a diagnostic machine called a dynamizer. A Rube Goldberg device if ever there was one, Abrams's dynamizer was designed to demonstrate his belief that every disease has a signature electronic vibration that could be measured. After putting drops of a patient's blood—first treated with a horseshoe magnet to cleanse it of untoward electronic squiggles—onto blotting paper, Abrams put the paper into the dynamizer.

Then things really got weird. A wire issuing from the machine was connected to the forehead of a second, healthy person (the "subject" or "reagent"), who stood on grounded metal plates. The reagent was stripped to the waist, facing west in dim light. As the machine passed the vibrational frequency of the patient's blood to the healthy reagent, Abrams or his surrogate tapped the reagent's abdomen. When they felt a dull area, it served to pinpoint the location of disease in the patient. The vibrational reading was known as the Electronic Reactions of Abrams, or

MANHOOD RESTORED

One of the chief uses to which self-applied electrical gadgets were put was restoring that vital spark of what contemporary accounts referred to as "lost manhood."

Pulvermacher's Galvanic Company was a leader in providing said spark, the loss of which company promotional literature attributed to masturbation, "the greatest outrage on Nature's sexual ordinances man can possibly perpetrate." Self-abuse, as Pulvermacher's saw it, was always visible, "especially those black and blue discolorations under the eyes . . . on faces by the millions." Pulvermacher's felt obliged to point out that "the male excretion embodies FORTY TIMES more vital force than an equal amount of red blood right from the heart."

The key to restored manhood was obvious: Pulvermacher's own products. The company approvingly quoted an unnamed writer who asserted that "in severe cases, one of Pulvermacher's Electro-Galvanic Belts should be worn for an hour or two daily round the hips and under each testicle."

Did the belts work? Eager testimonials said they did. Wrote G.W.T., from Virginia City, Nevada:

> I have worn the Belt and Suspensory for six weeks, and every symptom of the disease is gone. The night losses stopped altogether two weeks after putting the appliance on, and the old vigor has returned. I feel better in health and spirits; and can do a good man's work in the mines without fatigue. I was troubled for many years, and got medicines from half a dozen doctors in 'Frisco that did me no good. Several of the boys here were in my fix, and got cured by your belt and Suspensory.

E.R.A. for short. This convoluted procedure confirmed Abrams's departure from orthodox medicine to somewhere beyond the fringe.

But he wasn't done yet. After he perfected the dynamizer to diagnose disease, the erstwhile establishment doctor developed another electrical machine, called the oscilloclast. Abrams used the gadget, a boxlike device with electrodes that were placed on the patient's body, to duplicate—and thus neutralize—the signature vibrations of disease. He leased the machines to "electronic practitioners" and advertised heavily, thereby violating yet another mainstream canon.

In addition to enthusiasts among osteopaths and chiropractors, Abrams attracted support from the muckraking novelist Upton Sinclair, the poet George Sterling, and *Pearson's* magazine. At the peak of Abrams's popularity just after World War I, a San Francisco judge accepted electronic vibrational data as evidence in a paternity suit. Abrams established societies, journals, and a dozen schools to boost his theories. Sinclair served on the board of directors at one of Abrams's schools.

When Prohibition hit home, Abrams was ready. His gadgets could duplicate the vibrational frequency of alcohol, to produce an electric "jag." Abrams's latest fancy caused a San Francisco newspaper to break into verse one day in 1920: "Hail the Ohm cocktail! The highball hilarious—Turn on the switches, and fill me with jolts!"

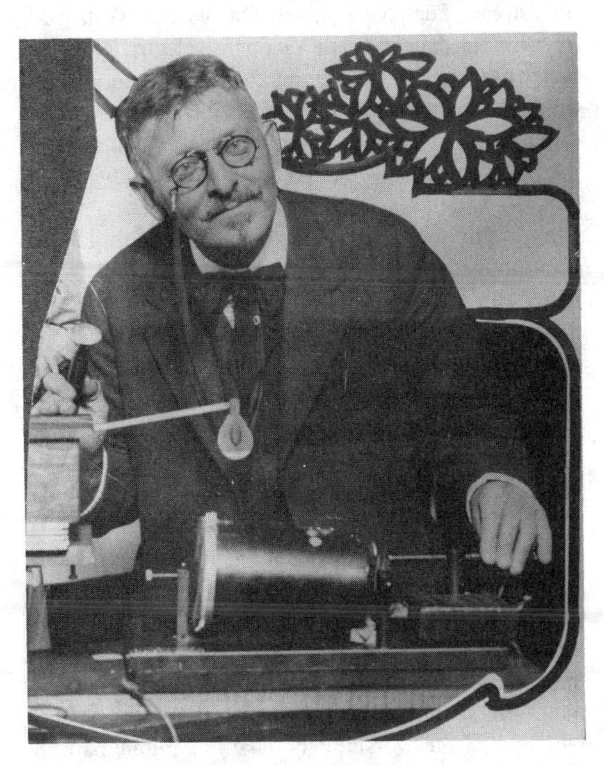

87. The AMA called Dr. Albert Abrams the "dean of twentieth century charlatans." *San Francisco Public Library.*

But a backlash wasn't long in coming. Abrams was attacked by the AMA, which concluded that he "easily ranked as the dean of twentieth century charlatans." Other skeptics also challenged Abrams and his followers. One prankster took chicken blood represented as human to an Abrams acolyte and, reported the AMA, "The Abramsite diagnosed the case as general cancer and tuberculosis of the genital-urinary tract."

Scientific scrutiny cast doubt on Abrams's bold claims. One investigator failed to detect any electric current passing from the oscilloclast to the patient. In 1923, R.A. Millikan, a Nobel Prize-winning physicist at the California Institute of Technology, concluded that Abrams's inventions "did not rest upon any scientific foundation whatever."

Scientific American magazine was conducting an intense, year-long investigation of Abrams when the doctor fell ill. On January 13, 1924, Abrams died at the age of 60 in his posh San Francisco home. The cause of death was pneumonia, one of the diseases that the oscilloclast was used to treat. Abrams passed away just two days before he was scheduled to testify in an Arkansas courtroom, where another Abramsite had made a diagnosis from chicken blood.

Abrams's front-page obituary in the *San Francisco Examiner* noted that "worry over attacks launched on his theories in all parts of the civilized world by the medical profession led to a breakdown in his health three months ago." The disgraced doctor left an estate valued at two to five million dollars. His money was earmarked for a school of electronic medicine, but relatives contested the will and the school never opened.

Eight months after Abrams's death, the *Scientific American* investigation was made public. The report, by a team of physicians and physicists, was scathing. According to the *New York Times,* the investigating committee noted that:

> Thousands of doctors and near-doctors have entered the electronic fold. They have gone about their work of diagnosing and treating that part of the public which seeks something new, in medicine, as well as in clothes and in automobiles.
>
> Many a small manufacturer has found a profitable field in turning out all manner of pseudo-radio devices called electronic diagnosis and treatment apparatus. And all of this actually

comes right down to the so-called electronic reactions to Abrams, which according to this committee, do not exist.

The newspaper of record itself was scarcely more charitable. A 1924 *Times* editorial commented acidly:

> Of all this country's many medical quacks and charlatans, he showed the most cynical confidence in the amount of credulity, of gullibility, characterizing a considerable fraction of its inhabitants, and for the exploitation of that fraction he devised a scheme of magnificent absurdity.

Noting that Abrams had cited the testimonials of apparently satisfied patients, the *Times* observed: "Every charlatan has his triumph; it is to be regretted that his victims cannot be buried in a special graveyard, where they could be counted."

Even these denunciations didn't end Abrams's influence right away. In the early 1960s the Food and Drug Administration seized a device called the Electro-Metabograph that was described as "patterned on the radionic theories" of Abrams. The gadget was used to "realign" the vibrations given off by diseased organs. The FDA sent the device to the National Museum of Medical Quackery in St. Louis.

SHORT CIRCUITS . . .

The novelty of electricity took several generations to wear off, but eventually it did. With the widespread introduction of radio and household appliances, electricity no longer seemed as miraculous. Moreover, electronic medicine was surpassed by other technological miracles, especially penicillin and other antibiotic drugs.

The federal government, which had long left the enterprising makers and sellers of electric medical devices virtually untouched, took a closer look. In 1938 the FDA began to regulate medical devices, although, notes the magazine *FDA Consumer,* the agency "had to prove that the product was fraudulent or unsafe. There was no way to keep unsafe or ineffective medical devices from reaching the market."

That is no longer true, at least on paper. In 1976, the Medical Device Amendments to the Food, Drug and Cosmetic Act placed the burden of proof on the manufacturer.

. . . AND POWER SURGES

It would be much more difficult for an Albert Abrams to thrive in the late twentieth century than it was in the early twentieth century. With the decline of the most blatant frauds, the legitimate uses of electricity in medicine have surged, especially with the discovery that, in one sense, the old hustlers were right: The human body houses detectable electrical "wiring."

Some of the most common medical instruments, such as the EKG (electrocardiogram), developed in the early twentieth century to measure the electrical activity of the heart, and the EEG (electroencephalogram), used to monitor the brain, tune into the body's circuitry.

That is not to say that all controversy over electricity in health care has ceased. There is a continuing battle over ECT (electroconvulsive therapy, better known as shock treatment). ECT patients are given general anesthesia, oxygen, and muscle paralyzers, and then juiced with 75 to 150 volts; a typical course is 6 to 12 treatments a month. Developed in 1938 by Italian psychiatrist Ugo Corletti, ECT's defenders promote it as an effective treatment for depression; detractors say it causes brain damage and memory loss.

Modern electric devices are used by doctors—usually not, as in the past, by patients themselves—to treat a surprising range of maladies. Orthopedists use currents of electricity to help bone to heal. In the early 1990s, studies of women wearing electric coils on their wrists to increase bone mass and prevent osteoporosis were underway. At the same time, a mainstream Pennsylvania hospital used a Tesla coil to surround patients with "halos of electricity," the better to stimulate endorphins to control pain. Superficially, such uses resemble the cruder approaches of a hundred years ago, although modern practitioners might reject any comparison with the plugged-in quacks of the past.

As for the quacks, they are nearly forgotten. Well-known though Pulvermacher's Galvanic Company may have been in its prime, the firm blew a fuse long ago in its showplace San Francisco "Galvanic Establishment." A visit to 513 Montgomery Street in 1990 revealed a site smothered by a high-rise building that housed law firms and banks.

Most traces of Albert Abrams have similarly vanished. His medical societies, journals, and schools are all gone. The house at 2151 Sacramento Street where Abrams died still stands, but Abrams is not visibly commemorated there. A charming, two-story private residence flanked by stolid apartments, the vintage 1881 building is marked with a brass plaque that commemorates the sojourn of a more famous man, Sir Arthur Conan Doyle. Across the street, where oiled sun-worshippers bake in a public park in 90-degree heat, the only electrical devices in sight are portable radios.

CHAPTER
· 20 ·

DIVINE HEALING: YA GOTTA BELIEVE

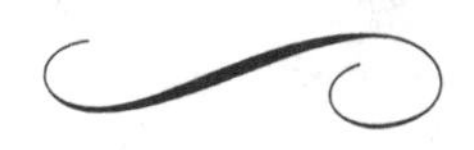

Oh, you who are down in the Shadowland of sickness and despair—whatever your hurt, whatever your need, there is health in His wings for you.

AIMEE SEMPLE McPHERSON, 1925

On a May afternoon in 1926, a dark-haired woman dove into the Pacific off Ocean Park Beach in Los Angeles. A strong swimmer, she had relaxed in the surf many times before and returned to her work refreshed and revived. This day turned out to be different. According to the woman's secretary, a nonswimmer who was watching from the shore, her boss swam out to the breakers and seemed to vanish beneath the waves.

One month later, the missing woman's mother received a ransom note demanding a half million dollars for her daughter's safe return. Stuffed in the envelope was a lock of what appeared to be her daughter's hair. Presumed drowned, the young woman was, in fact, alive. The next morning, the harried mother was awakened by a telephone call from her daughter, who said she was in Douglas, Arizona. She had been kidnapped and tortured, she said, and held prisoner in a shack in Mexico. While her abductors were out, she had managed to escape.

A skeptical press questioned the story. There were rumors that the victim had made up the whole thing, that she had actually run off with a gentleman friend to Carmel, an oceanside resort on the central California coast. Long after the heavily publicized investigation closed, the celebrated subject, Aimee Semple McPherson, founder and head of the International Church of the Foursquare Gospel in Los Angeles, insisted that she was telling the truth. The mysterious kidnappers were never found.

That summer of 1926, Sister Aimee was easily the most famous evangelist in America. Thousands packed into her church, waiting to get a glimpse of the woman who many believed had been resurrected from the dead. The press had a field day. "Every factor that goes to make up a motion picture thriller was to be found in the disappearance and resurrection of the pastor of Angelus Temple," wrote the San Francisco *Argonaut*. "Had Douglas Fairbanks, that athletic marvel of the screen, known the whereabouts of the shack, he would have crossed the desert in a few bounds, put the kidnappers to rout with a few well-directed blows, and in a few more leaps, have carried the evangelist back to civilization, that is, Hollywood."

Aimee Semple McPherson was not the first evangelist in America to gain celebrity status, nor would she be the last. Since the late nineteenth century, a stream of spiritual pitchmen and -women, most less flamboyant and glamorous than Sister Aimee, have mesmerized crowds with promises of a life free of

worry, pain, and disease. They call themselves "divine healers," conduits of the healing powers of God. "I am not a healer," said McPherson. "Jesus is the healer. I am only the office girl who opens the door and says 'come in.' "

"PREACH THE GOSPEL AND HEAL THE SICK"

In the years following the Civil War, a small but growing number of Protestants in Europe and the United States became interested in spiritual healing, setting up "faith homes" and "healing homes" (hospitals) where prayer was considered as important as medicine and surgery. By the late 1880s, more than 30 such healing homes were in operation in America.

Among American Protestants, this renewed interest in the power of prayer caught fire first among members of the Holiness Church, precursors of the twentieth-century Pentecostals.

One of the earliest nineteenth-century Holiness healers was a man named G.O. Barnes, who "received the call" in 1876 after hooking up with the evangelist D.L. Moody. Preaching in the hills of Kentucky, Barnes quickly earned a reputation for miracle cures, although initially he was concerned only with saving souls. Using a variety of methods, Barnes anointed the sick, answered requests for prayers through the mail, and visited patients who were too sick to travel. Barnes taught that not only disease, but medicine and herbs, were the work of the devil. "Avoid the medical profession," he warned his patients. "Just trust in the Lord."

Divine healing has a long, entrenched history in Christianity. "The faithful have believed that God provided physical as well as spiritual healing throughout most of Christian history," writes religion scholar David Edwin Harrell, Jr., author of a major biography of Oral Roberts, numerous articles on divine healing, and *All Things Are Possible,* the leading study of the post-World War II healing and charismatic revivals in America. "Few Christian rituals have a more legitimate ancestry than prayer for the sick."

It was the early Pentecostals at the turn of the twentieth century who thumbed through their Bibles and found evidence for the "gifts of the Spirit," including the "gift of tongues" (glossolalia) and the "gift of healing." An ex-slave named William Joseph Seymour brought Pentecostal teachings into the international spotlight out of his Asuza Street church in Los Angeles. Out of this movement came the traveling evangelists, whose down-home religion pulled many an ailing soul into the gospel tents. Although soul-saving was as important as curing the sick, it was the healing miracles that caught the public's imagination and brought the evangelists both converts and publicity.

According to Pentecostal theory, divine healing is possible through a variety of methods, all of which were practiced by Jesus at one time or another: by touch (the laying on of hands); by command ("Demons, out!"); by releasing the patient's sins; by praying from a distance; by anointing the patient with oil; through "prayer handkerchiefs" or other objects; or through good, old-fashioned praying in person. The devil evidently plays a leading role in sickness. As Robert Maples Anderson explains in his *Vision of the Disinherited,* "healing and 'casting out demons' were almost synonymous terms." Thus healing prayers often include a command, as, for example, to "the cancer demon" to "come out in the name of Jesus."

For most Americans, even those who have considered themselves religious or spiritual but have never been drawn to the likes of Aimee Semple McPherson or Oral Roberts, divine healing has remained a mystery, something quite alien to their own experience. Conjuring up images of Holy Rollers, fire-and-brimstone, Elmer Gantry-type figures preaching to ignorant rural folk, they have looked skeptically at the crowds packed into tents and auditoriums, who appear to be worshipping the evangelist on stage as much as God.

This image is understandable. For much like that very American institution the Hollywood star, many divine healers have won celebrity status from a public that has hungrily devoured news about their successes and failures and granted them whole chapters in American folklore. Even cynics have heard of Sister Aimee, whose name appeared in the popular press of the 1920s as often as that of any movie star. "Her fabulous evangelistic career put Hallelujah in the headlines," read her 1944 *San Francisco Chronicle* obituary. Whether packing them into auditoriums or the tents that became their trademark, these legendary men and women, whose own lives have often been unhealthy and short, have been masterful at convincing their audiences that miracles are indeed possible.

JOHN ALEXANDER DOWIE AND THE CITY OF ZION

In December 1906, Chicago-based healing revivalist John Alexander Dowie was laughed off the stage of Madison Square Garden. It seems that the New York City public found the man who proclaimed himself a

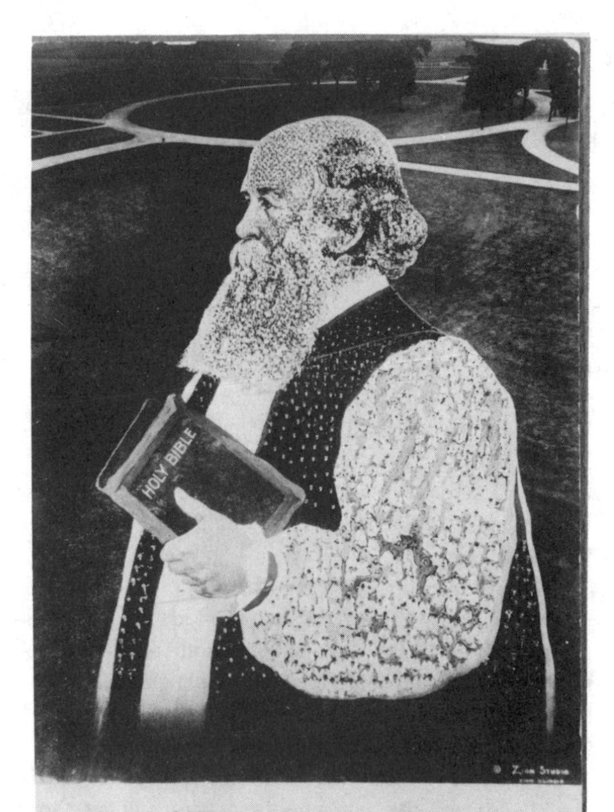

Living Picture of JOHN ALEXANDER DOWIE, Founder of Zion, Illinois. Made on Temple Site, of 3000 persons, July 14, 1921, the 21st anniversary of the Consecration of the Temple Site and land of the City of Zion.

88. *Photo by Mole and Thomas. ICHI-16310. Chicago Historical Society.*

reincarnation of the prophet Elijah to be more ludicrous than inspiring.

That Sunday afternoon's revival meeting at the Garden had promised to be uplifting and dramatic, for Dowie's reputation as a powerful speaker and spiritual leader had followed him east. At first the New York City crowd was not disappointed. Wrote *Harper's Weekly*:

> The chief musician of Zion, an accomplished artist, took his place at the key-board of a great organ that had been especially built in the Garden for the occasion, and presently there rolled out over the congregation and reverberated among the arches the strains of a noble old hymn. Now the surpliced choir of Zion appeared, chanting the hymn as it moved in solemn procession . . . . Dowie had grouped scores of little children at the head of the choir. Very slowly and reverently they marched, all clad in long white robes and black stoles . . . . Last of all marched Dowie, clad in the robes of a bishop, the big white balloon-sleeves swaying and rising as he walked. Beside him his wife, a gentle, beautiful woman of middle age with sad eyes, she, too, wearing a bishop's robes; then the son of these two, Gladstone Dowie, far heralded as the Great Unkissed. He was arrayed in the purple of an archbishop.

All went well until the end of the hymn. Then Dowie, clutching a large Bible, ascended the pulpit and began to speak. As the crowd strained forward, one could feel a ripple of disappointment through the great hall. They were not prepared for the high rasping voice that scolded and bullied them. Quickly and quietly they got up from their seats and left. "Sit down!" screamed Dowie. "You shall not go out!" The next day the press was calling him "Old Doctor Dowie" and predicting his demise.

It was an ironic response to a man who is considered the first nationally known divine-healing celebrity. Born in Scotland and raised in Australia, Dowie landed in San Francisco in 1888 after a short stint as a healer in his boyhood home. By the time he reached the United States, his reputation as a healer had spread. Making his way to Chicago, Dowie immediately leased three hotels and turned them into faith-cure homes, where he ministered to the sick and dying. He taught his patients to disregard "devil-worshipping" physicians and their medications and blamed failures to cure on his patients' lack of faith. Lack of faith or no, several of his patients died, causing the city authorities to investigate and charge him with manslaughter and practicing medicine without a license. When the higher courts decided in his favor, declaring the city ordinances unconstitutional, Dowie made legal history.

By the turn of the twentieth century, Dowie was attracting thousands of supporters and gaining a national reputation, the first of the healing revivalists to do so. He started his own church, the Christian Catholic Church of Zion, proclaimed himself the reincarnation of Elijah, and bought 6,000 acres of land between Chicago and Milwaukee. There he organized a utopian community he called the City of Zion.

In only two years over 10 thousand congregants were living in Zion, where the prophet ruled his flock with an iron hand. Like most healing revivalists that followed him, Dowie spread the word through his own magazine; this was called *Leaves of Healing*. Still condemning doctors and medicine, he lectured on "Doctors, Drugs and Devils; or the Foes of Christ the Healer."

Yet all was not utopian in Zion. By 1906, when his unsuccessful New York City campaign cost Dowie

500 thousand dollars, he was already in trouble for financial mismanagement, whispers of vaguely defined sexual misconduct, and a taste for worldly luxuries that turned away even his most loyal followers. Within a year he had suffered a stroke and Zion was declared bankrupt. Bedridden, alienated from his family, and ridiculed by the press, Dowie died in March 1907, a mere three months after his New York City debacle.

Despite his setbacks, John Alexander Dowie fixed healing revivalism in the eye of the American public. By the 1920s, while their contemporaries were bobbing their hair and chugging down bootleg whiskey, a growing number of Americans—mostly rural whites in the South and Midwest, urban blacks and Hispanics, recent immigrants to big cities, the poor and disheartened, and those forgotten by the Silent Generation—were discovering the healing crusades. They found the visiting Englishman Smith Wigglesworth, who prayed for audiences of thousands; F.F. Bosworth, who grew up in Alexander Dowie's City of Zion and pioneered radio evangelism out of Dallas; Charles Price, an English Oxford-educated lawyer-turned-evangelist; and Mrs. M.B. Woodworth-Etter, whose Indianapolis tabernacle drew thousands of believers from across the country. And they found the Canadian-born Aimee Semple McPherson in Los Angeles, offering entertainment and controversy not even Hollywood could surpass.

SISTER AIMEE: THE LADY IN WHITE

As the founder and head of Angelus Temple and her own sect, the International Church of the Foursquare Gospel, Aimee Semple McPherson had come a long way since her girlhood days on a farm outside Ingersoll, Ontario, where she was born in 1890. There her mother, Minnie Kennedy, a Salvation Army worker, reared Aimee on Bible stories and the Salvation Army drums and tambourines. Young Aimee, according to her major biographer, Lately Thomas, was a headstrong, extroverted girl who excelled at sports and preferred playing with farm animals to dolls.

Aimee Kennedy questioned everything and everybody—the evolutionary theory she was taught in school, her parents' religious beliefs, and the strict moral code by which she was raised. She was constantly exploring, searching, and even testing the waters of worldliness by reading novels, going to the movies, and dancing.

Then she discovered religion, not her mother's Salvation Army brand, but the Pentecostals' baptism of the Holy Spirit. Through the Pentecostals she also met her future husband, a tall, dynamic preacher named Robert Semple. It was Robert Semple who introduced the 17-year-old Aimee to the world outside rural Canada, when, as a newlywed, he took her to China, where he worked as a missionary. He also gave Aimee her first lessons in "taking the Lord as my Great Physician."

Aimee's sojourn in the Far East was to be short-lived, however. A little over a year later Semple died of what appears to have been malaria, leaving Aimee alone with their newborn girl, Roberta, whom Aimee named after her late husband. Destitute and depressed, Aimee sailed for the United States. Eventually young Aimee remarried, this time to a wholesale grocery clerk named Harold Simpson McPherson from Providence, Rhode Island. The couple had a son, Rolf.

Ever the restless spirit, Aimee soon set out on a full-time healing career. Packing the kids off to Canada to stay with her ever-patient mother—it would not be the last time Minnie Kennedy played Nanny—Aimee happily barnstormed up and down the East Coast of the United States, leaving a crumbling marriage behind. Aimee thrived on the gypsy life and quickly learned the fine art of preaching under the big top. Writes Thomas: "She was her own advance agent, business manager, and star of the show."

Soon she was the proud owner of a gospel car, an automobile painted with the slogan "Jesus Is Coming Soon—Make Ready." She scoffed at those who told her that preaching was no work for a woman, especially a mother of two: "Oh, don't you ever tell me that a woman can not be called to preach the Gospel!"

In October 1918, Aimee, her children, and Minnie, along with an entourage of volunteers, climbed into the gospel car and headed for southern California. With Aimee driving all the way, they arrived in Los Angeles just before Christmas. Within a week, the 29-year-old Aimee was conducting her first revival meeting under the auspices of the Assemblies of God. Shortly thereafter, her new converts presented her with a two-story bungalow.

By the early 1920s, Aimee Semple McPherson was known far beyond the City of Angels. Her healing sessions brought her international followers and publicity. In Denver; St. Louis and neighboring Alton, Illinois; Dayton, Ohio; Washington; Montreal; and San Diego, where she took over the city's Balboa Park, the deaf, blind, arthritic, and terminally ill crammed into her tent to hear "Sister McPherson." Known as "the lady in white," she wore an outfit resembling a nurse's, all white with a military cape, a preview of the many costumes she

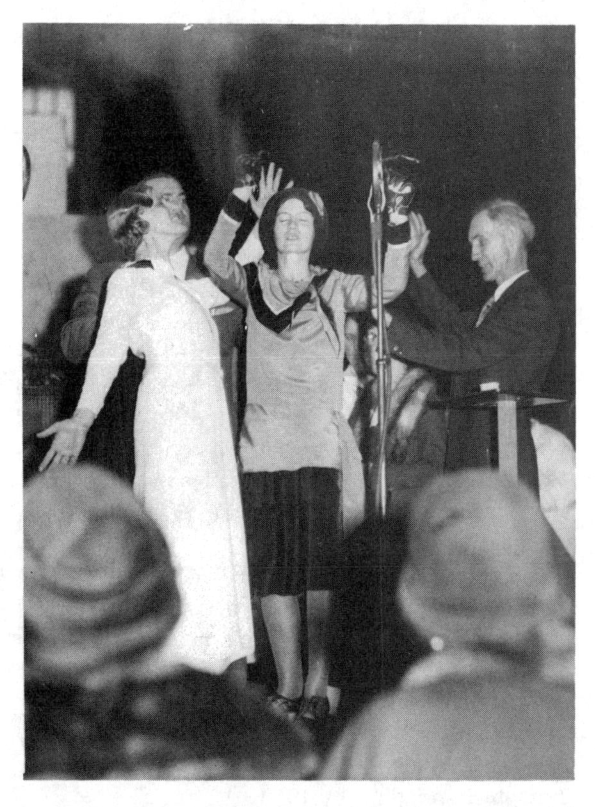

89. Aimee Semple McPherson, left, took her miracles on the road (Boston, 1931). *International Newsreel/The Bettmann Archive.*

would don for her "illustrated sermons" at Angelus Temple throughout the 1920s. One of the few women to reach celebrity status in the gospel world, Aimee Semple McPherson became the archetypal female evangelist for Americans of her day.

Angelus Temple was completed in 1923. It was McPherson's dream of an evangelistic center in the West. Built on Glendale Boulevard across from Oak Park, north of downtown Los Angeles, it was largely financed by her thousands of followers across the country, who also built Aimee and her family a mansion next door.

In the 1930s, a brochure issued by Foursquare Publications, the church's publishing arm, described Angelus Temple as "the church with the big heart." Written in the style of a travelogue, the pamphlet took the reader on a guided tour of the temple that seated 5,300 and included two balconies, a concrete dome, a Prayer Tower, and a baptismal pool with a painted backdrop of the Jordan River: "Entering the Temple through any of the 25 doors one is pleased with the soft tones in design of fixtures . . . . From the lighthouse and boat in the lower main foyer to the quiet dignified Council Chambers and the busy offices of the Church Secretary and City Sisters surrounding it, one is impressed by the atmosphere of serenity." The brochure went on to list the 57 departments of the church, including the publications department, radio station KFSG (Kall Foursquare Gospel), a Bible college and a nursery, four choirs, the Angelus Temple Symphony Orchestra, the Great McPherson String Ensemble, three bands, and a children's orchestra.

Aimee's taste for innovation and nonconformity brought her both praise and ridicule from her own church members as well as outsiders. Her 1926 disappearance tarnished her reputation among church leaders, who cringed at rumors that Aimee had concocted it to run away with her handsome KFSG radio engineer.

A year after that scandal, Angelus Temple's former band and choir leader criticized his ex-boss for bowing to fashion by bobbing her hair, charging the temple leader with "worldliness." Many of the organized churches looked down their noses at the "lady evangelist" and her theatrical sermons, labeling her a fraud and a menace. The secular Los

"THE ALMIGHTY OCCUPIES A SECOND POSITION"

Over the great lower floor and two balconies attendants are hurrying to seat the mob, a full hour before the entrance of the star. Men and women stand against the wall, they sit upon the steps of the aisles, and still, when the final whistle blows, there are thousands turned away, thousands who stand for two, three, four hours on the street and in the nearby park, to listen to the concert and the inspired utterances as they scream themselves forth from the loud speaker outside the building. . . . An hour of orchestral music, then the singers file in, from fifty to a hundred of them, ranging themselves in a loft over the speaker's platform. Their costumes, for this particular evening of nautical entertainment, are in sailor effect, navy and white, jaunty caps atilt. When at length the leading lady enters in the role of rear admiral, she is gallant in a swinging cape over a white uniform, her red-gold coils surmounted by an all-but-official cap . . . . Aimee Semple McPherson's power lies in the remarkable combination of showman and actress in her gifts which attracts and holds the multitude.

Harper's magazine
December 1927

Angeles press put her in the headlines an average of three times a week, but gave her mixed reviews.

By the late 1930s, a scandal-weary McPherson was suffering from nervous exhaustion, a common ailment among divine healers, who frequently neglected their own health. Her short-lived third marriage to a singing instructor named David Hutton made the gossip columnists sit up again, but the press soon turned to more urgent matters through most of the decade. The Depression saw a lull in healing revivalism and many divine healers had to pack up their tents forever. It was a time when "hobo evangelists" rode the rails and roamed the countryside, preaching to a dwindling audience.

But Aimee Semple McPherson held on, expanding her influence even as her health was deteriorating. By the early 1940s her International Church of the Foursquare Gospel had grown to include over 400 churches in the United States and 200 missionary stations abroad. The *San Francisco Examiner* referred to her as "the world's acknowledged mistress of hallelujah revivalism."

Had she lived to a ripe old age, Sister McPherson might have added a colorful touch to the healing revival of the post-World War II years. But that was not to be. On September 28, 1944, three days after she arrived in Oakland, California to begin a four-day revival campaign, the 53-year-old queen of divine healing was found dead in her hotel room. According to the coroner's report, she died from "shock and respiratory failure from an accidental overdose of barbital compound." More than 20 thousand people attended her funeral. Under the terms of her will, her 31-year-old son, Rolf McPherson, became head of Angelus Temple.

ORAL ROBERTS: "PRAY FOR THE SICK AND CAST OUT DEMONS"

After the earthly travails of World War II, Americans were ready, once again, to lift their eyes heavenward. Some sought out Kentucky-born "Brother Bill" Branham, who claimed to have raised a man from the dead. But the best known of the postwar healing mavericks was Granville Oral Roberts, whose paternal grandfather was among the first whites to settle in what was then called Indian Territory (present-day Oklahoma). Born in 1918 into a deeply religious Pentecostal family, the fifth son of Ellis and Claudius Roberts grew up believing that divine healing was a given.

As a youngster, Oral—known by his middle name—was given to bouts of restlessness and self-consciousness that were not helped by a serious stuttering problem. Oral developed a passion for basketball and baseball and dreamed of a career as a professional athlete. When he was in high school the preacher's son left home to play basketball on his favorite coach's team.

Young Oral's life took a dramatic turn when he collapsed in the middle of a basketball tournament in 1935. Diagnosed with tuberculosis, he returned home an invalid. Given his family's religious bent, it was perhaps inevitable that he would find his way to a revival meeting, where he claims to have been healed of his sickness. Roberts studied for the ministry and worked in a series of small Pentecostal Holiness churches. By 1947 he was out on his own, an itinerant preacher who "prayed for the sick and cast out demons."

Roberts found receptive audiences wherever he traveled. He proved to be an eloquent speaker and was widely regarded as a natural healer. In his first healing success, he claimed to cure a youngster of polio. Soon he was publishing his own magazine, called *Healing Waters,* and writing his first book, *If You Need Healing—Do These Things,* which went through six printings by 1950.

Like many evangelists, Roberts used the "healing-line" technique. As the sick and disabled filed past, Roberts touched the afflicted with his right

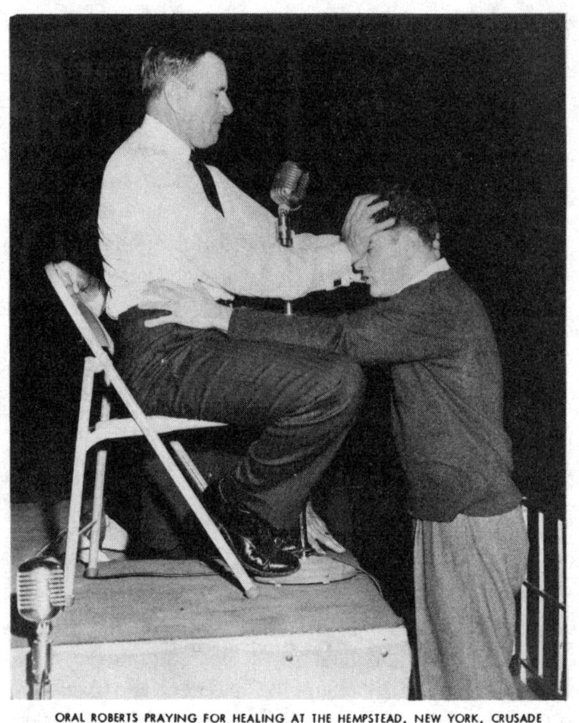

ORAL ROBERTS PRAYING FOR HEALING AT THE HEMPSTEAD, NEW YORK, CRUSADE

90. *The Bettmann Archive.*

hand. (Evidently, the left hand did not work.) His healing crusades, some lasting nearly three weeks, took him through much of the South and Southwest.

By the 1950s, Roberts headed a successful, tightly managed organization. In 1952 alone, a reported 1.5 million attended his tent campaigns. That same year Roberts prayed for 66 thousand people in his healing lines and was heard on 85 radio stations across the United States. In 1954, he began broadcasting over nine television stations, one of the earliest of the healers to use the new medium. By the late 1950s the former invalid from Oklahoma was the most successful healing revivalist in America.

BEWARE OF FALSE PROPHETS

Those outside the revival tents did not take too kindly to the more flamboyant evangelists. Among the leading critics were mainstream Christian churches and medical doctors.

In 1962, the United Lutheran Church in America appointed a committee of doctors and ministers to study divine healing. As reported in *Time,* that committee "warned the church's 2,500,000 members to beware of faith healers." The Lutherans were not alone, nor was it the first time mainstream churches had spoken out against faith healers. The *Christian Century* had labeled Oral Roberts a "Ringling press agent" in 1955, while the National Council of Churches challenged him to provide evidence that miracles had actually occurred at his revivals.

Orthodox doctors as well as public-health officials came down hard on divine healers, questioning their "cures" and pointing to their lack of proof. In 1956, the *Journal of the American Medical Association* warned, "The healing revivals were conducted with a woeful ignorance of public health measures" that allowed diseased people to mingle freely with the healthy.

Medical critics zeroed in on problem patients who quickly relapsed after supposedly being cured by divine healers. Dangers arose, said the doctors, when patients, falsely believing they were cured, avoided seeking medical care. But Aimee Semple McPherson blamed a patient's relapse on his or her own backsliding. Citing an Illinois man who went from a revival meeting straight to the gambling hall and discovered that his paralysis had returned, she wrote: "If instead of walking a holy, sober, God-fearing life with Jesus, he goes back to his theatre, dance hall, card party . . . this protection and abounding life and strength is not promised unto him."

The media eagerly joined the critics, questioning the healers' motives, investigating their finances, accusing them of lusting for power at the expense of naive followers, and challenging them to prove that their healings were genuine.

THE TROUBLES THEY'VE SEEN

The postwar years saw the rise and fall of two of the most colorful healers ever to pitch a tent. Their names were Jack Coe and A.A. Allen. Both were raised in poverty and appealed particularly to poor blacks and whites. Both ran into trouble with the law.

Coe, born and raised in Oklahoma and ordained as an Assemblies of God minister near the end of World War II, set out as an itinerant healer in 1947. Just as he was reaching the pinnacle of his career, Coe, who was set against using either doctors or medication, was arrested and charged with practicing medicine without a license. The charge was initiated by a Miami, Florida mother of a polio-stricken boy who complained that Coe had told her to remove her son's braces after the boy was allegedly healed, then never returned her phone calls when her son suffered a relapse. At his trial Coe argued that God, not he, was doing the healing. In a groundbreaking case that extended some measure of legal protection to healing revivalists, the charges were dismissed.

A year before Coe's arrest, another popular healing revivalist, Asa Alonzo Allen, was arrested in Knoxville, Tennessee for driving while intoxicated. In his own defense, Allen blamed the incident on "the devil," who he claimed was trying to "kill" his ministry. Like Coe, Allen preached against using medication. Known as the miracle man, he loved to take the toughest healing cases and even claimed to have raised the dead. In the late 1950s he moved to "Miracle Valley," Arizona, where he continued his "raise-the-dead" campaigns. Always a heavy drinker, he was found dead in his room at the Jack Tar (now the Cathedral Hill) Hotel in San Francisco in 1970 of an apparent heart attack. His death was blamed on "acute alcoholism." He was 59.

In his 1967 book *Faith Healing: Good or Fraud?*, Geroge Bishop wrote, "The people who enter the revival tent seek essentially the same suspension from reality as do their more conventional cousins under circus canvas.'' James Randi angrily observed in his 1989 book *The Faith Healers,* ''Reduced to its basics, faith healing today—as it always has been—is simply magic.'' Quoting his fellow investigator David Alexander, he wrote: ''Take these evangelists away from their silk suits, well-coiffed hair and fancy limousines and put them in animal skins with a few rattles and beads. You've got a Cro-Magnon shaman, complete and ready to go to work.''

''GIMME THAT OLD TIME RELIGION''

Despite the skeptics, healing revivalism was still going strong in the 1960s and 1970s. Oral Roberts was expanding his overseas work, visiting 54 countries by the end of the 1960s. Eventually, tiring of the road, Roberts folded up his tent and, to the shock of his Pentecostal supporters, joined a local Methodist Church. In 1962 he founded a university of evangelism, appropriately named Oral Roberts University and based in Tulsa. In addition to a stringent dress code—the first student handbook specified ''blouses, skirts and sweaters or simple dresses for classroom and casual wear'' for women and ''ties and coats, or sweaters when in the classroom, cafeteria, and chapel'' for men—ORU emphasized physical fitness as part of its curriculum and rejected anyone who was overweight.

In the 1970s, Roberts's organization also built a medical school and the City of Faith medical complex, where, as in the old ''healing homes,'' ministers who were trained as ''spiritual care-prayer partners'' worked alongside doctors. Both institutions quickly became Tulsa's leading tourist attractions. The medical complex was the result of Roberts's dream of turning out ''medical missions'' similar to those of the Seventh-day Adventists. (Roberts claimed to have received all of his instructions from God. The most publicized commandment was his 1980 report that a 900-foot-high Jesus had spoken to him.)

Critics questioned whether the medical school, controversial from its inception, could maintain high standards, given ORU's philosophical leanings. ORU's attempts to affiliate with local hospitals were met with stiff resistance from Tulsa doctors who argued that Oklahoma did not need another medical school, and especially not this one. In the mid-1980s, the school ran into financial difficulties. Despite Roberts's last-ditch campaign to raise money after allegedly being warned by God that He would strike Roberts dead if the preacher did not raise 8 million dollars, the medical school closed in 1989.

THE NEVER-ENDING MIRACLE

The divine-healing movement may have gone into eclipse and toned down its exuberant style, but it survived on the verge of the twenty-first century, though in somewhat changed form.

As of 1991, American law appeared to be on the side of divine healing. Although every state had laws against ''quacks,'' these laws specifically exempted divine healers because they were praying for healing, not performing a medical function. As of the late 1980s, 44 states permitted parents to refuse medical treatment for their children on religious grounds. According to a study done by the *Los Angeles Law Review* in 1984, cases that ended up in court usually resulted in overturned convictions.

In the early 1990s, Aimee Semple McPherson's Angelus Temple was very much alive and thriving. It was still the headquarters of the International Church of the Foursquare Gospel, which had grown to 1,300 churches in the United States and Canada and more than 20 thousand churches abroad. Radio KSFG/FM 96.3 was broadcasting 24 hours a day and Foursquare Publications continued to churn out literature for the church, including a slick bimonthly magazine called *Foursquare World Advance.* The temple, attracting an ethnically and racially mixed congregation, held two separate services, one in English and one in Spanish.

When one of the authors visited the temple one warm April morning in 1990, she was led to a seat by a friendly couple who introduced her to several of the congregants as ''Sister Liz.'' Sitting there at the back of Angelus Temple, she began to imagine what this place must have been like a half-century earlier, during one of Sister Aimee's illustrated sermons. Gone were the emotionally charged crowds packed into the auditorium to get a glimpse of the lady in white. This was a far quieter congregation that swayed and clapped to the gospel hymn ''Crown Him with Many Crowns.'' Even the healing line was a more subdued affair, as those who needed healing or saving came forward to talk in hushed voices to the church elders awaiting them.

While Sister Aimee was long gone, her family's presence was very much in evidence that day. Seated behind the pulpit was a grandfatherly-looking gentleman who rose and smiled when he was introduced as Rolf McPherson, the church's living link to its flamboyant founder.

CHAPTER
· 21 ·

Bernarr Macfadden and Physical Culture: "Weakness is a Crime"

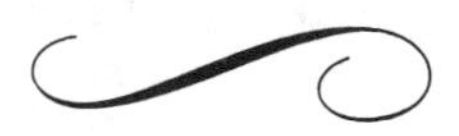

The Natural tonic of the healthful body is exercise.

BERNARR MACFADDEN, 1914

She was England's "most perfect woman." He was America's king of fitness. As part of his British tour in 1913, he instructed her to jump onto his stomach from a high table. As she had done many times before, 19-year-old Mary Williamson climbed up to her station and warily eyed her 44-year-old future husband, lying nude except for a breechcloth, below. "I could hear the audience take in its breath as I poised on my perch to step off feet first into a dead-weight fall," she wrote 40 years later. "A gasp came from the house when I left the table and a simultaneous 'oomph!' floated above the footlights as I landed smack on the crusader's belly button . . . . It was always received with applause as Bernarr, stretched out on the stage, leaped to his feet and sprang about bowing right and left, hugging the swinging spotlight."

It would not be the only time the controversial and daring Missourian would enjoy the spotlight as the founder of a twentieth-century version of Grahamism that he called physical culture, an anti-medicine, anti-doctor health regimen that included rules for eating, exercising, breathing, and bathing, and as the head of a publishing empire that provided him with a fortune worth 30 million dollars by the early 1930s. While he may not have fulfilled his dream of being the first physical-culture President of the United States, from the end of World War I to the early 1940s Bernarr Macfadden was a cult figure whose name was synonymous with health.

A MIDWESTERN BOYHOOD

Bernard Adolphus McFadden—he changed the spelling of his name as an adult—was born on August 16, 1868, near Mill Spring, Missouri. His father, William R. McFadden, was a farmer. By the time Bernard was 11, both his parents, now divorced, were dead, his father of alcoholism and his mother of tuberculosis. Taken in by relatives in Illinois, young Bernard spent the next two years working on their farm, a regimen that turned the weak, sickly child into a robust teenager.

Farm life was evidently not to his liking, however, and Bernard soon made off for St. Louis, where he worked at various jobs—as a delivery boy, bookkeeper, bill collector, and partner in a laundry business. "I had no chance to indulge in those exercises so necessary to the health of boys of that age," he reminisced in *Physical Culture* magazine in 1899, the first of his numerous publishing projects that would bring him fame and wealth. "At the age of 16 I was a complete physical wreck. I had the hacking cough of a consumptive, my muscular system had so wasted that I resembled a skeleton; my digestive organs were in a deplorable condition."

It was at this time that McFadden developed an intense dislike of both drugs and doctors. "Drugs seemed to be a delusion and a snare. They simply promised cures that they rarely if ever accomplished." After frustrating visits to several doctors in search of a cure, the teenager decided to shun all medical advice and rely only on his own instincts. He would preach his very American self-reliance message to his followers in the years to come. "Study your own body—your own peculiarities and tastes—and find out what is best for yourself," he advised. As for McFadden, he decided after visiting a gymnasium for the first time that what would be best for *him* was exercise.

After buying himself a pair of dumbbells, McFadden took up a rigorous daily regimen of gymnastics with the discipline that stayed with him for the rest of his life. Within a month his hollow cheeks began to fill out and his thin arms grew round and muscular. "The wild joy that thrilled my nerves when I began to feel that health and strength were surely within my reach no words can describe," he wrote. "I was literally dying for the need of exercise, and when that need was supplied day by day, month by month, I grew stronger."

By the time he was 18, McFadden was calling himself a "professor of kinesitherapy" and teaching gymnastics at military schools in Missouri and Illinois. He soon expanded his cure to include a preventive-health regimen of periodic fasting, 20-mile walks, quasi-vegetarian meals, fresh air, cold bathing, and minimal clothing even in winter, a philosophy he dubbed "physcultopathy," or "physical culture." He also worked as a professional wrestler for a brief time and demonstrated an exercise gadget at the 1893 Chicago World's Fair.

In 1892, Bernard McFadden changed his first name to "Bernarr" and his last name to "Macfadden." "He decided his name didn't have what he later called 'Adam Power,' " wrote Mary Williamson Macfadden in *Dumbbells and Carrot Strips,* the colorful and detailed story of her life with Macfadden. "My future husband reached the conclusion that if he could add length and strength to his last name it might be easier to put muscle in the first one . . . 'Mac' was substituted for 'Mc' and the big 'F,' which stuck out like a broken thumb in a wrestling match, was cut down to small size. The chesty last name that came out was Macfadden. It looked strong."

Like his new name, Macfadden emerged the model of the new American strongman so popular at the time. At five-feet-six-inches tall, he had a hairless brawny body and a large head covered by a mass of thick, wiry, long hair. Yet his perfect build could not make up for some apparent weaknesses, according to those closest to him. Mary Macfadden complained of his flat Missouri twang and mercurial and unpredictable personality. He appears to have been a man with a large and stubborn ego that would help him professionally, if not in his four marriages.

THE BICEPS CRUSADER

After spending several years in St. Louis, the ever-restless Macfadden decided to move his operations to Boston. But on a stopover in New York City, he liked the Big Apple so much that he decided to stay. There he set up an exercise studio for businessmen and married and divorced his first wife, Tilley Fountaine, whose relationship with him remains something of a mystery. He also found time to write a novel he called *The Athlete's Conquest,* a love story that preached exercise and condemned corsets. When it was turned down by several publishers, he published it himself, eventually serializing it in his new *Physical Culture* magazine, launched in 1898.

Physical Culture magazine, with its motto, "Weakness is a Crime: Don't be a Criminal," was an immediate success. By the 1930s Macfadden's publishing empire would include, among other titles, *True Story* (the idea came from third wife, Mary), *True Romances, Photoplay,* and the sensational tabloids *Midnight* and the *New York Graphic,* where young Walter Winchell and Ed Sullivan got their first breaks as writers.

Physical Culture was the heart of Macfadden's ventures. Starting as an instruction pamphlet for an exerciser Macfadden made and sold, *Physical Culture,* "Devoted to Subjects Appertaining to HEALTH, STRENGTH, VITALITY, MUSCULAR DEVELOPMENT AND THE GENERAL CARE OF THE BODY," first sold for a nickel. Within a year, Macfadden was bragging, "Our circulation is increasing from one to three thousand per month." By 1900, the magazine sold for 15 cents and was published by Macfadden's new Physical Culture Publishing Company, located at 25th and Broadway in New York City.

A TALE OF AN ATHLETE'S LOVE

"How have you been amusing yourself since I last saw you?" inquired Edith, after a silence of a moment.

"Athletics have been my principal amusement," he answered.

"What branch of athletics do you prefer?"

"I hardly know. I like everything in that line, though I believe wrestling and sparring are my favorite exercises."

"I like fencing the best. Did you ever try it?"

"Yes, once or twice."

"If you would thoroughly master it, I know you would like it. It keeps one interested every moment. I fence a great deal when at home, and I have missed it greatly since I have been here."

"Yes, it is a fine exercise. It's both recreative and healthful, and I am sure I should like it with you for a teacher. What do you say?" said he smiling.

"All right, if you will come to my home for your lessons."

from *The Athlete's Conquest*
by Bernarr Macfadden
Physical Culture Publishing Company, 1899

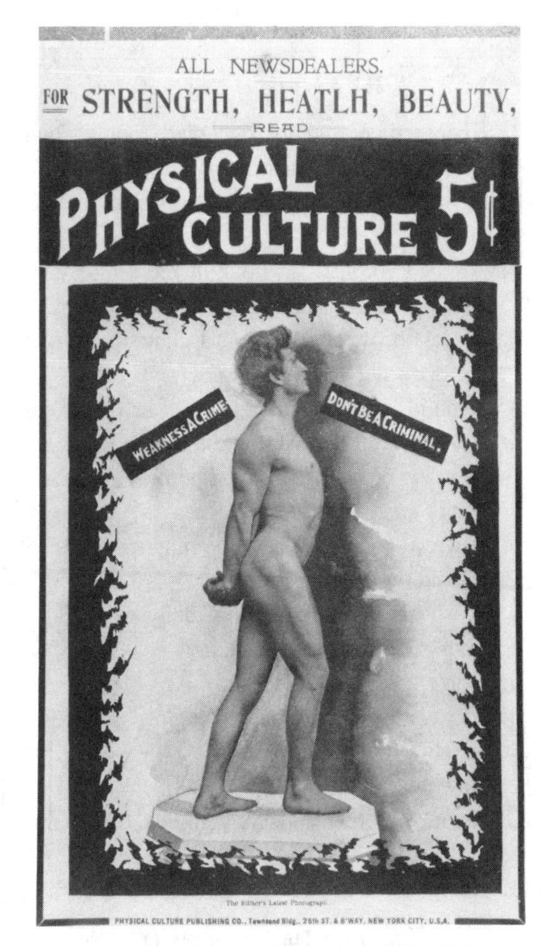

91. Cover boy Bernarr Macfadden, circa 1900. *Collection of Advertising History, Archives Center, National Museum of American History, Smithsonian Institution.*

Edited and largely written by Macfadden himself, *Physical Culture* ran the gamut of his health philosophy—the need for fresh air and sunshine, causes and cures of colds, physical beauty, women's health, exercise demonstrations, dietary rules, fasting, and the proper way to sleep, walk, and breathe. The November 1899 issue featured Macfadden's hero, Theodore "Rough Rider" Roosevelt, "a splendid specimen of physical manhood" who built up his muscles as Macfadden himself had—through exercise. Including women's fitness along with men's, Macfadden urged women to get in shape and toss out their corsets. Writing that physical culture was the key to longevity, he warned "both sexes—who are desirous of lengthening their days, try and 'postpone' the inevitable as follows: devote ten minutes at least to exercises which tend to strengthen the muscles of the abdomen and chest." While Macfadden advised against using drugs or doctors, he did not hesitate to seek out confirmation of his theories from mainstream medical practitioners, who wrote articles for nearly every issue.

Because many issues of the magazine contained photographs of men and women exercising in a minimal amount of clothing, *Physical Culture* magazine was considered rather steamy by early twentieth-century standards. So it was no surprise that the post office carefully monitored its contents. In 1907, Macfadden was arrested for mailing an issue of the magazine that contained an "obscene" feature on how one could transmit venereal disease. The angry publisher, who was convicted and fined 2,000 dollars, lambasted his critics, accusing them of prudery. In his own defense he argued that sex was both healthy and health-giving. Although in his writings he urged restraint, Mary Macfadden's descriptions of her husband's sexual appetite during the course of their marriage suggests that he did not always practice what he preached.

Soon after starting *Physical Culture* magazine, Macfadden also established a string of physical culture sanitaria in Kingston, New York; Spotswood, New Jersey; Battle Creek, Michigan (across from Kellogg's "San"); and Chicago, Illinois, the latter

HEALTH HINTS

1. Keep temperature of occupied rooms about 70 degrees Fahrenheit.
2. Always sleep with window open at top and bottom.
3. Air bed for half an hour in morning by removing all the bedding and hanging the same out of the window or on a chair in front of the open window.
4. A rapid mode of changing the air of a room is to open all the windows and then swing the door violently to and fro a number of times.
5. Never sleep with underclothes on.
6. Always hang up underclothing in front of a window at night to air.
7. Wash the whole body once daily.
8. Drink plenty of pure water.
9. Don't forget man needs a mixed diet.
10. Always breathe through the nose and never through the mouth.
11. Never ride when you can walk.
12. Avoid overcrowded and overheated cars, buildings, etc.
13. Exercise for at least 15 minutes each day.

J.H. Thompson, M.D.
Physical Culture, November 1899

ACTIVE EXERCISE IN MIDDLE AGE

Q. I enjoy the exercises you recommend for boys, such as turning handsprings, walking on my hands and a little horizontal bar work. I have experienced no bad results as yet. Do you think such active exercises beneficial to a man of my age, which is 41 years?

A. There is no reason in the world why a man of middle age should not be able to practice with pleasure and benefit the active sports of early youth. Indeed, this should enable one to retain his youthful vigor and elasticity. The reason why we commonly suppose that middle-aged men are incapable of such activity is because they habitually neglect such exercises and naturally in time become incapable of them.

Physical Culture, August 1907

turning out "graduates" of the Physical Culture Training School who became "doctors" of Kinesitherapy, Hydropathy, or Physcultopathy.

In 1907, *Physical Culture* magazine described the Bernarr Macfadden Health Home at Battle Creek, a "rendezvous for physical culturists and health seekers," as having 180 rooms, all "luxuriously furnished." It included "every conceivable appliance for giving natural treatment." As an incentive, those who worked in the building's special Physical Culture "subscription department" had a chance to earn all the expenses of their visit.

Mary Macfadden described the Chicago "healthatorium" as a big stone building where her husband was greeted "like a king at the door by a bowing, muscular flunky . . . . We were surrounded by the enthusiastic creatures who ran this Macfadden Kingdom of Health. Men and women in white uniforms, working together in the cause of the Master, they all looked like agile wrestlers with barrel chests, powerful hips, strong arms, and low foreheads."

Macfadden's Physical Culture Publishing Company published an impressive list of "health and sex books." These included books on marriage, muscular development, male diseases, and "vital power," the healthful state to which physical culturists aspired. Also on the list was a series of books on physical culture for babies, co-written with his second wife, Marguerite, a Canadian nurse he married in 1901. (They were divorced in 1911.)

Besides his publishing ventures and "healthatoriums," Macfadden started several physical culture restaurants, eventually numbering 20, where one could feast on vegetarian soup and beans, a chopped-nuts-and-vegetable steak, and other vegetarian delectables. These were forerunners of his Depression-era penny-and-nickel restaurants in Manhattan, Brooklyn, Chicago, and Washington, D.C.

In 1911–12, Macfadden published his widely read five-volume *Macfadden's Encyclopedia of Physical Culture,* subtitled "A Work of Reference, Providing Complete Instructions for the Cure of all Diseases Through Physcultopathy, with General Information on Natural Methods of Health-Building and a Description of the Anatomy and Physiology of the Human Body." This mammoth project that would become the physical culturists' bible covered everything from anatomy and physiology, dietary guidelines, exercises for building health, and critiques of modern medicine and drugs to health of the vocal chords and women's health and physical training.

By the time Macfadden traveled to England in 1913 to advertise his books and theories and hold his contest for England's most perfect woman, his future bride was already familiar with Macfadden's work

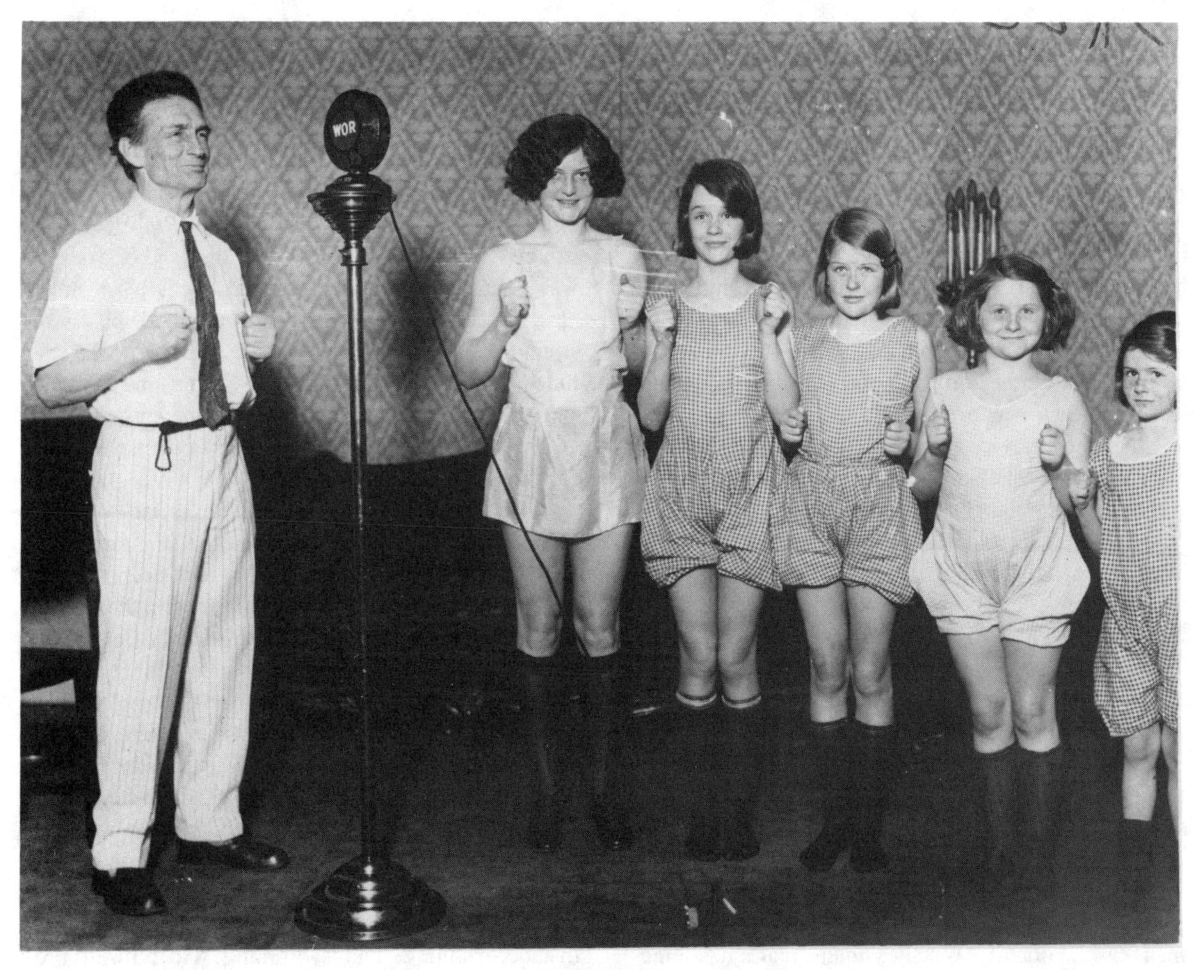

92. Macfadden's children got into the act on his radio fitness program (1925). *The Bettmann Archive.*

through the *Encyclopedia* and was impressed with his ideas. Little did she know that after she was to win the contest and marry its sponsor and judge (none other than Macfadden), she and her children would become his living laboratory, his very own "physical culture family."

"THE DRUG CURSE"

Macfadden's intense abhorrence of drugs and doctors permeated all his writings. In *Building of Vital Power,* written in 1904, he accused "medical science" of devising new and unnecessary surgical operations and useless remedies and tonics. "Drugs never cured anything or anybody unless you call death a cure," he wrote in the November 1899 issue of *Physical Culture.* In contrast to physical culturists, he wrote, "the dupes of medicine are still degenerating physically." In the August 1907 issue, Macfadden answered a letter questioning him on the use of drugs to cure catarrh. His answer: "All drugs are of a more or less poisonous character and depend upon this fact for their stimulating and other supposedly effective properties . . . . Drugs can only hinder the progress of the patient toward recovery and can never help."

For Macfadden, there was only one disease—impurity of the blood. Since there was only one disease, there was but one cure—fasting. According to Macfadden, during a fast the body knows to devour both useless fat and its diseased sections. However, fasting does not mean starvation: "As a general thing one can fast for a number of weeks before he reaches the point at which starvation begins."

Macfadden was no kinder to dentistry than to orthodox medicine. "He had no use for dentists," wrote Mary Macfadden. "His specific recommendation for a toothache was to bite the teeth hard, or chew upon a piece of wood with the aching teeth."

Although he never forced his tooth cure onto his wife, he did expect her to follow his anti-medicine rules. "You will have to remember, always, that doctors are taboo," he warned her in the early days of their marriage. "You must be a living example of everything that I teach and that I believe . . . . When you have your children, you cannot have a doctor. You will have only midwives . . . . Our children must never be vaccinated. If they're sick any time, I'll prescribe for them my knowledge of natural methods of curing people . . . . You will bring them up, but strictly under my regime of health." True to his orders, Mary gave birth to seven of his nine children (every one of their first names began with "B," according to Macfadden's wishes) without assistance from either drugs or medical doctors. None of his children was ever vaccinated.

No doctors were allowed to care for Macfadden's family. Mary Macfadden described a time in 1923 when her four daughters were sick with whooping cough: "Bernarr ordered them on a complete fast. They were not permitted to eat anything for three weeks. They could have water to drink, and after the first two or three days, were given orange juice. Toward the end of it they were emaciated and staggering from weakness. Bernarr did not relent and saw to it that they didn't have a mouthful of food until the twenty-second day of their fast. They were to go through the same ordeal with the measles, scarlet fever, and other diseases."

In a more tragic circumstance, when his first son Byron ("Billy") was shivering from convulsions, Macfadden plunged him into a hot bath rather than call a doctor. Whether mainstream medicine could have saved the child the family would never know, but within minutes Billy was dead.

THE ANNUAL 30-DAY FAST

To celebrate his fasting cure, in June 1906 Macfadden inaugurated an annual 30-day fast for his followers. This proved to be a perfect publicity stunt, since Macfadden would then publish the testimonials from fasters all through the year. One "well-known physician" from Belleville, Illinois, who broke his fast with a glass of malted milk, claimed to have lost 28 pounds. "There was little or no depreciation of physical strength," wrote Macfadden in September 1907, "as shown by the fact that at the termination of the fast, he lifted to elbow-height with one hand, weights of seventy-five and a hundred pounds with apparent ease." During the doctor's fast, the only thing he let touch his lips was "copious drafts of distilled water."

"FUNCTIONAL VIGOR"

The core of Macfadden's teaching was exercise, based on his own transformation as a teenager in St. Louis. Although he taught that exercise was not the "sole factor" in the true science of health, "without exercise," he wrote in *Building of Vital Power,* "there can be no physical culture." Yet the goal of exercise was not simply building external strength and muscles, but also developing what he called the "vital strength" of the internal organs, in particular the lungs, heart, stomach, intestines, liver, and kidneys. Thus his exercise regimen involved the entire muscle system, with special attention given to those muscles surrounding the vital organs.

His instructions for physical exercise were detailed and exacting, and he warned his readers to follow them accurately, continuing each exercise "until the muscles you bring into use are thoroughly fatigued." In Volume II of *Macfadden's Encyclopedia of Physical Culture,* readers were treated to more than 400 pages of these instructions, complete with illustrations, for proper breathing to strengthen the lungs, for relaxing, for doing floor calisthenics and wand, dumbbell, and Indian-club drill routines, and for exercising the face, vocal chords, and bust. Arguing that outdoor exercise was superior to the indoor variety, Macfadden encouraged his readers to take up outdoor sports, such as tennis, golf, long-distance running, and swimming. He himself preferred long-distance walking in the country and made it a point to walk to his office from wherever he was living: "Even under the most disadvantageous circumstances, a short brisk walk is always beneficial; but a long walk that will take from three to five hours of steady rhythmic movements, can hardly be improved upon."

Citing his own example, he described how he rose between four and six o'clock each morning and walked between 15 and 20 miles per day. His preferred method was going shoeless, "with hat in one hand and coat and shoes in the other. Thus equipped, when I arrive at some point where I again wish to enter the realms of so-called civilization, by stopping at a convenient brook by the road, it is an easy matter to remove the dust of travel and assume the articles of clothing that qualify one to become one of the conventional human sheep."

Every day of their married life, Mary watched her husband's morning routine, one that she was reluctant to join, especially during her pregnancies. "As I lay in bed watching him," she wrote of those months when she was pregnant with their first child, "I knew that this morning he would not ask me to do the torturous knee bends which he had reduced from 200 to half that number as my pregnancy developed. He was going a bit easier with me. He had taken me for a 15-mile walk the day before. We had dispensed with the jog trotting."

"THE SUPREME IMPORTANCE OF DIET"

Macfadden's rules for eating specified that one should eat only when hungry. "Eating without appetite or thorough enjoyment of food is a crime against the stomach," he wrote in 1899. "If one is not hungry at meal-times, one is recommended to wait until there is a genuine appetite." In *Eating for Health and Strength,* published in 1921, he told his readers that the "ideal plan" was to eat "just enough to maintain a feeling of strength and all around vigor and with the body in a well-muscled condition and without any visible evidence of surplus fat." Making special note of women's health, in the 1920s he criticized the then current ideal of feminine beauty, which, while promoting a more slender figure than during World War I, was still not the athletic type he preferred himself.

His dietary rules departed somewhat from those of Sylvester Graham, who had popularized a vegetarian diet a century earlier. Although Macfadden taught that a lactovegetarian diet (a meatless diet that includes dairy products) was ideal and warned his followers to stay clear of lamb, veal, and pork, he allowed for moderate quantities of meat, preferably beef. (He admitted that his favorite cut was the round of a steak, and Mary cites several examples of his meat-eating binges.) As for chicken and fish, they were, he claimed, "not as nourishing as beef." Like Graham, he was a true champion of greens and encouraged his readers to eat large quantities of green leafy vegetables.

Also like Graham, Macfadden taught the superiority of whole-wheat bread and whole-wheat products and recommended breakfast cereal over the meat, pancakes, and fried eggs still popular at the turn of the twentieth century. One of his inventions was a cereal aptly named "Strenthro," which evidently bombed on the market. However, in the days before cholesterol consciousness he also preached that fat was necessary to a wholesome diet, ideally "emulsified" fat from milk, cream, egg yolks, butter, and cheese.

The "torso king" had a high regard for milk, especially as a curing agent. In *The Miracle of Milk,* written in 1923, Macfadden wrote that the white liquid was "the greatest of all diet cures . . . ." Arguing that milk furnishes the elements necessary "to make new blood," he recommended drinking a milk-only diet for a variety of illnesses. This cure required drinking from five to six quarts of unpasteurized milk daily for three to four weeks.

Macfadden also preached the gospel of Horace Fletcher, the great masticator, who urged his contemporaries to chew each morsel of food until the taste disappeared, at which time this liquefied mess merely slipped down the throat. Writes Mary Macfadden, "He had increased our crunches at the table to one hundred and twenty per mouthful. We counted them dutifully."

He was against drinking at meals, unless one was thirsty. In true Grahamite fashion, Macfadden also shunned tobacco, spicy foods, and all alcoholic beverages.

Most of his life, Macfadden followed his own dietary advice. In 1921, Macfadden told his readers that he took only one "square" meal a day, down from his previous two, at which time he ate all he desired, usually raw or stewed fruit, cereal, eggs, and Graham gems (small, sweetened pieces of Graham bread). This feast was usually supplemented during the day by one or two oranges and nuts and raisins.

At times his family rebelled against the dietary regimen they were expected to follow. Mary Macfadden grew so weary of the vegetarian diet her husband had forced upon her during her first pregnancy that, when they were traveling in France after the birth of their child, she sneaked out to a French restaurant, where she dined on porterhouse steak, wine, and vanilla ice cream with whipped cream and liqueur.

"PURE VITALIZED AIR"

In Volume I of his *Encyclopedia,* Macfadden described how most of his fellow men and women had little regard for the value of fresh air, "the most essential necessity of life . . . . Walk through the streets, both of residence and business, in any of our large cities, except during the summer months, and you will invariably find the larger part of the windows closed as if the inmates of the houses, stores, shops and offices regarded fresh air as an enemy to be avoided." In contrast, he urged his readers to swallow huge goblets of fresh air year-round. "You cannot breathe too much pure air," he wrote in the March 1907 issue of *Physical Culture*. "If you want to enjoy life in every sense of the word, become a fresh-air crank." He instructed his readers how to breathe by drawing in deep, full breaths, filling the lungs to their greatest capacity, "being careful always to expand in the abdominal region."

He also criticized his fellow Americans for overheating their homes, arguing that the ideal indoor temperature should be 45 degrees to 55 degrees Fahrenheit. He paid particular attention to sleeping habits. Pooh-poohing the commonly held beliefs that night air, cold air, and damp air were injurious to one's health and that drafts could cause illness, he encouraged his followers to sleep with the windows wide open and to position their beds so that they would receive the fullest benefit of the ensuing ventilation. "All through the last cold winter I slept with my windows . . . as far as I could get them open, and I have two windows on each side of my bed," he wrote in *Building of Vital Power*. "The wind blew directly on over me, and I am far better able to do my work because I have pure oxygen to breathe."

Macfadden taught that the best way to enjoy the full benefits of fresh air was to wear as little clothing as possible, even in winter. "Have all your clothing so made that as much air as possible can reach the skin of all parts of the body. Don't be afraid of air—even of winter air. It is a life-saver, and a cleanser," he wrote in *Building of Vital Power*. He described how one recent winter, "for experimental purposes," he wore a summer suit and no underwear. Although at first he felt as if he had no clothes on at all and that the wind was blowing right through his body, gradually he became accustomed to it. "There is no need of a long outercoat," he wrote in 1907, "if one is capable of walking briskly or indulging in an occasional short run." As for underwear, Macfadden was against it, in particular the popular heavy woolen underwear of the day.

BATHING FOR A HEALTHY SKIN

Macfadden was a big advocate of baths—water baths, sun baths, air baths, and something he called "friction baths." Proper and frequent bathing, he claimed, was the best way to assure the healthy, clean skin so necessary for maintaining health. Like every other part of his regimen, there was also a proper way to bathe.

After exercising, Macfadden suggested a dry friction bath or rubbing a dry towel back and forth first across the neck and shoulders and then proceeding downward until every inch of skin is glowing from the "accelerated circulation." This ritual should be followed by a cold bath, "to awaken thoroughly the circulation and the functional and muscular systems." Macfadden did not recommend a direct cold plunge "unless a great deal of vital strength is possessed by the bather." Instead, he instructed his readers to dip their hands into the cold water and then rub them all over the body. In combination with these daily cold baths, he recommended one or two hot baths each week, at which time one should use soap.

"The skin requires air just as much as the lungs do," he wrote in 1904. And to satisfy this need, he recommended "air baths," a ritual that essentially involved removing one's clothing and going about the household naked. "One of the best times for the air bath is while going through forms of muscular exercise, and while resting between them," he advised. "Take one as often as you can; two or three every day will do you no harm."

Adopting the popular belief that the sun's rays were a curative agent, Macfadden also championed sun-bathing. "Accustom yourself gradually to the effects of the rays of the sun and, with the added habit of taking air baths, you will soon be the possessor of a well-tanned, healthy looking skin, strong enough to endure any change or condition in weather."

VIRILITY AND HEALTH

Of all Macfadden's writings, his most controversial were those about sex and marriage. Starting with *The Virile Powers of Superb Manhood: How Developed, How Lost: How Regained,* written in 1900, he fought a one-man battle against "that horrible curse of prudishness and the ignorance of sex." His campaign was, according to his critics, carried to extremes with his often lurid stories and photographs in the *New York Graphic*.

As for sex and health, Macfadden posited that sexual prowess is directly related to one's general physical and mental condition. "It is the barometer of the physical and nervous organism," he wrote in 1900. "Impotence sexually means impotence in everything . . . . Your powers are fast waning—you might just as well be laid away without further notice." One of his most bizarre inventions was an instrument for exercising the male genitals, called the "peniscope." Bernarr recommended it in particular to "harassed captains of industry."

As always, he included women in his teachings, encouraging his male readers to marry only women who "have sufficient stamina to be normal in this way . . . . Never marry a weak, sickly girl. Such women have not the slightest right to marry," he warned. "They become in every case a curse to themselves and to the man who marries them."

Yet he was no free-love advocate. Like many of his contemporaries, Macfadden was against masturbation, "that horrible curse," and what he referred to as "sexual excess" in marriage, which, following the popular belief of the times, he claimed "depleted" the body of its vital energy. "Many men appear to think and act as though their sexual powers were limitless. Week after week, month after month, and often year after year, they indulge in this way to the extreme limit. The ultimate result is always serious . . . . The muscles lose some of their elasticity, firmness, and symmetry; the various vital organs become gradually weaker, and if there is any physical defect or a tendency toward disease, the weakened condition of the body enables it easily to develop."

Macfadden believed that marriage was the normal state of man- and womankind, and that the only purpose of sexual intercourse was procreation. If his personal goal was to raise the perfect physical culture family, his long-term dream was to see a nation of physical culture families. Writes James C. Whorton in *Crusaders for Fitness,* "bearing and rearing robust babies was the sum of female existence in the physical culture world." It goes without saying that in Macfadden's scheme of things there was no need for birth control.

"PERNICIOUS PROPAGANDA"

Macfadden may have been able to attract a few allopathic doctors to write for his publications, but his anti-medicine diatribes won him few friends in the established American medical community.

In 1925, the editor of the *Journal of the American Medical Association,* Dr. Morris Fishbein, took on physical culture in his book *The Medical Follies.* At first glance, Fishbein appeared mainly to attack the "erotic appeal" Macfadden used in his teachings, accusing the physical fitness crusader of publishing magazines "reeking with sex." But the meat of Fishbein's criticism was Macfadden's attack on scientific medicine and alignment with such "borderline cults" as chiropractors, Abramsites (promoters of electrical gadgets to cure various diseases), and naturopaths:

> It does not suffice Mr. Mcfadden [sic] to prove that good health may be achieved through proper diet and proper exercise; he seems to feel that in promoting these desiderata he must attack those phases of the scientific care of the body that lie within the purview of the scientifically trained physician . . . . Macfadden's periodicals are devoted largely to an attack on scientific medicine and to discredit not only the modern treatment of disease but also the campaigns for the prevention of disease carried on by scientific medicine.

Eleven years later, Dr. Arthur M. Cramp, former Director of the Bureau of Investigation of the AMA, lambasted Macfadden's *Physical Culture* magazine in his *Nostrums and Quackery and Pseudo-Medicine*. He particularly took aim at a course heavily advertised in the magazine offered by Dr. W.H. Bates, "a graduate of a reputable medical school," and Macfadden for "a new course in eye training." This course promised its students that they could throw away their glasses. Bates's name was eventually dropped from the course, although the magazine continued to promote it.

Writers took their turns poking fun at the crusader. In May 1930, H.L. Mencken wrote in the *American Mercury:* "His chief intellectual possession, one gathers, is a vast and cocksure ignorance. He seems to be taken in by all of the transparent quacks who advertise in his magazines, as he postures as an authority upon the crimes of modern medicine without knowing anything more about the human body than any other gymnast."

FLEXING HIS MUSCLES

By the end of World War I, *Physical Culture* magazine had reached an impressive 500-thousand circulation, attracting, in addition to Upton Sinclair, writers George Bernard Shaw and H.G. Wells. With the physical fitness boom in the 1920s, Macfadden was on his way to earning a national reputation as both an unconventional publisher and a health crusader. In 1919, he launched *True Story,* perhaps his most successful publication (Mary Macfadden evidently approved every story before it went into the magazine), and, in 1924, the lurid Manhattan tabloid the *New York Graphic,* which lasted until 1932.

By the 1930s, Macfadden's magazines and newspapers were read by an estimated 35 to 45 million people and the bare-torso champ was living the comfortable life of a millionaire, winning free publicity by walking the 25 miles daily from his home in Nyack, New York to his Manhattan offices. He was doing his fair share of elbow-rubbing with celebrities as well, among them Henry Ford, with whom he once enjoyed a bag of nuts washed down with carrot juice.

In the early days of the Depression, Macfadden instituted the Bernarr Macfadden Foundation to spread further his physical culture philosophy and opened the Physical Culture Hotel in Dansville, New York, a

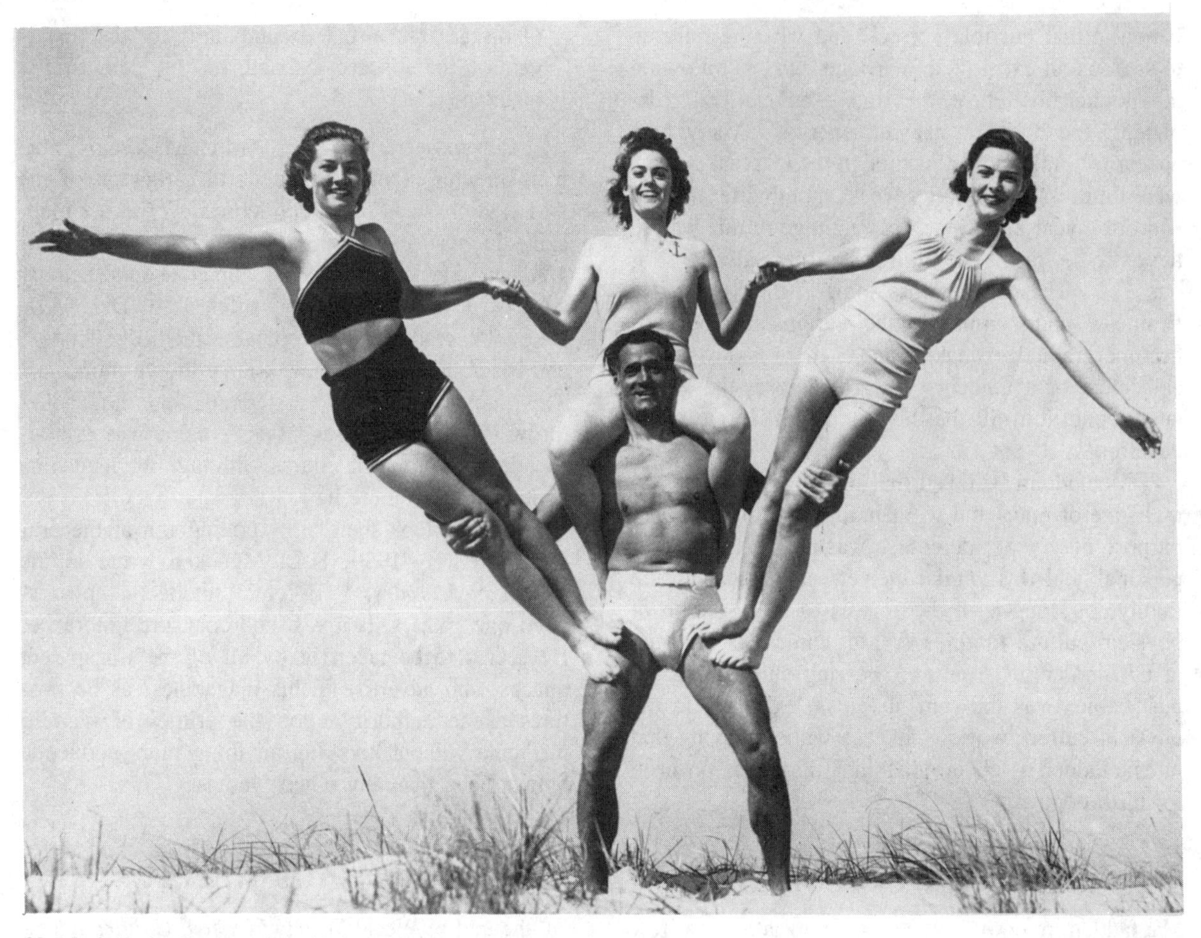

93. Macfaddenite Charles Atlas with friends (1936). *UPI/Bettmann News Photos.*

THE MAKING OF CHARLES ATLAS

One of Macfadden's most celebrated converts was an Italian-born former 97-pound weakling named Angelo Siciliano. Like Macfadden, young Angelo built himself up with exercise, using a daily regimen of isometrics. In 1922, he entered a competition sponsored by Macfadden's *Physical Culture* magazine, winning the coveted title of "The World's Most Perfectly Developed Man" along with a 1,000-dollar prize. After renaming himself Charles Atlas, he started his own muscle-building course. With the aid of an astute business manager, Charles Roman, who named Atlas's system "dynamic tension," the course eventually enrolled more than 70,000 students each year. In 1970, *Esquire* magazine featured a still-muscular 78-year-old Atlas, who had by then "made seven million weaklings into strong men in his lifetime and is now prepared to die." Two years later he died of a heart attack.

former water-cure establishment owned by James Caleb Jackson. Here, as *Time* magazine pointed out in 1936, one "might choose a Macfadden diet-&-exercise cure which is supposed to correct 150 human miseries, including acidosis, alcoholism, apoplexy, gout, impotence, lowered vitality, masturbation, ptomaine poisoning, sleepwalking, sterility and writer's cramp."

By the end of the 1930s the physical culturist's fortunes had taken a nose dive. First there were his unsuccessful campaigns to become the 1936 Republican presidential candidate, the governor of Florida, and the mayor of New York; then his public admiration of Mussolini brought the critics down hard on him; and finally his stockholders accused him of using corporate funds for personal ends, and in 1941 forced him out of Macfadden Publications. The new editors renamed *Physical Culture,* calling it *Beauty and Health.* By the end of the decade Macfadden had sold off all his magazines. Finally, after years of increasing marital tension, his marriage to Mary fell apart, leading to their separation in 1933 and divorce in 1946.

YOU'RE NEVER TOO OLD TO FLY

As a young man, Bernarr Macfadden had predicted that he would outlive his critics, and as he entered his sixties it appeared as if he were on his way to doing just that. At the age of 63, he earned his pilot's license. On his seventy-fifth birthday, he lectured to reporters on the benefits of physical culture while standing on his head. When he was 80 he married a 43-year-old interior decorator named Jonnie Lee. (Their marriage lasted until 1954.) And he celebrated his eighty-first, eighty-third, and eighty-fourth birthdays by jumping out of an airplane in a parachute.

As he neared his eighty-eighth birthday, Macfadden appeared to be in perfect health, still muscular and fit and still following his recommended dietary and exercise regimens. Except for the physical examinations necessary to get his pilot's license, he had never seen a doctor as an adult. Then in October 1955 Macfadden died in Jersey City, New Jersey. The cause was cerebral thrombosis, after Macfadden evidently tried to cure himself of jaundice by fasting.

He had come a long way from St. Louis, leaving behind guidelines for health and longevity that were carried on by his loyal followers, among them a young Californian named Jack LaLanne, whose physical feats and showmanship would easily match Macfadden's. In 1989, Macfadden Holdings, Inc., his corporate descendant, bought the G.P. Group, owner of the tabloids *The National Enquirer* and *The Star*. It seemed like a fitting match for a publishing giant whose founder had discovered early on that sensationalism sells just as well as health.

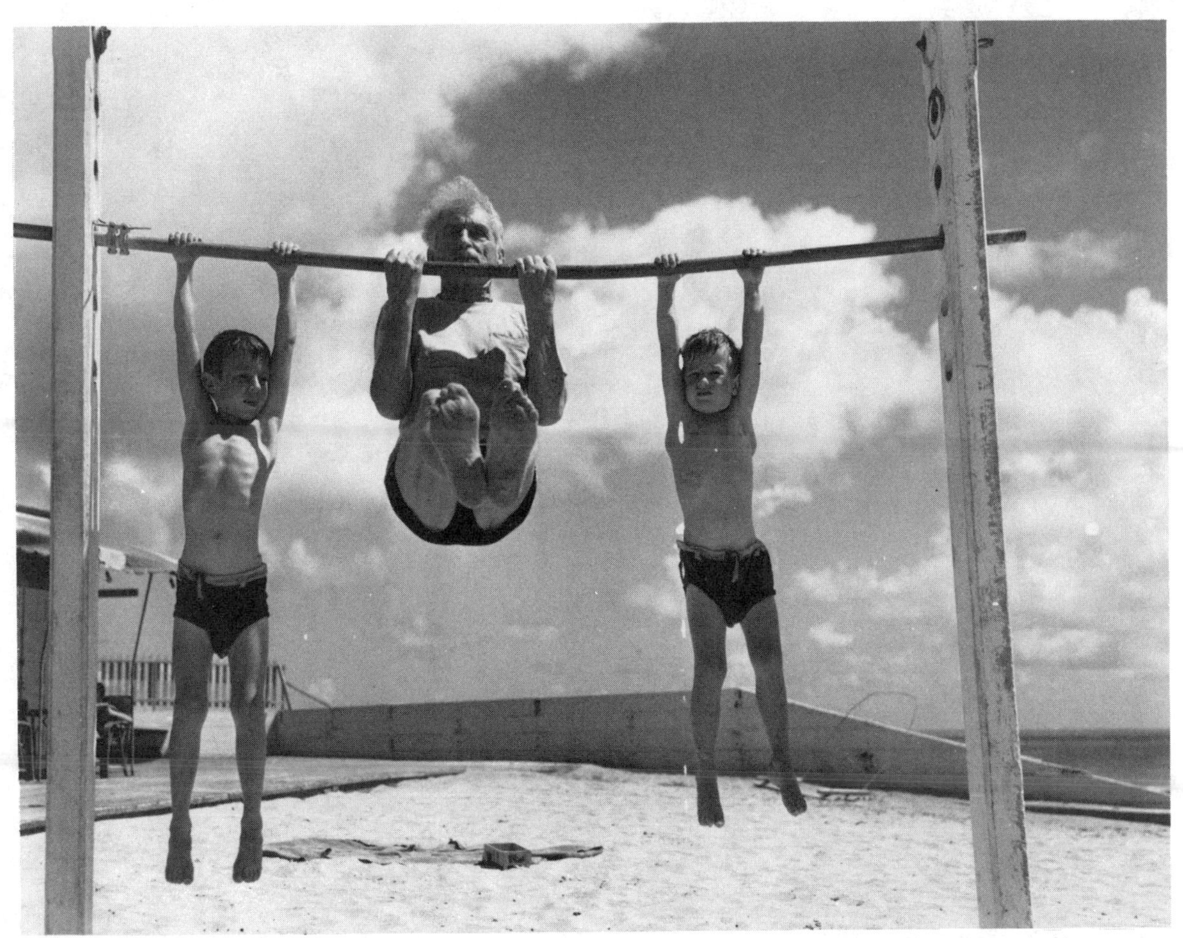

94. A daring young man of 77, Macfadden at his Miami Beach home (1945). *International News Photos/The Bettmann Archive.*

CHAPTER

· 22 ·

HOLLYWOOD: A CAST OF THOUSANDS

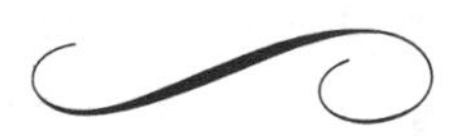

My students out in Hollywood . . . have breakfasts of fresh fruit juices—their delicious oranges and lemons and grapefruit. These health-giving and slenderizing fruit juices are served to the leading ladies of the screen before they dash off to the studio for the day's work. If you would be slim and healthy, too, follow their example.

GAYELORD HAUSER
Eat and Grow Beautiful, *1936*

Hollywood is more than the center of the American film industry. It is also the locus of the modern good-health movement—the place where bodies are sculpted, unwanted pounds are banished, sickly attitudes are readjusted, and clean-and-sober vitality is regarded as a birthright.

Actually, Hollywood—all southern California, really—was a health mecca even before the motion-picture industry colonized it. The popular notion of the region as a languorous but healthful Lotus Land was born in the 1880s, after the transcontinental railroad brought the area within reach of consumptives from back East who descended on spas and boarding houses to restore themselves in the hot, dry, sunny climate.

It didn't take long for philosophers and proselytizers alike to declare that southern California was a very special place—indeed, *the* special place as far as good health and good living were concerned.

The late-nineteenth-century author Joseph Pomeroy Widney, who moved to California for his health, helped to propagate the new myth. According to historian Kevin Starr, "A lifelong health faddist and physical culturist (no liquor, no tobacco, a raw onion in the morning to get the gastric juices flowing), Widney envisioned Los Angeles as developing into the health capital of the world, a heliopolis of holistic health culture, highly technological . . . but also devoted to natural living."

Greater Los Angeles was not the first seedbed of American health manias, to be sure. That distinction belonged, in the early nineteenth century, to New York City, where a resident writer and physician, David Meredith Reese, grumbled that "this is the theatre of humbugs; the chosen arena of itinerating mountebanks . . . . Here is found a motley population, multitudes of whom spend their 'time in nothing else but in searching for some new thing.' "

That may have been true in 1838, when Reese wrote his book *Humbugs of New-York*. But by the 1920s, the Big Orange had rolled over the Big Apple. In place of the wily old snake-oil salesmen were toothsome newcomers whose tanned good looks personified healthfulness. Some, like Gloria Swanson and Greta Garbo, were movie stars who radiated vitality on the big screen; another, fitness king Jack LaLanne, rose to stardom on small-screen TV; while still another, nutritionist Gayelord Hauser, worked behind the scenes.

THE VAMP AND THE "THREE-DOLLAR DOCTOR"

The scene: outside a Pasadena, California doctor's office so tiny and nondescript it doesn't even have a nurse or receptionist. A young woman, expensively dressed and with a look of apprehension, approaches the door, hesitates, and knocks. She is greeted by a kindly doctor of short stature. He is barely bigger than the woman, who stands just five-feet-two-inches tall. He bids her welcome, and then makes an unusual request. "Take off your earrings, please," he asks. Startled, the patient removes her costly earrings, and the physician nods in approval. "Long lobes indicate healthy adrenals," he says, "and you certainly have them."

The year was 1927. The patient was an actress, not yet 30, who had already made her reputation by portraying the vamps so popular in the twenties. Her name was Gloria Swanson. The doctor was Henry G. Bieler. He had, he said, cured himself of chronic asthma and kidney disease when he was a young medical student by turning to simple foods, simply prepared and consumed sparingly. In the process, he lost 60 pounds. Now he would cure Swanson, who worried that she was developing an ulcer.

"Then," recalls Swanson in her 1980 autobiography, "he prescribed a series of enemas and a modified fast of vegetable broth made of zucchini, celery, and string beans, and told me to come back in a week."

Swanson, who had visited Bieler on a friend's advice, did as she was told. On her return visit she felt marvelous: "My skin was glowing, my eyes were clear and sparkling, and my nerves were calm." Dr. Bieler had made an important convert. Swanson was a rich, worldly entertainer with an enormous following. She was to follow the doctor's orders for the rest of her long life, paying the same modest fee (three dollars) that he charged all his patients.

Born in Chicago in 1897 or 1899 (records are unclear), Gloria Swanson made her movie debut while still a teenager in 1914. The following year, she moved to Hollywood and made comedies for Mack Sennett, and then worked for Cecil B. DeMille. Petite, with dark hair, large blue eyes, and a generous mouth, she enjoyed the lifestyle of the rich and famous. She ate sinfully rich food, smoked, and stayed up to all hours of the night. "At the peak of her career," noted one of the countless articles about her, "she earned $25,000 a week and lived in a 24-room Beverly Hills mansion with eleven servants."

Swanson lived opulently even after seeing Bieler, but she cut way down on fatty food and began to exercise. In her seventies she insisted on having a second-floor dressing room so she could exercise by walking up the stairs. To the end of her life, she held the modest Dr. Bieler, who never became famous, in high esteem. She swore by his theory that there were not thousands of diseases, as popularly supposed, but just one, which he called toxemia. When people stopped poisoning themselves with artery-closing, high-calorie foods, Bieler believed, the body could heal itself. He didn't prescribe even simple drugs, not even aspirin.

Shortly after she met Bieler, Swanson recommended him to Joseph P. Kennedy, father of the future President. She suggested that Kennedy's daughter Rosemary, who was retarded, might benefit from Dr. Bieler's regimen. "His blue eyes turned to ice and then to steel," Swanson remembered. "He said he had taken Rosemary to the best specialists in the East. He didn't want to hear about some three-dollar

CALIFORNIA BUNCOMBE

California has long put East Coast writers in high dudgeon, especially when it comes to fringe medicine. A typical example is this lead-in to a critique of Pasadena medical charlatan Gaylord Wilshire, from a 1927 issue of *Hygeia*, a magazine published by the American Medical Association:

> . . . One expects big things from the Pacific coast—and usually gets them. The greatest piece of quackery of our generation came from San Francisco when Albert Abrams . . . capitalized [on] the public's ignorance of, and interest in, radio to exploit his so-called electronic reactions. California should have been satisfied with this superb piece of pseudo-scientific buncombe. Apparently she is not, for today we are being treated to another piece of electrical hocus-pocus that promises to eclipse, for the proverbial nine days, the electronic reactions and make Abrams look like a piker. It must be the climate.

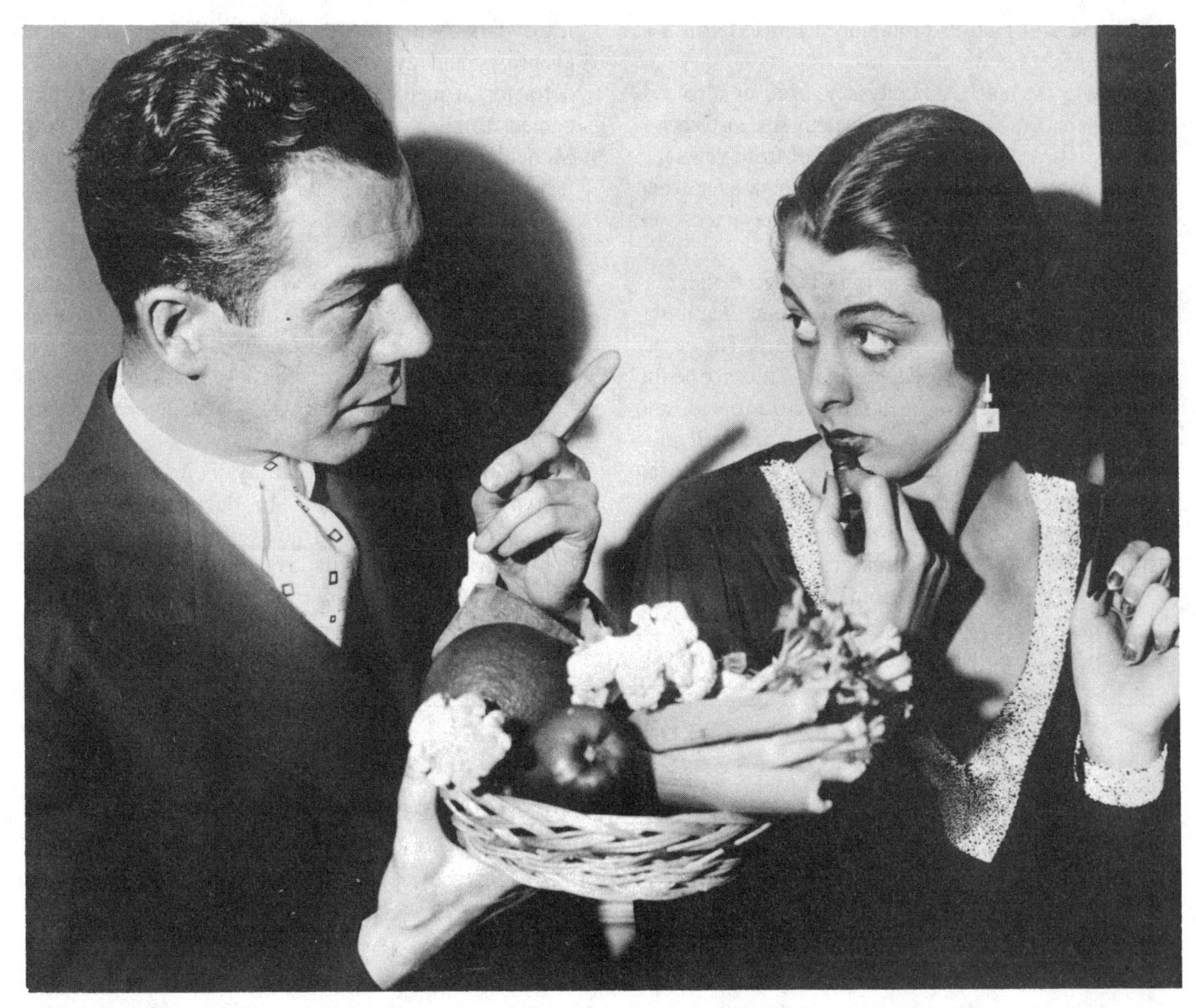

95. Health guru Gayelord Hauser tells Billie Ridgeway that fruits and vegetables, not lipstick and rouge, will enhance her beauty (1937). *San Francisco Examiner.*

doctor in Pasadena who recommended zucchini and string beans for everything . . . . People must think I was unhinged suggesting that grave illnesses could be treated with squash.''

Kennedy never did consult Bieler, but Swanson, the doctor's loyal student, metamorphosed decades later into one of the nation's most visible and forceful advocates of natural foods, physical fitness, and organic farming.

ENTER GAYELORD HAUSER

In 1927, the same year that Gloria Swanson met Henry G. Bieler, a young German immigrant by the name of Gayelord Hauser made his first visit to the film capital. Soon afterward, Hauser moved to Beverly Hills and became a dietary guru and companion of movie actresses—beautiful women with a professional stake in looking good for the cameras.

Hauser was born Helmut Eugene Bengamin Gellert Hauser in 1895. His home was Tübingen, a Black Forest town in southwest Germany. The eleventh of 12 children, Hauser emigrated to America in 1911, at age 16, to join an older brother in Milwaukee. But soon after his arrival he was felled by ill health, diagnosed as tuberculosis. Hauser developed an abscess on his hip and several operations failed to heal him. In Chicago's Evangelical Deaconess Hospital the doctors told him to go home and prepare to die.

Hauser was not yet ready to meet his maker, however. In the early 1920s, Benedict Lust, a German-born medical doctor and naturopath, introduced him to bathing cures, herbal teas, and clay packs. Hauser also journeyed to Basel, Switzerland, to visit his sister. There he met a monk named Brother Maier, who had him drink copious amounts of fruit juices and sup on herbs and broths. At Brother Maier's behest, he ate 36 lemons a day. The abcess on his hip closed and Hauser pronounced himself cured at last.

While on his health odyssey, Hauser also visited Carlsbaden Sanatarium, a health spa in Czechoslovakia. There he drank a daily pint of fresh vegetable juice, a habit he was to recommend years later when he became famous. Newly healed, he hastened back to America.

Hauser took a degree at the Chicago College of Naprapathy, which specialized in spinal manipulation related to chiropractic and osteopathy. The newly credentialed healer opened his own Chicago health clinic in 1922, teaching a hybrid of European and American fringe medicine. The clinic did well, and Hauser broadened his activities to include writing and lecturing. Fascinated by citrus fruits ever since his own lemon cure, Hauser journeyed to Los Angeles to see the city where citrus grew on trees.

He fit right into the boom town Hollywood of the 1920s. Hauser was tall (six-foot-three), trim (200 to 215 pounds, a weight range he maintained all his life), dark (with slicked-back black hair and dark eyebrows and eyes), and handsome. Although one detractor, a medical doctor, wrote that Hauser's accented English made him sound like Baron von Munchhausen, *Time* magazine was more complimentary, describing him as "a suave Continental with a provocative accent."

Hauser's new, elite clientele got highly irregular advice from their suave Continental counselor. In his first book, *Harmonized Food Selection*, published in 1930 under the name Bengamin Gayelord Hauser (he legally changed his name in 1923), the nascent nutritionist sounded more like a metaphysician than a physician of medicine.

Hauser classified people by their temperament, or types. "Mental types," he decided, "use up a good deal of phosphorus and sulphur" with all the brain work they do. Milk, Hauser declared, was just plain bad: "Among modern physicians, it is a widely demonstrated fact that milk uniformly causes two definite conditions within the human body: lowering

GAYLORD WILSHIRE: BOULEVARDIER . . . AND QUACK

Remembered best as the namesake of Los Angeles's Wilshire Boulevard, which he cut through a bucolic barley field in 1896, Gaylord Wilshire achieved notoriety in his lifetime for a different reason: He invented a cure-all electronic gizmo that outraged the medical profession.

Born Henry Gaylord Wilshire in Cincinnati in 1861, Wilshire dropped out of Harvard and emigrated to California in 1885. Although he made and lost several fortunes in billboard advertising and southern California real estate, the high-powered businessman converted to socialism and founded *Wilshire's Magazine*, an influential monthly that advocated nonviolent Fabian socialism. George Bernard Shaw, H.G. Wells, and Upton Sinclair were among his friends. Wilshire's wealthy second wife, Mary Reynolds Wilshire, was an early champion of Jungian psychology in America.

The literature on Wilshire doesn't explain why the cultivated parlor socialist became a medical charlatan. Maybe he secretly needed the money. In any case, he began marketing his I-ON-A-CO in 1925, pitching it as a sure-cure for, among other things, heart disease, cancer, diabetes, and prostate problems. Wilshire claimed that the device, an electric belt worn around the neck or waist, healed by magnetizing iron in the blood and zapping cells with electricity. According to one ad, "All you have to do is to place over your shoulders the Wilshire Ring or I-ON-A-CO. That's all. You may then light a cigarette and read your newspaper for 10 or 15 minutes . . . . Often patients at the first treatment, like Lazarus, arise well and whole . . . ."

Wilshire's grandiose claims attracted the Public Health League and Better Business Bureau in Washington State. According to their investigation, the I-ON-A-CO consisted of a large coil and a small coil of insulated wire; the large coil, when plugged into a wall socket, generated a weak alternating current. The American Medical Association commented that the gadget was as useful as "the left hind foot of a rabbit caught in a churchyard in the dark of the moon."

His pretentions punctured, Wilshire died in New York in 1927, a victim of heart disease— one of the ailments the I-ON-A-CO was supposed to cure. Popularly believed to be worth millions, he left only 17,000 dollars. His legacy, Wilshire Boulevard, runs 15.6 miles from downtown Los Angeles to the sea, ending in Santa Monica, and is one of the most prominent business addresses in the United States.

of the mentality and general clogging of the entire system.'' Hauser also observed that ''iodine is the perfecting chemical and stands for beauty, refinement, culture.''

All of these notions were wildly unscientific, a fact that did not escape the American Medical Association, which did not equate minerals with social status or intellectual prowess. The AMA labeled Hauser a charlatan. Meanwhile, the Food and Drug Administration impounded several food products sold under Hauser's name, among them Diabetic Tea, for misbranding.

In an era before the roles of dietary cholesterol or saturated fats were well understood, Hauser recommended fat-filled calorie bombs for everyone except dieters. For breakfast he suggested trying two egg yolks in a glass of orange juice; for lunch, a cream-cheese-and-pineapple salad or baked apple with cream; and for dinner, cream of tomato soup and a ''fresh vegetable plate with plenty of butter.''

Hauser's groaning board—he emphasized that healthy eating should be fun—especially appealed to the pleasure-loving, novelty-starved residents of the film capital. Among his followers were Clara Bow, Claudette Colbert, Mae West, Paulette Goddard, Billie Burke, Anita Louise, Barbara Hutton, and, most glamorous of all, the enigmatic Swedish-born star Greta Garbo.

''GARBO'S GAYELORD''

By the late 1930s, Hauser was living in what *Time* magazine called ''palatial Beverly Hills quarters.'' It was there that he met Garbo at one of his parties. Later, she came alone to dinner, and Hauser served her wild-rice hamburgers and broiled grapefruit. The menu must have been appetizing, because Hauser and Garbo were soon seen everywhere together, much to the delight of the press, which was as celebrity-hungry then as it is now.

''Gayelord Hauser put Garbo on a diet of his 'wonder foods,' such as yogurt, dried skim milk, brewer's yeast, blackstrap molasses and vegetable juices,'' wrote Garbo biographer John Bainbridge. ''Garbo . . . thrived on it.''

In 1939–40, Garbo and Hauser embarked on a long, high-profile tour. They lunched in New York with Mrs. Cornelius Vanderbilt in her Fifth Avenue mansion. Hauser was now so ubiquitous at Garbo's public appearances that the ever-attentive *Time* called him ''Garbo's Gayelord.''

Hauser decided to propose marriage, and was so sure Garbo would accept that he tipped pals at International News Service to await his call before

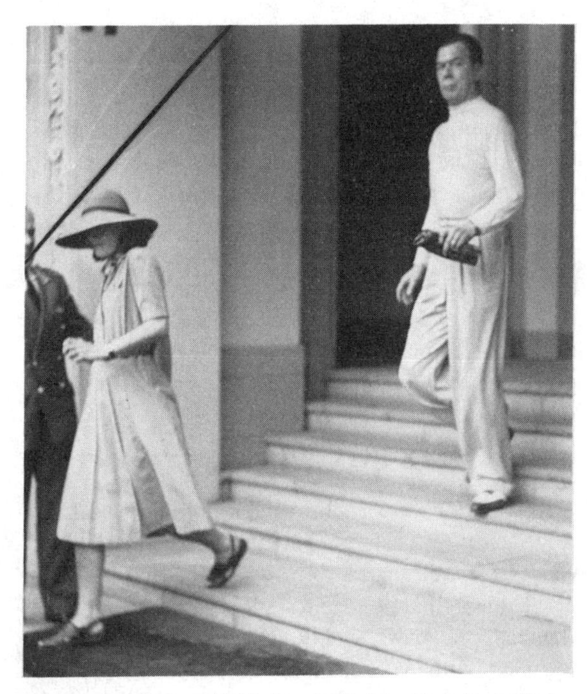

96. Gayelord Hauser with his favorite disciple, Greta Garbo (Palm Beach, Florida). *The Bettmann Archive.*

releasing a story that he had helped prepare. The call, to be placed from a luxury yacht where he and Garbo were sunning themselves, never came, and Hauser never married.

Garbo and Hauser's relationship apparently cooled, but the actress stayed on the diet that Hauser prescribed, even when she was with other beaus. *Time* caught up with the globe-trotting star in Italy, where she was traveling with conductor Leopold Stokowski: ''At the Hotel Caruso, where, until they were discovered, the couple had gone regularly to eat their vegetarian lunch, their waiter said: 'He certainly must love her to eat that stuff [carrots, beets, lettuce]. Before she came, he used to eat plenty of meat and spaghetti.' ''

Hauser had no shortage of clients. Through his books and lecture tours he expanded his audience from a few hundred influential insiders to the proverbial Hollywood cast of thousands.

In his 1936 book *Eat and Grow Beautiful*, Hauser spelled out the links between health and glamour that had been implicit in his earlier writing. Declaring that ''miracles have been performed with food,'' Hauser rhapsodized about ''Nature, the greatest Beautician of them all.'' Once again, Hauser's regimen was unorthodox. He recommended large doses of laxatives to help health- and beauty-seekers lose weight fast. Calling constipation ''the sin of sins,'' Hauser confided, ''I am convinced that you can never win a victory over your complexion if your intestines are against you."

Although he was obviously out of step with mainstream medicine, Hauser was in some ways ahead of his time. He emphasized diet as a key to health and personal responsibility as the key to wellness. He even anticipated, and helped to coin, catchphrases that would not enter general circulation until 30 years after *Eat and Grow Beautiful* was published. He exhorted believers to "Keep on keeping on!" and further admonished, "Never forget that you are what you eat!"

THE LONG GOODBYE

Gayelord Hauser was still dispensing nutritional advice nearly 60 years after trading the cold winds of Chicago for the balmy breezes of southern California. Although the specifics of his dietary regimen changed, the basis of his appeal did not. He was relentlessly upbeat, remained handsome well into his old age, and continued to woo followers with anecdotes about his famous friends. In the 1950s, when his popularity peaked, he titillated lecture audiences, usually crowded with older women of means, with references to Garbo.

Long a behind-the-scenes influence, Hauser became a star in his own right in 1950 with the publication of his best-selling book *Look Younger, Live Longer*. Selling nearly 500 thousand copies in the United States alone, the book, which was translated into 19 languages, topped *Publishers Weekly's* 1951 nonfiction best-seller list, edging out *Betty Crocker's Picture Cook Book*, which finished first in 1950. At 55, Hauser was a household word.

Hauser presented more sophisticated ideas in *Look Younger, Live Longer* than he had done in his earlier books. Drawing on expanding knowledge of cholesterol, he deemphasized butter and cream in his recipes. He also addressed the stress of modern life by endorsing a can-do attitude and placing new emphasis on vitamin and mineral supplements; he himself, Hauser wrote, took 100,000 international units of vitamin A every day for two-month stretches—20 times the daily U.S. Recommended Dietary Allowance.

Hauser once again stressed the efficacy of his five "wonder foods": blackstrap molasses, brewer's yeast, yogurt, wheat germ, and powdered skim milk. Hauser was especially enthusiastic about fresh vegetable and fruit juices, which he claimed to have introduced to America; he popularized fresh juices as tasty, easy-to-prepare and easy-to-digest sources of nutrients.

BEST-SELLER BLUES

Look Younger, Live Longer generated controversy as well as sales. Fifteen copies were seized by the FDA in a Rochester, New York health-food store in 1951, along with a 50-gallon shipment of Plantation brand blackstrap molasses. (The gooey residue of sugar refining, blackstrap retains the vitamins and minerals of raw sugar cane.) The FDA claimed that the book falsely called blackstrap a panacea and therefore constituted a misleading label for molasses sold in food stores that also sold *Look Younger, Live Longer*.

Hauser and his publisher, Farrar, Straus & Young, vigorously objected on First Amendment grounds. Hauser added that he didn't claim that blackstrap was a cure-all, only that it was nutritious, and that his book described "a way of life." After a flurry of publicity, charges were dismissed in federal district court and the book continued to be sold in health-food stores. Bookstores were not enjoined from selling Hauser's opus.

Having abandoned his most idiosyncratic flourishes, Hauser had a common-sense approach that anticipated trends of the 1970s and 1980s. He emphasized fresh raw or lightly cooked vegetables, variety in the diet, light consumption of red meat in favor of poultry or fish, and moderation in drinking and smoking. (He thought a long drag on a cigarette after a meal was relaxing.)

Hauser's vegetable juices, which he called "liquid salads" or "vegetable cocktails," proved immensely popular. "Hauser bars," where one could order a stiff vegetable cocktail straight up, sprouted in trendy restaurants (one of them owned by cosmetics queen Helena Rubenstein). Elizabeth Arden served Hauser's juice combinations at her chic "fat farm," the Main Chance Farm, in Maine. Hauser closed *Look Younger, Live Longer* by urging readers to establish Look Younger, Live Longer restaurants, food stores, and beauty shops and suggesting that ministers' wives, YWCA women, and retired schoolteachers would be ideal for operating franchises. "If necessary, take a course in tea-room management," he advised female readers.

The chain never materialized, but there were lucrative lecture tours, admiring profiles in mass-circulation magazines, and new writing assignments. Hauser published his diets in *Vogue* magazine, wrote a syndicated newspaper column, and even published his own magazine, *Diet Digest*.

During the years of his greatest triumphs, Hauser was an indefatigable self-promoter and shameless name-dropper. He dedicated *Look Younger, Live Longer* to Lady Elise de Wolfe Mendl, a 94-year-old high-society decorator. His recipe for "Royal Hashed Potatoes" was dedicated to Queen Alexandra of Yugoslavia and his "Four-Star Soya Muffins" to Paulette Goddard. Baron Philippe de Rothschild was his European distributor for private-label foods. The Duchess of Windsor was said to adore Hauser. A writer for the *Saturday Evening Post* noted of Hauser: "If testimonials from distinguished patients . . . constituted the sole qualifications, his only rival as a source of well-being would be the shrine at Lourdes."

Hauser's enterprises made him wealthy. He owned homes in Beverly Hills, Sicily, New York City, and Germany, bought expensive cars, hung Picasso and Renoir originals, and collected ceramic dishes shaped like fruits and vegetables. He also invested in real estate. He was Gucci's landlord on Rodeo Drive, the posh shopping street in Beverly Hills.

Hauser's advancing years and ostentatious ties to the stars of a fading era caused his popularity to wane in the informal, egalitarian 1960s. He did, however, live long enough to see the rise of the hippies and a new wave of health-food stores in North America and Europe. In 1972 Hauser wrote, "Today, after nearly 50 years of writing and lecturing and shouting from the housetops, my greatest reward lies in the fact that millions of young people in America are shouting with me."

JACK LALANNE: "TV'S NATURE BOY"

In 1951, the same year that *Look Younger, Live Longer* topped the bestseller list, a new kind of program jumped, pumped, and sprinted to prominence on television, the electronic toy that was then just beginning to challenge the hegemony of the movies. The program was the "Jack LaLanne Show," a half-hour exercise lesson aired from Los Angeles and hosted by a powerfully built 37-year-old man with a sunny disposition. The show's namesake, Jack LaLanne, stood only five-feet-five-inches tall and weighed about 160 pounds, but he possessed improbable 48-38-35 measurements. Atop this small but muscular package—*Sports Illustrated* called LaLanne "a dynamic pixie"—perched a wavy pompadour borrowed from Elvis Presley or maybe Ronald Reagan.

LaLanne was a homegrown Californian, born in San Francisco in 1914 and raised in nearby Oakland. He was a sickly child who was hooked on junk foods. "As a kid," remembered LaLanne, "I was stoned out of my mind on sugar. A freak. It made me weak. I had boils, pimples, fallen arches. I was nearsighted. Listen, little girls used to seek me out just to beat up on me."

LaLanne's tour of duty in nutrition hell ended when he was 14 years old. His parents took Jack to hear a lecture by Paul C. Bragg, an early fitness and diet crusader. The lecture hall was so crowded that Jack had to sit on the stage. Bragg, who claimed to be the son of a famous Confederate general and had the fire-and-brimstone style of a Southern preacher, galvanized young LaLanne. After the lecture, Jack prayed for divine guidance:

> I got on my knees and prayed to the Lord just to give me the intestinal fortitude to be able to give up these foods I was eating. I guess He listened, because in five days—five days!—it was like someone had pounded the demon out of me. I learned the truth, that two and two is four, not three, and I haven't compromised in all the years since.

Young Jack gave up junk foods and began working out in his backyard, using cement in paint cans for weights. He played sports for Berkeley High School and enrolled at the University of California, but dropped out to answer his one true calling: bringing health and fitness to the masses. In 1936, at the tender age of 22, he opened in downtown Oakland the first of what would eventually number more than a hundred health clubs bearing his name. He became a bodybuilder, winning the Mr. America title. In 1951, when the infant television medium beckoned, LaLanne was ready, beginning a 26-year run on TV that was to last until 1977.

LaLanne was perfect for TV's age of innocence. He was open, guileless, and corny. He performed on camera with his two German shepherds and a poodle; like him, the dogs were trim, as was LaLanne's wife Elaine, a TV talk-show producer whom he married in 1959. "It would blow my image to have a fat wife and fat dogs," LaLanne explained. His enthusiasm seemed boundless. *Look* magazine summed up his style by observing, "If Jack LaLanne felt any better, he'd explode."

LaLanne had reason to be happy. He was impossibly fit, looking great in his tapered jumpsuits and ballet slippers. He owned a home in the Hollywood hills. His company, Jack LaLanne, Inc., was grossing three million dollars a year by 1960 from his television show, health clubs, and health foods sold under his name. At its peak, around 1970, the "Jack LaLanne Show" was syndicated to 140 markets, with a potential audience of nearly half the American population.

Although he was mainly known for his pumped-up physique, LaLanne also stuck to a natural-foods diet, packed with literally hundreds of supplements. He favored raw fish ("man's primary food," as he called it), poultry, vegetables, and fruit ("nature's blood cleaner"). In 1979, a writer for *Family Health* magazine quoted LaLanne on his mind-boggling array of food supplements:

> "I take four hundred supplements," he confides. His kitchen cabinet contains every conceivable vitamin and mineral, all stacked in neat rows, in alphabetical order.
>
> "I take one hundred liver and yeast tablets, seventy-five kelp, plus zinc, potassium, dolomite, selenium, bonemeal, vitamins E, C, A and D. Plenty of iron—everyday! I put them in a blender with about eight ounces of warm water, and then I gulp the whole thing down . . . . Then, after I've had my vitamins, I fix a combination of half raw skimmed milk and half organic apple juice. And then I put from sixty to eighty grams of my high-protein mix (called Reduce) in it, and that's my breakfast."

LaLanne performed staggering public feats on or near his birthdays to demonstrate that health and fitness are ageless. On his forty-second birthday, in 1956, he did 1,033 push-ups in 20 minutes. On his sixtieth birthday, in 1974, he swam from Alcatraz Island, in San Francisco Bay, to Aquatic Park (about two miles)—handcuffed, with boats tied to his body. And on his sixty-second birthday, to celebrate the 1976 U.S. bicentennial, he pulled 13 boats filled with 76 YMCA youths one mile in Long Beach harbor.

All this won LaLanne oceans of publicity. But when the slick, cynical 1980s washed across America, LaLanne—hokey and undeniably aging—came to be seen as a likeable anachronism. His name still graced a chain of health clubs, but producers pulled the plug on his long-running TV show. LaLanne's jumpsuit gave way to spandex and Day-Glo colors and he was nudged aside by such younger fitness champions as Jane Fonda, who used her movie-star status to launch a best-selling line of exercise videotapes, and Arnold Schwarzenegger, who used his bodybuilding celebrity to become a movie star.

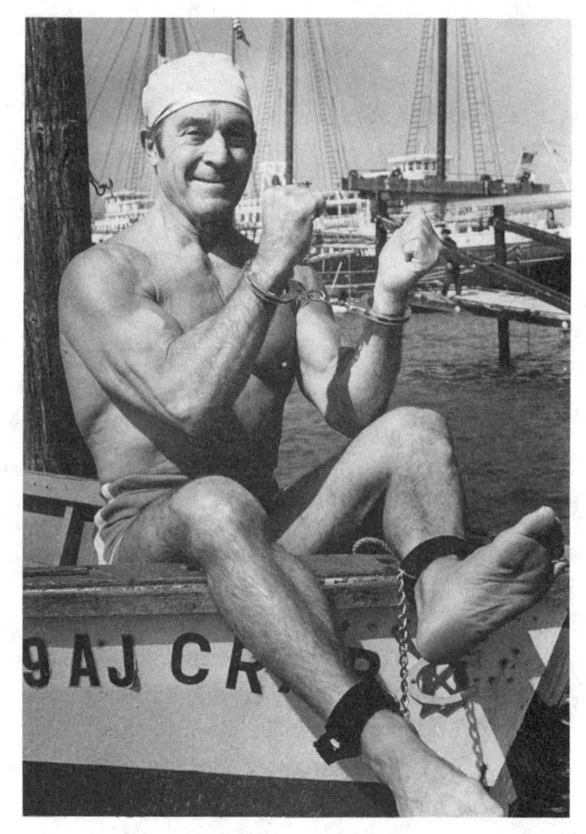

97. Jack LaLanne before his handcuffed birthday swim in San Francisco Bay (1974). *San Francisco Examiner*.

ENCORE

True to their expectations, the first generation of Hollywood health enthusiasts lived a long time.

Gloria Swanson was 84 or 86 before she expired in New York in 1983 of a heart ailment. Right up to the end, she was admired for her spirited style and a fresh appearance that belied her age. "People bring binoculars, even up close," Swanson said of theater audiences who saw her on Broadway in her seventies. "They want to know whether I'm retouched like a photograph or done up with wires. Well, it's not surgery . . . . But I am an organic food faddist. I'm better known for that than I am for my movies."

Indeed, Swanson's last years were distinguished by her crusade for pure foods and a restored natural environment. After lobbying in Washington to secure passage of the so-called Delaney Clause—a 1958 law limiting the use of known carcinogens in food—Swanson got a thank-you letter from Representative James J. Delaney that she called "my proudest possession." A woman of passionate beliefs, she told an interviewer in 1970 that "Americans are literally killing themselves with the foods they eat. The soil is sick from being covered with sprays and synthetics. The cattle are sick from eating the crops. The fish are dying. And the people are sick from eating this dead or dying food."

In 1976, Swanson's health crusades merged with her personal life. She married William Dufty, the author of *Sugar Blues*, a broadside against the nutritional shortcomings of sugar. Dufty dropped 85 pounds after switching to a diet of whole grains, vegetables, and nuts before he became Swanson's sixth husband. After exchanging their wedding vows, the couple went on the road, blaming social ills on malnutrition. "Kids hopped up on junk foods not only cannot learn," Swanson said, "they are out of control and become criminals."

When the celebrated couple traveled, they toted their food in suitcases and drank bottled water. According to *San Francisco Examiner* reporter Mildred Hamilton, their "typical day's fare . . . started with a breakfast of oatmeal . . . dusted with sunflower crunch . . . and substitute coffee made of barley, figs and chicory. The soup and salad lunch was split pea soup, salad of wilted onions, watercress, celery and scallions, and unleavened stoneground wheat bread spread with sesame seed butter . . . . Dinner was brown rice with onions sauteed in sesame oil, lentils, green salad, fruit."

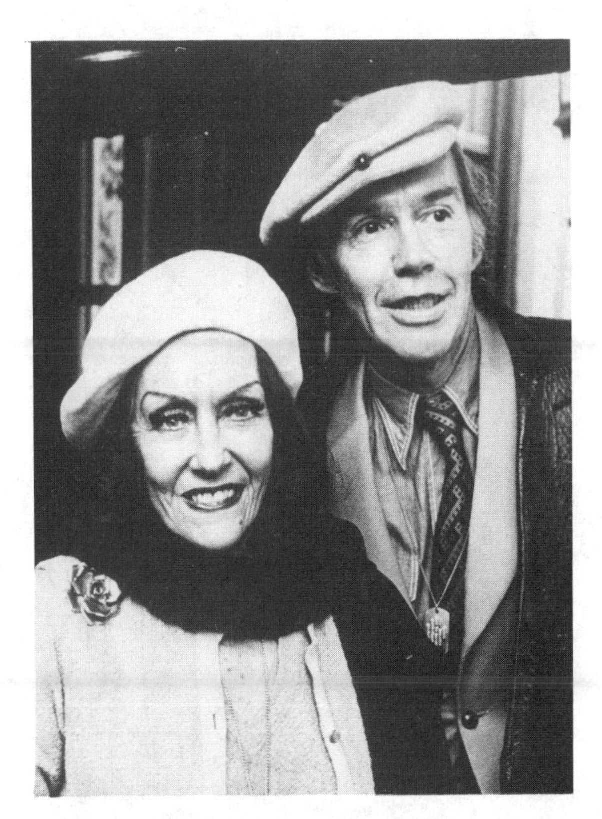

98. Gloria Swanson with *Sugar Blues* author William Dufty (1976). *UPI/The Bettmann Archive.*

Gayelord Hauser died at age 89 in North Hollywood in 1984 from complications of pneumonia, after selling 50 million copies of his self-help books around the world. Hauser wasn't often in the limelight in his last years, although he emerged from time to time in magazine feature stories about the art

**UPTON SINCLAIR:
HEALTH UTOPIAN**

Upton Sinclair, whose 1906 muckraking novel *The Jungle* spurred badly need reforms in the meatpacking industry, experimented during many of his 90 years with a variety of medical treatments and regimens from his Pasadena home.

Just after the turn of the twentieth century, Sinclair (1878–1968) lived on fruits and nuts to cure a dyspeptic stomach. Following what he called his "squirrel diet," Sinclair ate "no cooked food for five months." When that failed to effect a permanent cure, he simply switched to an all-meat diet and subsisted on Salisbury steak for a while.

Sinclair took his search for a healthy utopia to Battle Creek, Michigan, where he alighted in a sanitarium run by the physical culturist Bernarr Macfadden. Sinclair met his second wife, Mary Craig Kimbrough, in Battle Creek, where she was a patient at Dr. John H. Kellogg's famous "San."

Although Sinclair was friendly with Gaylord Wilshire, he was not involved with his pal's curious I-ON-A-CO scheme. He did, however, stoutly defend Dr. Albert Abrams, the electronic-medicine quack whose efforts preceded Wilshire's. Upton and Mary spent two weeks observing Abrams in his San Francisco clinic in 1921, emerging as believers. When the doctor was attacked in *Survey* magazine, Sinclair wrote a blistering letter to the editor. Sinclair noted that Abrams diagnosed patients partly by tapping their bodies and insisted that not all the "two or three million finger taps" the doctor made in his career could have been for naught.

Another of Sinclair's friends, the dyspeptic intellectual H.L. Mencken, castigated Sinclair for his susceptibility to medical follies: "He believes in every one of them, however daring and fadtoddish; he grasps and gobbles all the new ones the instant they are announced. But the man simply cannot think right."

of growing old gracefully. When he died, a *San Francisco Chronicle* editorialist observed:

> Generations of fitness enthusiasts owe a debt to the late Gayelord Hauser, a pioneer nutritionist who preached diet and intelligent eating long before it became fashionable and long before hippie gurus glorified granola . . . . Many will remember the nutritionist for his flamboyant lifestyle, but no one can fault the essence of his crusade: diet and exercise.

Hauser's friend Greta Garbo died in 1990, at age 84, of kidney disease in New York. The legendary actress followed Hauser's health regime well into her old age, half a century after her ocean cruise with the dashing dietitian.

Jack LaLanne and his wife Elaine left the fast lane in Hollywood for the backwater fishing village of Morro Bay, California in 1985. In the fall of 1990, Elaine LaLanne was leading fitness walks in shopping malls for senior citizens. Seventy-six-year-old Jack LaLanne still rose at 4 A.M. to pump iron in the couple's home gymnasium and worked the lecture circuit as an inspirational speaker. He told interviewers he hankered to get back on television.

And Hollywood? In 1966, Gloria Swanson told *Esquire* magazine that "Hollywood was a real postmark whose name became attached to a mythical kingdom which didn't exist. It had to be invented. We did our best. Our antics, our happenings, our way of life happened for a while to influence national style."

Swanson was too modest. Hollywood (and enclaves of greater Los Angeles such as Bel Air, Malibu, and especially Beverly Hills) still sets the pace in entertainment, diet, and physical fitness. Although it is choked with automobiles and baked in smog, Los Angeles maintains a paradoxical and very public love affair with good health and good looks. The area is dotted with health-food stores and juice bars. Natural food restaurants abound. Gym-toned bodies share the beaches with lean surfers.

Were he transported for a day to modern southern California, old Dr. David Meredith Reese would probably conclude that his strange new surroundings were awash in the rising tide of humbug. But to millions around the world, Hollywood is still the stuff that dreams are made of.

CHAPTER · 23 ·

ORGANIC AMERICA: RODALE & CO.

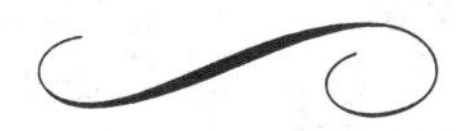

Wake up, scientists! Get your hands into Nature's soil. Don't be contemptuous of the natural ways. Help your fellowman. Please!

J. I. RODALE

My Own Technique of Eating for Health, *1969*

Do we dare to eat a peach? How about an apple ripened with a synthetic growth regulator, or a pear imported from a country where toxic pesticides and fertilizers are used with almost no oversight? By the 1980s, just as consumers were being firmly admonished to eat fresh fruit, whole grains, and vegetables instead of high-fat, high-cholesterol meat and dairy diets, such questions took on unprecedented urgency.

These questions are not new. They have long obsessed reformers who have been urging consumers to just say no to chemically dependent farming—and yes to organic agriculture. Indeed, the organic idea has been championed since the early years of the twentieth century by self-taught farmers, a handful of experts, and health crusaders, most notably publisher J.I. Rodale (1898–1971), the founder of *Prevention* magazine and Rodale Press.

Organic has been a fighting word in the public arena for decades; there is little agreement about the proper definition of the word. To chemists, ''organic'' means only that a substance contains a carbon compound, as many things do—from a plump, ripe strawberry to the banned pesticide DDT. To reformers, however, ''organic'' signifies something quite different. It is a catch-all label for farming and gardening that uses crop rotation, intertillage, natural fertilizers (such as manure), insect predators, natural insecticides (such as soap sprays), and other techniques in place of powerful chemicals that reformers

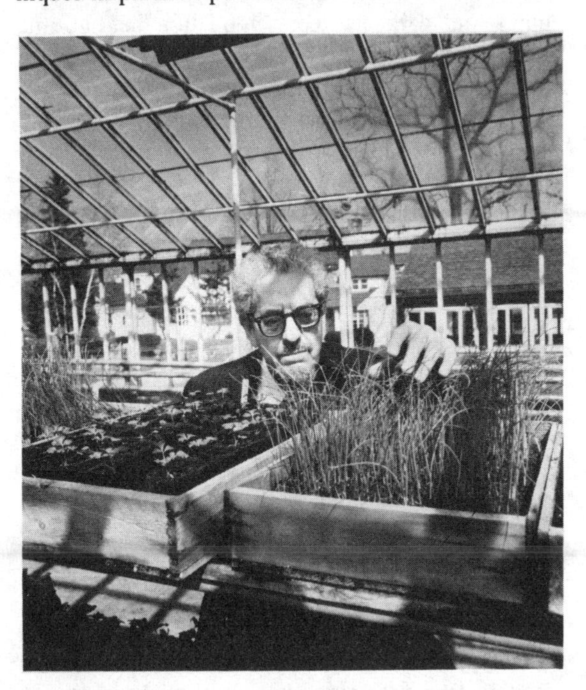

99. Organic food crusader J.I. Rodale (circa 1970). *Courtesy, Rodale Press.*

believe harm the soil, and, ultimately, hurt farmers and consumers.

In its purest, most modern form, organic agriculture not only uses radical techniques, it embraces a visionary philosophy. Indeed, organic philosophy exemplifies the popular saying "you are what you eat," making a direct connection between personal health and planetary well-being.

NO-NAME AGRICULTURE

The word *organic* is of relatively recent vintage. J.I. Rodale's son, Robert Rodale, himself a publisher and environmentalist, traced the word (in its reformist sense) back to British newspapers just after World War I. The term was popularized in North America by J.I. Rodale after he began publishing his monthly magazine *Organic Farming and Gardening* in 1942.

For centuries before the Rodales, peasant farmers practiced organic farming, although they didn't call it that. Indeed, they didn't call it anything; they just sowed the fields and harvested crops. They had no choice, since modern chemical aids didn't exist. Nevertheless, some agricultural peasant societies were very successful, among them the farmers of ancient China and Japan and the pre-Columbian masters of terraced farming in the mountains of South America.

A German chemist named Justus von Liebig changed all that. In the 1840s, von Liebig, considered a founder of the German chemical industry, developed a commercial fertilizer to take the place of humus—the dark, nutrient-rich mixture that old-time farmers spread on the land. Artificial fertilizers rich in nitrogen, von Liebig said, were easier to use than humus, and more effective. Many farmers, especially in Europe and North America, agreed.

But not all. "The reaction to von Liebig was the beginning of organic farming," observed Robert Rodale in a July 1990 interview in his office, just two months before his death in a traffic accident in Moscow. But, Rodale added, "Organic farmers started with a handicap; they didn't have nitrogen and microbes figured out."

Rodale meant that early organic farmers didn't know that the humus they spread on the soil contained living organisms. Moreover, they didn't realize that the legumes they planted drew nitrogen from the air to the soil. In short, organic advocates knew their methods bore fruit—and vegetables and grain—but couldn't explain how or why in scientific language.

Organic farmers gained indirect support from the work of Louis Pasteur, who identified bacteria in the soil in the late nineteenth century. Even before Pasteur, Charles Darwin wrote of benefits from the humble earthworm, which loosens the soil just by digging through it, allowing air and water to reach plant roots. However, intuitive, experiential organic growers were slow to exploit what scientific support they had.

By the early twentieth century, even as chemical farming was growing apace, a small counterforce was sprouting. One of its first champions was F.H. King, a University of Wisconsin professor and soil scientist at the United States Department of Agriculture. In his 1911 book *Farmers of Forty Centuries*, King praised traditional farmers in Japan, China, and Korea, whom he observed first-hand, for preserving the life of the soil. Their crop rotation, intertillage, and use of night soil and decaying plants ("green manure") helped microorganisms flourish, King wrote. King, who intended his book to be a warning, died before he could complete his closing chapter, "Message of China and Japan to the World."

King did not label the traditional farming of the Far East "organic." Nor did a later writer, Sir Albert Howard, a Briton who, in effect, took up where King left off; but in essence that's what the two men wrote about—King in *Farmers of Forty Centuries* and Howard in his 1940 book *An Agricultural Testament*.

Howard, a farmer's son who graduated from Cambridge and served as an advisor in the Indian state of Indore, operated a 75-acre farm based on age-old techniques. Like King, Howard praised traditional peasants. Their methods, he wrote, avoided reliance on soil-depleting monoculture, respected the role of earthworms and burrowing animals, and protected what he called "the mycorrhizal association,

---

A GLOSSARY

Several overlapping terms are used to describe related forms of alternative farming and gardening.

Organic, the oldest term, signifies chemical-free agriculture, which uses refinements of traditional techniques instead of synthetic pesticides and fertilizers.

Sustainable agriculture is designed to enable farmers to strike a balance with nature instead of becoming dependent on soil-depleting chemicals. It may or may not be fully organic, but nearly always emphasizes the reduced use of synthetics.

Regenerative agriculture seeks to enrich the soil and leave it healthier and more fertile than before farmers started working the land. It, too, may or may not be fully organic.

---

the living fungus bridge between humus in the soil and the sap of plants.''

Howard saw the developing, chemical-dependent agriculture of his day as a quick and temporary fix, born of war. ''The factories engaged during the Great War in the fixation of atmospheric nitrogen for the manufacture of explosives had to find other markets'' once peace broke out, he wrote.

Howard assumed, but did not spell out, a connection between the health of society's farms and the health of its citizens. ''Artificial manures,'' he wrote, ''lead inevitably to artificial nutrition, artificial food, artificial animals, and finally, to artificial men and women.'' Howard ended *An Agricultural Testament* with a bold prediction: ''At least half the illnesses of mankind will disappear once our food supplies are raised from fertile soil and consumed in a fresh condition.''

The chemical companies, and most farmers, paid little heed to Howard's erudite but somewhat technical treatise. But he found one unusually dedicated and resourceful reader in the quiet Lehigh Valley city of Allentown, Pennsylvania, 60 miles north of Philadelphia. His name was J.I. Rodale.

SON OF THE CITY

Rodale was no man of the soil—not in 1940, anyway. On the contrary, he was a native son of one of the biggest cities in the world. Born Jerome Irving Cohen in 1898 of Polish-Jewish immigrants, J.I. grew up on New York's famed Lower East Side. He was one of eight children in a family whose name in the old country was Lachofsky. The Cohens lived above the family grocery store, where young Jerry, by his own account, gorged on sweets and fretted about his health.

Like many health reformers, J.I. was sickly as a youngster. Years later, when he had achieved some degree of celebrity, he told *Time* magazine that he was ''the runt of a litter of eight, and not a healthy child.'' His family was evidently not healthy either. J.I.'s father died of a heart attack at age 51, and J.I.'s brothers and sisters died in their fifties and sixties, also of heart ailments.

But like a lot of health reformers, J.I. developed a can-do attitude, and he adopted an eclectic approach to health and fitness. As a young man, he fancied the bodybuilding regimens of Bernarr Macfadden; he and Macfadden even shared the same birthday, August 16. J.I. also devoured the uplifting books of Horatio Alger. ''I slept next to the kitchen stove where I read Horatio Alger stories by gaslight turned to halfmast,'' J.I. recalled. ''The sulphurous fumes drifting out of the coals would furnish vivid colors to the scene where the heroine is tied to the railroad tracks as the Chicago Flyer is bearing down with fiendish relentlessness. I had to watch out for two villains, the one in the book, and my father's heavy forewarning footsteps.''

For a city boy, J.I. had an unusual fascination with farming. But as a young man, he turned to practical matters, attending night school at New York University and Columbia University and later serving a brief stint in Washington, D.C. as an accountant for the Internal Revenue Service. At age 23, to sidestep antisemitism, he changed his surname to Rodale.

In 1930, J.I. Rodale changed cities and careers. He moved with his wife, the former Anna Andrews, and his brother Joe to Allentown, where the brothers ran an electrical manufacturing business in nearby Emmaus. That same year Robert, one of Anna and J.I.'s three children, was born.

Although J.I. was in business making electrical appliances, he never abandoned his fantasy of owning a farm and making himself into a robust man of the soil. In 1940, when he read Sir Albert Howard's book, the linkage between business, farming, and health was forged in Rodale's mind.

''The impact on me was terrific!'' he said of *An Agricultural Testament*. Of Sir Albert, Rodale said ''He changed my whole way of life. I decided that we must get a farm at once and raise as much of our family's food by the organic method as possible.'' That same year, 1940, J.I. bought a farm near Allentown and commenced teaching himself how to grow things.

With characteristic passion, Rodale decried factory-made fertilizers and the synthetic insecticides, rodenticides, fungicides, and herbicides beginning to flood the market. In 1945, in his book *Pay Dirt*, Rodale wrote: ''. . . chemical fertilizers are slowly but definitely killing off the earthworm population . . . strong insect sprays containing lead, arsenic, or copper; lime-sulphurs and tar-oil, etc. destroy earthworms . . . . Nature consists of a chain of interrelated and interlocked life cycles. Remove any one factor and you will find that she cannot do her work effectively. Remove the earthworm, and the bacteria fail to thrive.''

Once he converted to organic farming, Rodale converted completely. Even Sir Albert allowed for the use of chemicals in a pinch. Not Rodale. He struck up a correspondence with Howard, and the two men became friendly. Although they never met, Howard became Rodale's mentor in matters agricultural.

J.I. RODALE, PUBLISHER

With Howard as a long-distance associate editor, Rodale, who had published small newsletters, magazines, and books on the side while he ran the family electrical business, launched the first successful magazine in what would become a growing Rodale "family" of publications. Called *Organic Farming and Gardening*, the first 16-page issue (priced at 10 cents) appeared in 1942—just in time to instruct tillers of World War II "victory gardens." The magazine would prove instrumental in seeding organic gardening and nurturing it until it grew into a movement in the early 1970s.

Ironically, the same year that *Organic Farming and Gardening* appeared, the pesticide DDT came to prominence. DDT (dichlorodiphenyltrichloroethane) was not new; it had been synthesized back in 1874 and adapted as an insecticide in 1939. The Swiss chemist Paul Muller, who turned DDT into a pesticide, won a Nobel Prize for developing what seemed to be a wonderful new tool.

In 1942, the same year that Rodale urged gardeners to spare the sprays, DDT was used on American GIs to kill lice. After the war, DDT was sprayed on plants to kill predatory insects. Not until years later did scientists warn that DDT was stored in human body fat, where it had long-term cancer-causing properties. On January 1, 1973, DDT was banned in the United States, but many nations continued to use it.

While modern agribusiness was pledging allegiance to the " 'cide sisters," Rodale was trying to grow food in unusual ways. One of his ideas, electroculture, centered on J.I.'s belief that plants grew better if they were gently zapped with electricity. So Rodale set up metal cans and wire netting on his experimental farm, the better to jolt the corn and juice up the radishes. The idea never caught on, but there were plenty more where it came from.

Rodale's most productive brainchild, *Prevention* magazine, was born in 1950. Instead of focusing on healthy plants, as did *Organic Farming and Gardening* (called *Organic Gardening and Farming* and just plain *Organic Gardening* at various times), *Prevention* cultivated healthy people.

Prevention was published from a decidedly grassroots perspective. Remembered J.I.: "What *Prevention* soon became was a medical journal for the people, over 90 percent of the material being excerpted from medical journals and other orthodox medical sources, always the name and date of the sources being given, but written so the average person could understand it." Rodale had little truck with doctors. He assumed that people could be their own best doctors, a notion that did not sit well with M.D.s.

Sir Albert Howard died before Rodale got *Prevention* rolling, but J.I. found another cohort in his son, Robert, who went to work as an editor in the family business in 1949. Robert was then all of 19.

"*Prevention* has been a success since day one," Robert Rodale remembered. "When it started, *Organic Gardening* had less than 300,000 circulation. Fifty thousand of them wrote back with money for the first issue of *Prevention*. What's amazing is that no health magazine in America had over 10,000. *Physical Culture* [Macfadden's fitness magazine] had about 100,000, but that wasn't strictly a health magazine. Within a few years, *Prevention* was bigger than *Physical Culture*."

The younger Rodale opined that *Prevention*, which he took over after J.I.'s death in 1971, "has had a big influence on the health culture in America."

IT TAKES A CRANK

J.I. Rodale's personal health regimen was a mixed bag of his own ideas and other health fads.

Standing just over five-feet-six-inches tall, Rodale—who was an avid walker—waged war on flab, dropping his weight from over 200 pounds in early middle age to as low as 170 pounds. Although he was not a vegetarian, Rodale echoed Sylvester Graham by inveighing against smoking, alcohol, and white bread. Rodale, in fact, did not think wheat flour of any kind was healthy.

Like Graham 100 years earlier, Rodale had a long hit list of forbidden items, including milk (for adults), aluminum pots and pans, plastic utensils, food additives, and fluoridated water. Rodale favored raw seeds and vegetables. An obsessive man, he kept a detailed written "history of J.I. Rodale's pulse" in his personal papers. He took some 60 food supplements a day. Once, to test the efficiency of the bone-meal tablets he took to strengthen his frame, Rodale deliberately threw himself down a flight of stairs, bumping and bouncing all the way.

Called a crackpot, a crank, and worse by his opponents, Rodale had a pointed reply: "Even the critics admit it takes a crank to turn things," he said.

The magazine popularized the essential idea that preventing disease is much easier than treating illness once it develops, and went further, linking health to lifestyle. In 1951, *Prevention* published reports on the connection between salt and high blood pressure. In 1952, the monthly warned of the dangers of high-cholesterol diets. In 1954, it urged the health-minded to eat more fish. *Prevention* also warned about the health hazards of smoking at a time when most mass-circulation magazines were afraid to offend powerful tobacco companies that then, as now, bought substantial advertising. (*Prevention* didn't accept tobacco ads, though it did seek ads for other controversial products, such as vitamin supplements designed to be taken in extra-large doses.)

MOMENTUM . . . AND RACHEL CARSON

By the 1960s, *Prevention, Organic Farming and Gardening*, and Rodale's book-publishing arm, all gathered under the Rodale Press umbrella, were building momentum. J.I. Rodale was himself a prolific, self-taught writer who generally published his own books and sold them through mail order. Not all his books were about health or food. His 1947 book *The Word Finder*, designed to help readers digest the English language, was a long-term success. By 1990, the 1,344-page book was still in print, having sold 200,000 copies.

The energetic J.I. also wrote plays—33 of them, according to Rodale biographer Carlton Jackson—although only about 10 were produced. Again, Rodale often footed the bills himself. In the mid-1960s, he even bought his own theater in Manhattan, which he used to stage his plays. His great theme? Health, naturally.

Unfortunately for him, Rodale couldn't buy good reviews. *The New Yorker* judged his 1960 preachment on the evils of sugar, a play called *The Goose*, "perfectly awful," noting with unconcealed disdain that Rodale, having called Adolf Hitler "a sugar drunkard," seemed to blame the dictator's madness on diet. Wrote critic Donald Malcolm of *The Goose*: "It is supremely inept. It is magnificently foolish. It is sublimely, heroically, breathtakingly dreadful. It inspires a sacred terror. It is beyond criticism."

Success was not to come to J.I. Rodale in the world of the theater. In the early 1960s, however, Rodale's health agenda got a big boost, albeit indirectly.

Once again, the agent of change was a book, this time a lyrically written but tough-minded outcry against the dangers of pesticides. Published in 1962, Rachel Carson's *Silent Spring* galvanized American public opinion. Written by a woman with strong scientific credentials, and published by the Houghton Mifflin Company after being serialized in *The New Yorker, Silent Spring* became a classic of environmental literature in a way that Rodale's earnest and intelligent but plodding self-published books never could be.

A marine biologist for the U.S. Fish and Wildlife Service, Carson (1907–1964) was already well-known for her books about the web of life, such as *The Sea Around Us*. With *Silent Spring*, she helped make *ecology* part of the common vocabulary. Carson invested the book with a sense of drama that can be read in her chapter titles: "Elixirs of Death," "And No Birds Sing," and, in a distillation of her philosophy, "The Obligation to Endure."

Carson's prose was no less urgent. DDT and its chemical cousins were different from the crude pesticides of earlier times, she wrote; they were more powerful and more widely and indiscriminately used. She wrote of "new chemicals to which the bodies of men and animals are required somehow to adapt . . . chemicals totally outside the limits of biologic experience." They should, she declared, be called "biocides," since they killed so many forms of life.

Carson outlined the progressive degeneration of ground water, described the destruction of trees and birds, and told how humans were harmed by aerial spraying of suburban neighborhoods to eliminate insects: "It is ironic to think that man might determine his own future by something so seemingly trivial as the choice of an insect spray."

As alternatives to synthetic pesticides, Carson endorsed biological pest controls—in simple terms, setting "good" bugs, such as ladybugs, against "bad" bugs, such as aphids. That would prove more effective, she argued, and far less risky, than employing dangerous broad-spectrum pesticides to wipe out unwelcome insects like the fire ant, which kicked into evolutionary overdrive and adapted to the chemicals.

Just how perceptive Carson was could be seen in a 1990 *New York Times* dispatch about the fire ant:

> The ant's inexorable spread has occurred not only in spite of, but partly because of, nearly four decades of determined campaigns to eradicate it with chemical pesticides. Through it all, the fire ant has thrived because the pesticides destroyed its enemies and paved the way for far larger colonies . . . . An airborne pesticide assault in the 1960s and '70s, designed to eradicate the fire ant from American soil, has been

described by the Harvard biologist Edward O. Wilson as "the Vietnam of entomology."

Carson did not mention Rodale or adopt the term *organic* in her vision of a chemical-free future. But her work could be fairly read as a more sophisticated version of ideas that Rodale had been propounding, and practicing, for years. Rodale and Carson evidently never met. Carlton Jackson reports that Carson made a point of staying at arm's length from people she regarded as cultists and faddists who could compromise her credibility. Once, Jackson writes, Rodale booked himself and the author of *Silent Spring* for a joint lecture appearance and didn't tell Carson he would be there. When Carson found out, she canceled.

IN FROM THE COLD

Rachel Carson's apparent snub notwithstanding—and despite criticism from scientists and medical doctors who considered Rodale's notions of self-care to be quackery—Rodale intensified his crusade against the health establishment. Sometimes the establishment bit back.

In 1964, the Federal Trade Commission, which oversees the American advertising industry, took Rodale Press to court. The cause of the commotion was advertising for *The Health Finder*, an encyclopedia of alternative health treatments that J.I. had published in 1954. The FTC charged that Rodale's ads (which the company modified several years before the court action) falsely promised that the book could tell readers how to prevent and cure a variety of maladies, ranging from colds to cancer.

Rodale countered that the First Amendment to the U.S. Constitution threw a protective blanket of free speech over both the book and its advertising. The American Civil Liberties Union agreed, as did noted constitutional lawyer Thurman W. Arnold, who represented Rodale Press; it was Arnold's last case before he died. The battle dragged out for four years and cost Rodale 250 thousand dollars in legal fees. In 1968, a Federal District Court of Appeals in Washington, D.C. remanded the case to the FTC and the discouraged commission dropped the charges. Rodale had won.

The legal victory did not confer instant respectability on Rodale, but it did strengthen his resolve and drew media attention to his unorthodox, health-minded publishing house. Even as the case dragged on, the *Saturday Evening Post* published a profile of J.I., headlined "Apostle of the Compost Heap." The lengthy piece, though largely favorable, included this observation on J.I.: "Under the niceness, something sad is visible, the man who has had to reach his conclusions by himself, without the correction of more critical minds. He exists in the disabling isolation of the self-educated."

Rodale's isolation, however, was ending, not least because of the *Saturday Evening Post* article. Here was a health radical being accepted, after a fashion, by a magazine that showcased the four-square Americanism of Norman Rockwell and traced its ancestry, however tortuously, to Benjamin Franklin. Next to discover J.I. was the bible of the back-to-the-land counterculture of the 1960s and 1970s, the *Whole Earth Catalog*. Periodicals as disparate as *Barron's*, *Penthouse*, and the *Smithsonian* magazine soon followed. "Before the young people came to us, my magazines were being listened to by a very limited audience," J.I. told *Penthouse*. "Suddenly, these hippies and dropouts who had been making a lot of noise read my writings and found something real . . . . They are buying land and growing food organically."

Finally, in 1971, just a few months shy of his seventy-third birthday, full immersion in the mainstream media arrived. J.I. was the cover story in the *New York Times Magazine*. As with earlier articles in other publications, the profile was favorable, even if it made gentle fun of Rodale's obsessiveness. "Guru of the Organic Food Cult," as the piece was titled, included this quotation from J.I.: "In the old days, I used to get such a clobbering and insulting, you know, and if I wasn't so well-nourished, it would have affected me, but I stood up under it, because I had plenty of vitamin B, which is the nerve vitamin."

Producers of "The Dick Cavett Show" invited J.I. to appear on their popular American Broadcasting Corporation talk show, telecast nationwide. J.I. promptly accepted. The night before the *New York Times* profile appeared—and only two days before he went off to tape the Cavett show—J.I. gave a speech in Allentown. Carlton Jackson describes the scene: "He closed his speech by giving his play schedules for the upcoming month and announcing that soon he intended to take a long trip. Anna, from the front row in the audience, jokingly said 'Good-bye.' "

On June 7, 1971, Rodale was videotaping the Cavett show in ABC's New York studios. He had just finished showing the host a large organic goose egg and explaining how he used a special machine to absorb life-enhancing electricity. "I am so healthy," he told Cavett, "that I expect to live on and on." Just moments later, he was stricken with a massive heart attack. Efforts by doctors in the studio audience and firemen called to revive him failed. The tape was never aired.

The novel way Rodale died threatened to eclipse his life's work; but as his family pointed out, 72-year-old J.I. outlived his father and brothers by 10 to 20 years. His hard-charging style, the strain of sudden attention, and the burden of his advancing years all put great stress on Rodale. The man may have literally been killed by success.

Rodale's death left many things undone. *Organic Gardening and Farming* (as it was then known) noted that he left 40 file drawers filled with clippings he had kept, notes he had made, and books that he planned to read. J.I. was an organic Ben Franklin: a self-made man (almost certainly a millionaire in his later years), a clear and useful writer, a practical man, and an optimist in the American grain. Wrote Robert Rodale:

> I will always remember J.I. Rodale not only as my father, but as the man who taught me to think of myself as an organic person, trying to live in tune with nature, striving always to help improve the environment while working to improve myself, too. That was his message to me and to you, and it will live on for a long time.

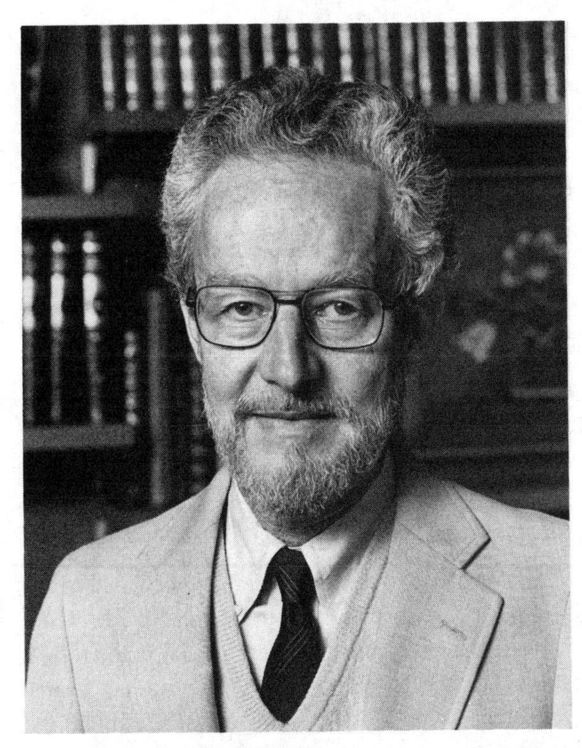

100. Robert Rodale refined his father's theories and extended the reach of Rodale Press. *Courtesy, Rodale Press.*

FATHER TO SON

At age 41, in 1971, Robert Rodale took over Rodale Press. A self-described "dutiful son," he had worked for his father since he was 12 years old. But Robert Rodale had a mind and style of his own. A well-read, well-connected world traveler, he proved to be far less isolated and eccentric than his father had been. Sitting in his modestly appointed office in July 1990, under a framed painting of a furrowed field with green plants stretching to the horizon, Robert Rodale said of J.I.: "He liked controversy. He used argument as a means of getting attention. He was very friendly, he loved people, but he liked to get a rise out of them." Robert, by way of contrast, described himself as "a natural-born soft person."

In his two decades at the helm of the good ship Rodale, Robert Rodale took down a lot of the vessel's odd rigging while staying his father's course. A prolific writer like J.I., Robert Rodale, unlike his father, had a low-key but sophisticated style.

Robert Rodale's death in September 1990 rocked the family-owned company and shocked the environmental movement. Consumer advocate Ralph Nader eulogized Rodale as "a great environmentalist . . . . He took old values and applied them to new technologies and took old technologies and applied them to new values."

Rodale Press survived both J.I.'s and Robert's deaths. Housed in a cluster of low buildings in a peaceful setting the company calls Organic Park, Rodale Press has let part of its lawn revert to meadow. A building that looks like a greenhouse is actually the corporate library. The commissary, located in a refurbished house on Main Street in Emmaus, is called Fitness House.

By 1990, *Prevention* was bigger than ever, with just over three million paid circulation and a total readership of eight million. The firm employed 1,000 people and published 40 to 50 book titles a year, generating 215 million dollars annually with magazines and books. Typically, Rodale books are about gardening, fitness, nutrition, crafts, and self-help; true to Rodale tradition, they are sold mainly through direct mail.

Rodale Press is a company with a mission, even without J.I. or Robert Rodale. In recent years, the historic rift between Rodale and medical doctors has been narrowed; indeed, *Prevention* lists a physicians' advisory board. Even Washington cooperated with Rodale Press in the 1990s. A *Prevention* index, commissioned annually, is used by the U.S. Department of Health and Human Services to evaluate American health habits.

A slender, graying man who seemed younger than his 60 years, Robert Rodale presided over his flurry of activity with soft-spoken authority. Talking to him just before his death, the authors got the impression that Rodale was a calming influence in the overheated world of agriculture, where calm is as rare as a field without weeds.

PANIC

Just as consumers showed signs of heeding doctors' orders to eat more produce, fish, and poultry, the Great Produce Scare of 1989 almost upset the apple cart.

DOWN ON THE FARM

Cynics who expect organic farms to be small and parched would be surprised by the Rodale Research Center, a lush, 305-acre spread in the rolling countryside of eastern Pennsylvania, near Kutztown.

Operated by the nonprofit Rodale Institute (started as the Soil and Health Foundation by J.I. Rodale in 1947), the research center features clean, well-maintained buildings surrounded by green fields and fragrant gardens. A nineteenth-century stone farmhouse graces the grounds near a creek and a 1906 schoolhouse that doubles as a bookstore and visitors' center. A large, solar-heated commercial greenhouse sits nearby, as does a much smaller greenhouse designed to grow vegetables year-round for a family of four.

An apple orchard sits atop a flanking ridge, and is protected by an electric fence to keep deer away. A tour guide takes pains to assure visitors that the fence gives off only the gentlest of jolts. Nearby, a tractor ploughs, bees buzz, and birds sing. It looks like a healthy farm.

Serious research is done at the center, consistent with Robert Rodale's conception of himself and his colleagues as "science writers who make science policy." A full-time scientist from the USDA's Low-Input Sustainable Agriculture project is in residence. The center has done extensive testing of amaranth, a drought-resistant grain. It also pioneers techniques to enable conventional growers to make a transition to organic farming and sponsors gardening workshops and produce tastings for the public.

The year had barely started when the Natural Resources Defense Council released a report asserting that 6,000 American preschool children would eventually develop cancer because of their high consumption of apples and apple products treated with Alar. Alar, the trade name for daminozide, was used to make apples red and firm. With actress Meryl Streep testifying before Congress on behalf of Mothers and Others Against Pesticides and the CBS-TV program "60 Minutes" highlighting the charges, school officials hurriedly pulled apples—even green ones, which weren't treated with Alar—from school menus.

Alar was consequently taken off the market by its maker in 1989. In May 1990, Alar was banned for all food uses by the Environmental Protection Agency. That November, Washington State apple growers, insisting that Alar was safe, sued CBS and the Natural Resources Defense Council, claiming damages of 100 million dollars.

Consumers had barely simmered down when traces of cyanide were found in two red seedless grapes in Philadelphia. The grapes had been imported from Chile, where thousands of laid-off farmworkers complained bitterly about the ensuing U.S. boycott of Chilean fruit. Although the cyanide was apparently injected by an unknown party described in news reports as a would-be terrorist—and was not a residue of pesticides or fertilizers—the discovery again had consumers worrying about the safety of their food.

Their concern was understandable. Statistics on the use of chemical farm aids are staggering. American farmers spend eight billion dollars yearly on fertilizers and five billion more on pesticides. Yet, according to *Newsweek*, "Since the 1950s, insecticide use has increased ten-fold . . . . During the same period, the amount of crops lost to pest damage has doubled." Meanwhile, the World Health Organization reported, one million people around the globe have been poisoned by pesticides and 20 thousand have died—many of them farmworkers in the Third World, where environmental laws are looked upon as indulgences.

The panics of 1989 called food-safety regulations into question. The EPA sets acceptable limits for chemical residues, called "tolerances," but hadn't tested many older chemicals. The Food and Drug Administration, which tests food for contamination, asserted that America's food supply is eminently safe. But the FDA examines only one percent of the nation's food, down from 20 percent in the mid-1970s, before the deregulation fever of the Reagan years struck Washington.

All this has given a powerful boost to organic farming. In a 1989 opinion poll conducted before the Alar and cyanide scares, 84 percent of American consumers quizzed by the Lou Harris Organization said that they would buy organic food if it were available. Forty-nine percent said they would pay more for it.

BETTING THE FARM

On the cusp of the 1990s, organic agriculture was more popular than ever before in the modern era, and was expected to become still more popular if certain problems could be resolved. These included the reluctance of bankers to grant loans to organic farmers, traditional disregard of organic farming by agricultural colleges, the absence of consistent standards for what, exactly, constitutes organic food, high retail prices, and a weak distribution system. (In 1990, demand for organic food outstripped supply by a factor of 10 to 1.)

Its problems notwithstanding, the organic-food industry was worth an estimated 1.25 billion dollars in 1989, up from only 174 million dollars in 1980—and scientific support was growing. In a landmark 1989 study, the National Academy of Sciences concluded that organic farming is viable. Crop yields might be lower, the NAS decided, at least while farmers learned unfamiliar organic methods; but expenditures would also be lower, profits would be about the same, and the health of the soil would be enhanced.

Skeptics still doubt that organic farming can work on the huge scale needed to feed a teeming, hungry world. Moreover, enthusiasts' claims that organic food is tastier and more nutritious than conventionally grown edibles remain unproven. But debate has been joined over this once-scorned and obscure philosophy, and that alone is progress for the agricultural heirs of J.I. Rodale, Rachel Carson, and Sir Albert Howard.

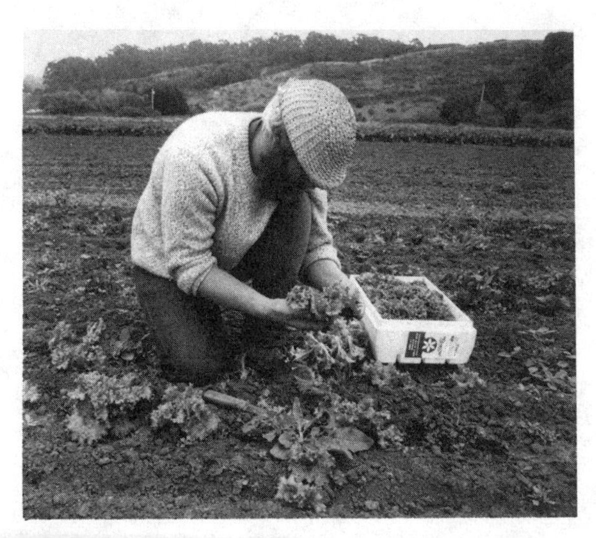

101. Part of the billion-dollar organic food industry, a Bolinas, California grower (1985). *Photo by Chris Hardy,* San Francisco Examiner.

BONNIE PRINCE CHARLIE

In 1990, Prince Charles of Great Britain—who has publicly endorsed organic farming—went into business, marketing bread called Wholemeal Highgrove, after the prince's Highgrove Home Farm in Cornwall. Sold in a British supermarket chain, the bread was made from wheat grown without pesticides at Highgrove and on organic farms in Canada.

CHAPTER
· 24 ·

VITAMINS: THE NEW PATENT MEDICINES?

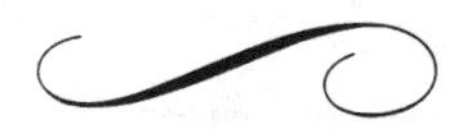

The old-fashioned tonics, which depended for their kick on the content of alcohol, have been replaced by combinations of vitamins and minerals which depend for their kick on the psychological stimulation resulting from professional advertising.

AMERICAN MEDICAL ASSOCIATION,
Hygeia *magazine, 1944*

They're all-natural pep pills. They're miracle cures. They help a body shape up and slim down. They're pumped into such staples as bread and milk, and blended into luxuries such as cosmetics. They're omnipresent on the shelves of supermarkets, drug stores, and health-food stores. Skeptics call them the successors to the old patent medicines. They are, in short, vitamin supplements.

Vitamins—in pills, powders, lotions, oils, and gels—generate half the sales in the three-billion-dollar-a-year U.S. food-supplement industry. Vitamin supplements generate big money for pharmaceutical companies, health practitioners, and advertising agencies. According to the trade publication *Advertising Age*, Miles Laboratories spent 5.8 million dollars to advertise its Flintstones vitamins for children in 1984. Vitamins have been staples of advertising for several generations. In 1944, *Hygeia*, published by the AMA, compared vitamin salesmen to "high-pitch men operating from the radio tailboard."

There are important differences between modern vitamin products and the tonics, bitters, and snake oil of old, to be sure. Vitamins are essential to proper nutrition, even to life. And vitamin supplements, unlike the nostrums sold by ersatz "Indians," "Quakers," and "professors" in the gaslight age, are free from alcohol and narcotics. Vitamins are rarely toxic, especially water-soluble vitamins.

Still, there are distinct similarities in the way patent medicines and vitamins are marketed: Both are sold through appeals to fear (What if I have a terrible disease?) and hope (Product Z can save me). Both are mysteries to most consumers. And both are sold with extravagant claims. So powerful is the vitamin mystique that even unrelated substances are marketed as vitamins. Chief among these is Laetrile, an extract of apricot pits falsely labeled "vitamin B_{17}" and used in unorthodox cancer treatments (and judged worthless by most medical authorities).

Despite all the hyperbole, vitamins are necessarily less than magical. Vitamins are organic com-

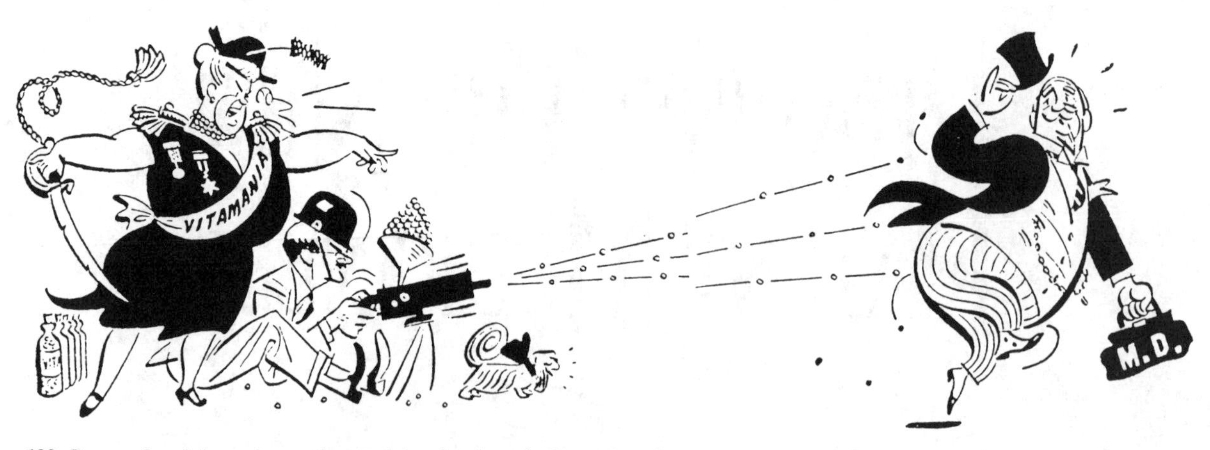

102. Doctors found themselves under attack by vitamin enthusiasts. *From* Hygeia *magazine, April 1942. Courtesy, Office of Publishing, American Medical Association.*

pounds found in plants and animals and are involved in the absorption of nutrients, such as fats, carbohydrates, and proteins. They also take part in the manufacture of hormones, blood cells, and other elements of body chemistry. The water-soluble vitamins—the B-complex and C—are excreted in the urine. The fat-soluble vitamins—A, D, E, and K—are stored in the fatty tissues of the body. There are 13 recognized vitamins, all discovered between 1911 and 1943. In over-the-counter preparations, vitamins are often sold in combination with their inorganic chemical cousins, minerals. Although vitamins are popularly believed to be sources of energy, they're not, because they lack calories.

Scattergun self-care is anathema to most medical doctors, who look down on vitamin crusaders, much as their nineteenth-century predecessors dismissed unlettered Thomsonian herbalists. Thomsonianism, however, is dead, and the vitamin boom is very much with us. As physician/author Michael Halberstam noted, wistfully remembering life before everyone seemed to be gulping vitamin pills:

> Those were the days, the lovely days, when we could sit around the doctors' dining room and tell about examining some nutty woman who was taking 800 units of vitamin E daily, and not have to worry that some colleague across the table would reply that he took 1,600 units and had never felt better.

THE AGE OF DISCOVERY

Long before scientists, doctors, and merchants got into the act, European explorers made important discoveries about vitamins, even without knowing what they were. Back in 1593, British admiral Richard Hawkins gave his men orange and lemon juice and found that scurvy—a vitamin C deficiency disease that causes bleeding gums, swollen limbs, paralysis, and, finally, death—went way down. Unfortunately, Hawkins's example was not widely copied.

Another Briton, eighteenth-century navy physician James Lind, rediscovered lemon juice. The juice again effected cures—until sailors, displaying the light British touch with fresh food, boiled their juice, thereby destroying its vitamin C. Deciding there was nothing to this rubbish about lemons curing scurvy, the gobs stopped using them.

Not for more than a century did scientists unlock the secret of vitamin C and other vitamins. No single researcher discovered vitamins; rather, they were isolated and synthesized through a decades-long international research effort.

In 1906, after Japanese and Dutch researchers had traced beriberi to a lack of protective nutrients in white, fluffy, polished rice, an Englishman, Sir Frederick Gowland Hopkins, healed sick laboratory rats by giving them whole milk. Hopkins hypothesized that a shortage of mysterious substances essential for health—he called them "accessory food factors"—were responsible for some diseases, but he didn't know what the factors were or how they worked.

The mystery substance was finally discovered in 1911 by Casimir Funk, a Polish scientist working at London's Lister Institute. Funk, a brilliant man who wrote and spoke five languages, precipitated rice polishings to get a crystalline substance that, when given to sick birds in very small amounts, restored them to health. The substance was thiamine, (vitamin B_1). Funk used a ton of rice polishings, the discarded hulls and skin of whole rice, to come up with one-sixth of an ounce of crystal.

Then Funk made an intuitive leap, hypothesizing that scurvy, beriberi, rickets (a disease that causes deformed bones), and pellagra (which causes skin discoloration and listlessness) were caused by a lack of vital substances in the diet. Time was to prove him correct. Years later, one of his associates called Funk's insight his "grand generalization," saying Funk had an "imagination more like that of a poet than a scientist."

Funk had something else, too: a gift for language more like that of a public relations wizard. He called the newly discovered substance a "vitamine" —*vita*, for life, and *amine* because he thought it belonged to a class of chemical compounds containing nitrogen. It turns out that Funk was wrong about one thing: The new vital factors weren't amines after all. So scientists knocked off the final letter E. Funk may have been remembered for using the wrong word, but that didn't bother him. "I coined the word to make the whole subject more popular," he told *Newsweek* in 1962.

Following Funk, the American chemist Elmer V. McCollum, a Kansas farm boy with a Yale Ph.D., made more major discoveries. Working at the University of Wisconsin in the 1910s, he found what he dubbed "fat-soluble A" in butter. Scientists now knew there were different types of vitamins.

As new vitamins were discovered, they were given letters, to keep them from bumping into one another in the minds of scientists and nonscientists alike. On the Johns Hopkins University campus in 1922, McCollum pinpointed vitamin D. That same year, at the University of California at Berkeley, Herbert McLean Evans discovered a substance that laboratory rats needed to reproduce: vitamin E.

In another major step, Albert Szent-Gyorgyi synthesized vitamin C in 1934. A Hungarian scientist with a Cambridge Ph.D., Szent-Gyorgyi found the vitamin in the adrenal cortex of cattle and later in fruits and paprika. It was called ascorbic acid, from the Latin for "no-scurvy."

Szent-Gyorgyi won a Nobel Prize for his work on vitamin C, and his was not the only one. A group of researchers won a Nobel in 1934 for their work on vitamin B_{12}. Another Nobel went in 1943 to American biochemist Edward Doiry, Sr., who isolated vitamin K.

As knowledge spread, so did commercial exploitation. Vitamins became faddish. What were once confined to chemists' flasks made their way into health-food stores and drugstores (supermarkets came later), where people who just weren't feeling up to par could buy them in supplement form. As early as 1921, when most vitamins were still to be discovered, an American book called *The Vitamine Manual* noted: "Today in magazines, newspapers and street car advertisements people are urged to use this or that food or medicament on the plea of its vitamine content."

"VITAMANIA"

Like eager advertisers, health practitioners in the margins of mainstream medicine were quick to see the potential of food supplements in general and vitamins in particular—and to use the new food factors in their practice.

One such practitioner was an Iowa chiropractor by the name of Forrest C. Shaklee. Shaklee, whose family name is perpetuated in the Shaklee Corporation's line of vitamins, minerals, cosmetics, and household goods, was a renaissance man of alternative medicine. Born in 1894 on a farm near Carlisle, Iowa, Shaklee was, by age 24, owner and operator of a 15-bed clinic that included under one roof chiropractors, osteopaths, and surgeons. He was also a liberal dispenser of food supplements, one of the first practitioners in any discipline to make heavy use of them.

Before going into business for himself, Shaklee was a fan of Bernarr Macfadden, devouring Macfadden's *Physical Culture* magazine and swearing by his books. In 1912, as a lad of 18, Shaklee went to work for Macfadden, then touring the heartland performing feats of strength in lyceums, Grange halls, and theaters. Shaklee pulled down five dollars a week, plus room and board. One of his duties on stage was to grunt and grimace as he lifted a heavy-looking iron ball that was, in fact, hollow.

After toiling for Macfadden, Shaklee traveled with a Professor Santinelli, who pretended to hypnotize him before rapt backcountry audiences while Shaklee pretended to be hypnotized. But Shaklee was not a simple charlatan. He had heard touring Chautauqua lecturers as a boy—the populist orator and failed presidential candidate William Jennings Bryan was a Shaklee houseguest—and he proceeded to blend self-improvement and show business.

When he was in his twenties, Shaklee claimed to have been cured of appendicitis by a chiropractor and decided to become a chiropractor himself. He studied in Davenport, Iowa under B.J. Palmer, the irascible son of chiropractic's founder, D.D. Palmer. Shaklee brought his show-business flair to his new profession, piloting his own two-seat Curtiss airplane to house calls in far-off towns. At Palmer College's annual lyceum in 1919, Shaklee's plane buzzed a big parade that featured a 50-foot-long replica of a spine.

As early as 1915, Shaklee hawked food supplements. He called them Vitalized Minerals—extracts from legumes that he made into tablets high in iron and calcium. He corresponded with Casimir Funk to learn everything he could about the exciting new vitamin discoveries. According to Georges Spunt's biography of Shaklee, *When Nature Speaks*, the eclectic young chiropractor used vitamin- and mineral-rich foods to cure himself of a skin cancer that he believed he had gotten from diagnostic X-rays. Doctors in the Mayo Clinic, writes Spunt, had given Shaklee up as a hopeless case.

That was in 1921–22. In 1931, Shaklee moved with his family to California, where he opened a new clinic in Oakland. Again, he used supplements—alfalfa pills and the like—which he made by enlisting his young sons, Forrest, Jr. and Raleigh, to fill capsules after school. Eventually, the elder Shaklee decided to dispense with doctoring altogether and just sell the supplements, along with doses of his self-improvement philosophy, which he called by the trademarked name Thoughtsmanship.

In 1956, the Shaklee Corporation was founded in Oakland with five salespeople on the payroll, plus Shaklee's sons and their wives. Fusing faith in supplements and the chance to earn money by selling supplements door-to-door, Shaklee laid the foundation for a lucrative business.

Science and technology made empires like Shaklee's possible, even though scientists knew little about how vitamins worked in the body. But precisely because so little was known, much could be claimed (or at least implied).

A Sunkist advertisement for California oranges, published in the *Saturday Evening Post* in 1924, emphasized that oranges had "vitamines and rare salts and acids in most attractive form." The ad copy didn't name any vitamin (vitamin C hadn't been discovered yet), but extolled the health-giving properties of oranges and even hinted that the fruit would prove useful in winning friends and influencing people.

Once vitamin supplements became available, the novel little pills were seen as near-magic. A 1932 *Scientific American* article cited a study purporting to show that vitamin A halved lost time in the workplace. In 1942, union members demanded of the Empire Ordinance Corporation of Philadelphia that they be supplied with vitamin pills on the job—

MEGASTATS

Virtually all the statistics associated with the modern vitamin industry are big numbers:

- In 1990, U.S. sales estimates for vitamin supplements ranged from 1.3 billion dollars to 1.7 billion dollars a year.
- Forty percent of adult Americans in the late 1980s took vitamin supplements. White, middle-class women were the heaviest users.
- A 1987 Gallup Poll estimated that 12 million American adults take vitamin C for colds.
- Devotion to vitamins and other supplements doesn't stop with regular folks. In a 1988 survey, 60 percent of the registered dietitians in the state of Washington said they took nutritional supplements of some kind.
- Earl Mindell's *Vitamin Bible*, a self-help book written by a former pharmacist, sold 3.5 million copies in the United States by 1990 and was translated into 12 languages.

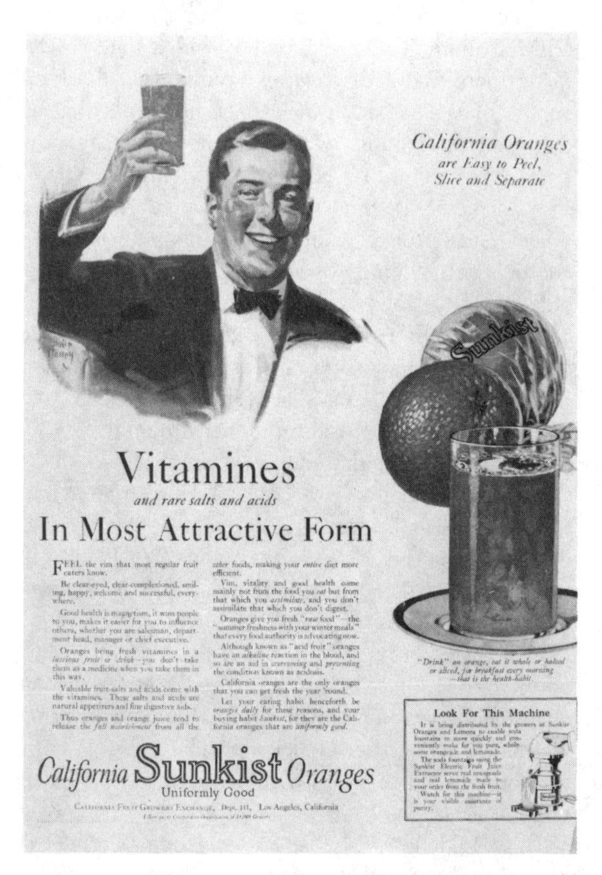

103. One of the first advertisements for vitamin-rich foods. *From* Saturday Evening Post, *1924. Reproduced with permission from Sunkist Growers, Inc.*

and the company agreed to provide them. That same year, *Time* magazine reported that vitamins "are now the largest single class of products handled by wholesalers" serving pharmacies.

Early on came warnings that the new food factors should come from a balanced diet alone. According to a 1921 issue of *Harper's Monthly*: "The daily diet of the average American family seems to provide a sufficiency of vitamins, although as a nation we are backward in gustatory culture, and some of us are no less than feeble-minded in the selection of our food . . . . It is better to buy our vitamins of the greengrocer than the apothecary."

That such advice was rarely heeded is evident from this comment in the *New Republic*, which briefly turned its attention in 1939 from politics to health:

> The list of products that can be bought with vitamins lengthens every day: milk, soap, chewing gum, garlic, yeast, cosmetics, mineral oil, candy and Lydia Pinkham's Vegetable Compound . . . . That there is a big element of voodoo in the public passion for vitamins goes without saying, as an astonishingly large proportion of the American public doesn't feel very well and are looking for some magical elixir of youth.

Not surprisingly, medical doctors deplored the search for an elixir of youth, and virtually equated vitamins with discredited patent medicines. In a *Hygeia* article puckishly headlined "Vitamania," the writer remarked, "Why the patent medicine men don't get wise . . . and sell their stuff by its chemical designation instead of using patent medicine names is hard to see."

But not all doctors shared the AMA's concerns about vitamins, or its caution in using megadoses.

HEART OF THE MATTER: THE DOCTORS SHUTE

One of the first sustained uses of vitamin megadoses to cure chronic diseases—not just to wipe out deficiencies—was spearheaded by Canadian medical doctors Evan V. Shute and Wilfred Shute. Starting in the 1930s, the Shutes (who were brothers) used vitamin E to treat rheumatic fever, traumatic burns, acne, and—most controversial of all—heart disease.

Vitamin E is a strange vitamin, in part because there is no apparent deficiency disease associated with it. Nevertheless, it has an important role in normal body development. Vitamin E helps form red blood cells and protects vitamin A and essential fatty acids from oxidation. It eases leg cramps, and its antioxidant properties help prevent blindness in newborn infants who require extra oxygen. In addition, vitamin E attacks free-radical particles, believed to be the key components in aging.

But while mainstream medicine recognizes some uses of vitamin E, most physicians did not, and do not, accept it as a treatment for heart disease, holding that reputable scientific studies have not established vitamin E's utility as a heart-saver.

The Shutes believed otherwise. Maintaining that vitamin E sends oxygen to the heart, the brothers used vitamin E to treat their mother's angina attacks. When *Time* wrote about the Shutes in 1954, interest in their work soared. They began lecturing widely and welcomed a stream of visitors to their clinic in London, Ontario. But when tests didn't support their claims for the vitamin, the Shutes were barred from addressing major medical conferences. The headaches didn't end there: The U.S. Post Office barred vitamin E literature with unproven claims from the mails.

Medical and governmental opposition did little, however, to slow public interest in vitamin E. One of the visitors to the Shutes' clinic was J.I. Rodale, the millionaire organic farmer and publisher. Rodale was impressed. He began taking 1,200 International Units of E every day (24 times the 1990 Recommended Dietary Allowance) to control pain from angina attacks and treat a heart murmur. "I am sure the Shutes saved my life," Rodale wrote in his 1969 book *My Own Technique of Eating for Health*.

Indeed, Rodale was avid, writing "my mental capacity . . . has improved at least 300 percent since I began taking vitamin E . . . ." Rodale, who was to die of a heart attack at age 72, also wrote of vitamin E: "I am sure it is keeping me from having a heart attack." He claimed, perhaps correctly, that glowing articles about vitamin E in his *Prevention* magazine helped "several millions of persons" to learn about the unorthodox uses of the vitamin.

By 1972, sales of vitamin E had soared 500 percent in just a year or two, rivaling even sales of vitamin C, which Linus Pauling extolled for treatment of colds in those same years. "It's the most versatile vitamin," Evan Shute, a gynecologist by training, said of vitamin E to *Newsweek* in 1972. He added, "It provides better circulation and enhances the power of the muscles. Almost nothing in the body wouldn't be improved by a large intake of vitamin E." Wilfred Shute's book, *Vitamin E for Ailing & Healthy Hearts*, became a fixture in health-food stores at about the same time.

The Shutes' Ontario clinic experienced a boom in the 1970s. When American journalist John J.

Fried visited the Shutes in the mid-1970s, he dismissed vitamin E as "snake oil for the heart," but noted that the thriving clinic had by then treated some 30 thousand patients.

It was no wonder. Shortly before Fried's visit, vitamin E and the Shutes got a timely endorsement by a prominent nutritionist whose own popularity was on the upswing. The nutritionist—impressed by the Shutes' vitamin E work with burn victims—extended her enthusiasm to the vitamin's anti-cancer potential. "Vitamin E, mark my word, will be recognized as very important in prevention of cancer," she told the press in 1972, and the press duly marked her words. The nutritionist was a controversial health crusader named Adelle Davis.

"VITAMIN DAVIS"

Adelle Davis was born in 1904, on a Union Township, Indiana farm. As a Purdue University undergraduate, classmates gave her the nickname "Vitamin Davis." Transferring to the University of California at Berkeley, she earned a degree in dietetics in 1927, adding a master's degree in biochemistry from the University of Southern California.

After college, Davis drew up personalized nutritional programs at Bellevue Hospital in New York City. Later, she became a private consultant, treating some 20 thousand clients, one of whom was the cigar-smoking comic actor W.C. Fields.

But while Davis's academic and early professional background were mainstream, she adopted unconventional views on nutrition, and it was her forceful articulation of those views that won her popular acclaim.

Davis wrote four best-selling books: *Let's Cook It Right* (1947), *Let's Have Healthy Children* (1951), *Let's Eat Right to Keep Fit* (1954), and *Let's Get Well* (1965). The books were as determinedly upbeat as their titles; *Let's Eat Right to Keep Fit* was dedicated "to the perfection that is you." They were also filled with hair-raising descriptions of vitamin deficiencies and written in a style that blended can-do philosophy with a desire for academic respectability; *Let's Get Well* had 2,042 footnotes. Even so, Davis's critics, many in academia, complained that she oversimplified scientific studies cited in her books.

Such complaints didn't stop the public from snapping up Davis's writings, stuffed as they were with recipes and recommended megadoses of vitamins, minerals, and other nutrients. Parents of young children, older people looking for rejuvenation, and college students were Davis's staunchest supporters. Although Davis was not a vegetarian and sometimes scolded health-food proprietors for scientific shortcomings, her books were big sellers in their stores.

Finally, in the early 1970s, when Davis was in her late sixties, the journalistic establishment discovered her. Reporters journeyed to her home overlooking the Pacific in Palo Verdes Estates near Los Angeles, where Davis and her husband, a retired accountant, nurtured an organic garden and fruit trees, played tennis, and swam in their backyard pool.

Davis became so ubiquitous that the *New York Times Magazine* said of her in 1973: "Like Elijah, the Passover prophet, she is an unseen presence at the dinner table, advising us and admonishing us on every morsel we swallow." *Look* magazine described the short, somewhat plump, blue-eyed, gray-haired nutritionist by observing, "the voice fits the woman: gravelly, direct, punctuated by an indignant laugh."

Davis thrived on idiosyncrasy. She experimented with the mind-expanding drug LSD when it was still legal, writing a book about her experiences, *Exploring Inner Space*, under the pseudonym Jane Dunlap. A veteran of psychoanalysis, Davis was quick to comment when she believed disease had a psychosomatic dimension. But she blamed most illness on malnutrition—and her prescriptions were irregular indeed.

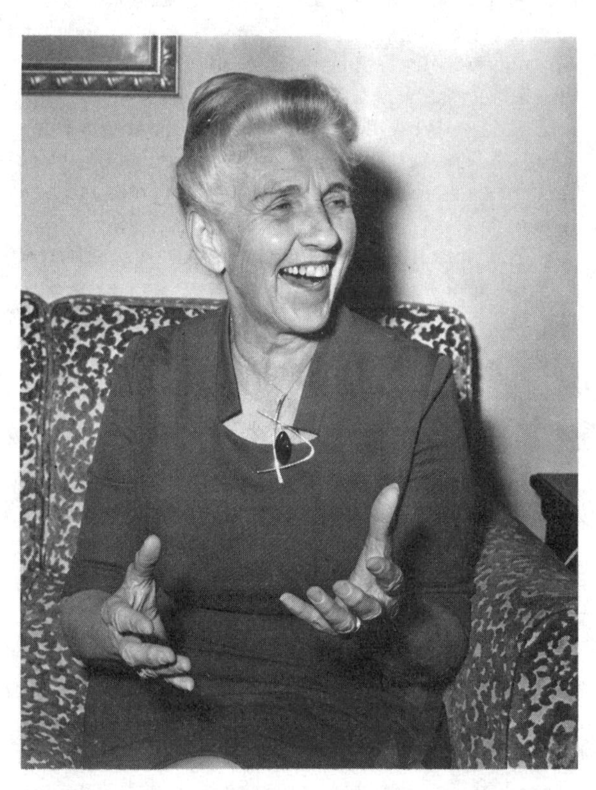

104. Adelle Davis in San Francisco (1971). *Photo by Walt Lynott,* San Francisco Examiner.

In 1962, the *San Francisco Examiner* reported that Davis had said that "normal breasts have developed after flat-chested women from 20 to 35 have conscientiously followed an excellent nutrition program." Three years later, in *Let's Get Well*, Davis endorsed the notion that Germany conquered France in World War II because unrefined German rye bread and vitamin-rich beer were nutritionally superior to refined white French bread and wine. In the same book, Davis wrote of curing a nurse of cancer when the patient took 600 daily international units of vitamin E.

Davis herself practiced a regimen believers dubbed "supernutrition." She took nine vitamin and mineral supplements per day and started each morning with a liquid booster called Pep-up. Whipped in a blender, Pep-up included egg yolks, lecithin, yogurt bacteria culture, and powdered magnesium oxide, among other things, and was dominated by the unforgettable taste of brewer's yeast.

At the peak of her popularity in the early 1970s, Davis's outspoken views and crusty personality made her a sought-after lecturer and television talk-show guest. But as her popularity rose, her standing among academic colleagues nose-dived in almost direct proportion.

STAR POWER

Vitamins, like other consumer goods, have long been sold through their identification with celebrities.

The already-popular vitamin C got another boost in 1979 when writer Norman Cousins published his best-selling book *Anatomy of an Illness*, in which he recounted his use of vitamin C megadoses (plus heaping helpings of humor) to cure his arthritis-like disease back in 1964.

During the vitamin boom of the 1970s and 1980s, the public prints were full of celebrity nutritional tips. Pop poet Rod McKuen told *People* magazine he just had no energy without his vitamins in a 1980 spread on star nutrition. Seven years later, *People* reported that the latest fad was snorting vitamin B_{12} gel for a fast, natural high.

In a reversal of this trend, some people became celebrities because of vitamins. In the 1980s, Dr. Harry B. Demopoulos, who packaged vitamin- and amino-acid supplements to reverse the aging process, was cast in *Sudden Impact* and *The Dead Pool* by one of his "name" clients, Clint Eastwood.

In the spring of 1973, Davis met critics face-to-face in a nutritional summit conference in Washington, D.C. Press reports characterized the meeting as confrontational. Some critics lambasted Davis for her recommendation of vitamin megadoses for a range of maladies. Others let her have it for endorsing commercial health-food products.

Matters came to a head later in 1973, when 20 University of California faculty members signed a letter protesting Davis's scheduled speech at the university's centennial bash. The professors castigated Davis for "perverting her training in the science of nutrition for her own personal gain with complete disregard for scientific truth."

Davis spoke as planned and fired back at her critics, accusing them of being trapped in their ivory towers and laboratories: "I have seen inflammation of blood vessels disappear with the help of vitamin E. And I have seen vitamin E help varicose veins. My critics wouldn't know because they never looked at anyone's legs, except a rat's."

Only a few months after the Berkeley controversy, Davis was diagnosed with cancer.

"I was dumbfounded," she said. "I just couldn't believe it. Cancer is one disease I was sure I would never get." But, Davis informed her shaken followers, she had eaten junk food after leaving the family farm and before adopting a healthy lifestyle in the 1950s. She had also been exposed to environmental toxins and extensive medical X-rays. "Whether I have cancer or not doesn't for one moment nullify the validity of my work," she insisted.

Hospital chemotherapy failed to arrest the spread of the disease. In 1974, about a year after the diagnosis, Davis died of bone cancer. She was 70 years old. At the time of her death, her books had sold nine million copies.

LINUS PAULING AND VITAMIN C

Despite her renown, even Adelle Davis was eclipsed in the pop nutrition field by one immensely influential figure: Linus Pauling. It was Pauling who, nearly single-handedly, made vitamin C a bestseller, first for treatment of colds and later for almost everything else.

Pauling is a two-time Nobel Prize winner, his first prize awarded in 1954 for chemistry (he studied the chemical bonding of atoms) and the second, in 1962 for peace. A long-time foe of nuclear-bomb testing, he warned about the health dangers of radioactive fallout; in 1957, he enlisted 2,000 scientists to sign a petition opposing atomic tests. After Albert Einstein, Pauling is probably the best-known scientist of the twentieth century.

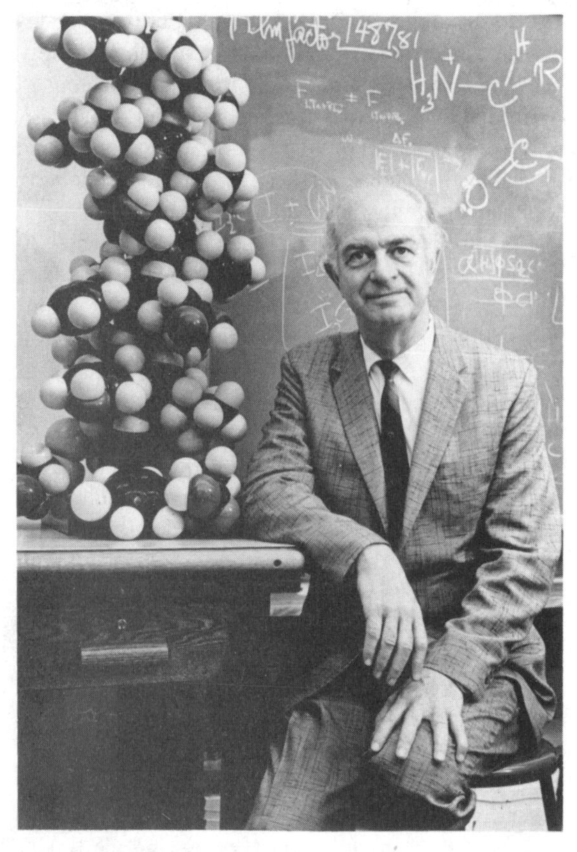

105. Nobel Prize-winning chemist Linus Pauling in his prime (1950s). *Linus Pauling Institute of Science and Medicine.*

Long before he championed vitamin C, Pauling was interested in health issues. In 1960, he called for a five-billion-dollar crash program to switch scientists from military to health research. In 1964, he called cigarette smoking a greater health hazard than nuclear testing. Perhaps Pauling's interest in medical matters was inherited; his father, a druggist, sold a product called Pauling's Pink Pills for Pale People. "I don't know what was in them," Linus admitted years later.

The future famous chemist was born in Portland, Oregon in 1901. He attended Oregon State University, did graduate work in Europe, and spent most of his adult life as a college professor, notably at the California Institute of Technology.

Pauling was 65 and rich with honors when he turned his attention to vitamin C. His interest was piqued in 1966 when biochemist Irwin Stone told him about the vitamin's magical powers. Stone wasn't the first to think that way; the *Ladies' Home Journal* had called vitamin C the "Mystic White Crystal of Health" in 1936.

Pauling and his wife, Eva, began taking three grams of vitamin C per day—50 times the RDA. They decided they felt marvelous and, oddly, never seemed to get colds. Pauling began to think hard about vitamin C.

Vitamin C is essential in the production of collagen fibrils, the long chains of protein that strengthen the intercellular cement of the body. It also helps prevent the oxidation of other vitamins and helps maintain teeth and bones. Vitamin C is found naturally in greens, peppers, potatoes, and, as James Lind might have guessed, in citrus fruits.

Although Pauling became fascinated by what vitamin C could do for the body, he first concentrated on what it might do for the mind. The vitamin had been used by a handful of psychiatrists to treat mental illnesses such as schizophrenia since the 1950s. In his 1968 book *Orthomolecular Medicine*, Pauling reasoned that mental illness might be caused by insufficient vitamin C or B vitamins in the brain, producing "cerebral scurvy" or "cerebral pellagra."

His thesis caused a stir in scientific circles, but it was nothing compared to the fuss Pauling kicked up with his book *Vitamin C and the Common Cold*, published in 1970 (and revised to include influenza). Pauling recommended taking one gram per hour at the first sign of a cold, and continuing for several days after symptoms disappeared. Such tactics would make colds obsolete, Pauling said. "I foresee the achievement of this goal, perhaps within a decade or two, for some parts of the world," he told the *San Francisco Chronicle*.

Mass-circulation magazines, always barometers of a changing cultural climate, declared the consumer demand for vitamin C to be a bona fide phenomenon. ". . . Vitamin C is one of the fastest-growing diet fads in the nation," *Newsweek* reported in 1970. Indeed, sales of vitamin C jumped 20-fold in the East and Midwest that winter, challenging vitamin makers to keep up with demand. When manufacturers turned to unlabeled sodium ascorbate, the Food and Drug Administration recalled 105 million tablets, saying they were dangerous to people on low-sodium diets.

Pauling's endorsement launched a flurry of studies, most of which concluded that vitamin C lessens the severity and duration of colds but does not prevent them. "People who think vitamin C cures colds," said one researcher, "will continue to use it, regardless of the scientific data. Americans today are a medication-taking public, for whom strong emotional appeals often override scientific facts."

Pauling dropped another bombshell at the end of the decade, in a 1979 book he wrote with Scottish physician Ewan Cameron. In *Cancer and Vitamin C*, Pauling and Cameron wrote that megadoses of vitamin C—10 or more grams a day—helped many cancer patients in Cameron's Scottish hospital and cured some, especially when combined with radiation and surgery.

Pauling and Cameron argued that vitamin C works by activating the body's immune system. According to Pauling and Cameron, vitamin C inhibits the production by tumors of the enzyme hyaluronidase, which eats away at nearby normal cells. In other words, vitamin C may fight cancer by isolating diseased cells rather than by blasting them.

That argument is considered unproven at best by conventional oncologists, who criticize Pauling and Cameron for failing to conduct double-blind studies, in which one group of patients is given vitamin C while another group gets a placebo.

In 1979, the Mayo Clinic concluded that vitamin C was of no value in fighting cancer, but Pauling protested that "nearly all of the patients in the Mayo Clinic control group had extensive courses in chemotherapy, while only four percent of Dr. Cameron's patients took anticancer drugs. We believe that chemotherapy suppresses the immune system." The Mayo Clinic did a second test, again concluding that the vitamin was of no value. Again, Pauling objected, saying that the Mayo doctors hadn't given patients vitamin C for a long enough time.

Scientists blasted Pauling for daring to leave his field of expertise. Pauling received exceptionally harsh treatment. His papers were rejected by important journals. His requests for government funds to study vitamin C and cancer were rejected. It was rough going indeed for a man whom the respected British magazine *New Scientist* had named as one of the 20 most important scientists of all time. To make tough times sadder, Eva Pauling was diagnosed with cancer. She had been taking three grams of vitamin C a day before the disease was diagnosed. Given six months to live, she upped her dose to ten grams and survived for five years. She died of cancer in 1981.

Pauling got some support from prominent vitamin researchers. At a Stanford University symposium, Albert Szent-Gyorgyi, the man who discovered vitamin C, revealed that he took four grams per day—but not to fight colds. He took wheat germ for that. In a 1978 interview, Szent-Gyorgyi said of his discovery: "Ascorbic acid is not a special remedy for colds. What it does is make your machinery work better, so that your body is stronger and healthier."

Despite the general lack of support in scientific circles, Pauling stood by his increasingly unconventional conclusions. "All progress is heresy," he said in 1981. "My earlier work in chemistry was just as unconventional . . . . Always, I have tried to stick close to nature, stick close to the facts, but not be constrained by conventional wisdom."

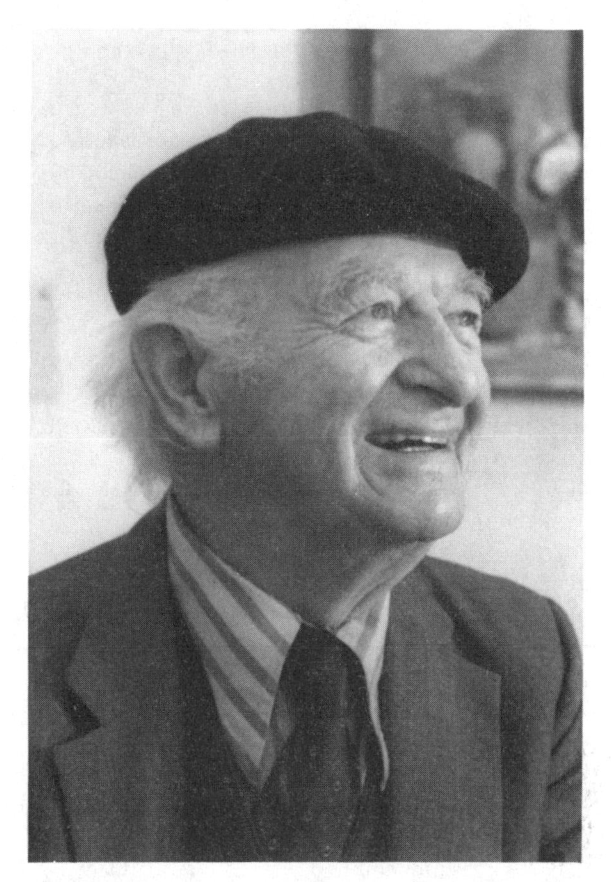

106. Linus Pauling posits vitamin megadoses as key to longevity (1980s). *Linus Pauling Institute of Science and Medicine.*

If anything, Pauling's ideas became more unconventional with the passage of time. In his 1986 book *How to Live Longer and Feel Better*, Pauling revealed that he took 18 daily grams of his favorite vitamin—300 times the RDA. He also recommended megadoses of vitamins A, B-complex, and E, along with exercise and no smoking, in his recipe for longevity, which was published when the author was 85.

SLOW DANCE OF THE REGULATORS

All these dizzying developments did not go unnoticed by government regulators.

Washington first tried to impose order on the vitamin boom in 1941, when the Recommended Daily Allowances were inaugurated. The RDAs were given fresh impetus during World War II, when authorities decided that a well-nourished citizenry was a weapon in the national arsenal. Fortification of foods was also pushed hard during wartime. Vitamin B_1 lost in refined flour was replaced in "vitaminized" bread, and vitamin C destroyed by pasteurization was put back in milk.

In 1962, the FDA decided to impose new regulations on the vitamin industry. Special claims for ingredients not recognized as essential in human nutrition could not be made on product labels, for example. But industry opposition short-circuited the rules.

In 1966, the FDA tried again. This time, it proposed regulations that would establish minimum and maximum amounts of essential nutrients and require a statement on labels acknowledging that sufficient vitamins could be obtained from food, except in special cases. The Pharmaceutical Manufacturers Association sued in federal court and the regulations were aborted.

In 1972, the FDA decided to establish maximum amounts of vitamins in over-the-counter supplements. "These regulations have been compared to the Volstead Act," said one commentator, alluding to the ill-fated prohibition of alcohol. "And when you take away a man's beer and his vitamins, you're in for some real trouble."

Just how much trouble soon became evident. After the FDA decided, in 1973, that large amounts of vitamins A and D would be available only with a doctor's prescription, 15 lawsuits—one of them by Linus Pauling—challenged the agency. Well-organized resisters, supported by the pharmaceutical and vitamin industries and consumer groups such as the American Association of Retired Persons, flooded Congress with angry letters. At a time when the Vietnam war was raging and the Watergate scandal was seeping into the news, Senator Edward Kennedy's office reported receiving more mail about the vitamin restrictions than on any other issue.

In 1975, a federal judge ruled that the FDA regulations were basically sound, but ordered more public hearings. Rather than face still more opposition, the FDA rescinded the prescription-only rule.

The bitter battle divided consumer groups. The Public Citizen Health Research Group, founded by consumer advocate Ralph Nader, had supported the regulations. "Vitamins are the patent medicines—the snake oil—of our age," said a Public Citizen spokesman, reviving the oft-made comparison. "And the FDA has backed down under terrific pressure . . . ."

After 1962 and 1966, 1972–75 was strike three, and federal regulators were out, at least for a while.

FUTUREAMA: HOPE AND HYPE

At the start of the 1990s, vitamins were still seen in hyperbolic terms, marketed by high-powered commercial interests, regarded by millions of consumers as alternatives to conventional medicine—drugless drugs, in a sense—and derided as the tools of quacks by many physicians.

The Shaklee Corporation was healthy, although its colorful founder, Forrest C. Shaklee, Sr., was gone; he died in 1985 of a heart attack, at age 91. The "doctor," as he was known, had steadily built the family business, taking it public in 1973. Even after the Shaklee company hired outside managers and sold stock, it held annual sales conventions where go-getters listened to the doctor's quasi-religious talks (he was an ordained Church of Christ minister) and sang songs like "I Can, You Can, We Can, the Shaklee Way."

The Shaklee Corporation went the way of many American businesses in 1989, when it was purchased by a large Japanese concern, the Yamanouchi Pharmaceutical Corporation, and took to running ads in the lucrative Japanese market that featured a 355-pound sumo wrestler. The American division, which left Oakland in the 1960s, was headquartered in a high-rise building sheathed in sleek silver aluminum in San Francisco.

Twenty years after J.I. Rodale's death, Rodale Press continued to ply *Prevention* subscribers with direct-mail appeals replete with testimonials and exhortations to buy mail-order books that promised the inside scoop on a "supervitamin," a "miracle substance," or a "smart pill." "Take 2 each day," trumpeted one Rodale mail-out, "and call me when you're 100!"

Pop nutrition books continued to discuss vitamins in near-religious terms. A 1990 book entitled *All Women Are Healers* declared "the patriarchy's tampering with Goddess Earth makes supplementation necessary."

Medical science is still debating who needs supplements and how much is enough. Enthusiasts believe the need for vitamins varies widely from person to person, while most medical authorities insist that only minute amounts are needed by all but very sick people. The anti-vitamin forces argue that a balanced diet provides all the essential vitamins, making supplements a waste of money. But vitamin boosters say that supplements provide nutritional insurance for dieters, fast-food addicts, and people who skip meals. Gradually, vitamins are being found to be useful in preventing and controlling disease, but in very specific situations and under medical supervision, not in self-administered megadoses. A 1989 study of 23 thousand pregnant women showed that folic acid (a B vitamin) and iron supplements reduced the rate of neural-tube birth defects by three-fourths. Other studies showed that injections of vitamin A were very effective against measles, a major killer of children in the Third World.

The brilliant first generation of laboratory explorers passed into history when the last survivor, Albert Szent-Gyorgyi, died of kidney failure at age 93 in 1986. True to form, the discover of vitamin C was productive to the end. Just days after his death, he earned a U.S. patent for chemical compounds designed to stabilize the immune system.

In 1991, Linus Pauling was 90. With his wispy white hair, bushy eyebrows, alert, amused eyes, and trademark black beret, he looked like the popular conception of a genius. Pauling headed a staff of 50 and oversaw a budget of three million dollars, much of it devoted to vitamin research, at the Linus Pauling Institute of Science and Medicine in Palo Alto, California. In the fall of 1990, he announced test results, unconfirmed by other researchers, that suggested vitamin C may play a key role in the fight against AIDS.

CHAPTER · 25 ·

DIETING CRAZES: REDUCTIO AD ABSURDUM

History furnishes us with an amazing succession of dietary cranks. Some of them have been possessed with a fanatical sincerity; others have been motivated largely by the opportunity for pecuniary gain; but the one thing that has, as a rule, characterized fanatic and charlatan alike, has been the basic lunacy of their systems.

CARL MALMBERG
Diet and Die, *1935*

William Banting loved to eat; he also suffered from a lifetime fear of fat. As the London undertaker approached his middle years, he watched his bulging midsection with horror. Desperately, he tried every reducing cure he knew—rowing, bathing, horseback riding, Turkish baths, diuretics, and purgatives—all to no avail. By the time he was 65 years old, he packed 202 pounds on his five-foot-five-inch frame and could barely walk up the stairs.

Then a surgeon specializing in diabetes put him on a diet of lean meat, dry toast, and vegetables. Banting lost 35 pounds in nine months. A year later he had trimmed off another 15.

Eager to share his success with the world, Banting wrote a book about his regimen that, to the delight of his readers, encouraged daily nips of alcoholic beverages. The year was 1863. By 1902, Banting's *Letter on Corpulence* had gone through 12 editions and proved as popular in America as in England. On both sides of the Atlantic, ''banting'' became the popular term for dieting.

In Banting's day, the majority of Americans still preferred a bit of meat on their bones; slimness too often signaled the dreaded consumption, and fat was equated with health and vigor. These were the days before bathroom scales and ready-made clothes that would automatically identify consumers by weight and clothing size, before calorie-counting would become a national obsession, and before slim was in and stout was out.

Yet by the turn of the twentieth century, banting was beginning to attract many a figure-conscious American, particularly upper-class women, for whom slimness was a sign of status. By the end of World War I, the craving for a svelte body had crept into the middle classes as well, and the dieting culture as we know it today became as American (and at times, ironically, as fattening and unhealthy) as apple pie.

FASHION VERSUS HEALTH

The first modern diet faddists in the United States were the Grahamites, followers of Sylvester Graham, who, in the years before the Civil War, advocated a diet of whole-wheat bread and meatless, fat-free meals. Unlike most twentieth-century dieters, the Graham-

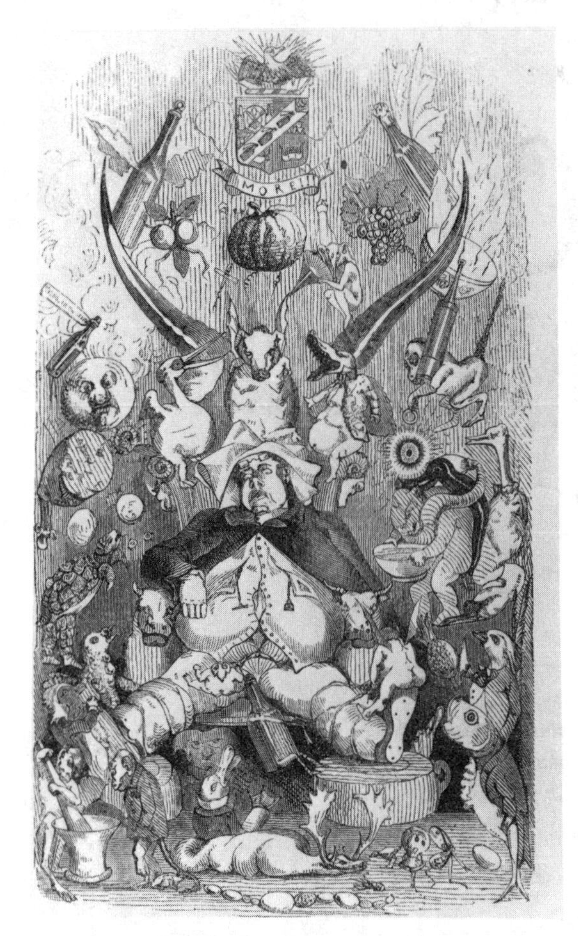

107. An overstuffed man is plagued by nightmarish visions of gluttony. *From Sydney Whiting,* Memoirs of a Stomach. *London, 1853. National Library of Medicine.*

BANTING'S OBESITY DIET

Breakfast

8:00 A.M.	5 to 6 oz. meat or broiled fish (not a fat variety of either); a small biscuit or 1 oz. dry toast; a large cup of tea or coffee without cream, milk or sugar.

Dinner

1:00 P.M.	Meat or fish as at breakfast, or any kind of game or poultry, same amount; any vegetables except those that grow underground, such as potatoes, parsnips, carrots or beets; dry toast, 3 oz., cooked fruit without sugar; good claret (10 oz.), Madeira or sherry.

Tea

5:00 P.M.	Cooked fruit, 2 to 3 oz.; one or two pieces of zwieback; tea (9 oz.) without milk, cream or sugar.

Supper

8:00 P.M.	Meat or fish, as at dinner (3 to 4 oz.); claret or sherry, water (7 oz.); fluids restricted to 35 oz. per day.

from *Practical Dietetics*
by Alida Frances Pattee, 1927

ites were obsessed with dyspepsia, not obesity, and with health rather than slimness.

The Grahamites looked odd to their contemporaries because they were too thin by the standards of the day. Medical theorists at the end of the Civil War claimed that a little heftiness was even a sign of *good* health. Fortunately for the general populace, the rounded look was also fashionable, popularized by the curvy actresses of the day, such as Lillian Russell, known as the American beauty of her era. Even the tall, long-limbed Gibson Girl, who first appeared in *Life* magazine in 1895, was allowed to grow plump as she aged.

For women in particular, concerns with fashion rather than health turned the twentieth century into the age of dieting. In the 1920s, the first decade when plumpness was considered unfashionable as well as unhealthy, most women dieted to emulate their favorite film stars, flat-chested, slender young women who popularized the flapper look of that era. By the mid-1960s the thin, androgynous look was taken to its starvation-dieting extreme, made fashionable by the English fashion model Twiggy. The 1920s also set the stage for the diet-industry boom, which did quite well even decades later when such film celebrities as Jane Russell and Marilyn Monroe represented the female ideal for many an American man.

As Americans have fought the battle of the bulge, reducing-cure fads have come and gone. By the 1990s the American diet industry was as healthy as ever. Unfortunately, too many dieters have learned that dieting may not only be useless, but dangerous to their health.

FAT IS OUT

At the same time American men and women were searching for ways to trim their waistlines, mainstream medical doctors were starting to suggest that obesity was, in fact, bad for health. In the 1920s life-insurance companies, with their ideal height-and-weight tables, helped produce a mania for weighing—in doctors' offices, on public penny scales, and eventually in the privacy of the home. (Insurance companies had been charging heftier premiums for their bulky clients since the 1830s.) And as medical examinations became mandatory for insurance and more middle-class families began to buy policies, Americans became obsessed with how much their weight deviated from the ''ideal.''

The obesity ''experts'' were ready to help them out, offering visions of slenderness to the first generation of Americans who would suffer through cycles of dieting fads, often to the detriment of their health. Among the array of diet regimens available in the late nineteenth and early twentieth centuries, Hillel Schwartz, author of *Never Satisfied: A Cultural History of Diets, Fantasies and Fat,* writes of obesity tablets containing arsenic, milk diets (also used to put on weight), Banting's lean beef diet, a ''No-Breakfast Plan,'' calisthenics, massage, electrotherapy, vinegar, lemon juice, reducing belts, Turkish baths, tobacco cures, fasting, calorie counting, thyroid medication, and Fletcherizing—chewing food until it turned into a liquid pulp. ''People set out to lose weight anyway they could . . . and they mixed everything up. They dieted one way, exercised another, dosed themselves with this and that, gave themselves pep talks or learned to relax.''

The American Medical Association's *Nostrums and Quackery* series, first published in 1912, detailed the most blatant examples of fraudulent obesity cures that lured overweight men and women with images of a new skinny life. From Battle Creek, Michigan, Kellogg's Safe Fat Reducer promised to turn fat into muscle, while Dr. Turner's Triplex System of Flesh Reducing, of Syracuse, New York, assured dieters they could ''eat what you want and whenever you want.'' Turner claimed to have discovered ''the most wonderful treatment for obesity'' after he himself ballooned to 254 pounds. At a cost of 25 dollars consumers received instructions to:

1. Shun carbohydrates, sweets, and fatty meats and substitute Dr. Turner's saccharin tablets at 50 cents a bottle. (Saccharin had been available since the 1880s.)
2. Swallow Dr. Turner's chocolate-flavored cathartic pills (one dollar for 100 tablets) to clean out the system.
3. Exercise regularly.
4. Supplement their diet with Dr. Turner's Concentrated Food Tablets (offered at no charge), whose chief ingredients were evidently milk and sugar.

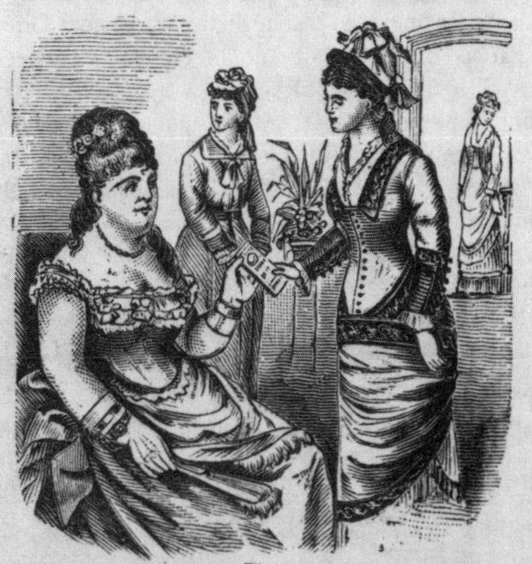
[April 27, 1878.
ANTI-FAT
The Great Remedy for Corpulence
ALLAN'S ANTI-FAT
is composed of purely vegetable ingredients, and is perfectly harmless. It acts upon the food in the stomach, preventing its being converted into fat. Taken in accordance with directions, it will reduce a fat person from two to five pounds per week.
"Corpulence is not only a disease itself, but the harbinger of others." So wrote Hippocrates two thousand years ago, and what was true then is none the less so to-day.
Before using the Anti-Fat, make a careful note of your weight, and after one week's treatment note the improvement, not only in diminution of weight, but in the improved appearance and vigorous and healthy feeling it imparts to the patient. It is an unsurpassed blood-purifier and has been found especially efficacious in curing Rheumatism.
CERTIFICATE.—I have subjected Allan's Anti-Fat to chemical analysis, examined the process of its manufacture, and can truly say that the ingredients of which it is composed are entirely vegetable, and cannot but act favorably upon the system, and is well calculated to attain the object for which it is intended. W. B. DRAKE, Analytical Chemist.
Sold by all druggists, or sent, by express, to any address, upon receipt of $1.50; quarter-dozen $4.00, or half-dozen for $7.50. Address,
BOTANIC MEDICINE CO.,
Proprietors, Buffalo, N. Y.

108. Diet remedies with ''magic ingredients'' are nothing new. *From* Harper's Weekly, *April 27, 1878. National Library of Medicine.*

Marjorie Hamilton's Quadruple Combination System of Fat Reduction promised to "remove double chin or excess fat without medicines. There are no drugs to ruin the stomach, no horrible dieting, no ridiculous fasting, no nerve-racking or harmful physical culture exercises, no poison internal remedy, no Turkish baths, no sweating. . . . By my system of treatment you may eat all you desire." This treatment also included a long list of recommendations, such as exercise with Indian clubs, twice-weekly rectal enemas, lemon juice in water, and "a good long walk each day." In addition, consumers were sent Majorie Hamilton's Healthtone Obesity Bath Powder, which was supposed to dissolve fat away if one bathed in it twice a day. The cost for the cure was a weighty 15 dollars. Ads for this "drugless fat reduction" method promised that fat would vanish, "one pound a day."

Mechanical devices promised effortless weight loss for consumers and fat profits for medical doctors. A letter mailed to doctors in 1916 from the manager of the Chicago manufacturer of the Gardner Reducing Machine assured the physician that "installing a Gardner Reducing Machine in your office will enlarge your practice and increase your income, for the Gardner Reducing Machine gives a treatment which is greatly in demand."

Early diet books were as popular as the cures. Near the end of World War I, weight-conscious Americans eagerly devoured Dr. Lulu Hunt Peters's *Diet and Health With Key to the Calories,* which by 1925 had gone through five printings. Writing in a conversational, personal tone, Peters, who dedicated her book to Herbert Hoover and ended it with the motto "Food Will Win the War. WATCH OUR WEIGHT!," admitted that her normal weight was 150 pounds and that "at one time there was 70 pounds more of me than there is now." Summing up America's wartime attitude toward fat people, she wrote: "Now fat individuals have always been considered a joke, but you are a joke no longer. Instead of being looked upon with friendly tolerance and amusement, you are now viewed with distrust, suspicion, and even aversion. How dare you hoard fat when our nation needs it? You don't dare to any longer."

Warning her readers against anti-fat medications unless used under the supervision of a doctor, Peters urged consumers to eat what they wanted but in small quantities and to count their calories: "Hereafter you are going to eat calories of food. Instead of saying one slice of bread, or a piece of pie, you will say 100 calories of bread, 350 calories of pie." Peters was among the first to encourage group therapy, in the form of "weight clubs" that even included regular weigh-ins. To pressure members to lose weight, she suggested that anyone who did not take off at least one pound each week would be fined, with the proceeds going to the Red Cross.

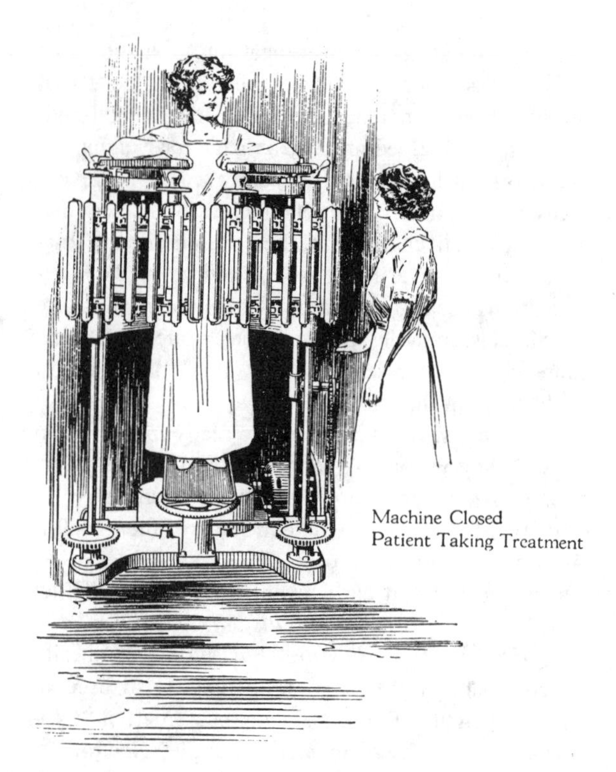

109. The Gardner Reducing Machine promised to roll flesh away (1915). *Collection of Advertising History, Archives Center, National Museum of American History, Smithsonian Institution.*

SLENDERIZE!

In 1927, an article appeared in the *Saturday Evening Post* called "Get Rid of That Fat," by Samuel G. Blythe. Written as a first-person account of the author's struggle to lose weight, Blythe's article lamented the new tyranny of slimness: "Back in the year 1912 . . . the world seemed to be populated mostly by persons belonging to one of two classes—fat persons who were trying to get thin and thin persons who were trying to get fat. . . . Now I find that the world is populated largely by fat people trying to get thin and by thin people trying to get thinner."

For women in the 1920s, this craving for an ever trimmer figure was determined more by fashion than by a concern for their health. The new short hemlines, along with the dropped waist, looked best on thin women with narrow hips, flat chests, and slender legs. The new bobbed hair could not hide double chins and thick necks. To achieve the flapper look, many voluptuous women struggled to transform themselves by flattening their breasts with bands of material stretched across their chests and squeezing into girdles to narrow their hips.

Hollywood helped accelerate the slimness mania. With the rising popularity of such slim flapper film stars as Clara Bow, Louise Brooks, Lillian and Dorothy Gish, and Mary Pickford, women could hardly afford to remain voluptuous and still appear fashionable.

As the pressure to reduce expanded in the 1920s, so did the diet industry. Warned Blythe in his *Saturday Evening Post* article, "Many things are being proffered, sold and used in the name of fat elimination and the attainment of slenderness that are bogus, are dangerous and, in a number of instances, are criminal."

Hillel Schwartz describes the increasing popularity of the surgical removal of fat in the 1920s (first performed in 1889). Bath salts with names like Every Woman's Flesh Reducer and Lesser Slim-Figure Bath, along with reducing soaps, were all the rage. Tobacco companies grabbed the attention of the figure-conscious woman who was no longer afraid to smoke in public with promises to "satisfy the appetite without harming the digestion." Meanwhile, chewing-gum companies took advantage of the gum-chewing rage with products that promised to take off the pounds—Slends Fat Reducing Chewing Gum, Silph Chewing Gum, and Elfin Fat Reducing Gum Drops. For the Hollywood crowd, a four-foot, eight-inch, 100-pound masseuse named Sylvia massaged away the fat from such stars as Jean Harlow and Gloria Swanson.

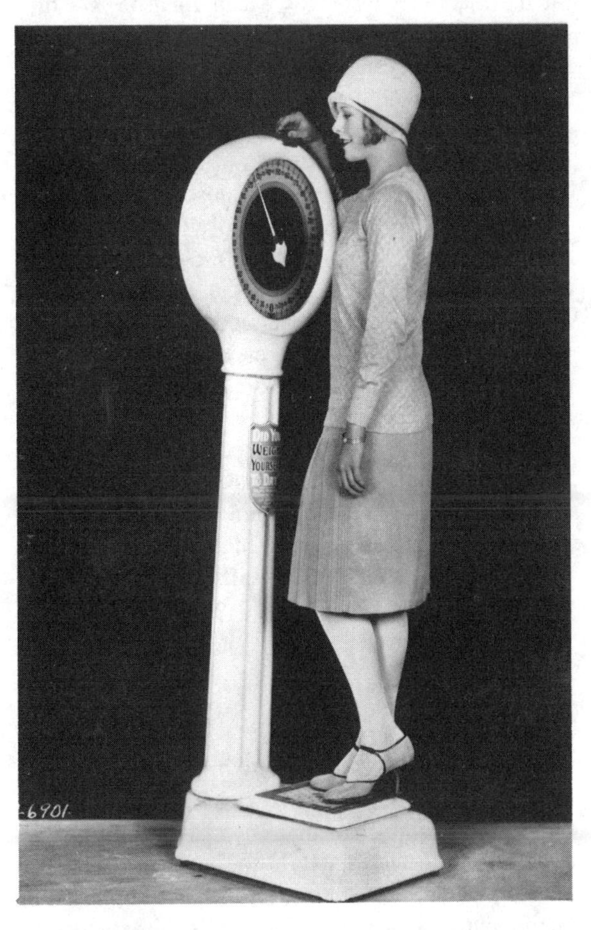

110. A flapper weighs in with the new look for beauty and health (1920s). *The Bettmann Archive.*

Even at the height of the Depression, the diet industry continued to flourish. In Hollywood, Marlene Dietrich and Greta Garbo may have brought back the shapely figure to the silver screen, but Americans continued on their great search for the perfect reducing cure.

With the growth of the advertising industry in the 1920s and 1930s, the diet industry took off, much of it offering useless, fraudulent, even dangerous cures. The third volume of *Nostrums and Quackery and Pseudo-Medicine,* published in 1936, described a laxative called Jad Salts, advertised as a kidney cure in the 1920s and then as an obesity cure beginning around 1930. At a cost of two cents a day, consumers could allegedly lose a pound a day and still eat three full meals. Another laxative, Sleepy Salts, promised to make "fat go fast . . . without starving—no exercise!" Dieters also had their choice of early liquid diets—food powders to be mixed with water, like Stoll's Diet Aid, a concoction made of milk chocolate, starch, and an extract of roasted whole wheat and bran, to replace breakfast and lunch.

A new miracle drug called dinitrophenol, meant to stimulate metabolism, promised dieters they could lose two to three pounds a week. The drug might have speeded up metabolism, but in some cases it also caused fevers, rashes, loss of taste, and blindness. It also ended up killing a number of its users, who literally cooked to death from dangerously high fevers before it was banned in 1938.

Critics of the diet industry voiced their concern. Carl Malmberg, in his *Diet and Die,* published in 1935, warned his readers that "it is better to be fat than dead" and lambasted nearly every diet fad on the market—fasting, Fletcherism, pills, soap, laxatives, vegetarianism, low protein and mucous-free diets, banana and skimmed milk diets, and the popular Hollywood Eighteen Day Diet, a 600-to-700-calorie-per-day regimen during which time the dieter consumed as many as 22 grapefruits per day. He added, "In addition to these there is a multitude of mechanical contraptions, belts, girdles, and harnesses of all sorts that chafe and injure the skin, machines which bruise and damage the tissues, and electrical devices which may burn and disfigure beyond hope of remedy.''

Amphetamines, first introduced as a diet cure in the late 1930s, were evidently a big hit among soldiers during World War II, who gobbled up 180 million tablets, not for their appetite-suppressing power, but to keep alert during combat. In 1943, *Time* magazine described a new appetite-suppressing drug called dextroamphetamine (a form of benzedrine): When a group of 300 men, women, and children tried the new drug, they each lost an average of two pounds a week. By the end of the war, amphetamines had become the diet drug of choice, particularly among overweight men. Others, like long-haul truck drivers, downed them to stay awake.

A NATION OF DIETERS

In 1952, the National Institutes of Health told Americans that obesity was the number-one health problem in the United States and that fat people stood a greater chance of suffering from chronic heart disease, diabetes, and cerebral hemorrhage.

But the American public didn't have to be reminded that it was better to be skinny than fat. For whatever the reason—health or fashion—dieting had already turned into a full-fledged national pastime. In 1959, *Time* magazine's Gerald Walker wrote, ''Never, it seems, have so many worked so hard to lose so little weight.'' Like Carl Malmberg 24 years earlier, Walker set up a red flag for those desperate dieters who would try any new diet fad that came down the pike. For Walker, the solution seemed simple: ''In an era of compulsive calorie counting the dieting public seems gullibly eager to try any scheme, however zany, except the very one that has any lasting effect—eating less.''

Walker cited Gallup Poll findings that would waver very little in later years: one out of every three adults was planning to go on a diet, and twice as many women as men worried about their weight. Citing some of the more popular cures, he described a ''reducing off the record'' long-playing disk produced by Columbia Records and *Good Housekeeping* magazine; the successful Slenderella International reducing salon chain, which had already attracted 300 thousand women since its inception in 1951; and Tasti-Diet, the first low-calorie food line that included 1,000-calorie frozen meals.

A month after Walker's article appeared, *Newsweek* warned its readers about ''Fat Frauds—fraudulent reducing aids [that] are slimming American pocketbooks by $100 million a year. Otherwise they are leaving people as fat as ever.'' The article was prompted by the previous week's release by Secretary of Health, Education and Welfare Arthur S. Flemming of a list of 27 reducing fads that had been suppressed by the government for false advertising or labeling. Among these were 22 vibrators, four reducing pills, and one phonograph record.

Postwar dieters joined programs like Take Off Pounds Sensibly (TOPS), created by Esther Manz of Milwaukee, the first of the national diet group therapies that would blossom in the 1960s. By the late 1950s, TOPS had attracted 30 thousand women. (Overeaters Anonymous was started in 1960, Weight Watchers in 1961, and Diet Workshop in 1965.) The new group dieting would appeal particularly to women, as a way of coming to grips with the social isolation and ridicule they experienced in a society that seemed to be more tolerant of fat men than of fat women.

In the new supermarkets, low-fat diet foods were moved from their segregated dietetic shelves into the main aisles, boosting sales by millions. Then, in 1959, a new liquid lunch called Metrecal hit the market. Created by Mead Johnson & Company, makers of Pablum for babies, Metrecal had been originally designed as a liquid meal for hospital patients who could not eat solid food. According to a 1960 *Time* magazine article, Metrecal ''has already spawned some 40 imitators from Sears, Roebuck's Bal-Cal to Quaker Oats's Quota, just out this week.''

In 1960, one of the hottest-selling diet books, Herman Taller's *Calories Don't Count,* found an eager audience. Taller raised the eyebrows of the medical community when he recommended that dieters cut back on carbohydrates but eat unlimited quantities of protein and fat and take six safflower-oil capsules every day. After his book sold over two million copies, Taller was fined 7,000 dollars for violating the federal Food, Drug, and Cosmetic Act and for mail fraud and conspiracy. As it turns out, he had been receiving a percentage of the profits from the manufacturer of the safflower capsules.

DIETS, DIETS, AND MORE DIETS

By the mid-1970s, a few diet experts began to emphasize healthy eating as well as slimness. Dieters were introduced to Nathan Pritikin's dietary regimen at the Longevity Research Center in Santa Monica, California. Pritikin, an engineer, had been diagnosed as having clogged arteries in the late 1950s. Rather than take it easy, as his doctors advised, he read up on nutrition and exercise. From his studies he created a program for himself that consisted of

FAT KIDS

• In 1924, popular diet author Dr. Lulu Hunt Peters published the first diet book for kids, *Diet for Children (And Adults) and the Kalorie Kids.*

• In 1951, Dr. Benjamin Sandler, in an address at Los Angeles Children's Hospital, warned that polio often attacked children who were overweight and recommended that parents reduce the amount of starch and sugar in children's diets.

• In 1975, William Dietz of Tufts New England Medical Center reported that an estimated 20 percent of kids between the ages of six and 17 were overweight. Dietz blamed television viewing and the fast-food lifestyle.

• In the late 1980s, a study of San Francisco children conducted by the University of California, San Francisco, found that 50 percent of nine-year-olds and 80 percent of ll-year-olds were on diets.

• In 1990, the Associated Press reported that new studies showed that sedentary, overweight five- and six-year-olds stood a good chance of suffering from high blood pressure or heart disease as adults.

running and a diet low in protein and fats and high in carbohydrates. Pritikin decided that if it worked for him, it would work for others. When his program hit the market in 1976, it was an immediate success.

The Pritikin 26-day program—at a cost of 4,600 dollars, which included a lifetime follow-up by the center's staff—allowed for eight small meals a day high in carbohydrates but forbade fats, oils, salt, sugar, caffeine and alcohol. Pritikin's followers swore by the success of his regimen, but the man who is often credited with creating one of the most successful diet programs in America did not live long enough to see the long-term results. In 1985, at the age of 69, Pritikin committed suicide in Albany, New York, where he was being treated for incurable leukemia.

Recent adherents of Pritikin's program have modified his regimen. One Pritikin successor, Ann Louise Gittleman, changed the no-fat rule to include "essential fats" such as unprocessed vegetable oils.

In spite of the popularity of Pritikin's diet, many dieters were still drawn to the get-skinny-quick cures. At best these placed little or no emphasis on health; at worst, they proved to be unsafe. In the early 1980s, Americans grabbed onto "starch blockers," a diet aid marketed as a food. Starch blockers were supposed to stop the digestion of starches, thus leaving the consumer free to gobble up all those yummy carbohydrates on many diets' "no-no" list. "If you like potatoes, pasta and bread," read an ad from General Nutrition Corporation, "but you want to lose weight, you need STARCH BLOCK." In 1982, a federal judge in Chicago determined that "starch blocker" was a drug subject to FDA regulation and ordered supplies destroyed.

Diet pills helped turn out a new generation of "diet doctors." In 1968, Susanna McBee, a writer for *Life* magazine, testified before the U.S. Senate Subcommittee on Antitrust and Monopoly that she had been given diet pills from each of 10 diet doctors she visited across the country when she posed as a prospective dieter. By the end of her research, the five-foot-three-inch McBee, who at 125 pounds was told by several of these same doctors that she was not even overweight, ended up with almost 1,500 pills in her bag, most of them amphetamines.

As of 1986, a concerned FDA allowed only two drugs to be used in nonprescription diet aids, phenylpropanolamine, an "appetite suppressant" known as PPA, and benzocaine with caffeine, which numbs the tongue to reduce the sense of taste. (In 1991 some medical doctors were still questioning the safety of phenylpropanolamine and the FDA was

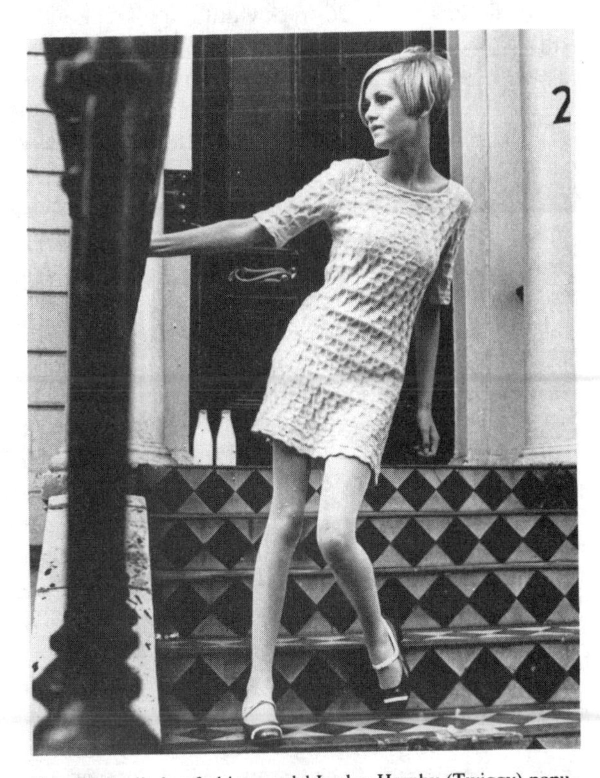

111. England's hot fashion model Lesley Hornby (Twiggy) popularized the underweight but not necessarily healthy look (London, 1966). *UPI/Bettmann Newsphotos.*

expected to decide on the drug's fate by the end of the year.)

Ever on the lookout for fast, effortless reducing magic, in the late 1970s the weight-conscious gulped down a new generation of liquid diets, until the fad cooled down after 60 people died from drinking the stuff.

By the early 1990s, liquid diets, such as Optifast, Health Management Resources (HMR), Medifast, and the over-the-counter Slim Fast, made a strong comeback after television talk-show host Oprah Winfrey lost 67 pounds on Optifast. (Like many others who have tried quick-weight-loss programs, she regained much of this weight over the next year. In 1991 Winfrey told *People* magazine, "I'll never diet again.")

Recommended for only those at least 40 pounds overweight, physician-monitored diets with daily caloric intake as low as 420 calories were considered safer than their 1970s predecessors, which were deficient in basic nutrients. Yet since 1984, the FDA has required low-calorie protein diets (those with fewer than 400 calories a day) to include a warning that they can cause serious illnesses and need medical supervision. The price of the medically supervised programs was enough to squeeze anybody's savings account. In 1990, hospitals were charging 2,500 to 3,000 dollars for the 26-week Optifast program. "It's little wonder," reported *Newsweek,* "that well over 1,000 hospitals and clinics have signed up with one of the three programs; the added outpatients can turn a losing year into a profitable year for some fiscally strapped centers."

Besides Pritikin, starch blockers, and the liquid diets, late-twentieth-century dieters were offered an array of programs. Many were new, many were not so new, and many were reruns of the old obesity cures—the ever-popular Weight Watchers, purchased by H.J. Heinz Corporation in 1978 from its founder, Jean Nidetch; The Diet Center Program, founded in 1971 by Cybil Ferguson; the Kempner Rice Diet, a rice and fruit diet supervised at Duke University and begun in 1939; Nutri/System, offering prepackaged diet foods since the early 1970s; retreats and spas (formerly called "fat farms"); and Jenny Craig Weight Loss Centre, started by Sid and Jenny Craig in Australia in 1983 and in the United States in 1985, with a diet consisting of prepackaged main courses, supplemented by fruits, vegetables, and low-fat milk.

Then there was liposuction, surgery that literally suctioned out flabby arms and thighs and extended tummies. First used in Europe in the 1960s, by the late 1980s 55,900 liposuction surgeries were reported to the American Society of Plastic and Reconstructive Surgeons. (Some ads for the procedure place that figure as high as 250 thousand.) By 1990, the allegedly safer laser process was introduced as a way to zap unwanted fat.

As always, the diet market continued to attract the usual array of questionable and unsafe remedies. The magazine *FDA Consumer* listed such gimmicks as skin patches, herbal capsules, grapefruit diet pills, and Chinese magic weight-loss earrings in its October 1989 report.

The following spring, the U.S. House of Representatives' Committee on Small Business presented a devastating series of reports on the American diet industry. "Many diet programs do little or nothing to inform patients of the health and safety risks of rapid-weight-loss dieting," reported the committee. "Untrained staff at diet programs are being held out as 'nutritionists,' or 'counselors,' or 'supervisors' with direct responsibility for overseeing patient care, though they know little about nutrition." The reports blamed a "lack of Federal oversight plus a total lack of industry self-policing . . . losing the balance between patient safety and making a profit."

By the early 1990s, Americans found themselves inundated with not only a plethora of diet products and programs, but also an equally massive array of reducing information from the media. More than 200 diet books were in print, reported the *San Francisco Examiner,* and each year 25 new diet books were crammed onto bookstore shelves.

Even so, consumers were warned not to believe everything they read. Reported United Press International, "nutrition professionals from coast to coast are warning the recent rash of fad diet books is not only an opportunity for the frustrated to waste money but a threat to the health of those who actually follow the eating plans." As an example, the story cited *Fit for Life,* the hottest-selling diet book of all time, written by Harvey and Marilyn Diamond. The American Dietetic Association warned that the Diamonds' recipes, based on the principle that the body can handle only one type of food at a time, were "inadequate in several nutritional ingredients." The ADA criticized another big seller, *The Rotation Diet* by Martin Katahn, for supposedly setting calorie levels far too low.

Ironically, despite all this advice, dieters seemed to be putting the pounds on as fast or faster than they were losing them. "Yo-yo dieting—repeatedly taking off weight only to put it back on—may actually promote weight gain in the long run," reported the *Washington Post* in 1988.

In late 1989, Marketdata Enterprises in Valley Stream, New York estimated that Americans would spend 33 billion dollars on diets and diet-related products the following year. As *Newsweek* magazine put it so well: "That's bad news for the well-upholstered of the world. But for American business it represents the marketing opportunity of the century: the chance to sell the same programs to the same people over and over again."

BREAKING A NEVER-ENDING CYCLE

In 1982, William Bennett, M.D. and Joel Gurin came out with a controversial book called *The Dieter's Dilemma*, arguing that diets don't work: "With rare exceptions, dieters lose weight temporarily and then, despite great determination, gradually regain it." Bennett and Gurin offered a rationale they called the "set point theory," suggesting that everyone has a natural weight. When dieters try to alter this set point, the body fights the process. Bennett and Gurin suggested that it was possible to lower the set point, and that the best and healthiest way was through physical activity.

Five years later a group of scientists at Stanford University suggested that exercising was better than dieting for losing weight. Bemoaning the neglect of exercise in many dieting programs, one researcher concluded that the best way to lose weight was through "moderate dieting and gradually increasing exercise." Cross-country skiing was rated as the best sport for burning calories by the *Lose Weight Naturally Newsletter* from Rodale Press. "Two hours' worth will burn more than 1,000 calories and help elevate your metabolism to use still more calories over the rest of the day." Swimming, vigorous cycling, handball, and singles tennis also rated highly. Such recommendations were a far cry from Banting's Obesity Diet—no midday Madeira or sherry, just less food and more time at the gym.

DIETING IN AMERICA, 1990

- 34 percent of Americans weigh 10 percent more than their recommended weight and 25 percent are considered "obese," defined as 20 percent or more over the accepted weight for their age and build. Approximately 15 percent are considered underweight for their weight, age, and build.
- Between 35 and 44, 16 percent of men and 14 percent of women become overweight. By the time Americans reach 50 years of age, one-third are overweight.
- One-half of women and one-fourth of men are dieting at any given time.
- For every 100 Americans who shed pounds, 90 to 95 percent will regain as much as they lost.
- Artifical sweetener sales doubled from 1980 to 1990.
- Between 1980 and 1990, two dozen new diet and fitness books hit the *Publishers Weekly* top-15 best-sellers list.
- Americans will spend an estimated 50 billion dollars on diets and diet-related products and services by 1995.

CHAPTER · 26 ·

FITNESS: THE ULTIMATE CURE

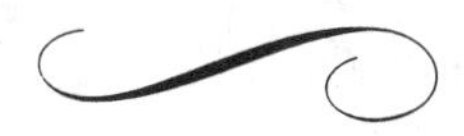

Throughout the United States the atmosphere is being churned about by gyrating, grunting, and perspiring bodies. Hundreds of thousands of arms, legs, and middle-aged torsos are bending, straining, pushing, and pulling to this monstrous rhythm: one-two-three-four, one-two-three-four. Exercise! Exercise! More! More!

PETER J. STEINCROHN, M.D.
You Don't Have to Exercise!
Rest Begins at Forty, *1942*

When running guru and author Jim Fixx died of a heart attack at the age of 52 while on a 10-mile run in Vermont, sedentary Americans nodded their heads and settled back. No matter that the author of the runaway bestseller *The Complete Book of Running* had been a 220-pound, two-pack-a-day smoker until he was 35, and no matter that his father had died of a heart attack at the age of 43. Fixx's death was proof enough that exercise can be dangerous to your health.

Fixx's death in 1984 set off a national debate about the health benefits of exercising, particularly for the middle-aged. Had his rigorous daily workout prolonged or shortened the runner's life? Given his family history, should the man who is credited with popularizing jogging in the 1970s even have taken up the sport? Is exercise necessary? Is it harmful?

To exercise or not—the debate was nothing new. Back in the 1890s, advocates of cycling, America's first full-scale fitness fad, argued that riding a bicycle would cure consumption and nervousness and make women more fit for childbearing, while critics of the "wheel" pointed to the dangers of permanently curved spines and displaced uteruses. In 1925, one writer, horrified by the boom in golfing, argued that middle-aged folks should indulge in nothing more strenuous than lawn bowling; and in 1942, Dr. Peter J. Steincrohn told his readers, "learn to be lazy."

Notwithstanding the critics, since the end of the nineteenth century an increasing number of middle-class adult Americans have been leaping onto the exercise bandwagon. For many fitness buffs, exercising has been the elixir to end all elixirs, as well as a means of taking control—of their shape, their weight, their looks, and their lifelines.

Perhaps more than any other health fad, fitness has had strong ties to the state of the national health. In the post-Civil War years, it promised to solve the problems of an increasingly urban and sedentary

America; in the early twentieth century, to guarantee against "race suicide"; and in the cold war years, to provide ammunition against communist aggression. After all, a nation of fit citizens could never be called "wimpish."

BODILY VIGOR

In the years before the Civil War, physical exercise appealed to only a small group of people. Before the German–American *Turnverein* movement, which helped popularize gymnastics and public gymnasiums in the United States, the most outspoken advocates of physical exercise were a handful of Philadelphia doctors who started the *Journal of Health*, America's first consumer health magazine, in 1829.

Utopian visionaries and educators, the physician/editors of the *Journal of Health* advocated sports and fitness for all ages, a radical view at a time when most of their colleagues neglected adult fitness for that of children. The journal encouraged its readers to take up outdoor exercise—games, sports, walking, running, leaping, or gardening—in addition to gymnastics and calisthenics. They recommended calisthenics, imported primarily from France and England, specifically for girls and women, "best calculated to develope the physical powers . . . without detriment to the perfecting of their moral faculties."

THE BENEFITS OF WALKING

In the month of June, 1830, I made a pedestrian excursion of about 300 miles, ascending in the course of it, Mount Anthony, near Bennington, Saddle Mountain, in Massachusetts and some other eminences. . . . Amongst the many important advantages that I feel I have derived from combined regular, and, in some instances, severe exercises with study, is the enjoyment of almost uninterrupted good health. I am now, and always have been, entirely free from those debilitating affections, under which so many of our literary men have sunk, and are fast sinking. I know nothing of that fashionable disorder, called dyspepsia, except the name.

from Captain Partridge, 45 years old
Letter to the *Journal of Health*, December 22, 1830

Educators like Dr. William Alcott and his cousin Bronson Alcott stressed physical exercise as a way of teaching moral development to the nation's children. William Alcott, a follower of Sylvester Graham, campaigned for outdoor exercise in large,

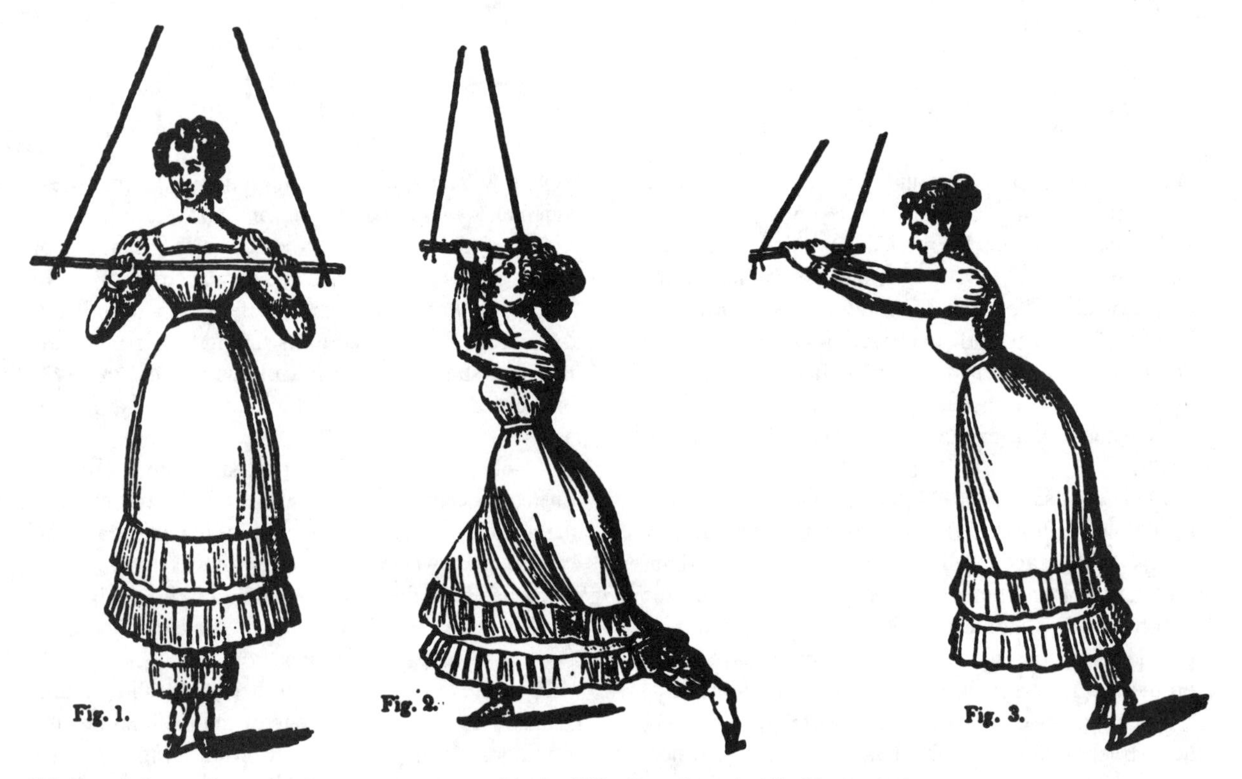

112. Even "vigorous" exercises for women were genteel in the 1830s. *From* Journal of Health, *April 27, 1831.*

fenced-in playgrounds, a suggestion that the progressives of the early twentieth century would turn into a cause célèbre. For reformers, like the Alcotts, fresh air and exercise went hand in hand, twin antidotes to the crowded, unventilated rooms of America's growing cities. Educators stressed the importance of physical education for girls as well as boys, although for their own female students, Emma Willard and Catharine Beecher rejected the more rigorous and "dangerous" German gymnastics in favor of gentler calisthenics.

Catharine Beecher was a prolific writer as well as an educator, and her advice books were popular before the Civil War. Among them was her *Physiology and Calisthenics,* written in 1856, and still available on the shelves of many university libraries. This book makes for fascinating reading. Written "for schools and families," Beecher gave her readers a crash course in human physiology as well as instructions for teaching "a system of physical training, to promote grace, health, strength, and beauty."

Edward Hitchcock started the first college physical education program in the United States at Amherst College in 1830. After that date, American colleges began to integrate physical education and physiology into their curricula. While Harvard built the first college gymnasium in the United States in 1826, adult Americans did not begin to flock to public gymnasiums until the 1850s. By 1860, New York City alone had seven public gyms.

Before the Civil War, fitness was only one facet of the larger popular-health movement. It offered yet another drugless therapy that appealed to the growing numbers of disillusioned consumers turning away from the heroic methods of bleeding, calomel, and surgery.

As Harvey Green writes in his *Fit For America,* a major source for the history of fitness and sports in the United States, physical exercise offered a preventive-health method rather than a cure. Offered as a painless therapy, "calisthenics and gymnastics joined with other new cures—vegetarianism, water cures, animal magnetism, electromagnetism, and electricity—to lay the ground work for a new era of health reform that began after the Civil War ended."

WORKING OUT

By the eve of the Civil War, more and more Americans were discovering the need to get up and exercise. Most converts were middle-class people who had migrated to the urban areas of the Northeast and settled into sedentary jobs that required more "brain work" than muscle work. They still represented a small minority; to be sure; most Americans still lived in rural areas and small towns and worked long, hard, physically taxing days.

By the 1860s, the fitness buffs were echoing the health reformers' belief that physical training and sports improved their health as well as helped build muscles. One example was the 1880 *Manual of Instruction in the Use of Dumb Bells, Indian Clubs and Other Exercises,* written by M. Bornstein (who confided to the reader that this was "his first book and probably his last"). The author wrote, "I may conscientiously say, a few moments' exercise with a light pair of clubs will accomplish more than all the medicines and tonics in the world." In his section "To the Ladies," the author recommended a "good, brisk walk for an hour in the morning: it gives a vital tone to the system, causes the blood to circulate, imparts a rosy hue to the cheeks and has a tendency to give health and strength to the whole body."

There was also a growing belief that getting and staying in shape was somehow a Christian duty. "Muscular Christianity," a movement originating in England in the early nineteenth century, had by the mid-nineteenth century reached the United States. Writes James Whorton in his *Crusaders for Fitness,* a major study of the nineteenth-century American fitness and alternative-health movements, "An age enchanted by athletics and action could interpret Muscular Christianity to mean a spiritual obligation to cultivate the body, and suppose that morality could be measured with a tape and weighed by athletic trophies."

The most famous fitness celebrity of the Civil War era was a former physician and temperance crusader turned physical-education instructor named Dioclesian "Dio" Lewis. The German-style gymnastics of the day built muscles, Lewis argued, but not necessarily a healthy body. Lewis created his own system of exercises while trying to cure his wife of tuberculosis. Known as the "New Gymnastics," Lewis's regimen combined calisthenics with games, using bean bags, wooden rings, rubber balls, and lightweight dumbbells and Indian clubs. In 1862, he outlined his system in a book called *New Gymnastics for Men, Women, and Children,* which, through its ten editions, was the standard physical-education text for the next quarter of a century.

Lewis's system was considered radical for its time because he encouraged girls and women to take part. When he opened his Institute of Physical Education in Boston in 1861 to train physical education instructors, half of his first graduates were women. (He even gave women a 25-percent break in tuition.)

Then in 1864 he opened the Family School for Young Ladies in Lexington, Massachusetts, designed for teenage girls of a "delicate nature." The students were given healthy doses of Lewis's exercise system each day in addition to fresh air and sunshine. By the time the school burned down in 1867, 300 girls had been trained there.

The Civil War helped further the fitness movement, adding popular military drills to a widening repertoire that now included German and Swedish gymnastics, Lewis's system, calisthenics, walking, riding, rowing, swimming, fencing, and skating.

While the sons and daughters of the middle and upper classes were building up their muscles in college gyms, young working-class men and women were sweating it out in the popular new "Y's." (The term "shaping up" referred to preparing cattle hides; not until the 1920s did the expression "being in shape" mean being physically fit.) Adult men, meanwhile, flocked to the new public gyms, which for many also served as social centers and places to make and break business deals. For those who preferred to work out in the privacy of their own homes, the "parlor gymnasium," designed for people in sedentary occupations, provided state-of-the-art devices one could use anywhere. Essentially they were pulleys one could either attach to a wall or use alone, designed to help stretch tired muscles. Those who could afford it could also buy a parlor rower, not too different from the high-tech rowing machine of today, and the "health lift," which resembled the modern step machine. One company, Peck and Snyder of New York, even offered a "complete home gymnasium," including bars, ropes, rigs, and weights.

Two groups of fitness theorists were vying for the exercise-minded consumer: those who pushed gymnastics and calisthenics workouts and those who advanced sports, or "athleticism." The former, mostly educators and physicians, argued that workouts were more "scientific," and that they alone provided a systematic exercise for all of the muscles of the body. The latter claimed that games and sports helped develop self-reliance and cooperation and built courage and character, a theme that would carry into twentieth-century physical-education classes. Although the debate would continue into the twentieth century, by the end of the nineteenth century organized sports seemed to be winning out.

In the years following the Civil War, yet another school, led by body-building "professors," was also doing a brisk trade. Solely a male pastime, "physical culture," which in the nineteenth century

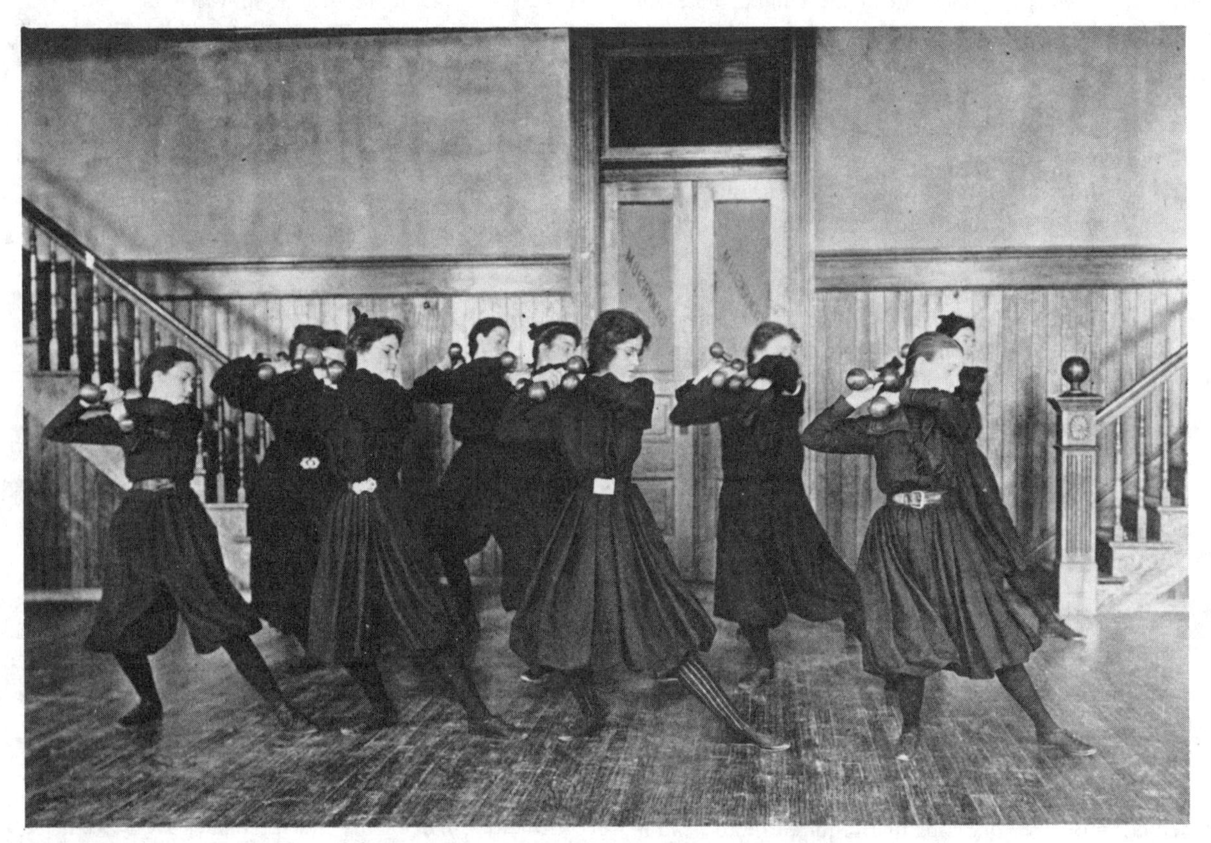

113. A girls' gym class, Western High School, Washington, D.C. (1898). *Photograph by F.B. Johnson. Culver Pictures.*

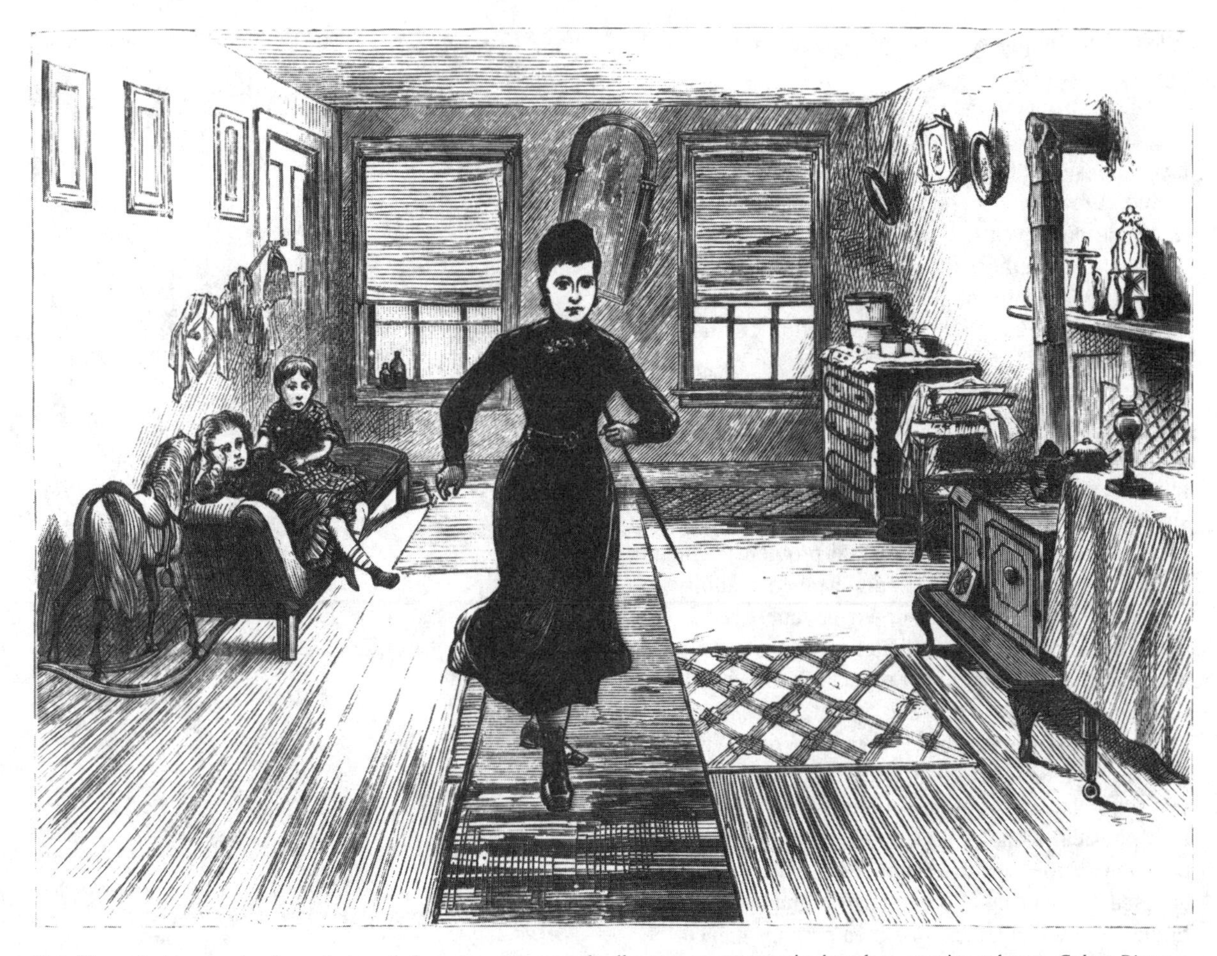

114. The pedestrian mania: An early twentieth-century tenement dweller uses an extemporized track to exercise at home. *Culver Pictures.*

emphasized muscular strength rather than health, featured pulleys and weights and 40-pound dumbbells to strengthen and accentuate the muscles. By the early twentieth century, the man whose name would become synonymous with physical culture, Bernarr ''Body Love'' Macfadden, was expanding his regimen to include healthy eating and deep breathing, jogging, and walking.

HOT WHEELS AND BICYCLE FACE

By the end of the nineteenth century, the champions of fitness had reached a large, ready audience in America, but for most the choices still remained limited. Calisthenics routines could get boring after a while; gymnastics appealed to the limber, strong, and well-coordinated; and one had to be young and in fairly good shape to participate in most competitive sports. Fitness was still a male pursuit. With the exception of doing light calisthenics, most middle- and upper- class women did not work out.

It remained for bicycling to become America's first unisex fitness fad. Bicycles cost about 75 dollars in the 1890s, still beyond the reach of many people, but a surprisingly large number of middle-class Americans plunked down their savings to buy one. The young, old, fat, thin, men, and women—everyone took to the wheel.

The earliest cycle was a contraption called a ''celeripede.'' Originating in the 1830s, it resembled a hobbyhorse on wheels. Dangerous to maneuver (it had no pedals and no brakes), it was also out of reach for everyone but wealthy hobbyists. At least one could ''drive'' the crank-driven ''velocipede'' of the 1860s, but it was barely an improvement. By the 1870s, some bicyclists, mostly men, were learning how to peddle the ''ordinary,'' with its large front wheel and small back wheel. Yet it, too, had no brakes and was difficult to control.

The ''safeties,'' first appearing in the 1880s, were the first modern bicycles. They had the advantage of having two wheels of the same moderate size, as well as brakes. Once safeties were mass produced for the first time in 1889 and equipped with the much-improved pneumatic tires (rubber tires filled with compressed air), the price came down and the craze was on.

Like any new fad, bicycling had its proponents and opponents. Health claims took on "cure-all" proportions. Peddling converts promised that the wheel would cure nervousness, consumption, obesity, anemia, varicose veins, curvature of the spine, and diabetes, strengthen the voluntary muscles, make women more fit for childbearing, stimulate the lungs and the heart, and cure drug addiction. Critics argued that bicyclists risked the dangers of a permanently strained expression called "bicycle face" and "bicycle throat," caused by gasping for air as the rider rode through the dirty streets and trails. Some physicians claimed that bicyclists, particularly women, suffered from overstimulation of the genitals and that men would fall victim to prostate problems. Others argued that cycling would ruin women's ability to bear children; still others urged anyone over 21 to retire from the sport immediately.

Women were particular objects of derision, since the bicycle allowed them to travel unaccompanied and shed their much-maligned corsets. Writes Whorton: "It seems undeniable that uneasiness about the social implications of feminism fed doctors' suspicions of a physical pathology of female cycling. The very costume of the wheelwoman, a Bloomer-type outfit adopted for reasons of comfort and safety, seemed to brand her a suffragette." Women perhaps gained the most from the bicycling craze, for the wheel gave them their first opportunity to become as fit as their husbands and brothers. Feminists, such as temperance reformer Frances E. Willard, eagerly took to the wheel; Willard, who learned to ride a bike at the age of 53, wrote of her experience in a best-selling book, *How I Learned to Ride the Bicycle,* in 1895.

Yet for many who took up pedaling, the bicycle was less a vehicle for fitness than a fast way to get around town. Therein lay its eventual decline. Ultimately, the new, speedier automobile took over, and the bicycle joined other relics in the attics of America, relegated until the second bicycling boom of the 1980s to the reduced status of a childhood toy.

THE DAILY DOZEN AND THE BODY BEAUTIFUL

After World War I, calisthenics enjoyed a resurgence with Walter Camp's "daily dozen." According to writer Paul Lancaster, Camp, a famous Yale University football coach, got the idea for the workout from watching lions stretch at the zoo. His daily dozen, resembling a modern jogger's warmup, was actually a ten-minute routine whose dozen movements were given names easy to recall: "hands, hips, head; grind, grate, grasp; crawl, curl, crouch; wave, weave, wing." Advocates of Camp's routine touted it as a cure for sluggish livers, constipation, and the ever-nagging dyspepsia.

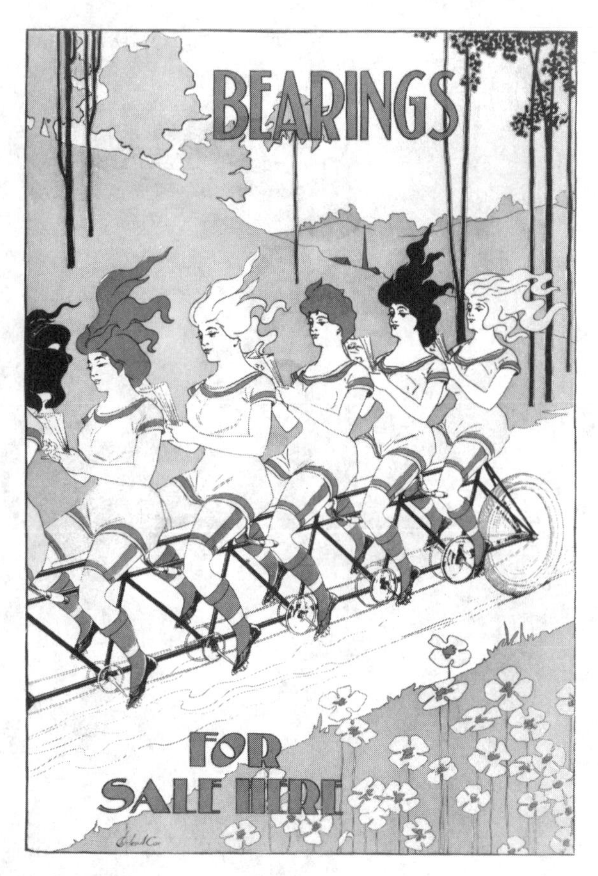

115. This bicycle built for many made cycling a breeze for these fitness-conscious women. Bearings *magazine cover. Courtesy of the Library of Congress.*

Radio created the perfect medium for popularizing the daily dozen and other calisthenic workouts. First on the air in 1923, radio exercise programs, in 15-minute intervals between ads, took their listeners through bends, twists, and turns every morning. Observed *Hygeia* magazine, published by the American Medical Association:

> What proportion of white collar workers and housekeepers get to recreation centers within a reasonable length of time after work to enjoy whatever exercise they can afford? What about the weather that makes impossible any outdoor sports for days at time? Under these conditions a well balanced calisthenic drill seems to be the only daily exercise available to these people. . . . When the alarm clock rings, one can rise to exercise with the "World's Largest Gymnasium Class."

While the debate over sports versus exercises persisted, commentators also argued over whether morning exercises were beneficial or useless. In 1929, a *New York Times* writer bemoaned the early-morning exercise "fiend" who dared to disturb others in the house by jumping out of bed, bright and cheery, turning on the early-morning radio exercise program and doing his (or her) daily dozen. That same year the *Times* ran a story about a physical-education professor at Teachers College, Columbia University, who argued that "setting up exercises before breakfast followed by the traditional cold plunge" were "silly, superstitious and artificial."

The late 1920s also saw the beginnings of a new fitness fad that would have pleased Dio Lewis, a game called "Hoover ball." Popularized by President Herbert Hoover, the game, using tennis rules, consisted of playing catch over a net with a "medicine ball," a stuffed, leather-bound, weighted ball. Hoover evidently played the game every day with members of his cabinet as a way to keep his weight under control. (Over 50 years later, "Hoover Ball" made a comeback in Iowa, with 50 teams competing for the national championship.)

Women in the 1920s took as their role model competitive-swimming champion Sally Kellerman, known as the "most perfectly formed woman." Kellerman helped popularize the new tight-fitting knitted swimsuit, which showed off a woman's contours better than the old-fashioned bloomer and provided the perfect excuse for toning up. This new sportswoman ideal fit in well with the boyish, independent-minded flapper, who had finally shunned the constraining corsets of the previous decades. Looking good was becoming as important as feeling good.

EASY DOES IT

Not everyone yearned to be fit. By the 1920s, a growing number of physicians and health writers were sending up red flags. Dr. C. War Crampton, one of the first physicans to sound the alarm over the growing number of heart attacks in the early years of the twentieth century, recommended a daily walk of 64 steps as sufficient exercise for anyone. A proprietor of a New York gym warned Americans to stay away from strenuous sports like bicycling, rowing, handball, and tennis.

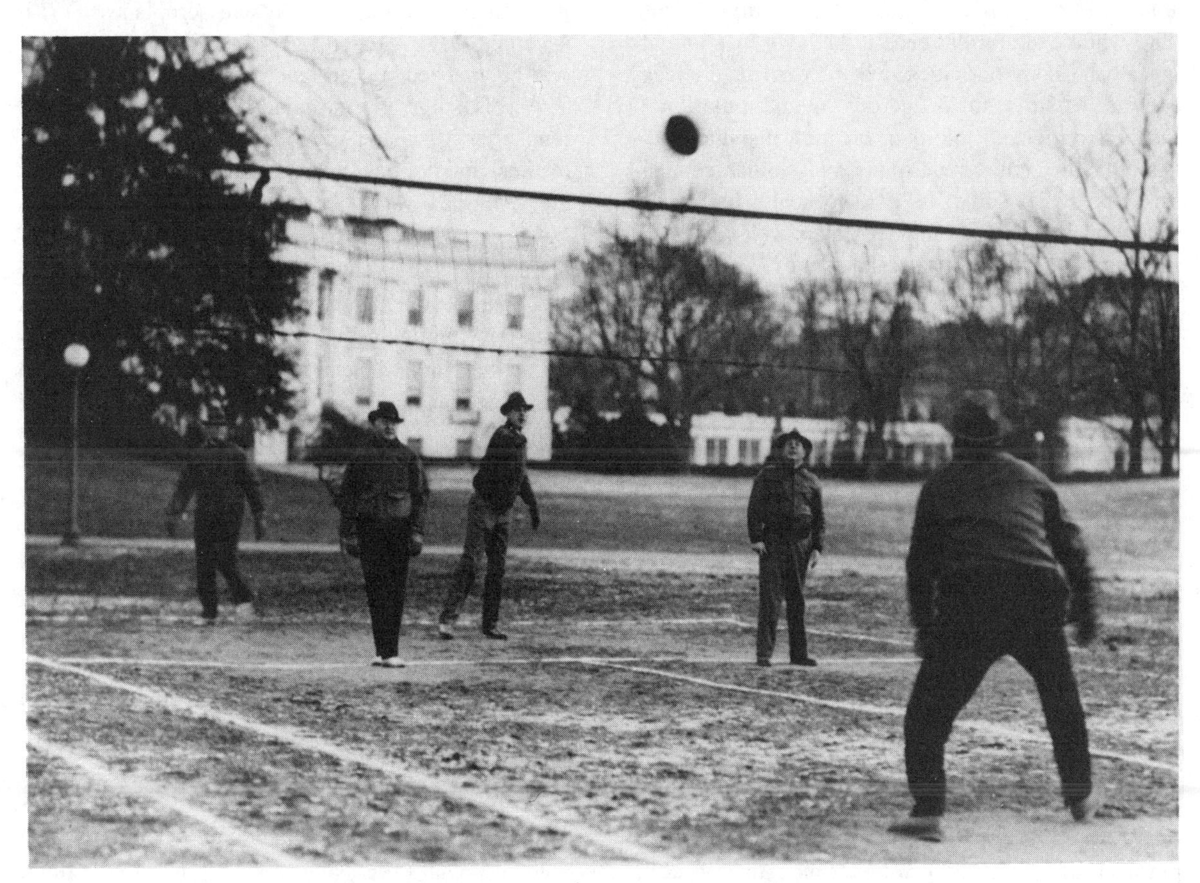

116. President Herbert Hoover, second from left, shapes up with a game of Hoover Ball on the White House lawn (1933). *Herbert Hoover Presidential Library-Museum.*

The common belief at the time, writes Paul Lancaster, was that everyone was supplied with a limited amount of "vitality." Strenuous exercise, the critics argued, would deplete a person of this vitality prematurely. Whenever an athlete died at a young age, the critics used the vitality theory to buttress their arguments.

Writer Samuel G. Blythe, author of "Too Much Exercise," which appeared in the *Saturday Evening Post* in 1925, was particularly concerned about those over 50. Comparing the amount of vitality of the human heart to money in a bank account, Blythe wrote, "You have a certain sum to start with. If you make reasonable drafts the capital continues to be useful for a long period, but if you make great drafts the time comes when the capital is exhausted." Blythe recommended rest over exercise: "I know one man who never stood up when he could sit down, never walked when he could ride, never climbed a flight of stairs when he could possibly stay on the ground floor, never sat down when he could recline at full length, and he lived to be 85 years old and was a leader in his profession to the end."

Five years later, Morris Fishbein, editor of the *Journal of the American Medical Association,* wrote that, while exercise did benefit the body by stimulating all the body activities, when "carried to excess exercise results in dangerous overstimulation." Fishbein criticized "out-door fanatics, marathon runners, hundred-mile pedestrians and similar enthusiasts who believe that the road to health lies in the exceptional performance rather than in well-conducted and suitably regulated physical activities." He warned that anyone over 30 who takes part in "serious overactivity" runs the risk of doing "more damage than good. . . . Calisthenics, daily dozens, and similar exercises are valuable within limitations, but our tendency is to become exercise fanatics if we do not become fanatics about something else."

But others believed that Americans needed to exercise even more. In a 1933 article in *Hygeia,* one writer complained that with all the talk about exercise and health, Americans were still not a healthy lot. "In spite of our gymnasiums, swimming pools, golf courses, municipal beaches, Olympic champions and professional athletes . . . we have not been able to overproduce the supply of sparkling eyes and glowing cheeks."

Throughout the late 1930s, writers in *Hygeia* continued to warn those "millions of sedentary Americans" who were giving up exercise for the "soft physical life" that they were ruining their health. Anticipating the advice of the 1990s, a writer in 1937 recommended "regular daily exercise in moderation," particularly walking and bicycling in the country. "One does not need to belong to expensive clubs or to become an expert sportsman. Adequate exercise can be procured by the simple process of walking or cycling at least part of the way to work or school."

Concern with worldwide flabbiness was evident in the fall of 1937 when the Health Committee of the League of Nations made plans for a world campaign to improve physical fitness. By the end of the decade, their work was cut short by the more pressing matter of the Second World War.

A NATION OF SOFTIES

In early 1940, as the world watched Hitler's armies storming through Europe, President Franklin Roosevelt proclaimed that "America is soft." Army physical examinations were showing an alarming number of rejections; draft-board results were no better. "We Americans think we're fit," wrote one major in the army's medical reserve corps just months before Japan attacked Pearl Harbor and the United States entered the war. "We are not. We are as far behind in physical fitness as in tanks and aeroplanes. . . . It is certain that if we don't get ourselves fit to fight we will be attacked and enslaved as France is now."

This surge in muscular nationalism continued long after VJ-Day. At the height of the cold war, medical and political leaders again sounded the alarm that America was indeed a nation of wimps. In 1955, the *New York State Journal of Medicine* reported that American children scored way below their European counterparts on basic physical fitness tests for "minimum" flexibility and strength. Studies at the Harvard School of Public Health showed that Americans were growing fatter because of a lack of physical activity. That same year, President Dwight D. Eisenhower created the Presidential Council on Physical Fitness.

Ike was particularly concerned about the flabbiness of the nation's children. When he was informed at a conference in 1957 that many American children were not exercising enough to be physically fit, it hit him "on a tender nerve," reported *U.S. News and World Report*. Ike was "shocked." His new Council on Youth Fitness, headed by Vice-President Richard M. Nixon, would try to reverse this trend.

American children and their parents were becoming softer because they were becoming more sedentary than ever, leading what one writer called, "push-button lives." Wrote Bonnie Prudden, author of the 1957 book *Is Your Child Really Fit?:* "Obviously, children no longer have to perform many of the active household chores of bygone years. There are no ashes to lug out. The groceries are delivered, or brought home, in the car . . . walking, working, using their bodies for recreation has kept the European children fit. There is no discernible equivalent in Europe of the suburban life."

Not that *some* adult Americans weren't sweating it out. The physical-fitness business was as hot as ever. At New York City health clubs in the late 1950s, clients were shelling out an average of 150 dollars a year to work out at paddle-ball courts and soak in steam baths. And as of the early 1950s, thanks to the new medium of television, Americans were tuning into Jack LaLanne's exercise show from Los Angeles. In 1957, a physiology professor at George Williams College suggested that sedentary adults integrate exercise into ordinary moves throughout the day: "Pull in your abdomen whenever the phone rings. . . . Reach while filing. . . . Sweep and dust with brisk movements. . . . Move vigorously. Reach where possible, as in bedmaking."

American consumers had their choice of physical-fitness gadgets and machines, some legitimate and some questionable. There was, for example, a combination muscle-toner and weight-reducer called the RelaxAcizor. Popularized in the early 1950s, it promised to stimulate the nervous system and control the metabolism by means of electricity. At New York City's RelaxAcizor Salon, clients sat back as an attendant placed several flat, round, wet objects onto the muscles of their arms, legs, and elsewhere that were electrically connected by wires to a generator. When the attendant switched on the juice, customers felt a slight electrical charge that tensed and then relaxed their muscles.

In 1970, *Newsweek* described Sauna Belts for sweating off inches, Tensolators to build up muscles, vibrator massage machines, treadmills, trampolines, vibrating belts, electric bicycles, and the Tone-O-Matic, a belt filled with 10 pounds of lead, designed to tone up the wearer's tummy muscles. As the jogging craze got off to a running start, the Executive Jogger, a device for indoor use, promised all the benefits of running no matter what the weather.

RUN FOR YOUR LIFE

At the turn of the twentieth century, Teddy Roosevelt jogged every night from the White House to the Washington Monument and back to help stay in shape. Presidential runs may not seem like a big deal these days, but until recently any adult, famous or not, who ran through the streets was considered either a robbery suspect or someone who had "gone round the bend."

But, in the late 1960s, the most widespread adult fitness movement in American history was off and running. By the 1970s it seemed as though everyone was jogging—baby boomers, college students, senior citizens, athletes, and would-be athletes.

Those early years of this latest exercise boom introduced millions to "aerobics," a term coined by a former Air Force senior flight surgeon named Dr. Kenneth H. Cooper, who developed the Aerobics Point System and started the Aerobics Center in Dallas, Texas. Described in his first book, *Aerobics,* published in 1968, his system was based on the amount of oxygen the circulatory system takes in and uses during exercise, with the goal of keeping the heart working at 70 percent of its maximum rate. Cooper was the first mainstream medical doctor to advocate preventive medicine through regular aerobic exercise.

By the end of the 1970s, an estimated 25 million Americans were jogging, the most popular aerobic exercise. Through the streets, around the tracks, and up and down forest trails, throngs of joggers turned the morning run into a national mania. Even those who had never participated in competitive sports were signing up for the 5-kilometer and 10-kilometer races held nearly every weekend. (In the nineteenth century, long-distance competitive running was called "pedestrianism.")

Others dusted off their bicycles, joined aerobics and Jazzercize classes, gave up their business lunches for a midday swim or game of squash or racquetball, huffed and puffed to Jane Fonda's workout videos, toned up at Nautilus machines, lifted weights, and hired personal trainers. In 1987, a Gal-

HOW FIT IS YOUR KID?

"A boy or girl is in GOOD SHAPE if able to—
climb four flights of stairs without puffing
walk 10 miles
carry one fifth of his body weight for two miles
run one mile in 10 minutes
do 50 knee bends
do 10 push-ups
do 30 sit-ups from supine position
chin a bar—five times for boys, three for girls"

from *Is Your Child Really Fit?*
by Bonnie Prudden, 1957

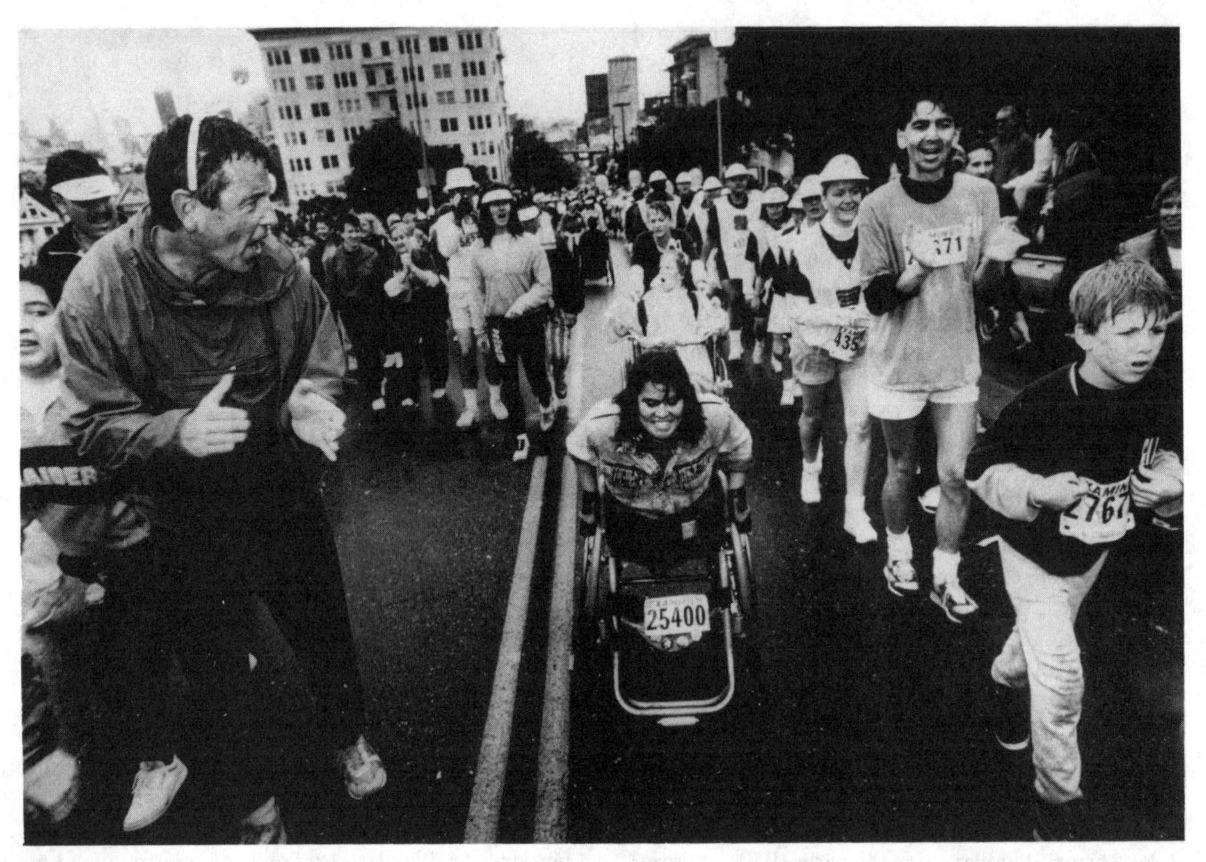

117. Some of the 100 thousand runners in San Francisco's annual Bay to Breakers race (1990). *Photo by Chris Hardy,* San Francisco Examiner.

lup survey showed that 69 percent of Americans exercised regularly.

Corporate America discovered that employees who exercised regularly not only took fewer sick days but proved to be long-term, loyal workers if they could work out on the job. It wasn't a new insight. Back at the turn of the twentieth century, John H. Patterson's National Cash Register Company in Dayton, Ohio had a fully equipped gym for its male employees; both male and female employees did calisthenics as part of their daily routine. In 1982, Tenneco, of Houston, Texas, opened an 11-million-dollar exercise complex that included a four-lane jogging track, racquetball and handball courts, and weight-lifting equipment.

Even so, Jim Fixx's sudden death in 1984 set exercise advocates scurrying to defend the benefits of the regular workout. Experts continued to recommend vigorous aerobic exercise for 25 to 35 minutes regularly, but also cautioned consumers to listen to the warning signs. Referring to Dr. Cooper's *Running Without Fear,* written after Fixx's death, health writer Jane Brody reminded her readers that one cannot take up jogging and expect to be healthy without also giving up unhealthy habits such as smoking and a high-fat diet. Nor should one ignore family medical history. Others spoke out against "fit-aholicism," an emotional disorder, according to a California psychiatrist, that literally means addiction to exercise.

WALK, DON'T RUN!

By the late 1980s, fitness proponents were discovering that sometimes working out could do more harm than good. A Harris Poll showed that 1 in 10 exercisers experienced a yearly sports-related injury. Just as joggers were racking up knee and back problems, the experts were telling them that it was time to slow down. Instead of "no pain, no gain," consumers were told that even moderate physical activity done regularly made a huge difference.

Exercisers may have slowed down, but they continued to work out. Instead of jogging 5 or 10 miles every day, they turned to "cross-training," combining several kinds of sports, such as cycling, swimming and walking; they gave up high-impact aerobics for the less stressful low-impact variety; and they traded in their jogging shoes for walking shoes.

Walking, in fact, turned into the most popular substitute for running, even generating a magazine aptly named *Walking*. ''Start a regular walking program and stay with it,'' advised *Prevention* in 1990. ''Even a low to moderately intense level of physical activity—such as walking—can reduce your odds of falling victim to a whole host of life-threatening diseases.'' As the testing director at the University of Michigan Fitness Research Center reported to Detroit's *Metro Times,* ''Walking is becoming more popular, especially for individuals who shouldn't or don't necessarily want to run: people who haven't exercised in a long time, the thirty-five-and-up crowd, or people who tried jogging and were frustrated or got injured.''

THE GREAT AMERICAN GENERATION GAP

As the twenty-first century edged closer, advocates of fitness continued to worry about American youngsters. In 1990, the National Association for Sport and Physical Education reported that 40 percent of American kids from five to eight years old were obese, inactive, or had high blood pressure or cholesterol levels. While middle-class baby boomers were sweating it out at the gym, the next generation was settling in front of the television.

America's children may be growing softer, but their parents continue to search for the perfect workout. In the late 1960s, adult bicycling came into its own again as part of the larger fitness boom. Bicycle enthusiasts could be seen racing through the streets on their new lightweight, thin-tired, 10-speed bikes that replaced the heavier, balloon-tired bikes they had ridden as kids. (Those thick-wheeled bicycles were first developed in 1933 by Frank W. Schwinn.)

But America's second bicycling craze didn't really take off until the invention of the mountain bike, first created in the 1970s by a group of San Francisco Bay Area bicyclists experimenting with a sturdy, fat-tired bike they could ride on mountain trails. With their knobby, thick tires, and handlebars designed to allow the rider to sit up rather than bend over, the bikes have proved more popular than their thin-wheeled cousins, because they are not only more versatile, but easier to ride. In 1990, two out of every three bicycles bought in the United States were mountain bikes.

That same year a special ''Good Health'' supplement to the *New York Times Magazine* published two articles that beautifully illustrated the current state of American physical fitness: One article described how kids were ''turned off'' by fitness; the other, how millions of adults were discovering the joys of mountain biking, the latest great American fitness fad.

SELECTED BIBLIOGRAPHY

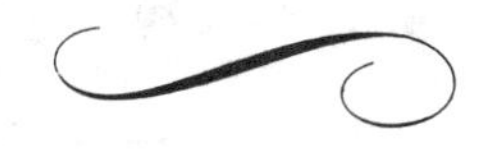

Adams, Samuel Hopkins. *The Great American Fraud: Articles on the Nostrum Evil and Quacks.* Reprinted from *Collier's Weekly,* 1905.

Aero, Rita. *The Complete Book of Longevity.* New York: G.P. Putnam & Sons, 1980.

"Aimee Is Dead." *San Francisco Chronicle.* 20 September 1944.

"Aimee's Bobbed Hair Wrecks Congregation." *San Francisco Chronicle.* 26 April 1927.

Altman, Nathaniel. *The Chiropractic Alternative: A Spine Owner's Guide.* Los Angeles: J.P. Tarcher, 1981.

Anderson, Robert Maples. *Vision of the Disinherited: The Making of American Pentecostalism.* New York: Oxford University Press, 1979.

"Animal Magnetism or Suggestion." *The Electrical World.* 27 April 1889.

"Are We Becoming 'Soft'?" *U.S. News and World Report.* 26 September 1955.

Armstrong, David. *The Insider's Guide to Health Foods.* New York: Bantam, 1983.

Bach, Marcus. *The Chiropractic Story.* Austell, Georgia: Si-Nel Publishing and Sales Company, 1968.

Banner, Lois. *American Beauty.* Chicago: University of Chicago Press, 1983.

Barnum, P.T. *The Humbugs of the World: An Account of Humbugs, Delusions, Impositions, Quackeries, Deceits and Deceivers Generally, in All Ages.* New York: Carleton, 1866.

Beecher, Catharine E. *Physiology and Calisthenics for Schools and Families.* New York: Harper and Brothers, 1856.

Begley, Sharon; Wright, Lynda; and Marshall, Ruth. "Can Water 'Remember'?" *Newsweek.* 25 July 1988.

Bennett, Linda A., and Ames, Genevieve M. *The American Experience with Alcohol: Contrasting Cultural Perspectives.* New York: Plenum Press, 1985.

Bennett, William, M.D., and Gurin, Joel. *The Dieter's Dilemma: Eating Less and Weighing More.* New York: Basic Books, 1982.

Berger, Michael. "How Shaklee Adapted to the Japanese Market." *San Francisco Chronicle.* 29 October 1990.

Berman, Alex. "The Thomsonian Movement and Its Relation to American Pharmacy and Medicine." *Bulletin of the History of Medicine.* September–October, 1951.

"Big Jocks." *Esquire.* April 1970.

Binger, Carl, M.D. *Revolutionary Doctor: Benjamin Rush, 1746–1813.* New York: W. W. Norton, 1966.

Bishop, George. *Faith Healing: God or Fraud?* Los Angeles: Sherbourne Press, 1967.

Bjorkman, Frances Maule. "Horace Fletcher and Fletcherism." *Independent.* 19 March 1908.

Blythe, Samuel G. "Too Much Exercise." *Saturday Evening Post.* 4 July 1925.

———. "Get Rid of That Fat." *Saturday Evening Post.* 23 April 1927.

Boand, Alfred C. "The Radio Gymnasium Class." *Hygeia.* June 1933.

Brody, Jane E. "How Exercise Keeps You Healthy." *New York Times.* 14 August 1985.

———. "Personal Health." *New York Times.* 9 March 1989.

———. "Intriguing Studies Link Nutrition to Immunity." *New York Times.* 21 March 1989.

———. "New Research Bolsters Long-Held Beliefs That Vitamin E Can Provide an Array of Benefits." *New York Times.* 27 April 1989.

Brooks, Douglass, and Copeland, Candice. " 'No Pain, No Gain' Is No Longer Gospel for Getting in Shape." *San Francisco Chronicle.* 1 January 1989.

Brumberg, Joan Jacobs. *Fasting Girls: The Emergence of Anorexia Nervosa as a Modern Disease.* Cambridge, Massachusetts: Harvard University Press, 1988.

Burnham, David. "FDA Eases Rules on Some Vitamins." *New York Times.* 28 May 1975.

Burns, Delores, ed. *The Greatest Health Discovery.* Chicago: Natural Hygiene Press, 1972.

Burros, Marian. "A Growing Harvest of Organic Produce." *New York Times.* 29 March 1989.

Burton, Jean. *Lydia Pinkham Is Her Name.* New York: Farrar, Straus, 1949.

Busch, Noel F. "You Can Live to Be a Hundred, He Says." *Saturday Evening Post.* 11 August 1951.

"C is for Controversy." *Newsweek.* 6 December 1971.

Cahalan, Don. *Understanding America's Drinking Problem: How to Combat the Hazards of Alcohol.* San Francisco and London: Jossey-Bass, 1988.

Cameron, Ewan, and Pauling, Linus. *Cancer and Vitamin C.* Menlo Park, California: Linus Pauling Institute of Science and Medicine, 1979.

Carson, Gerald. *Cornflake Crusade.* New York: Rinehart & Co., 1957.

———. "Sweet Extract of Hokum." *American Heritage.* June 1971.

———. "Who Put the Borax in Dr. Wiley's Butter?" *American Heritage.* August 1956.

Carson, Rachel L. *Silent Spring.* Boston: Houghton Mifflin, 1962.

Castleman, Michael. *The Healing Herbs.* Emmaus, Pennsylvania: Rodale Press, 1991.

Cayleff, Susan. *Wash and Be Healed: The Water-Cure Movement and Women's Health.* Philadelphia: Temple University Press, 1987.

Clemens, Samuel [Mark Twain]. *Christian Science.* New York: Harper and Brothers, 1907.

"Coffee Linked to Frisky 60s." *San Francisco Examiner.* 18 January 1990.

Cohen, Lester. *The New York Graphic.* New York: Chilton Books, 1964.

Collier, Peter, and Horowitz, David. *The Rockefellers.* New York: Holt, Rinehart, 1976.

Comstock, Sarah. "Aimee Semple McPherson." *Harper's.* 27 December 1927.

Cook, James. *Remedies and Rackets: The Truth about Patent Medicines Today.* New York: W.W. Norton, 1957.

Cooper, Gregory. "The Attitude of Organized Medicine Toward Chiropractic: A Sociohistorical Perspective." *Chiropractic History* 5 (1985).

Cost, Bruce. "Seasonings Have Roots in Folk Medicine." *San Francisco Chronicle.* 16 November 1988.

Coulter, Harris L. *Divided Legacy: The Conflict between Homoeopathy and the American Medical Association.* Richmond, California: North Atlantic Books, 1973.

Cousins, Norman. "Linus Pauling and the Vitamin C Controversy." *Saturday Review.* 15 May 1971.

Cramp, Arthur J., M.D. *Nostrums and Quackery and Pseudo-Medicine*, Volume 3. Chicago: Press of the American Medical Association, 1936.

Creemers, Debbie. Scripps Howard News Service. "Chiropractic Therapy Patients Believe, Even if Others Don't." *San Francisco Examiner.* 13 May 1985.

Crisp, Kathleen A. "Chiropractic Lyceums: The Colorful Origins of Chiropractic Continuing Education." *Chiropractic History* 4 (1985).

Davies, John B. *Phrenology Fad and Science: A 19th-Century American Crusade.* New Haven: Yale University Press, 1955.

Davis, Adelle. *Let's Eat Right to Keep Fit.* New York: Harcourt, Brace, 1954.

———. *Let's Get Well.* New York: Harcourt, Brace & World, 1965.

DeCarlo, Tessa. "The Dry Wine-Country Kingdom." *San Francisco Chronicle.* 15 July 1987.

Deford, Mirriam Allen. *They Were San Franciscans.* Caldwell, Idaho: Caxton, 1947.

Deutsch, Ronald M. *The New Nuts Among the Berries: How Nutrition Nonsense Captured America.* Palo Alto, California: Bull Publishing, 1977.

Dibner, Bern. *Early Electrical Machines: The Experiments and Apparatus of Two Enquiring Centuries That Led to the Triumphs of the Electrical Age.* Norwalk, Connecticut: Burndy Library, 1957.

Donegan, Jane B. *Hydropathic Highway to Health: Women and Water-Cure in America.* New York: Greenwood Press, 1986.

Donovan, Richard, and Whitney, Dwight. "Painless Parker, Last of America's Tooth-Plumbers." *Collier's.* 5 January 1952.

———. "Painless Parker Buys A Circus." *Collier's.* 12 January 1952.

———. " 'I Got A Toothache, Mister.' " *Collier's.* 19 January 1952.

Dooley, Nancy. "Critics Attacked by Adelle Davis." *San Francisco Examiner.* 29 March 1973.

Drew, Glen. "A Primer on Medical Device Regulation." *FDA Consumer.* May 1986.

Duke, James A. "Unlocking the Doors on the Tropical Medicine Chest." *Earth Island Journal.* Winter 1988.

Eberlein, Harold Donaldson. "When Society First Took a Bath." *Pennsylvania Magazine of History* 67 (1943).

Eddy, Mary Baker. *Miscellaneous Writings, 1883–1896.* Boston: A.V. Stewart, 1909.

———. *Science and Health With Key to the Scriptures.* [1875] 1971. Reprint. Boston: Christian Science Board of Directors.

Eddy, Walter H. *The Vitamine Manual: A Presentation of Essential Data About the New Food Factors.* New York: Williams and Wilkens, 1921.

Edstrom, David. "Medicine Man of the '80s." *Reader's Digest.* June 1938.

Ehrenreich, Barbara, and English, Deirdre. *Complaints and Disorders: The Sexual Politics of Sickness*. Old Westbury, New York: The Feminist Press, 1973.

———. *Witches, Midwives and Nurses: A History of Women Healers*. Old Westbury, New York: The Feminist Press, 1973.

Emboden, William A., Jr. *Bizarre Plants*. New York: Macmillan, 1974.

Farley, Dixie. "Setting Safe Limits on Pesticide Residues." *FDA Consumer*. October 1988.

Farmer, Jean. "The Rev. Sylvester (Graham Cracker) Graham: America's Early Fiber Crusader." *Saturday Evening Post*. March 1985.

Farmer, Laurence, M.D. "Mosquitos Were Uncommonly Numerous." *American Heritage*. April 1956.

"FDA Fights the Vitamin Craze." *Business Week*. 15 July 1972.

Fields, Wayne. "The Double Life of Hot Springs." *American Heritage*. April 1991.

Fishbein, Morris, M.D. *The Medical Follies*. New York: Boni and Liveright, 1925.

"Flesh Sculptors: Screen Players Find It's Fun to Keep Healthy—Here's How." *Literary Digest*. 6 March 1937.

Fletcher, Horace. *The A, B,–Z of Our Own Nutrition*. New York: Frederick A. Stokes, 1903.

———. *The New Glutton or Epicure*. New York: Frederick A. Stokes, 1903.

———. "What I Am Asked About Fletcherism." *Ladies' Home Journal*. October 1909.

———. "How I Feel at Sixty-Five." *Ladies' Home Journal*. May 1914.

Fletcher, Robert Samuel. "Bread and Doctrine at Oberlin." *The Ohio State Archaeological and Historical Quarterly* 49 (1940).

"Fletcherism in Europe." *New York Times*. 26 December 1914.

Flexner, Abraham. *Medical Education in the United States and Canada*. New York: Carnegie Endowment for the Advancement of Teaching, Bulletin No. 4, 1910.

Flexner, James Thomas. "The Death of a Hero." *American Heritage*. December 1969.

Fowler, Gene, and Crawford, Bill. *Border Radio*. Austin: Texas Monthly Press, 1988.

Fried, John J. *The Vitamin Conspiracy*. New York: Saturday Review Press/E.P. Dutton, 1975.

Funk, Casimir. "Who Discovered Vitamines?" *Science*. 30 April 1926.

"Garbo's Gayelord." *Time*. 16 February 1942.

Garraty, John A., ed. *Dictionary of American Biography*. Supplement Five, 1951–55. New York: Charles Scribner's Sons, 1977.

Gevitz, Norman. *The D.O.s: Osteopathic Medicine in America*. Baltimore: Johns Hopkins University Press, 1982.

———, ed. *Other Healers: Unorthodox Medicine in America*. Baltimore: Johns Hopkins University Press, 1988.

Gilbert, Susan. *Medical Fakes and Frauds: The Encyclopedia of Health, Medical Issues*. Edited by Dale C. Barell, M.D. New York: Chelsea House, 1989.

Gleason, Philip. "From Free Love to Catholicism: Dr. and Mrs. Thomas L. Nichols at Yellow Springs." *Ohio Historical Quarterly* 70 (1961).

Goldberg, Leslie. "The Fitness Boom Fallout." *San Francisco Examiner*. 30 May 1989.

Goode, Erica. "Exercise Beats a Diet, Researchers Say." *San Francisco Chronicle*. 2 April 1987.

Gorman, Tom. "Medicine Man of San Diego." *Los Angeles Times*, in *San Francisco Chronicle*. 15 January 1984.

Gottleib, Leon S., M.D. *Gold-Mining Surgeon*. Manhattan, Kansas: Sunflower University Press, 1985.

Graedon, Joe, and Graedon, Teresa. *Joe Graedon's The New People's Pharmacy*. New York: Bantam, 1985.

Green, Harvey. *Fit for America*. New York: Pantheon, 1986.

Green, Robert Montraville, M.D. *Commentary on the Effect of Electricity on Muscular Motion*. Cambridge, Massachusetts: Elizabeth Licht, 1953.

Griggs, Barbara. *Green Pharmacy*. New York: Viking Press, 1981.

Groh, George. "Doctors of the Frontier." *American Heritage*. April 1963.

Gromala, Theresa. "Women in Chiropractic: Exploring a Tradition of Equity in Healing." *Chiropractic History* 3 (1983).

———. "Broadsides, Epigrams, and Testimonials: The Evolution of Chiropractic Advertising." *Chiropractic History* 4 (1985).

———. " 'Bees in His Bonnet': D.D. Palmer's Students and Their Early Impact." *Chiropractic History* 6 (1986).

Gronowitz, Anton. *Garbo: Her Story*. New York: Simon & Schuster, 1990.

Grover, Kathryn, ed. *Fitness in American Culture: Images of Health, Sport, and the Body, 1830–1940*. Amherst, Massachusetts: University of Massachusetts Press and the Margaret Woodbury Strong Museum, Rochester, New York, 1989.

Gumpert, Martin. *Hahnemann: The Adventurous Career of a Medical Rebel*. Translated by Claud W. Sykes. New York: L.B. Fischer, 1945.

Halberstam, Michael, M.D. "The A, B-12, C, D and E of Vitamins." *New York Times Magazine*. 17 March 1974.

Haldeman, Scott. "Almeda Haldeman, Canada's First

Chiropractor: Pioneering the Prairie Provinces, 1907–1917." *Chiropractic History* 3 (1983).

Hall, Trish. "A New Temperance Is Taking Root in America." *New York Times*. 15 March 1989.

Halstuk, Martin. "Prayer Is His Only Medicine." *San Francisco Chronicle*. 25 April 1988.

Hamilton, Mildred. "The Jog Is Up." *San Francisco Examiner*. 21 November 1977.

Harrell, David Edwin, Jr. *All Things Are Possible*. Bloomington, Indiana: Indiana University Press, 1975.

———. *Oral Roberts: An American Life*. Bloomington, Indiana: Indiana University Press, 1975.

Harrow, Benjamin. "Funk, Father of the Vitamin." *Nation*. 16 December 1944.

Hauser, Bengamin Gayelord. *Harmonized Food Selection*. New York: Tempo, 1930.

———. *Eat and Grow Beautiful*. New York: Tempo, 1936.

———. *Look Younger, Live Longer*. New York: Farrar, Straus, 1950.

Hawke, David Freeman. *Benjamin Rush: Revolutionary Gadfly*. Indianapolis: Bobbs-Merrill, 1971.

Hendrick, Burton. "Some Modern Ideas on Food." *McClure's*. April 1910.

Hendrick, Ellwood. "Vitamines." *Harper's Monthly*. 21 March 1921.

Holbrook, Stewart H. "Bell, Book and Hatchet." *American Heritage*. December 1957.

———. *The Golden Age of Quackery*. New York: Macmillan, 1959.

Homewood, A.E. *The Neurodynamics of the Vertebral Subluxation*. St. Petersburg, Florida: Valkyrie Press, 1962.

Homola, Samuel. *Bonesetting, Chiropractic, and Cultism*. Panama City, Florida: Critique Books, 1963.

Howard, Sir Albert. [1943] 1979. *An Agricultural Testament*. Facsimile. Emmaus, Pennsylvania: Rodale Press.

Howard, Jane. "Earth Mother to the Foodists." *Life*. 22 October 1971.

Hubbard, Elbert. "The Gentle Art of Fletcherizing." *Cosmopolitan*. December 1908.

"Idyl." *Time*. 14 March 1938.

Inglis, Brian. *Fringe Medicine*. London: Faber and Faber, 1965.

"Inside America's Hottest Diet Programs." Five-part series. *Prevention*. January–May 1990.

"Is American Youth Physically Fit?" *U.S. News and World Report*. 2 August 1957.

Jackson, Carlton. *J.I. Rodale: Apostle of Non-Conformity*. New York: Pyramid, 1974.

Jacobs, John. "Meaty School Dispute Has Adventist-land in a Stew." *San Francisco Examiner*. 15 August 1982.

James, Henry. *The Bostonians*. 1886. New York: Bantam Classic edition, 1984.

James, William. *The Varieties of Religious Experience* [1901–02]. Introduction by John E. Smith. Cambridge, Massachusetts: Harvard University Press, 1985.

Josselyn, John. [1672] 1972. *New-Englands Rarities Discovered*. Facsimile with foreword by H. L. S. Boston: Massachusetts Historical Society.

Kaufman, Martin. *Homeopathy in America: The Rise and Fall of a Medical Heresy*. Baltimore: Johns Hopkins University Press, 1971.

Kelley, Thomas P., Jr. *The Fabulous Kelley: Canada's King of the Medicine Men*. Don Mills, Ontario: General Publishing, 1974.

Kellogg, John Harvey. *The Natural Diet of Man*. Battle Creek, Michigan: Modern Medicine Publishing, 1923.

Kett, Joseph F. *Formation of the American Medical Profession: The Role of Institutions, 1780–1860*. New Haven: Yale University Press, 1968.

King, F.H. [1911] *Farmers of Forty Centuries*. Facsimile. Emmaus, Pennsylvania: Rodale Press.

Kloss, Jethro. *Back to Eden: A Human Interest Story of Health and Restoration to Be Found in Herb, Root and Bark*. Loma Linda, California: Back to Eden Books, 1939.

Kolata, Gina. "Sharp Cuts in Serious Birth Defects Is Tied to Vitamins in Pregnancy." *New York Times*. 24 November 1989.

Kremer, Edward. *History of Pharmacy*. Revised by Glenn Sonnedecker. Philadelphia: J.B. Lippincott, 1963.

Krieger, Lisa M. "State Warns of 'Dangerous' Asian Remedies." *San Francisco Examiner*. 15 July 1988.

———. " 'Cal-Ban' Diet Pills Ordered Recalled." *San Francisco Examiner*. 27 July 1990.

Kronholm, William. "State Challenges Some 'Health Expos' as Modern-Day 'Snake Oil.' " Associated Press in *San Francisco Examiner*. 29 May 1985.

Lally, Steven. "The Doctor's Walking Prescription." *Prevention*. March 1990.

Lancaster, Paul, "Inhale! . . . Exhale! . . . Inhale! . . . Exhale! . . . ." *American Heritage*. October/November 1978.

Lane, M.A. *Dr. A.T. Still: Founder of Osteopathy*. Chicago: Osteopathic Publishing Co., 1918.

Langone, John. "Linus Pauling: Vim, Vigor, Vision and Vitamins." *Discover*. November 1982.

Leary, Warren E. "America's Young Women Getting Fatter." *New York Times*. 24 February 1989.

Leavitt, Judith Walzer, and Numbers, Ronald L. *Sickness and Health in America: Readings in the History of Medicine and Public Health*. Madison: University of Wisconsin Press, 1978.

Lender, Mark Edward, and Martin, James Kirby. *Drinking in America: A History*. New York: Free Press, 1982.

Levenstein, Harvey A. *Revolution at the Table: The Transformation of the American Diet*. New York: Oxford University Press, 1988.

Levi, Debra. "Oakland Chiropractor Chosen for Olympics." *San Francisco Chronicle.* 7 July 1988.

Lewis, Peter H. "Mighty Fire Ants March Out of the South." *New York Times.* 24 July 1990.

Lewis, Robert. Newhouse News Service. "America's Kids Are Getting Fat." *San Francisco Chronicle.* 1 August 1990.

Lewis, Sinclair. *Elmer Gantry.* New York: Harcourt, Brace, 1927.

Linhart, Gordon. "Selling the 'Big Idea': B.J. Palmer Ushers in the Golden Age, 1906–1920." *Chiropractic History* 8 (1988).

"Liquid Diets Make You Thinner But May Pose Big Fat Health Risks." *People.* 25 April 1990.

Lloyd, Barbara. " 'User-Friendly' Medicine Balls." *New York Times.* 30 April 1990.

"Local Lady Took Natex Year Ago—Had Good Health Ever Since," Advertisement in (Allentown, Pennsylvania) *Call Chronicle.* 27 May 1935.

Long, Patricia. "Fat Chance." *Hippocrates.* September/October 1989.

"The Losing Formula." *Newsweek.* 30 April 1990.

Lyons, Albert S., M.D., and Petrucelli, R. Joseph, II, M.D. *Medicine: An Illustrated History.* New York: Harry Abrams, 1978.

MacBride, Thomas Huston. *In Cabins and Sod-Houses.* Iowa City: The State Historical Society of Iowa, 1928.

Macfadden, Mary, and Gauvreau, Emile. *Dumbbells and Carrot Strips: The Story of Bernarr Macfadden.* New York: Henry Holt, 1953.

"Macfadden's Family: He Wages War on Weakness." *Time.* 21 September 1936.

Maddocks, Melvin. "Whither the Fitness Fad." *Christian Science Monitor.* 16 December 1984.

Major, Nettie Leitch. *C.W. Post: The Hour and the Man.* Washington, D.C.: Judd & Detweiler, 1963.

"The Making of a Milestone in Consumer Protection, 1938–1988." *FDA Consumer.* 30 October 1988.

Malcolm, Donald. "Sugar and Spites." *New Yorker.* 26 March 1960.

Malmberg, Carl. *Diet and Die.* New York: Hilman-Curl, 1935.

Maples, Glynn. "In Swansea, Wales, There's a Sucker Born Every Minute." *Wall Street Journal.* 9 September 1989.

Mayer, Jean. "Muscular State of the Union." *New York Times Magazine.* 6 November 1955.

McCormick, Sharon. "Fat People Fight for Self-Esteem." *San Francisco Chronicle.* 5 July 1989.

McNamara, Brooks. *Step Right Up.* Garden City, New York: Doubleday, 1976.

"The Medicine Show." *American Mercury.* June 1925.

Melville, Herman. *Moby-Dick, or the Whale.* New York: Harper and Brothers, 1851.

Meyer, Donald. *The Positive Thinkers: A Study of the American Quest for Health, Wealth and Personal Power from Mary Baker Eddy to Norman Vincent Peale.* Garden City, New York: Doubleday, 1965.

Millman, Marcia. *Such a Pretty Face: Being Fat in America.* New York: W.W. Norton, 1980.

"Miracle Woman." *Time.* 14 September 1970.

Mitchell, Barbara. "Sylvester Graham: The Genuine Name Behind the Not-So-Genuine Cereal and Crackers." *Vegetarian Times.* November 1989.

Morgan, Wayne H. *Drugs in America: A Social History.* Syracuse: Syracuse University Press, 1981.

Moskowitz, Milton. "Bottled Water Sparkles in Role as Wave of the Future." *San Francisco Chronicle.* 10 June 1985.

"Mr. Post's Perfect Town." *American Mercury.* March 1957.

"New Product of General Foods: The Physically Fit Employee." *New York Times.* 30 May 1977.

"New Ways to Make Walking Fun." *Prevention.* February 1990.

Nissenbaum, Stephen. *Sex, Diet, and Debility in Jacksonian America: Sylvester Graham and Health Reform.* Westport, Connecticut: Greenwood Press, 1980.

Nolan, Dick. "He Had Moxie." *San Francisco Examiner.* 30 July 1985.

Nostrums and Quackery: Articles on the Nostrum Evil and Quackery Reprinted with Additions and Modifications, from the Journal of the American Medical Association. Chicago: American Medical Association Press, 1912.

Numbers, Ronald L. *Prophetess of Health: A Study of Ellen G. White.* New York: Harper & Row, 1976.

Okie, Abraham Howard. *Homeopathy: With Particular Reference to a Lecture by O.W. Holmes, M.D.* Boston: Otis Clapp, 1842.

"The Omnipresent Oscilloclast." *The Survey.* 15 January 1923.

O'Neill, Molly. "How Fat Is Fat? The Rounding of the Body Beautiful." *New York Times.* 2 January 1991.

Orbach, Susie. *Fat Is a Feminist Issue: A Self-Help Guide for Compulsive Eaters.* New York: Paddington Press, 1978.

"Orthomolecular Minds." *Time.* 3 May 1968.

Ottum, Bob. "Look, Mom, I'm an Institution." *Sports Illustrated.* 23 March 1981.

Paley, Maggie. "Gloria Swanson Is Back, and Full of Organic Beans." *Life.* 17 September 1971.

Palmer, David D. *The Palmers: Memoirs of David D. Palmer.* Davenport, Iowa: Bawden Brothers, 1970.

Pauling, Linus. *Vitamin C and the Common Cold.* San Francisco: W.H. Freeman, 1970.

"Peddling Youth Over the Counter." *Newsweek.* 5 March 1990.

Perenyi, Eleanor. "Apostle of the Compost Heap." *Saturday Evening Post.* 16 July 1966.

"Perrier Loses Its Fizz." *Newsweek*. 26 February 1990.

Peters, Lulu Hunt, A.B., M.D. *Diet and Health: With Key to the Calories*. Chicago: Reilly and Lee, 1918.

"Physicians Defend Morning Exercises." *New York Times*. 9 April 1929.

"Pills in the Contract." *Business Week*. 16 May 1942.

Pogash, Carol. "The Great Gadfly." *Science Digest*. June 1981.

Poppy, John. "Adelle Davis and the New Nutrition Religion." *Look*. 15 December 1970.

Powell, Horace B. *W.K. Kellogg: The Original Has This Signature*. Englewood Cliffs, New Jersey: Prentice Hall, 1956.

Power, Keith. "Railroad Was Built to Reach Calistoga's Mineral Waters." *San Francisco Chronicle*. 27 March 1986.

Randi, James. *The Faith Healers*. Buffalo: Prometheus Books, 1989.

"Ready, Set . . . Sweat!" *Time*. 6 June 1977.

Reed, Dudley B., M.D. *Keep Fit and Like It*. New York: Whittlesey House. McGraw-Hill, 1939.

Reif, Rita. "It Had Fat Tires and Fenders You Could Polish." *New York Times*. 4 November 1990.

"Religious Quackery." *Time*. 9 February 1962.

"Return of the Leeches." Associated Press in the *San Francisco Chronicle*. 6 January 1989.

Roan, Shari. "Liquid Diet Safety Questions." *San Francisco Chronicle*. 6 June 1990.

Rockwell, A.D., M.D. *The Medical and Surgical Uses of Electricity*. New York: E.B. Treat, 1903.

Rodale, J.I. *My Own Technique of Eating for Health*. Emmaus, Pennsylvania: Rodale Press, 1969.

———. "Why I Started Organic Gardening." *Organic Gardening and Farming*. September 1971.

Rodale, Robert. "Celebrating Forty Years of Prevention." *Prevention*. July 1990.

Root, Waverly, and deRochemont, Richard. *Eating in America: A History*. New York: Ecco Press, 1981.

Rosen, Marjorie, et al. "Big Gain; No Pain." *People*. 14 January 1991.

Rosenberg, Charles E. *The Cholera Years: The U.S. in 1832, 1849 and 1866*, rev. ed. Chicago: University of Chicago Press, 1987.

Rubin, Sylvia. "In Praise of Oat Cuisine: Even Fit Folks Are Joining This Bran-New Trend." *San Francisco Chronicle*. 14 December 1988.

Rublowsky, John. *The Stoned Age: A History of Drugs in America*. New York: G.P. Putnam's Sons, 1979.

Sandburg, Carl. *Always the Young Strangers*. New York: Harcourt Brace, 1952.

Schaefer, Richard A. *Legacy: The Heritage of a Unique International Medical Outreach*. Mountain View, California: Pacific Press Association, 1977.

Schmid, Randolph E. Associated Press. "Alcohol Still Prominent in Many Medications." *San Francisco Examiner*. 21 January 1985.

Schneider, Keith. "Weaning Chemical Use: Seeds of Change on Farms." *New York Times*. 11 September 1989.

Schwartz, Hillel. *Never Satisfied. A Cultural History of Diets, Fantasies and Fat*. New York: Free Press, 1986.

Shealey, Tom. "A Fresh Look at Chiropractic Care." *Prevention*. May 1986.

Sietsema, Tom. "Fat's Back." *San Francisco Chronicle*. 2 January 1991.

Sifikis, Carl. "Body Love Macfadden," in *American Eccentrics*. New York: Facts on File, 1984.

Silberger, Julius, Jr. *Mary Baker Eddy: An Interpretive Biography of the Founder of Christian Science*. Boston: Little, Brown, 1980.

Simson, Eve. *The Faith Healer: Deliverance Evangelism in North America*. St. Louis: Concordia Publishing, 1977.

"The Snap, Crackle, Pop Defense." *Forbes*. 25 March 1985.

Sokolow, Jayme A. *Eros and Modernization: Sylvester Graham, Health Reform, and the Origins of Victorian Sexuality in America*. Rutherford, New Jersey: Fairleigh Dickinson University Press, 1983.

Spunt, Georges. *When Nature Speaks*. New York: Frederick Fell, 1977.

Stage, Sarah. *Female Complaints: Lydia Pinkham and the Business of Women's Medicine*. New York: W.W. Norton, 1979.

Starr, Kevin. *Inventing the Dream: California Through the Progressive Era*. New York: Oxford University Press, 1985.

Starr, Paul K. *The Social Transformation of American Medicine*. New York: Basic Books, 1982.

Steele, Robert [Lately Thomas]. *Storming Heaven: The Lives and Turmoils of Minnie Kennedy and Aimee Semple McPherson*. New York: Morrow, 1970.

Stein, Diane. *All Women Are Healers: A Comprehensive Guide to Natural Healing*. Freedom, California: Crossing Press, 1990.

Steincrohn, Peter J. *You Don't Have to Exercise! Rest Begins at Forty*. Garden City, New York: Doubleday, Doran, 1942.

Stern, Madeleine B. *Heads and Headlines: The Phrenological Fowlers*. Norman, Oklahoma: University of Oklahoma Press, 1971.

Still, Andrew Taylor. [1897] 1972. *Autobiography of Andrew T. Still*. Facsimile. New York: Arno Press, 1972.

Stuller, Jay. "Cleanliness Has Only Recently Become a Virtue." *Smithsonian*. February 1991.

Suits, Adelaide. *Brass Tacks: Oral Biography of a 20th Century Physician*. Ann Arbor: Halyburton Press, 1985.

Swanson, Gloria. "Hollywood Sunset." *Esquire*. August 1966.

———. *Swanson on Swanson*. New York: Random House, 1980.

"T.V.'s Nature Boy." *Look*. 30 August 1960.

"Two Hundred Years Ago." *American Heritage*. April 1988.

Tyrrell, Ian R. *Sobering Up: From Temperance to Prohibition in Antebellum America, 1800–1860*. Contributions in American History, No. 82. Westport, Connecticut: Greenwood Press, 1979.

Ullman, Dana. *Homeopathy: Medicine for the 21st Century*. Berkeley: North Atlantic, 1988.

Underwood, Henry. "Downfall of a Prophet: How New York, the Relentless, Shattered Boastful Dowie." *Harper's Weekly*, 22 December 1906.

U.S. Congress, House of Representatives, Committee on Small Business. *Hearing Before the Subcommittee on Regulation, Business Opportunities, and Energy: Deceptions and Fraud in the Diet Industry, Parts I and II*, 101st Congress, 2nd sess., 26 March and 27 May 1990.

"Vitamin E, Anyone?" *Newsweek*. 27 March 1972.

"The Vitamin Man." *Newsweek*. 31 December 1962.

"Vitamins Reduce Lost Time in Industry." *Scientific American*. December 1932.

"Vitamins, Vitamins." *New Republic*. 11 January 1939.

Vogel, Virgil J. *American Indian Medicine*. Norman, Oklahoma: University of Oklahoma Press, 1970.

Von Haller, Albert. *The Vitamin Hunters*. Translated by Hella Freud Bernays. Philadelphia: Chilton, 1962.

Walker, Gerald. "The Great American Dieting Neurosis." *New York Times Magazine*. 23 August 1959.

Wardwell, Walter I. "The Cutting Edge of Chiropractic Recognition: Prosecution and Legislation in Massachusetts." *Chiropractic History* 2 (1982).

———. "Before the Palmers: An Overview of Chiropractic's Antecedents." *Chiropractic History* 7 (1987).

———. "Chiropractors: Evolution to Acceptance," in *Other Healers: Unorthodox Medicine in America*. Edited by Norman Gevitz. Baltimore: Johns Hopkins University Press, 1988.

Waters, Christina. "Back to Basics: A Brief Look at the Chiropractic World." *Santa Cruz Express*. 2 February 1984.

Weber, Malcolm. *Medicine Show*. Caldwell, Idaho: Caxton, 1941.

Weil, Andrew, M.D. *Health and Healing*. Boston: Houghton Mifflin, 1983.

Weiner, Michael A. *Earth Foods: Plant Remedies, Drugs, and Natural Foods of the North American Indians*. New York: Macmillan, 1972.

Weisberger, Bernard A. "The Paradoxical Doctor Benjamin Rush." *American Heritage*. October 1975.

Weiss, Harry B., and Kemble, Howard R. *They Took to the Waters: The Forgotten Mineral Spring Resorts of New Jersey and Nearby Pennsylvania and Delaware*. Trenton, New Jersey: The Past Times Press, 1962.

———. *The Great American Water-Cure Craze*. Trenton: Past Times Press, 1967.

Wenner, Cheryl. "Patients Are Taught to Relieve Chronic Pain." (Allentown, Pennsylvania) *Call Chronicle*. 20 December 1988.

White, Paul Dudley. "Walking and Cycling." *Hygeia*. April 1937.

Whorton, James C. " 'Tempest in a Flesh Pot': The Formulation of a Physiological Rationale for Vegetarianism." In *Sickness and Health in America: Readings in the History of Medicine and Public Health*, edited by Judith Walzer Leavitt and Ronald L. Numbers. Madison: University of Wisconsin Press, 1978.

———. *Crusaders for Fitness: The History of American Health Reformers*. Princeton: Princeton University Press, 1982.

Wilstein, Steve. Associated Press. "Bad Backs Are Big Concern for Employers and Doctors." *San Francisco Examiner*. 10 October 1988.

Yergin, Daniel. "Supernutritionist." *New York Times Magazine*. 20 May 1973.

Yoder, Jon A. *Upton Sinclair*. New York: Frederick Ungar, 1975.

Yoder, Robert M. "Vitamania." *Hygeia*. April 1942.

Young, James Harvey. *The Toadstool Millionaires: A Social History of Patent Medicines in America Before Federal Regulation*. Princeton: Princeton University Press, 1961.

———. *American Self-Dosage Medicines: An Historical Perspective*. Lawrence, Kansas: Coronado Press, 1974.

Bibliographical Notes

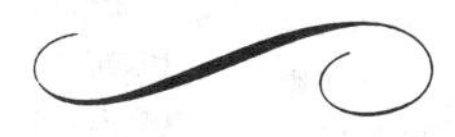

Chapter 1: *Pilgrims' Progress: Early American Medicine*

David Freeman Hawke's *Benjamin Rush: Revolutionary Gadfly* gives valuable details on Rush's life and medical training and includes an appendix of Rush's remedies. Carl Binger's *Revolutionary Doctor* provides the fullest biographical portrait and conveys Rush's tragic side, especially in the great yellow-fever epidemics. Paul K. Starr's *The Social Transformation of American Medicine* is an excellent source for medical knowledge of the eighteenth and nineteenth centuries, the sorry state of medical education, and the impact of the Flexner Report. Abraham Flexner's *Medical Education in the United States and Canada* is a sardonic dissection of North American medical education in 1910. A cluster of articles in *American Heritage* provide vivid and readable accounts of early American medicine. They include Laurence Farmer's April 1956 account of the Philadelphia yellow-fever epidemic of 1793; George Groh's piece on frontier doctors in the April 1963 issue; James Thomas Flexner's gripping December 1969 story about the death of George Washington; Bernard Weisberger's October 1975 exploration of Benjamin Rush's medical philosophy; and Jack Larkin's September/October 1988 excerpt from his book *The Reshaping of Everyday Life in the United States, 1790–1840*. Charles Rosenberg's superb *The Cholera Years* is a definitive account of the inadequate state of medicine during the contagions of 1832, 1849, and 1866. The surprisingly persistent legacy of early American medicine can be seen in colorful detail in the 1921 encyclopedia *Health Knowledge*, a 1,527-page, two-volume set, edited by J.L. Cornish, M.D., generously given to the authors by Barbara and Donald Yost of Harrisburg, Pennsylvania.

Chapter 2: *The Herbalists: Green Medicine*

An authoritative account of classical and medieval medical theories is provided in the sumptuous volume *Medicine, An Illustrated History*, by Albert S. Lyons, M.D., and R. Joseph Petrucelli II, M.D. Barbara Griggs's *Green Pharmacy* is a major source on the historical roots of herbal medicine, especially in England, North America, and China. John Josselyn's *New-Englands Rarities Discovered*, published in 1672, is a useful and delightful source, available in facsimile edition by the Massachusetts Historical Society. William G. Rothstein's article "The Botanical Movements and Orthodox Medicine" in *Other Healers*, edited by Norman Gevitz, gives well-researched information on herbal medicine in colonial America. Carl Binger's *Revolutionary Doctor* details the crude and often amusing use of early pharmaceutical drugs. The pamphlet "Shaker Medicinal Herbs," available at Hancock Shaker Village, Pittsfield, Massachusetts, illuminates the widespread use of herbs by this important religious sect. A copy was kindly given to the authors by Margarette Armstrong of Harrisburg, Pennsylvania. *Health and Healing*, by Andrew Weil, M.D., is a knowledgeable and sympathetic account by a physician trained in both allopathic and alternative medicine. Bruce Cost, a contributor to the *San Francisco Chronicle*, has written knowledgeably about the links between herbal medicine and cooking in Chinese cuisine. Virgil J. Vogel's *American Indian Medicine* is the major text on Native American health practices, which centered on the use of herbs and other plants. Michael Weiner's *Earth Foods* is another erudite account of Native American herbal expertise. The growing importance of endangered plants to modern medicine is widely covered in leading newspapers, such as the *Boston Globe* and *New York Times*. USDA researcher James Duke contributed an important overview in the Winter 1988 *Earth Island Journal*. Michael Castleman's *The Healing Herbs* is an informative and engaging modern herbal.

Chapter 3: *The Thomsonians: Every Man His Own Doctor*

The Francis A. Countway Library of Medicine, Harvard Medical School, Boston, is a motherlode of primary source material on botanic medicine. The library has bound volumes of the *Boston Medical and Surgical Journal*, forerunner of the *New England Journal of Medicine*, and the long-defunct *American Eclectic Medical Review*. The journal includes critiques of botanical healers, including Samuel Thomson himself. Also at Countway are bound volumes of the *Philadelphia Botanic Sentinel and Thomsonian Medical Revolutionist*, which includes case studies by Thomson. Thomson's own writings are available in the Boston Public Library. They include his autobiography, *A Narrative of the Life and Medical Discoveries of Samuel Thomson*, and his poetic broadside, *Learned Quackery Exposed*. Thomson's life is outlined in the *Dictionary of American Biography*, Volume Nine, 1935, published by Scribner's. The Boston Public Library also has microfilm copies of 1840s newspapers, including the *Boston Courier* and the *Boston Daily Advertiser*, which carries Thomson's obituary. Useful secondary sources include Alex Berman's two-part 1951 series in the *Bulletin of the History of Medicine*. Berman also wrote on neo-Thomsonianism in the April 1956 issue of *Journal of the History of Medicine*. Barbara Griggs's *Green Pharmacy* provides a valuable overview of botanical medicine. Paul K. Starr's *The Social Transformation of American Medicine* recounts Thomsonianism's threats to established medicine and its character as a counterculture in Jacksonian society. Barbara Ehrenreich and Deirdre English emphasize Thomson's debt to "the widow Benton" in their feminist histories *Complaints and Disorders* and *Witches, Midwives and Nurses*. Edward Kremers's *History of Pharmacy* outlines the Eclectics' contributions to modern pharmaceutical medicine.

Chapter 4: *Homeopathy: The Law of Similars*

Harris L. Coulter's *Divided Legacy* provides the most comprehensive history and analysis of American homeopathy through the beginning of the twentieth century, with particular emphasis on the movement's conflicts with the American Medical Association and the battles between the "highs" and "lows" within the movement. Martin Kaufman's *Homeopathy in America* is an excellent source for tracing the history of American homeopathy and is particularly useful for seeing how homeopathy permeated nineteenth-century American urban and intellectual society. Dana Ullman's numerous writings on homeopathy, and particularly his book *Homeopathy*, are essential for understanding the basics of homeopathy and provide a perceptive look into its role in the future of medicine. Martin Gumpert's biography of Hahnemann gives a detailed and very human look at the life of homeopathy's founder. The following individuals interviewed in the fall of 1988 were indispensible resources: Michael Quinn, head pharmacist and proprietor of Berkeley, California's Hahnemann Medical Clinic; Dana Ullman, author, educator, and proprietor of the Homeopathic Educational Services in Berkeley, California; Dr. George Guess, a medical doctor practicing homeopathy in North Carolina; Latifa Tabachnick, a student of homeopathy living in San Francisco; and Neda Tomasovich, administrator at Berkeley's Hahnemann Medical Clinic. Additional information on modern-day homeopathic clinics came from the Evergreen Clinic in Seattle, Washington and the Turning Point Family Wellness Center in Watertown, Massachusetts. Materials about current homeopathic education came from the National Center for Homeopathy in Washington, D.C.

Chapter 5: *Temperance: Exorcising Demon Alcohol*

A chief primary source, bound volumes of the *Journal of Health*, from 1830, are available in the University of California, Berkeley Library. Berkeley also has Henry Ward Beecher's 1871 sermon "Common Sense for Young Men," a well-reasoned exemplar of the anti-alcohol argument. Also at Berkeley is Leslie A. Keeley's "A Treatise on Drunkenness" from 1892 and the 1897 Sears, Roebuck catalogue that advertises patent-medicine drunkenness cures. Additional temperance arguments can be read in the *American Phrenological Journal*, from 1833, available in the Francis A. Countway Library of Medicine, Harvard Medical School, Boston. The University of California at San Francisco Library has the delightfully dyspeptic *Humbugs of New-York: Being a Remonstrance Against Popular Delusion, Whether in Science, Philosophy or Religion*, an 1838 polemic by David Meredith Reese, M.D. The most readable and comprehensive popular book, Mark Edward Lender and James Kirby Martin's *Drinking in America*, makes a surprisingly strong case for prohibition. Other useful scholarly books include Linda A. Bennett and Genevieve M. Ames's *The American Experience with Alcohol*; Ian R. Tyrrell's *Sobering Up*; Don Cahalan's *Understanding America's Drinking Problem*; and H. Wayne Morgan's *Drugs in America*. Carl Binger's *Revolutionary Doctor* gives a detailed account of Benjamin Rush's early efforts against alcohol. Stuart H. Holbrook contributes a useful profile of Carry Nation in the December 1957 *American Heritage*. Present-day new temperance efforts are widely covered in the popular press.

Chapter 6: *Sylvester and the Grahamites: "Put Back the Bran"*

The best secondary sources for understanding the Graham system and how it fit into nineteenth-century American health reforms are Stephen Nissenbaum's *Sex, Diet, and Debility in Jacksonian America* and Jayme A. Sokolow's *Eros and Modernization*. Both are also very helpful for tracing Graham's life. Additional sources for Graham's biography include Mildred Naylor's "Sylvester Graham, 1794–1851" in *Annals of Medical History*, Russell Thatcher Trall's "Biographical Sketch of Sylvester Graham" in *The Water-Cure Journal*, and Jean Farmer's "The Rev. Sylvester Graham" in the *Saturday Evening Post*. Both Nissenbaum's and Sokolow's works give detailed descriptions of Graham's followers. Robert Samuel Fletcher's "Bread and Doctrine at Oberlin" in the *Ohio State Archaeological and Historical Quarterly* gives the most detailed history of the Oberlin College experiment with Grahamism. Sylvester Graham's own *Science of Human Life* is the best source for understanding, first hand, Graham's views on bread and breadmaking, while Waverly Root and Richard de Rochemont's *Eating in America* gives a fascinating history of breadmaking and bread eating in the United States. *The Graham Journal of Health and Longevity* is a rich source of testimonials, advertisements, and Grahamite philosophy. Bound volumes are located at the Francis A. Countway Library of Medicine, Harvard Medical School, Boston. Newspapers from the period, in particular the *Boston Courier* and the *Evening Transcript*, published announcements of Graham's lectures, first-hand coverage of the riots surrounding Graham's Boston lectures, and reactions of readers. They are located on microfilm in the Boston Public Library.

Chapter 7: *Vegetarianism: "Hog Versus Hominy"*

Waverly Root and Richard de Rochemont's *Eating in America* is an outstanding secondary source for dietary habits from the colonial times to the present. For secondary sources on the history of vegetarianism, Gerald Carson's *Cornflake Crusade* presents an excellent account of the nineteenth-century American movement beginning with the Bible Christians, and James C. Whorton's "Tempest in a Fleshpot" in *Sickness and Health in America* presents a thorough account of the transformation of vegetarian arguments into Graham's physiological vegetarianism. Graham's arguments are also covered in Stephen Nissenbaum's *Sex, Diet, and Debility in Jacksonian America* and Jayme A. Sokolow's *Eros and Modernization*. Whorton's *Crusaders for Fitness* and Harvey Green's *Fit for America* are good sources for the aggressive vegetarianism of the Progressive Era. The *Vegetarian Messenger* and *Vegetarian Magazine* are excellent sources for evaluating the late-nineteenth-century vegetarian movement. Issues from the late nineteenth and early twentieth centuries are located in the Francis A. Countway Library of Medicine, Harvard Medical School, Boston. For the modern-day vegetarian movement, the *Vegetarian Times* is indispensible, as was a 1989 telephone interview with Jay Dinshah of the American Vegan Society.

Chapter 8: *Phrenology: Bonehead Medicine*

Two helpful secondary sources on phrenology are Madeleine B. Stern's *Heads and Headlines*, a detailed story of the Fowler and Wells family and business empire, and John B. Davies's *Phrenology Fad and Science*, which describes the history of phrenology and how the new pseudoscience permeated American culture. Stephen Nissenbaum's *Sex, Diet and Debility in Jacksonian America* and Jayme Sokolow's *Eros and Modernization* are good sources for understanding the connection between phrenology and Grahamism. *The Boston Medical and Surgical Journal*, available at the Francis A. Countway Library of Medicine, Harvard Medical School, Boston, shows how the regular medical establishment viewed phrenology and the *American Phrenological Journal*. The best primary source for understanding American phrenology as a practical method is the *American Phrenological Journal*. Bound volumes are located at both the Countway Library and the Boston Public Library.

Chapter 9: *Hydropathy: Wash and Be Healed*

Two superb secondary works on American hydropathy, focusing on women's health, are Susan E. Cayleff's *Wash and Be Healed: The Water-Cure Movement and Women's Health* and Jane B. Donegan's *Hydropathic Highway to Health: Women and Water-Cure in Antebellum America*. *The Great American Water-Cure Craze* by Harry B. Weiss and Howard R. Kemble is an essential source for a history of the water cure in the United States, including state-by-state descriptions of the major water-cure establishments. Harvey Green's *Fit for America* provides useful material on the water cure and its basic divergence from the mineral-spring champions. Useful primary sources on water-cure theory and descriptions of the treatments include Russell Trall's *The Hydropathic Encyclopedia* and Marie Louise Shew's *Water Cure for Ladies*. *The Water-Cure Journal* (1844 through 1913, published under different titles) is the best primary source for understanding the American hydropathic movement. With some later issues missing, the journal in bound volumes is located at the Francis A. Countway Library of Medicine, Harvard Medical School, Boston. The *Boston Medical and Surgical Journal*, also located at the Countway Library, is a wonderful source for gauging orthodox medicine's reactions to hydropathy. Harold Donaldson Eberlein's "When Society First Took a Bath" in the *Pennsylvania Magazine of History* gives an entertaining history of bathing habits in the United States. Two rich sources on hydropathy's most controversial couple, Thomas and Mary Gove Nichols, are Philip Gleason's "From Free Love to Catholicism: Dr. and Mrs. Thomas L. Nichols at Yellow Springs" in *The Ohio Historical Quarterly* and Bertha-Monica Stearns's "Memnonia: The Launching of a Utopia" in *The New England Quarterly*.

Chapter 10: *Mineral Water: Cure-All for the New American Nervousness*

One useful secondary source for the history, theoretical background, and detailed descriptions of the bottled mineral-water craze and mineral springs, particularly in the Northeast, is Harry B. Weiss and Howard Kemble's *They Took to the Waters*. Harvey Green's *Fit for America* includes an informative chapter on the new American nervousness and also provides an outstanding description of the rise and fall of the mineral-water craze. George Beard's 1881 *American Nervousness*, available at the University of California at San Francisco Library, gives a wonderful account of the new American nervousness by its leading nineteenth-century theoretician. Numerous primary sources provide colorful details about American mineral springs: Martha Norwood's *The Indian Springs Hotel as a Nineteenth-Century Watering Place* is an entertaining history of Georgia's most famous springs; F.C.S. Sanders's *California as a Health Resort* takes the reader on a tour of the springs he found in the Golden State in the early twentieth century and can be found at the University of California at Berkeley, Bancroft Library; and George Walton's *The Mineral Springs of the U.S. and Canada*, written in the 1870s, provides a guide to the major springs, along with their chemical analyses and alleged cures. The Bancroft Library has an outstanding collection of booklets from railroad companies and brochures advertising the springs in the West at the end of the nineteenth and beginning of the twentieth centuries.

Chapter 11: *Seventh-day Adventists: Holy Healers*

A detailed, church-authorized account of Ellen G. White and her medical heirs is found in Richard A. Schaefer's *Legacy*. The major critical, though respectful, history is *Prophetess of Health: A Study of Ellen G. White* by Adventist-trained scholar Ronald L. Numbers, who delineates White's influences, especially the writings of Dr. Larkin B. Coles. Stephen Nissenbaum forges links between early Adventists and Sylvester Graham in *Sex, Diet, and Debility in Jacksonian America*. Present-day press accounts detail the church's material prosperity and medical legacy. An account of the Baby Fae controversy can be found in the December 20, 1985 *Journal of the American Medical Association*. Statistics on modern-day Adventist care are available from Adventist Health Systems in Arlington, Texas. Pat Benton and Bill Redder of the St. Helena Hospital and Health Center in California gave the authors a first-hand look at a modern Adventist health-care facility.

Chapter 12: *The Cereal Revolution: The Brothers Kellogg and C.W. Post*

Dr. John Harvey Kellogg's book *Plain Facts* gives a lengthy and detailed sample of his thinking. The doctor's brother, William Keith Kellogg, is the subject of a biography, *W. K. Kellogg: The Original Has This Signature*, by Horace B. Powell. Nettie Leitch Major has written a useful, if worshipful, biography, *C.W. Post: The Hour and the Man*. The most insightful and engaging popular account of the cereal kings is Gerald Carson's 1957 book *Cornflake Crusade*. The Kelloggs and Post are the subjects of a detailed though unrelentingly sarcastic chapter in Ronald M. Deutsch's *New Nuts Among the Berries*. Harvey Green contributes a well-researched section on Battle Creek in *Fit for America*. Post's exploits and health problems were tracked in major publications including the *New York Times*. Post and the Kellogg brothers received prominent obituaries in the *Times*. Their corporate successors are frequently written about in the business press, especially *Forbes* and *Business Week*. The Historical Society of Battle Creek is an excellent source for, among other things, vintage pictorial records of the cereal wars. The Kellogg Company and the Battle Creek Adventist Hospital maintain archives filled with primary materials on the cereal heroes.

Chapter 13: *Horace Fletcher: The Great Masticator*

Fletcher, a prolific writer, is perhaps best encountered in his own work: His book *The A.B.–Z. of Our Own Nutrition* includes scientific papers supposedly boosting his theories and an eyewitness account of his marathon bicycle ride in France. Fletcher's book *New Glutton or Epicure* includes fan letters from John Harvey Kellogg. Fletcher also wrote for the *Ladies' Home Journal* and *Cosmopolitan* in the first two decades of the twentieth century and was profiled by magazines such as *World's Work, McClure's*, and the *New England Monthly*. Harvey Levenstein's *Revolution at the Table* gives a vivid account of America's "gobble, gulp and go" table manners and Fletcher's experiments at Yale. Biographical backgrounds can be gleaned from James C. Whorton's *Crusaders for Fitness* and Harvey Green's *Fit for America*. Green's book includes excerpts from Henry James's letters to Fletcher.

Chapter 14: *Christian Science: "Heal the Sick, Raise the Dead"*

Christian Science philosophy is best imbibed from the source, Mary Baker Eddy's classic *Science and Health With Key to the Scriptures*. Her additional thoughts, musings, personal history, and assorted testimonials are available in her book *Miscellaneous Writings*. William James constructs an intellectual framework for Christian Science in his *Varieties of Religious Experience*. Eddy is the subject of several recent biographies, notably Julius Silberger, Jr.'s *Mary Baker Eddy*, an interpretive biography by a psychiatrist who argues that she made creative use of illness to become an independent person. A similar point is made in George White Pickering's *Creative Malady* and Donald Meyer's *The Positive Thinkers*. Mark Twain's corrosive book *Christian Science* and Georgine Milmime's 14-part series in *McClure's* in 1907 and 1908 are critical contemporary accounts. Major modern newspapers regularly report on Christian Science's legal battles over its healing practices. The First Church of Christ, Scientist in Boston provides a counterpoint in its pamphlet "A Century of Christian Science Healing." Church spokesperson Thomas C. Johnsen's article in the January/February 1986 *Medical Heritage* and Noreen C. Frisch's article on Christian Science nursing in the January 1989 *Journal of Holistic Nursing* are articulate explanations of Christian Science practice. Testimonials are published weekly in the *Christian Science Sentinel*.

Chapter 15: *Osteopathy: The "Lightning Bonesetters"*

Andrew Taylor Still's *Autobiography of Andrew T. Still* gives the founder's account of the origins of the profession. A favorable early interpretation of Still's teachings is M.A. Lane's *Dr. A.T. Still, Father of Osteopathy*. Morris Fishbein dissents in his *The Medical Follies*. The major scholarly source is Norman Gevitz's *The D.O.s: Osteopathic Medicine in America*, which analyzes osteopathy's birth and *de facto* absorption by mainstream medicine. Fascinating artifacts can be viewed and authorized histories obtained at the Still National Osteopathic Museum on the campus of the Kirksville, Missouri College of Osteopathic Medicine. Statistics and licensing information are issued by the American Osteopathic Association in Chicago.

Chapter 16: *Chiropractic: The Spine Adjustors*

A readable primary source on the Palmers that provides colorful and entertaining anecdotes is David D. Palmer's *The Palmers*. Marcus Bach's *The Chiropractic Story* offers an additional first-hand look at B.J. Palmer at home and at the Davenport Lyceum. Daniel D. Palmer's *The Chiropractor*, published in 1914, provides an excellent background to the founder's philosophy. The Archives at the David D. Palmer Health Sciences Library at Palmer College of Chiropractic in Davenport, Iowa has an excellent collection of primary source materials covering the early history of chiropractic. The journal *Chiropractic History* is an invaluable resource, with articles covering a wide range of subjects: Walter Wardwell's "Before the Palmers" provides a detailed chronology of chiropractic's antecedents and "The Cutting Edge of Chiropractic Recognition" describes the legal history of chiropractic in Massachusetts; Gregory Cooper's "The Attitude of Organized Medicine Toward Chiropractic" provides a clear, well-documented history of the tension between orthodox medicine and chiropractors; Kathleen Crisp's "Chiropractic Lyceums," Gordon Linhart's "Selling the 'Big Idea,' " and Theresa Gromala's "Broadsides, Epigrams, and Testimonials" provide detailed and colorful descriptions of B.J. Palmer's advertising genius. For a fascinating anti-chiropractic point of view from the early 1960s, read Samuel Homola's *Bonesetting, Chiropractic, and Cultism*. Drs. Maria Merritt and Norlin Merritt of Greenbrae Chiropractic, Greenbrae, California, interviewed in 1990, were a valuable resource for books on chiropractic and rebuttals to chiropractic's present-day critics. The American Chiropractic Association and the International Chiropractic Association provide current information on chiropractic. Both are located in Arlington, Virginia.

Chapter 17: *Patent Medicines: "It Will Cure You at Home Without Pain, Plaster or Operation"*

The best, most detailed secondary source on the history of American patent medicines before 1906 is James Harvey Young's *The Toadstool Millionaires*. Young also updates the story in his excellent *American Self-Dosage Medicines* from the perspective of the 1970s. Stewart H. Holbrook's *The Golden Age of Quackery* is a less balanced story but is filled with a lot of colorful, detailed anecdotes. For comprehensive descriptions of the nostrum makers and their medicines before 1905, the most important primary source is Samuel Hopkins Adams's *The Great American Fraud*. The book reprints the original investigative series that appeared in *Collier's Weekly* beginning on June 3, 1905. The American Medical Association's three-volume *Nostrums and Quackery* provides a critical look at the medicine makers after the 1906 Pure Food and Drug Act. For an excellent article on the background of the Pure Food and Drug Act see Gerald Carson's August 1956 *American Heritage* article "Who Put the Borax in Dr. Wiley's Butter?". Jean Burton's *Lydia Pinkham Is Her Name* is an indispensible biography of the first lady of patent medicines, as is Sarah Stage's *Female Complaints*. Nineteenth-century almanacs are immensely useful, showing the widespread advertising for patent medicines. A large collection can be found at the Bancroft Library at the University of California at Berkeley. We located several bundles in an antique store in Kahoka, Missouri.

Chapter 18: *Medicine Shows: Pitch Doctors Take to the Road*

Nevada Ned (AKA Dr. N.T. Oliver) gives a tangy, first-person account in "Alacazam—The Story of Pitchmen High and Low" in the October 19, 1929 *Saturday Evening Post*. Nostalgic memoirs appeared throughout the 1920s and 1930s in *American Mercury, Reader's Digest*, and others. Painless Parker holds forth in a three-part series in January 1952 issues of *Collier's Weekly*. Age-old scams are limned with humor and insight in P.T. Barnum's 1866 book *Humbugs of the World*. The best modern overview is Brooks McNamara's illustrated 1976 volume *Step Right Up*. John Harvey Young contributes a characteristically authoritative chapter on medicine shows in his *The Toadstool Millionaires*. Stewart H. Holbrook's *The Golden Age of Quackery* is a useful text. The Museum of American History, at the Smithsonian Institution, Washington, D.C., has an entertaining collection of medicine-show memorabilia and bottles of patent medicines.

Chapter 19: *The Body Electric: Future Shocks*

Brochures from the Pulvermacher Galvanic Co. are in the collection of the Bancroft Library, the University of California at Berkeley. Valuable bound volumes of nineteenth-century issues of the *Electro-Clinical Record* and *Electrical World* are in the main library of the University of California, Berkeley. David Meredith Reese's 1838 *Humbugs of New-York* skewers the mesmerists, as does Charles Mackay's classic 1843 *Extraordinary Popular Delusions and the Madness of Crowds*. A.D. Rockwell's 1903 textbook *Medical and Surgical Uses of Electricity* gives a mainstream view of the topic. *Early Electrical Machines*, by Bern Dibner, details the great scientific discoveries. The American Medical Association gives close, unflattering attention to Albert Abrams in its three-part *Nostrums and Quackery* book series. Abrams is also attacked in a 1924 *Scientific American* series. He is profiled in Miriam Allen Deford's *They Were San Franciscans* and given detailed, bemused attention in the San Francisco dailies, including the now-defunct *Bulletin*. Morris Fishbein's *The Medical Follies* continues the assault on Abrams. James Harvey Young's "Device Quackery in America" is a useful survey from Elisha Perkins to Abrams, appearing in Leavitt and Numbers's *Sickness and Health in America*. Modern uses of electricity in medicine make news in newspapers and consumer magazines such as *In Health*. In 1990, the authors saw a sampling of electrical devices confiscated by the FDA at the St. Louis Science Center in St. Louis, Missouri.

Chapter 20: *Divine Healing: Ya Gotta Believe*

The most comprehensive, scholarly secondary works on divine healing are by David Edwin Harrell, Jr. His *All Things Are Possible* not only tells a clear and comprehensive story of the post-World War II healing revival movement but gives an excellent theological and historical background for the late-nineteenth- and early-twentieth-century healers. His article "Divine Healing in Modern America" is a compactly written piece that provides a valuable framework for further investigation. His biography of Oral Roberts is a balanced and fascinating story of the most successful modern-day revivalist. Robert Maples Anderson's *Vision of the Disinherited* is a good sociological study of the followers of the divine healers at the beginning of the twentieth century. Most secondary works about Aimee Semple McPherson have emphasized her celebrity escapades. Robert Steele's *Storming Heaven* is more a study of the stormy relationship between Aimee and her mother than a biography as such, but provides excellent biographical material on the evangelist. Excellent sources for studying the healing revivalists are contemporary newspapers and magazines, although most take a cynical view of the healers. Archival materials on Aimee Semple McPherson are located at Angelus Temple in Los Angeles; however, use of these materials is heavily restricted by the Foursquare Gospel Church. A small collection of primary source materials on Sister Aimee is also located at the Bancroft Library at the University of California, Berkeley. For criticism of divine healing, see George Bishop's *Faith Healing* and James Randi's *The Faith Healers*.

Chapter 21: *Bernarr Macfadden and Physical Culture: "Weakness is a Crime"*

Primary source material on Bernarr Macfadden is plentiful and accessible. Particularly helpful for biographical information is Mary Macfadden and Emile Gauvreau's *Dumbbells and Carrot Strips*, co-written years after Mary and Bernarr went their separate ways. It provides an endless supply of honest and amazing tales about his personal habits and family life. Also useful is the *Dictionary of American Biography*, Supplement Five, 1951–55. Obituaries in both *Time* and *Newsweek*, while useful, were not as complete or suffered from some inaccuracies. Also useful for Macfadden's own point of view are the early issues of *Physical Culture* magazine. The St. Louis Public Library has the entire set of the magazine, from 1899 to 1942. *Physical Culture* is also an excellent source for Macfadden's theories and provides testimonials and letters from his loyal followers. For detailed descriptions of specific areas of Macfadden's teachings, his own writings are the best sources. Fortunately, they are easily found in many university and medical libraries. Particularly helpful for this chapter were *The Virile Power of Superb Manhood, The Miracle of Milk, Eating for Health and Strength,* and *Building of Vital Power*. Macfadden's five-volume *Encyclopedia of Physical Culture* provides an endless source of material on physical-culture philosophy and teachings. We found Volumes I and II in a used bookstore in San Francisco.

Chapter 22: *Hollywood: A Cast of Thousands*

Kevin Starr constructs an intellectual framework for the history of Southern California health movements in *Inventing the Dream*. Gayelord Hauser's books are a gold mine of primary material, especially *Harmonized Food Selection, Eat and Grow Beautiful,* and *Look Younger, Live Longer*. Karen Feldman generously provided copies of Hauser's books to the authors. Hauser's adventures were widely covered in west-coast newspapers and in *Time* and *Newsweek*. Noel F. Busch wrote a major profile of Hauser in the August 11, 1951 *Saturday Evening Post*. Greta Garbo's biographers include John Bainbridge, author of *Garbo*, and Anton Gronowicz, author of *Garbo: Her Story*; both men were publicly challenged by the movie star for alleged inaccuracies. Gloria Swanson wrote in detail about her health regimens in her autobiography *Swanson on Swanson*. Garbo, Swanson, and Hauser all received prominent obituaries, as befitted their celebrity status. Upton Sinclair's health experiments were chronicled in his *Autobiography of Upton Sinclair* and Jon A. Yoder's biography *Upton Sinclair*. Jack LaLanne received important profiles in *Newsweek* and *Look* in 1960, *Family Health* in 1978, and *Sports Illustrated* in 1981.

Chapter 23: *Organic America: Rodale & Co.*

Loamy source material can be unearthed in F.H. King's *Farmers of Forty Centuries* and Sir Albert Howard's *An Agricultural Testament*. J.I. Rodale expounded in his book *My Own Technique of Eating for Health*. Rodale's biography *J.I. Rodale: Apostle of Nonconformity* by Carlton Jackson is a sympathetic and fact-packed volume. J.I.'s publishing battles were tracked in *Publishers Weekly*. He was profiled in the *Saturday Evening Post* in 1966 and in the *New York Times Magazine* in 1971 and received a post-mortem tribute in the September 1971 *Organic Gardening and Farming*. Robert Rodale's philosophy was given monthly exposure in his column in *Prevention* and in his 1987 book *The Healing Garden*. He was interviewed by the authors on July 13, 1990 in Emmaus, Pennsylvania. After his September 20, 1990 death, Robert Rodale received affectionate tributes in the November and December 1990 *Prevention* and the December 1990 *Smithsonian* magazine. The most comprehensive of his obituaries appeared over several days in September 1990 in the Allentown, Pennsylvania *Call Chronicle*. Rachel Carson's superb *Silent Spring* laid a sophisticated intellectual groundwork for later environmentalists. Organic farming received voluminous coverage after the 1989 food scares, including cover stories in *Time* and *Newsweek* and major pieces in the *Wall Street Journal, New York Times, FDA Consumer, Consumer Reports,* and *California* magazine. The Rodale Institute is an excellent, ongoing source of information about regenerative farming, exemplified by its model farm near Kutztown, Pennsylvania, which is open to the public.

Chapter 24: *Vitamins: The New Patent Medicines?*

Linus Pauling's books *Vitamin C and the Common Cold* and *Cancer and Vitamin C* are rich primary sources. Pauling was profiled in the *New York Times Magazine* in 1974 and is a frequent subject in *Time, Newsweek*, and such popular magazines as *Science* and *Science Digest*. He critiqued the Mayo Clinic's study of vitamin C in a telephone interview with David Armstrong in 1979. The Linus Pauling Institute of Science and Medicine in Palo Alto, California is a continuing source of information. Adelle Davis's books *Let's Eat Right to Keep Fit* and *Let's Get Well* beg to be quoted. Davis was a popular profile subject in the early 1970s in *Life, Harper's Bazaar, Look*, and the *New York Times Magazine*. She received informative obituaries in the *New York Times* and *Los Angeles Times*. Forrest C. Shaklee, Sr. is the subject of an admiring authorized biography by Georges Spunt, *When Nature Speaks*. Stories about the Shaklee Corporation in *Forbes*, the *Wall Street Journal*, and *Business Week* have been more critically inclined. Albert von Haller's engaging and authoritative *The Vitamin Hunters* is a major source on the early history of vitamin research. Other excellent sources are *Scientific American* in the 1910s and 1920s and *Time, Newsweek*, and *Business Week* in the 1930s and 1940s. *Consumer Reports* and the *New York Times* covered the continuing battles over regulation of sales. John J. Fried's *The Vitamin Conspiracy* is a tough but fair-minded modern look at "vitamania."

Chapter 25: *Dieting Crazes: "Reductio Ad Absurdum"*

The most comprehensive secondary source on the subject of dieting is Hillel Schwartz's *Never Satisfied*, a beautifully written, entertaining, and exhaustive work. For the history of images of female beauty (there is one chapter on men) and the beauty industry in the United States, Lois W. Banner's excellent *American Beauty* is extremely helpful. It also includes much detailed information on the history of dieting cures up to the early twentieth century. Joan Jacob Brumberg's powerful *Fasting Girls* gives valuable and mind-opening information about the history of anorexia nervosa and bulimia. Dr. William Bennett and Joel Gurin's *The Dieter's Dilemma* presents a convincing and powerful critique of dieting. Marcia Millman's *Such a Pretty Face* is very helpful for understanding the degradation and discrimination fat people have suffered in America. Susie Orbach's *Fat Is a Feminist Issue* presents an enlightening argument for how dieting is, indeed, a dilemma for women. Diet books are an outstanding primary source for the history of dieting. Lulu Hunt Peters's hot-selling *Diet and Health*, written in 1918, is particularly useful for understanding World War I-era attitudes toward fatness and dieting. Karen Feldman kindly provided a copy of Peters's book to the authors. The most accessible primary sources are contemporary newspapers and magazines. In addition to the daily press, news magazines and women's magazines provide a steady flow of articles on dieting and diet-related issues. Additional articles can be found in health magazines, such as *In Health* and *Prevention*.

Chapter 26: *Fitness: The Ultimate Cure*

Two outstanding secondary sources for a history of fitness and sports in America, particularly for the nineteenth and early twentieth centuries, are Harvey Green's *Fit for America* and James C. Whorton's *Crusaders for Fitness*. Both are major sources for the early history of the bicycle and the late-nineteenth-century bicycle craze. Paul Lancaster's October/November 1978 piece "Inhale! . . . Exhale! . . . Inhale! . . . Exhale! . . ." in *American Heritage* gives an excellent analysis of trends in American fitness. *Fitness in American Culture*, edited by Kathryn Grover, includes very useful theoretical articles. The most helpful for this chapter were Donald J. Mrozek's "Sport in American Life: From National Health to Personal Fulfillment, 1890–1940" and Roberta J. Park's "Healthy, Moral, and Strong: Educational Views of Exercise and Athletics in Nineteenth-Century America." Exercise manuals of the times can be found in major university libraries. For this chapter we used M. Bornstein's 1880 *Manual of Instruction in the Use of Dumb Bells, Indian Clubs and Other Exercises*. For trends and debates in the 1920s and 1930s we found health books, *Physical Culture* magazine, *Hygeia* magazine, the *Saturday Evening Post*, and the *New York Times* rich in information. Throughout the middle and late 1950s *Newsweek*, the *New York Times*, and *U.S. News and World Report* published a large number of articles about the sorry state of the American physique. Daily newspapers as well as *Newsweek, Time*, and *Prevention* provide volumes of articles covering the late-twentieth-century fitness revolution.

INDEX

Company names, brand-name products, and publication titles are *italicized*. Page references in *italics* represent illustrative material. **Boldface type** refers to boxed material.

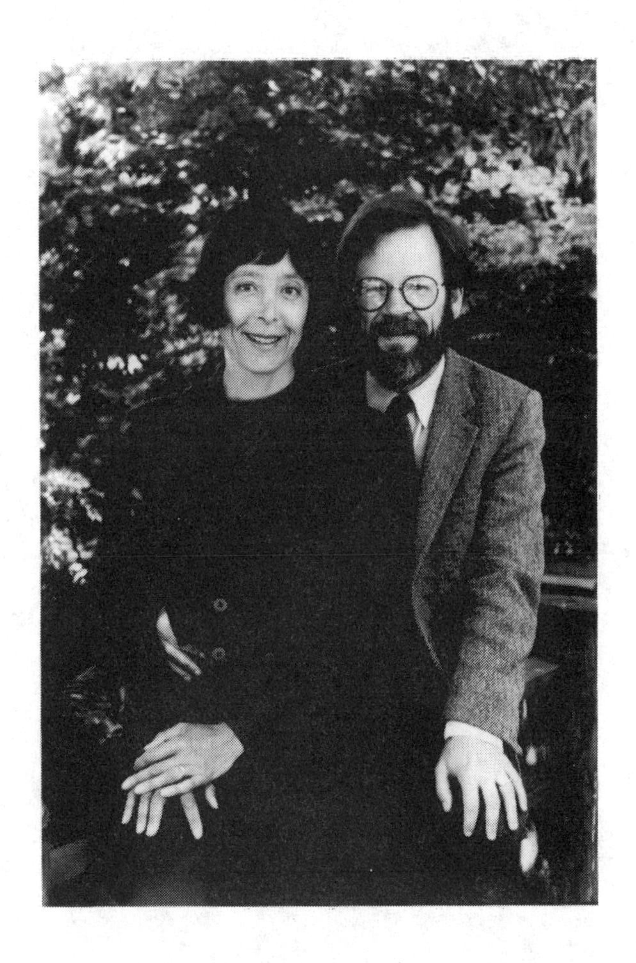

ABOUT THE AUTHORS

San Francisco writers David Armstrong and Elizabeth Metzger Armstrong have written four books between them.

David Armstrong is also author of *The Insider's Guide to Health Foods*, published by Bantam Books in 1983, and *A Trumpet to Arms: Alternative Media in America,* published in hardcover by J.P. Tarcher/Houghton Mifflin in 1981 and in a revised trade paperback edition by South End Press in 1984. He is presently an entertainment feature writer and critic for the *San Francisco Examiner*.

Elizabeth Metzger Armstrong has an M.A. in U.S. History from the University of Missouri and has worked as a college history instructor. She is the author of *The Breakfast Book: Where to Find the Best Breakfasts and Brunches in Northern California*, published by Chronicle Books in 1979. She currently works as a free-lance writer for software and textbook publishers.